Selective Toxicity

CHART OF SIZES

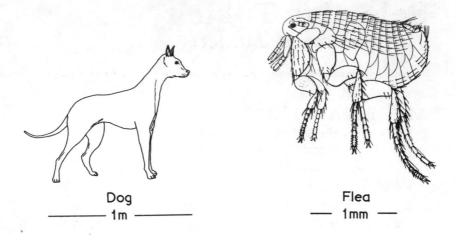

Dog
———— 1m ————

Flea
— 1mm —

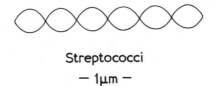

Streptococci
— 1μm —

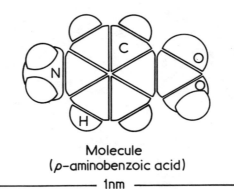

Molecule
(*p*-aminobenzoic acid)
————————— 1nm —————————

This chart is to help one remember the relative sizes of Mammals, Insects, Microbes, and Molecules. In each case an example of medium size has been chosen (e.g. Dog and not Whale). Each object is drawn with a magnification 1,000 times greater than the object preceding it.

Selective Toxicity
The physico-chemical basis of therapy

ADRIEN ALBERT
D.Sc. (Lond.), Ph.D. Medicine (Lond.),
Fellow of the Australian Academy of Science

Professor Emeritus, Research School of Chemistry,
Australian National University, Canberra ;
Research Professor, Department of
Pharmacological Sciences, State University
of New York, Stony Brook, N.Y.

Sixth Edition

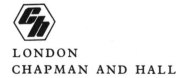

LONDON
CHAPMAN AND HALL

A Halsted Press Book
John Wiley & Sons, New York

First published 1951
Second edition 1960
Third edition 1965
Fourth edition 1968
Reprinted once
Fifth edition 1973
Sixth edition 1979
Published by Chapman and Hall Ltd
11 New Fetter Lane, London EC4P 4EE
© 1979 Adrien Albert

Printed in Great Britain by
Richard Clay (The Chaucer Press) Ltd., Bungay, Suffolk

ISBN 0 412 15650 4

Distributed in the U.S.A.
by Halsted Press, a Division
of John Wiley & Sons, Inc., New York

Library of Congress Cataloging in Publication Data
Albert, Adrien, 1907-
   Selective toxicity.

   Bibliography: p.
   Includes index.
      1.   Chemotherapy.   2.   Chemistry, Pharmaceutical.
      3.   Drugs–Physiological effect.   I.   Title.
RM262.A5   1979   615'.7   78-15491
ISBN 0-470-26482-9

Contents

Contents   ix

Preface to the Sixth Edition

This is a book about selectively toxic agents, namely those substances which affect certain cells without harming others, even when both kinds are close neighbours. The toxicity can be reversible, as with general anaesthetics. The subject covers an immense field: most of the drugs used for treating illness in man and his economic animals, as well as all of the fungicides, insecticides, and weed killers that he uses in agriculture. This book is concerned with the physical and chemical means by which selectivity is accomplished; essentially it is a study in molecular pharmacology.

Selective Toxicity began as a course of postgraduate lectures that Professor F. G. Young encouraged me to give at University College (London) in 1948, and again in 1949. The first edition appeared in 1951, a very small book because little was known about the factors that provide selectivity. Since then, the subject has grown in stature and aroused much interest in many countries. At first, the drug industry was unreceptive to the word 'toxicity', however qualified. It was not denied that Paracelsus (1493–1541) wrote, 'All things are poisons, it is only a matter of the dose', but the modern drug was a highly purified substance. There was some fear that the word 'toxicity', although selective in the patient's favour, could create a bad image, not conducive to good public relations.

A tremendous change has since occurred within that industry. Side-effects, which used to be thought almost unmentionable, have come to be presented with commendable frankness, and accepted for what they are by a better-informed public. Two events of the 1960–1962 period marked a turning-point. One was the realization that the sedative thalidomide, administered to expectant mothers after what was then considered adequate testing, had caused permanent deformities in about 10 000 children. The other event was the demonstration that our environment was becoming contaminated through unrestrained use of the chlorinated insecticides.

Since that turning point, have we become overcautious? Each year, the use of several familiar chemicals is condemned, often on insufficient grounds. It may be hard for us, but it is very necessary, to hold a judicial frame of mind while solid evidence is being collected and discussed. Drugs, and other agents, must be used with all the skill that arises from an intimate knowledge of their mode of action. Above all, an acceptable level of hazard has to be defined, one comparable with the many other risks that life in a community imposes. More education is called for. Enquiring young minds are aware, as never before, of the complexities that pervade medication and the use and abuse of drugs.

In 1976, I had the fortune to be invited to give a course of 30 lectures on 'The Selectivity of Drugs' in the State University of New York at Stony Brook, and to repeat it in the following years. The class was made up of fourth year (Honours) undergraduates plus graduate students in the first year of a PhD course. The prerequisites were: two years of (University) chemistry and biology, the latter commencing with cell biology. As a text, I offered a 64 page introduction *The Selectivity of Drugs* (Albert, 1975), but the class demanded heavier fare. In the end they did creditably with the 5th edition of *Selective Toxicity*.

This experience of teaching and examining has led to changes in the present edition, although the general structure is unaltered. *Part One* of the book, arranged to form a nucleus of a course, now has an additional chapter, on the correlation of structure with biological action (Chapter 2). Teaching experience has shown that these correlations must be understood *before* the more difficult study of how to make them selective is commenced. *Part Two* presents, in greater depth, topics that have been referred to earlier. These can usefully be sampled during the course, depending on its intensity and main interests; they also have independent value as reference material for the research worker.

The rapid thrust of discovery has furnished many new and exciting data which have been incorporated in space vacated by material of less current relevance. At the end of *Part Two*, a new chapter has been added on the perfection of a discovery, regardless of whether the latter was chanced upon, or found by the exercise of logic (Chapter 16). The chapter on selectivity through comparative cytology has been largely rewritten with special attention to cell de-differentiation and cancer (Chapter 5). The chapter on pharmacodynamics has been more usefully restructured (Chapter 7). The former, very short chapter on free radicals has been dismantled, and its contents distributed to more relevant chapters.

New sections have been added on psychotherapeutic agents and their receptors, the repair of membranes by biologically active agents, partition coefficients and the current trend to replace π-values by fragmental constants (**f**) (also a Table of these constants), and the properties of *robust* metal chelates.

Other topics whose treatment has been rewritten or greatly expanded include: receptors and the mutual conformational changes of drug and receptor, the metabolic alteration of drugs, the continuing history of chemotherapy, the Singer-Nicolson model of membranes, steric factors, intercalation, sustained release, pharmacokinetics, drug resistance, drugs that act by interference with DNA synthesis or use, analogous enzymes, tropical diseases (including epitomes of the life-cycles of parasites), opioid receptors, enkephalins and endorphins; quinine and the new anti-resistance antimalarials, cardiac glycosides, adrenergic amines, catecholamine receptors, prostaglandins, ionophores, plant hormones, biologically-active metals in Nature, anticoagulants, antihistamines, drug resistance, antiviral chemotherapy, cancer therapy, tetrahydrocannabinol, and all the anti-biotics in current use. Important new information is also included on: pharmacogenetics, aspirin and other anti-inflammatory drugs, lethal synthesis, n.m.r. in biology, the Hammett and the Taft sigma values, inhibitors of microtubule formation, antidotes for inorganic poisons, the mode of action of isoniazid.

There are hundreds of new references. Throughout the emphasis is on selectivity, with more examples and explanations than before. It is hoped that this book will be enjoyed by all researchers who combine chemical and biological interests. Any reader who feels a need to brush up the essentials of organic chemical nomenclature, can get help from the small and inexpensive book by Jepson and Smith (1974).

In conclusion, I want to thank Professor Arthur P. Grollman, MD, Head of the Department of Pharmacological Sciences, School of Basic Health Sciences in the State University of New York at Stony Brook, for faith, stimulus, and encouragement. I also thank Drs D. F. Waterhouse, FRS, and J. N. Phillips of CSIRO (Canberra) for current information on insecticides, fungicides, and herbicides. I thank, too, Mr D. Light for drawings and the Wellcome Historical Medical Museum (London) for the photograph of Ehrlich and Hata.

A. A.

PART ONE

Topics of general interest

1 Selectivity in the service of man

Throughout the countless millenia of evolution and under the strong pressure of natural selection, nature has evolved many small, highly selective molecules to do the work of the cell. They govern its nutrition, growth, and reproduction. They are the vitamins and coenzymes, hormones and neurotransmitters, inorganic ions (some light, some heavy), metabolic fragments (such as acetyl), and the pigments (respiratory and photosynthetic). Even more remarkably selected are the polyaza-heterocycles: adenosine triphosphate which, in every kind of living cell, stores the energy provided by the breakdown of nutrients and releases it on demand; and the purine and pyrimidine bases of DNA, which encode all needed information for regulating the cell's moment-by-moment metabolism, and also define its character and heredity.

These molecules interact with their complementary biopolymers to generate every response needed for the cell's continuity both as an individual and as a species. Collectively they are *the natural agonists*.

1.0 What is 'selectivity'?

A remedy is said to have selectivity if it can influence one kind of living cell without affecting others, even when these cells are close neighbours. Man has found many selective agents for treating his diseases and those of his farm animals and field crops. Most of the chemical substances that man uses in therapy differ from those evolved by nature, and yet are often related to them because both kinds may act on the same receptors. The substances employed by man are called *drugs* when used for the treatment of human beings or farm animals, and *agricultural agents* when designed to suppress weeds, insects, or fungi in crops. Collectively they are known as biologically active agents, or simply *agents*, and the principles governing their actions are identical. Most of what is written about drugs in this book is applicable to agents generally.

Man's therapeutic agents are of three kinds. A few, such as vitamins, hormones, and minerals, are simply used for *replacement* when depletion has taken place. The replenishment of phosphorus and calcium during pregnancy provides an example. The second kind is the *agonist*, one of Nature's controlling substances, but modified to form depots for longer action, or to be less susceptible to wastage, or to act locally rather than generally. The therapeutic steroids furnish several examples of these agonistic drugs. Most agonists are made by effecting a change, usually a very small one, in hormones and neurotransmitters.

The vast majority of drugs, however, are *antagonists*, designed either to eliminate invading organisms (this is *chemotherapy*) or to suppress sensations of pain or counter metabolic events when these have gone out of balance (*pharmacodynamics*). Antagonism, provided it is selective, enlists toxicity into the service of man, and provides the benefits of 'selective toxicity'. Selective toxicity means the injury of one kind of living matter without harming another kind with which the first is in intimate contact. Either reversible or permanent injury may be chosen to suit the problem in hand. The living matter which is to be injured is conveniently referred to as the *uneconomic species*, and the matter which is to remain unaltered is the *economic species*. These may be related to one another as parasite and host; alternatively uneconomic and economic cells may be two tissues in the one organism.

General anaesthetics admirably illustrate the selective use of toxicity. The more toxic the anaesthetic, the more valuable it is, but only if the toxicity is selective for the central nervous system and completely reversible with time. Morton's success with ether as a general anaesthetic in 1846 was an early and convincing demonstration of selective toxicity. The accepted general anaesthetics combine a high toxicity for the central nervous system with negligible toxicity to other tissues; *all* toxicity rapidly and completely disappears when administration is halted. So, too, with local anaesthetics, muscle relaxants, and (but less rapidly) the antagonists of histamine and of neurotransmitters. Antiparasitic agents, on the other hand, although they must be selective against the parasite and sparing to the host, are preferable irreversible.

It is an achievement of prime importance for man that selectively toxic agents have been found not only for many of his ills, but also for use in his animal husbandry, fields, and forests. The continuance and even expansion of these benefits requires continuous discovery of improved selectively toxic agents.

Whereas the task of chemotherapy is to rid the host of bacteria, viruses, fungi, protozoa, worms and insects, pharmacodynamics has a more difficult programme because the uneconomic cells are part of the organism of the economic species. For example, the uneconomic form may be an endocrine gland that has hypertrophied and upset the balance of metabolism of an otherwise healthy body; it may simply be some part of the nervous system which has become overactive and has disrupted the harmony in which bodily functions normally work. Moreover, all selectively toxic agents for pharmacodynamic use are required to have a graded and temporary action. For instance, the abolition of the ability to feel pain in a circumscribed area is one of the great triumphs of pharmacodynamic practice; but it would be no triumph if the local anaesthesia were to persist throughout the remainder of the patient's life.

Chemotherapy and pharmacodynamics together constitute the science of *pharmacology*.

Selective drugs are usually synthetic and of low molecular weight ($<$ 500). Sometimes, however, they are of natural origin, but used outside their natural context (examples being, alkaloids, antibiotics and overdoses of steroids). Immunochemicals, as in vaccines and sera, are separated from our subject by their enormous molecular weight.

Overdoses of vitamin C, so popular at the present time, should not blind us to the fact that replacement substances can be toxic in excess, either through a side-effect, or by exerting their normal action more strongly. Thus calciferol (vitamin D) in excess causes calcification of arteries and kidneys, and an excess of vitamin A has repeatedly proved lethal. A small dose of ferrous sulphate has often killed young children. A slight overdosage of the pituitary antidiuretic factor increases the blood-pressure unpleasantly; thyroid hormones in small excess cause muscular tremor; and adrenaline, injected before a dental extraction, can precipitate tachycardia. Steroid hormones are often used in unphysiologically large doses; e.g. oestrogens and progestogens for the prevention of conception, and cortisone for arthritis and the atopic diseases. While it has not been thought necessary to review all replacement substances in this book, their borderline character has earned them a place in many of the discussions.

Food, too, is not free from toxicity. Through millenia of enforced experimentation, man has gradually learnt to avoid eating acutely toxic species. However, choice or necessity can restrict the diet to foods whose feeble toxicity may not otherwise be apparent. Chronic toxicity can then arise, as from the natural goitrogens of cabbage and cauliflower, the liver-injuring pigment lycopene in tomatoes, the convulsant alkaloid in yams, the biotin-depleting whites of eggs, and calcium deprivation from the phytic acid of oatmeal. (For many other hazardous factors in common foods, see National Academy of Sciences, 1967.)

The main theme of this book is selective toxicity in its scientific aspects. Many applications will be discussed because they provide familiar examples on which to hang the scientific discussion. However, the main emphasis is on the scientific principles, because of their value in interpreting known examples of selectivity; also it is expected that study of principles leads to important developments which might otherwise be overlooked.

A much-discussed alternative to selective toxicity is *biological control*.

Thus economic species can be bred, or trained, to become more disease-resistant. Also, specific parasites can occasionally be found for the uneconomic species. For example, the cactus known as prickly pear, which deprived Australian farmers of great areas of valuable pasture, was eliminated in the 1930s by the release of a beetle (*Cactoblastis*) which attacked no other form of life. Again the Japanese beetle, which became a serious pest to crops on the Atlantic seaboard of the USA in about 1916, has been kept in check by the introduction of a parasitic wasp (*Tiphia vernalis*) from China and a bacterium (*Bacillus popilliae*), both of which are harmless to earthworms, birds, mammals, and plants. The predacious mosquito *Toxorhynchites inornatus* was used in Fiji in 1931 to control another mosquito *Aedes polynesiensis* which spreads the disease filiariasis. Also, the unicellular fungus *Coelomomyces stegomyiae* was used against the same species of *Aedes* in the Tokelau Islands (Western Pacific) in 1958. Algae and nematode worms are also being investigated for controlling mosquitoes. However, the only established biological weapon against mosquitoes is the release of fish to feed on their larvae in stagnant water (WHO, 1971). The possibilities of virus infections are exemplified by the strong killing action of myxomatosis in rabbits following its liberation in Australia (in 1950) and France (1952). An insecticidal virus, called Viron H, was released in the United States in 1971 to kill bollworms (*Heliothis*) in cotton plants. In general, however, the use of viruses for biological control is out of favour because of a risk of adding malignant genes to the chromosomes of economic species, including man. *Genetic control*, which differs from biological control in that no new species is introduced, will now be exemplified.

Swamping numbers of (a) sterilized males or (b) incompatible males (as far as fertilization is concerned) have been released. By the first method, the screw-worm (a serious pest of livestock) has been exterminated from large areas, also tropical fruit flies have been exterminated from some islands. Sterilization can be effected by X-rays or by agents selectively toxic for spermatogenesis. Concerning the expansion of genetic control from these modest beginnings, WHO recorded the opinion: 'The possibilities are for the distant future and have no operational significance at the moment' (WHO, 1971). If genetic control could be perfected, it would have the advantage of endangering no other type of living organisms, whereas ordinary biological control is much riskier. (For chemosterilizants, see Borkovec, 1966.)

It is most unfortunate that, for the most part, the search for biological controls has been very expensive of time and money, and has not often yielded a practical result. Selective toxicity, on the other hand, is solving a high proportion of the problems of disease in plants, domestic animals, and human beings. At present, the most successful examples of biological control are those effected with selectively toxic agents. Thus trypanosomiasis, a protozoal disease of man and cattle, is controlled by chemical defoliation of those areas of the African jungle where tsetse flies breed, and then spraying organophosphorus insecticides on the exposed breeding sites. In this way, by attacking the insect vectors, which transfer trypanosomes to their mammalian hosts with every bite, the biological life cycle of these parasites is broken. For the same reason, houses in malarial areas and swampy grounds which harbour anopheline mosquitoes are regularly sprayed with insecticides to kill these insect vectors of plasmodia (the protozoa which, transmitted to humans by the mosquito's bite, produce the disease malaria). Needless to say, drainage of the swamps where practicable has helped to control this disease. Another example of the use of selectively toxic agents to break a life cycle is the spraying of streams with molluscicides to kill snails that are the inter-mediate host to the worm that causes bilharziasis in man (see Section 6.4). Although these three examples are of tropical diseases, the principle of exterminating the vectors of disease by selectively toxic agents is also fundamental to maintaining good health in temperate climates. Two universally dreaded diseases are kept in check only by constant vigilance over rats and insects: typhus (rat → louse → man) and bubonic plague (rat → flea → man).

Another way of combining biological and toxic methods is to use phero-mones (the natural insect sex-attractants) as lures to bring insects to poisoned baits (for pheromones, see Section 4.7). This method, not yet very successful, looks promising. Another contemporary search is for substances which could make crops unattractive to insects, or impair their appetites.

I.I Beneficial results from the use of selectively toxic agents

Ability to resist change is inherent in even the simplest physical system, such as a cup of water, as Le Chatelier showed in 1880. Any external effect, such as heat or pressure, always displaces the equilibrium in the direction that tends to restore the original state. Small wonder, then, that living organisms resist change, particularly as they have stores of energy to apply to the task. This homeostasis of living cells enables them to fight man's best efforts to control them, and though he has won some notable victories, some of these have been only temporary. This is not surprising because even the humblest species of prokaryote has been in existence much longer than man and, in the course of that time, has built into its genome much information on how to survive almost every imagin-able type of catastrophe. The real surprise, then, is that man has, in many cases, discovered how to influence, injure, or even eliminate a pathological form of life without endangering his own. These remarks are particularly applicable to selective toxicity.

An annual record of what selectively toxic agents have accomplished, where they have lost ground, or what they have yet to do, can be found in the *Annual Report of the Director-General to the World Health Assembly and to the United Nations*, issued separately or bound annually in *The Work of WHO*, and abstracted and supplemented in the monthly *WHO Chronicle* (all are published in Geneva, Switzerland). The following account owes much to this source (WHO, 1976, 1977).

Infectious diseases. Malaria is still the disease that causes the greatest amount of debility, illness, and death in the whole world. WHO has long given top priority to advising nations on the elimination of this disease by draining and spraying to eliminate the insect vector, and by medication, both prophylactic and curative. WHO also labours constantly to find improvements in all these approaches. Projects approved for a country by WHO can expect to be funded internationally.

Malaria is a chronic illness characterized by periodic attacks of high fever. It is caused by various species of protozoa of the genus *Plasmodium*. The complex life cycle of the parasite begins when a biting female mosquito ingests human blood containing the sexual form (gametocytes) of the parasite. These mate inside the mosquito, and the progeny (sporozoites) reside in the salivary glands and so enter man when he is bitten. The sporozoites multiply in the human liver and their progeny (merozoites) enter red blood corpuscles where they mature to schizonts, which later burst the corpuscles and escape into the host's blood stream (this erythrocytic cycle usually takes about 48 hours). Most of the escaped schizonts migrate to other erythrocytes and repeat the cycle, but a few become gametocytes. Only partial immunity is acquired after repeated attacks.

Malaria has been eliminated from Europe and the U.S.A. within living memory. For example Italy had 8407 deaths from this disease in 1919, but none since 1948. WHO's worldwide programme, begun in the late 1940s, had, by 1976, eradicated malaria from about 20 countries with the result that about 436 million people are now freed from the risk of infection. Moreover, the incidence of the disease has been greatly reduced in areas inhabited by another 1260 million. Unfortunately, about 350 million other people live in areas where malaria is still freely transmitted, and there are countries which at first had the disease under good control but have since lost ground through diminished vigilance (Noguer *et al.*, 1978). In 1966, WHO estimated the world's annual death rate from malaria as one million. Thanks to adequate spraying and drainage, to widespread prophylaxis with daraprim tablets, and the high rate of cure with chloroquine, deaths are now quite rare in developed and developing countries; in undeveloped countries there still seem to be many deaths, but exact figures are hard to obtain.

After malaria, trypanosomiasis, leishmaniasis (kala-azar), and ameobiasis (amoebic dysentery) are the most serious of the diseases caused by *protozoa*.

Whereas malaria is endemic in the majority of tropical countries, trypanosomiasis is confined to Africa (in a wide belt between latitudes 10°N and 25°S) and Latin America. In Africa, trypanosomes are transmitted during bites of the tsetse fly to man in whom the smaller crithidial form becomes the elongated trypanosomal form, which reverts to the crithidial when taken up by flies in subsequent bites. The Rhodesian species of this protozoon often causes death within one year, but the Gambian species produces chronic infection lasting many years. In both types, the central nervous system is affected giving rise to extreme lassitude, hence the popular name 'sleeping sickness'. About 50 million Africans are infected, and their horses, cattle, and camels die of related trypanosomal infections. Although there is some drug-resistance, several effective remedies are known (see Section 6.3c). The factors which prevent the wider use of these selectively toxic agents, and the control of the vector flies, are largely economic, and the incidence is not decreasing.

In America, from Mexico down to the Argentine, a different species (*T. cruzi*) is transmitted by a face-biting nocturnal bug. The result, Chagas' disease, is caused by trypanosomes lodging in the heart muscle, leading often to sudden heart failure, especially in children. About 12 million cases a year occur and no completely effective drug has yet been found. Chagas' disease is confined to under-developed areas, and is complicated by under-nutrition. In fact nutrition must always be considered alongside medication as a prime requirement for health in countries where food is not adequate.

Visceral leishmaniasis is caused by a trypanosome-like protozoon transmitted by sandfly bites in China and India and the Eastern Mediterranean. With enlarged spleen and liver, the patient becomes increasingly listless and soon dies. A cutaneous form of the disease is caused by another species of *Leishmania*. Both forms, together affecting 12 million, respond to selectively toxic drugs.

Amoebiasis, common in many tropical countries but not confined to them, responds well to drugs, particularly metronidazole (Section 6.3c).

Concerning *bacterial* diseases, it is interesting to contrast conditions today in the developed countries with those encountered by a medical student in the 1930s. The medical wards always had several patients severely ill, and others dying, with pneumonia; there were special wards for patients with tuberculosis, and at the outskirts of the city there were special TB hospitals. In the surgical wards, severe and disabling bacterial infections of the hands and limbs were common and difficult to treat, bacterial infection of the bladder was almost inevitable in elderly men with prostatic enlargement, and peritonitis was a dreaded complication of abdominal surgery for which little could be done. Mothers, in childbirth, often acquired septicaemia from which very many died. In the children's wards osteomyelitis was an intractable disease, and there were always cases of severe middle ear infection. After the discovery and application of sulphonamides, penicillin, the tetracyclines, and isoniazid, these severe bacterial infections almost completely disappeared because chemotherapy either prevented or cured them. Bacterial epidemics are now less dreaded; children are no longer immunized against scarlet fever (a streptococcal infection) because penicillin so rapidly cures it. Similarly, although travellers can be immunized against typhoid and paratyphoid fevers, treatment of the non-immune with chloramphenicol is simple and rapid.

The least-controlled bacterial diseases in the world today are cholera, trachoma, leprosy, tuberculosis, brucellosis, gonorrhoea, and the treponematoses. Indonesia, North Africa and (especially) the Indian subcontinent are most severely afflicted with cholera, but thanks to the aeroplane, no part of the world is safe. Cholera is easily cured with chloramphenicol and intravenous saline. Cholera epidemics begin through poor hygiene, and spread explosively where the number of sufferers exceeds the nursing resources. Trachoma, which is simply infection of the eyes by a minute bacterium of the psittacosis group, has 400 million sufferers at the present time, as reported by WHO, and is the greatest cause of blindness in the world. It readily yields to the local use of antibiotics, but reinfection is common because this disease occurs mainly in lands where water is scarce and hygiene poor.

The WHO estimate of the number of lepers in the world is 12 million, many of whom have no access to treatment. The most effective remedy is dapsone (diaphenylsulphone), but recovery takes about 7 years and this drug can cause haemolysis.

It is amazing that such a well understood and readily prevented (and cured) disease as tuberculosis should still be rampant in Latin America, Africa, Asia, and the Western Pacific, but in these countries it is a public health problem of the first order. WHO reports: 7 million infectious cases in the world, and half a million deaths annually.

Brucellosis is a very worrying disease in all countries. Cattle, sheep, pigs, and goats are commonly infected and in turn infect the men who handle them; also whole families can be stricken through drinking the unsterilized milk of an infected animal. Treatment with tetracycline is effective in man, but prophylaxis still presents a problem. This disease is a typical zoonosis, i.e. a disease transmitted to man by animals (there are many of these zoonoses). The incidence of gonorrhoea (about 1% where health facilities are good and up to 20% elsewhere in the developed countries) is rapidly increasing, and highly drug-resistant strains are emerging. The main cause of the increase is failure to seek treatment, rapid and painless though this is. Fifty per cent of all cases occur in the age-group 15 to 24. Of the treponematoses, syphilis (about 40 times less prevalent than gonorrhoea) is slightly increasing, and yaws (mainly affecting children in the less hygienic of the tropical countries) is diminishing; penicillin remains the best treatment for both diseases. Louse-born typhus, caused by a very small bacterium called a rickettsia, has declined greatly through the use of DDT and rodenticides: two African countries (Ethiopia and Burundi) have 95 per cent of the world's cases, according to WHO.

Of *virus-caused* diseases smallpox, formerly the most prevalent and damaging, has been wiped out through the widespread use of vaccination as a prophylactic. Only in very recent years have promising clues been found for drugs against viral diseases (see Section 6.3b), and a few of them (notably herpes) are being successfully treated with selectively toxic agents. Meanwhile, immunotherapy remains the cornerstone of prevention, and is seldom successful for treatment. Hence selectively toxic agents are needed against hepatitis, yellow fever, rabies, dengue fever, mumps, influenza, and the common cold.

Fungal diseases of man, even when superficial, are being treated more successfully than before by internal medication. There is still great scope for improved remedies.

The position regarding diseases caused by *worms* is as follows. Of parasitic diseases in man, schistosomiasis is second only to malaria in causing prolonged, debilitating illness and economic loss. Of the 600 million people at risk in Egypt, China, and their neighbouring countries, about 200 million are severely infected. The disease occurs also in Brazil, Venezuela, and the Caribbean. Schistosomiasis is caused by the parasitic flatworm *Schistosoma mansoni* in hot, dry countries wherever sanitation is poor. New irrigation schemes, population growth, and poverty all increase the prevalence of infection. The life cycle begins with a larval stage, in freshwater snails, which penetrates the skin of anyone working or bathing in the same stream. The larvae mate, then lay eggs in the victim's intestinal veins. The eggs, due to an immunochemical effect, are intensely irritating and cause large, painful swellings. Eggs, passing out in the faeces, hatch in the streams, releasing embryos called miracidia. Magnesium ions, emitted by the snail, attract these embryos which enter the snail's liver where they give rise to larvae. Bilharziasis, a genito-urinary form of the disease, is caused by *S. haemotobium* which has a similar life cycle.

In worms, as in most protozoal diseases, the host's immune response is not only ineffective, but sometimes counterproductive. Moreover, adult schistosomes attract enough host material to their surfaces to become immunologically undetectable. Selectively toxic drugs for treatment of schistosomiasis are now available (see Section 6.3e) although better prophylactic drugs are needed. The use of molluscicides against the infected snails is helping. Greatly improved hygiene would work wonders, but is hard to enforce in those parts of a hot country where the population is large relative to the amount of water available.

Filariasis, a tropical mosquito-borne worm infection, responds well to mass medication with diethylcarbamazine combined with spraying against larvae. WHO estimates that there are 100 million sufferers, many with elephantiasis (grossly enlarged limbs). Onchocerciasis, a worm disease transmitted by biting flies in tropical Africa, often leads to a total loss of sight known as 'river blindness', sometimes affecting 20% of the population. Drugs are available for treatment but not for prophylaxis, and a new lead is required. Meanwhile spraying with DDT is eliminating the larvae of the insect vector. Hookworm, which penetrates the skin in about 500 million agricultural workers in the tropics, is grossly debilitating. The worms become attached to the host's intestinal wall, from which they suck his blood. Common in Africa, Asia, and South America, children are most often the victims. Fortunately, it responds well to drugs.

Roundworms, common in the tropics, with about 650 million sufferers, have an interesting life cycle shared between intestine and lungs. They are easily killed by anthelmintic drugs, and so are the universally-occurring tapeworms and threadworms. Two worm infestations of temperate climates that are difficult to treat are trichinellosis, which starts in undercooked pork and ends up in the sufferer's muscles, and hydatid disease, which often follows the course sheep → dog → man; promising drugs are available.

Many farm animals suffer from severe worm diseases which sap their vitality and decrease their market value. In most cases, effective anthelmintics are known, but many good ones are too uneconomic to use. This state of affairs illustrates the well-known fact that veterinary remedies have to be inexpensive or they cannot be afforded.

Over and over, in the above account, it can be seen that even more important than good selective agents to prevent infectious diseases is a good water supply and waste-disposal system. At present about three-quarters of the world's population lacks an adequate and safe water supply and are depending on the most primitive methods for sewage disposal. In March 1977, the United Nations Water Conference, meeting in Mar del Plata (Argentina), proposed an international drinking water and sanitation decade, commencing 1980. It was agreed that the health problems of undeveloped, and even of many developing, countries cannot be solved until their water resources are efficiently managed (Falkenmark and Lindh, 1977). The cost of providing an adequate and pure supply of drinking water to all nations who lack it has been estimated at sixty thousand million dollars.

Meanwhile the fight against infections must be waged with selectively toxic agents. In 1976, WHO's World Health Assembly, meeting in Geneva, resolved to intensify the attack on the following tropical diseases: malaria, schistosomiasis, trypanosomiasis (both African and American), leishmaniasis, leprosy, and filariasis. With resistant strains in mind, they urged the search for new chemotherapeutic agents against malaria, trypanosomiasis, leprosy, and schistosomiasis.

Non-infectious diseases. Whereas in under-developed countries most cases of illness stem from infectious diseases which require chemotherapeutic agents, most of the illness in the more prosperous countries is metabolic in origin and hence requires pharmacodynamic agents. In the latter countries, the principal causes of death are (in decreasing order of frequency); heart disease, cancer, and stroke. Altogether these form 70 per cent of all deaths. In most of these highly industrialized countries, the mortality from arteriosclerotic and degenerative heart disease is continually rising. Mental ill-health and rheumatoid diseases account for a high percentage of incapacitating illness. Common diseases in industrialized countries, but almost unknown in communities untouched by Western urbanization and Western dietary habits are: coronary heart disease, cancer of the large bowel, diabetes, gallstones and obesity. For each of these diseases some pharmacodynamic agents are available, but still more effective ones are sought.

Yet the versatility of pharmacodynamic medication is remarkable. Patients can be relieved of pain of all types and degrees of severity, put to sleep or made more alert, prevented from having convulsions or caused to have them for their therapeutic value. All of these things can be done with simple selectively toxic agents. Similarly, the patient's temperature can be raised or lowered, his sympathetic or his parasympathetic nervous system can be selectively stimulated or depressed, his basal metabolic rate raised or lowered, and the clotting power of his blood can be made greater or less. Moreover, deficiency or hyperactivity in the action of muscles (including the heart) has come under control, and so have the activities of several of the endocrine glands. Excessive secretion of histamine, the cause of so many distressing symptoms, can be counteracted, and Parkinson's disease (an error of brain metabolism arising in middle age) now yields to medication.

The last 20 years have seen severe mental illness treated far better by medication than by psychological treatment; many otherwise hopeless cases have been able to return to their homes, and to employment, on maintenance doses of new drugs. More and more, biochemical research on mental illness is suggesting that many cases are caused by purely biochemical changes in the central nervous system (schizophrenia by over-methylation, for example). Hence the hope for more specific drug-based treatments is very bright.

Cancer, a collective name for about 100 diseases characterized by unrestrained growth, began in 1942 to yield more and more to medication. Cancers are of two major kinds, (a) solid tumours and (b) the leukaemias and lymphomas of the blood and lymphatic systems respectively. In the Western nations, lung cancer is the largest cause of cancer-related death, followed by colonic and rectal cancer, breast cancer coming third. At any time in the USA, with its population of a little over 200 million, about 650 000 new cases of cancer are diagnosed each year (for the whole world,

WHO estimates 5 million new cases each year). No correlation between human cancer and viruses has ever been demonstrated, although known in other mammals.

Usually some 50% of malignant tumours in man initiate colonies in remote sites. Hence chemotherapy, which used to be reserved for terminal cases, is now introduced at the beginning of treatment, as soon as the mass of a solid tumour has been removed by surgery or radiation. This is done because drugs can reach out, far beyond the surgeon's knife and radiotherapist's rays, to destroy metastatic colonies of cancer cells anywhere in the body. Some 50 anti-cancer drugs have now been established as clinically useful (see Sections 5.0 and 6.3f).

Chemotherapy is effective against Burkitt's lymphoma, testicular carcinoma, muscle cancer, bone cancer, histiocytic lymphoma, and melanoma. Moreover, choriocarcinoma, a womb tumour of young, pregnant women which used to be 90% fatal within a year, now has a 90% chance of complete cure, thanks to two selectively toxic drugs. The leukaemia of childhood, which until recently was almost always fatal within two years, now yields to a combination of selective drugs, and more than half the children who have received this therapy are alive and well 5 or more years later (see Section 9.3c). Both Hodgkin's disease (a lymphoma) and lymphosarcoma are responding well to a combination of radiation and chemotherapy. In early cases of Hodgkin's disease there is now an 80% chance of cure. Wilms' disease, a kidney cancer of children, is being cured in 80% of cases by using a combination of surgery, radiation, and chemotherapy. Several other solid tumours of children can be similarly cured. The foregoing information was obtained from the American Cancer Society in 1977, and reflects American practice.

About 20% of cases of advanced breast cancer respond to hormone therapy and another 48% to antimetabolites such as 5-fluorouracil and cyclophosphamide (Brulé et al., 1973). But here, as in the chemotherapy of ovarian cancer, the figures refer to survival time rather than cure. Current interest centers on (a) prevention of the recurrence of postoperative breast cancer with a combination of methotrexate, fluorouracil, and cyclophosphamide (Bonadonna et al., 1976), and (b) in the clinical trials now being conducted on this and other epitheliomas, most dreaded of all solid tumours, with adriamycin and the retinoids (see Sections 4.0 and 5.0 respectively).

Clinical trials.   As soon as a substance has shown it is both promising and harmless in two laboratory species, nothing short of its administration to man can give useful new information. Many a seemingly specific and potentially useful substance, chosen on the basis of animal trials, has had to be rejected in the clinic for such reasons as: too brief an action, not absorbed from the gut, or serious side-effects not shown earlier. (Parenthetically, the member of a series of new compounds that turned out best in man has not always been the member that excelled in laboratory experiments.) The following study is illustrative.

Six much-used drugs, with different pharmacological actions, were tested for toxic side-effects during several months on dogs and rats. The results were compared with the case records of 500 patients for each drug. It was found that, when the rat was used as a basis for predictions, only 18 out of 53 (i.e. 34 per cent) of the physical signs observed in man were predicted correctly, and even dogs gave only 53 per cent agreement. These figures indicate that one should not expect too much from animal experiments as a guide to clinical trials. The latter are indispensable (Litchfield, 1961).

When different test-species are compared, little connection can be found between dosage and activity, but activity is usually well correlated with blood level. Hence the first task of a clinical unit is cautiously to find what dose in healthy human beings will produce the blood level found effective in laboratory animals. From kinetic data, obtained from the analysis of blood and urine samples as described in Section 3.6, a safe and effective probable dose for patients can be calculated.

The next step, provided that the drug is unquestionably more promising than any existing remedy, is to introduce it to a selected group of volunteer patients, using the necessary precautions of placebos and cross-over tests. Where any element of risk exists, much can be done on (a) human post-mortem material, (b) excised samples (biopsy, or necessary surgery), and (c) tissue cultures. However, human trials (where possible) are preferable, and should be conducted within the strict ethical framework laid down by the Declaration of Helsinki made by the World Medical Association in 1964.

1.2 The physical basis of selectivity: the three principles

Regular consideration of the available data during the last three decades has convinced the present author that there are three main principles by which a selective agent can exert its favourable effect. It can be accumulated principally by the uneconomic species, *or*, utilizing comparative biochemistry, it may injure a chemical system important for the uneconomic (but not for the economic) species, *or* it may react exclusively with a cytological feature that exists only in the uneconomic species. Often two or all of these principles can be seen functioning together, but with one preponderating.

Selectivity through accumulation is sometimes only a matter of gross morphology. Thus the comparative hairiness of weeds in a crop of grain, or the comparatively large surface area (per unit weight) of an insect resting on a mammal, brings about a greater retention of sprayed material by the uneconomic species. In other cases, selective accumulation is achieved in a more positive way. This topic is developed in Chapter 3.

Selectivity through comparative biochemistry. It used to be thought that all living matter, whether animal, plant, or microbial, had a common biochemistry which, if universal, would offer no biochemical basis for selective toxicity. Some of the more important items in this common ground-plan are as follows. Life, in all its aspects, depends on the cell as a unit (even viruses require cells to parasitize, to effect their reproduction). All forms of life have nucleic acid on which is encoded the genetic information required for the functioning of the particular organism. Agents, such as colchicine, which can interfere with mitosis do so at one particular stage in *all* the species examined, and this indicates a universal biochemical pathway of cell-division.

Moreover, a great resemblance in catabolic processes is shown by all cells. There is no essential difference between glycolysis in such a lowly form of life as yeast, and in some of the most highly organized tissues such as human muscle and liver. This has been shown conclusively by the use of inhibitors and by the actual isolation of enzymes and intermediates. Adenosine triphosphate, too, is an almost universal 'currency' by which cells exchange large increments of energy between the various parts of the metabolic cycle, balancing anabolism against catabolism. Certain vitamins, notably thiamine, riboflavine, and nicotinamide, form essential parts of coenzymes in all living cells.

Yet, remarkable as these similarities are, the very fact that one species functions differently from another indicates that there must actually be marked biochemical differences, and many of these are now known. Similarly, marked differences in the biochemistry of various tissues within a single organism have been found. The most striking biochemical differences between species are present not in degradative processes, but in the choice and biosynthesis of enzymes and smaller substances used in growth and division. A discussion of selectivity through biochemical differences constitutes Chapter 4.

Selectivity through comparative cytology. It has long been known that plants and animals have outstanding cytological differences. Thus cell walls and photosynthetic apparatus are found in plants but not in animals; likewise nerve and muscle cells are found in animals but not in plants. In the last three decades, with the help of the electron microscope, it has been found that the cell itself is full of component parts (called organelles) and that each kind of these components displays strong species differences; also there are differences between cells from different tissues in the same species. How these differences can assist selectivity in toxic agents is discussed in Chapter 5.

A classification (very condensed) of animals and plants, from the simplest to the most highly evolved, is given in Tables 1.1 and 1.2 respectively. Alternative taxonomic systems exist. The phrase 'higher animals' usually refers to the vertebrates, and 'higher plants' to the spermatophytes, but many of the physiological characteristics of higher forms are already well developed lower down in the scale of evolution. Bacteria are recognized as a form of life that stands apart from the plant and animal kingdoms, by reason of its structural and functional simplicity. Lacking a nucleus, they are spoken of as *prokaryotes*. Other prokaryotes are the cyanophyta ('blue-green algae'), actinomycetales (for example, *Streptomyces*), and mycoplasms. Protozoa, fungi, and all higher organisms, being nucleated, are known collectively as *eukaryotes*. Viruses present an even simpler form of life than bacteria in so far as they lack a metabolism of their own and do not exist in the form of cells.

Table 1.1

EPITOME OF ANIMAL CLASSIFICATION
(see also Clark and Panchen, 1971)

Sub-kingdom 1: Protozoa
Unicellular animals (for example, amoebae)

Sub-kingdom 2: Porifera
Multicellular animals without a nervous system (for example, sponges)

Sub-kingdom 3: Metazoa
A   Coelenterates (for example, jellyfish)
B   Platyhelminthes (flat worms, occasionally segmented)
    (a) Cestodes (tapeworms, for example, *Taenia*, *Echinococcus*)
    (b) Trematodes (for example, *Schistosoma*, *Fasciola*)
C   Nematoda (round worms, unsegmented; for example, *Ascaris*, *Nippostrongylus*, *Haemonchus*, *Litomosoides*, *Wucheria*, *Trichuris*)
D   Annelida (the typical segmented worms)
    (a) Polychaeta (for example, lugworms)
    (b) Oligochaeta (for example, earthworms)
    (c) Hirudinea (for example, leeches)
E   Mollusca
    (a) Gastropoda (for example, snails, slugs)
    (b) Lamellibranchia (for example, clams)
    (c) Cephalopoda (for example, squids)
F   Arthropoda
    (a) Crustacea (for example, crabs, barnacles)
    (b) Insecta (for example, flies, lice, fleas, beetles, roaches)
    (c) Arachnida (for example, spiders, mites, ticks)
G   Echinodermata (Five-rayed animals, for example, starfish, sea urchins, *Arbacia*, *Echinus*)
H   Chordata
    (a) Urochordata (for example, tunicate sea-squirts, ascidians)
    (b) Craniata (Vertebrates)
        (i)   Pisces (fish)
        (ii) Amphibia (for example, frogs)
        (iii) Reptilia (for example, turtles, lizards)
        (iv) Aves (birds)
        (v)   Mammalia (including man)

Table 1.2

EPITOME OF PLANT CLASSIFICATION

A   Phycophyta (green, brown, and red algae)
B   Mycophyta (fungi)
C   Bryophyta (mosses, liverworts)
D   Pteridophyta (ferns, lycopodia)
E   Spermatophyta (seed plants)
    (a) Gymnospermae (conifers and allies)
    (b) Angiospermae (flowering plants)
        (i)   Monocotyledons
        (ii) Dicotyledons

2 Steps in the correlation of structure with biological action

The three best known sources of selectivity that are available for controlling uneconomic cells were outlined at the end of Chapter 1. Before going on to an expanded treatment of these principles, the narrative must pause to review, in this Chapter, the means by which a foreign substance can influence living matter, whether selectively or not. Experience has shown that to neglect this step and proceed straight into discussion of the principles of selectivity is an unreasonably large jump, as a result of which too many independent variables compete for attention at the same time. It seems better to begin with a simple examination of the sources of foreign molecules' biological activity, which can assume many forms. This activity is, in fact, the primary force, one that can be tamed in the service of man by application of the principles of selectivity. Ill advised is the investigator who, esteeming his new candidate drug 'too toxic' (meaning, really, 'insufficiently selective') changes the molecule in a way that extinguishes the toxicity, and thereby loses the force that could have been made selective by thoughtful molecular modification.

Fundamental to any study of correlations, between structure and biological activity, is knowledge that the messengers and coenzymes of each organism depend strongly on small details of their chemical structure without which their characteristic biological effect is lost. If these details are varied, even slightly, the degree of action is usually radically changed. For example, the vitamin activity of thiamine (*2.1*) (tested on pigeons) drops to 5 per cent if the methyl-group is removed from the pyrimidine ring, and to < 1 per cent if the methyl-group is removed from the thiazole ring (Schultz, 1940). Finally, if an extra methyl-group is inserted into the thiazole ring (between nitrogen and sulphur), the vitamin activity completely disappears (Bergel and Todd, 1937). This rule of the essential nature of every part of a molecule need not apply to a side-chain. For example, the long aliphatic side-chain in the 3-position of vitamin K_1 (2.2) can be pruned without affecting the principal action of this vitamin. In such a case, it is evident that the side-chain lacks every atom responsible for adsorption of this vitamin.

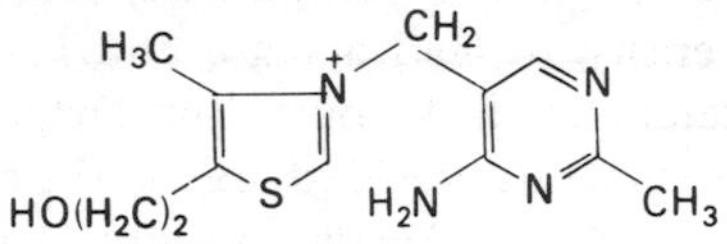

Thiamine
(2.1)

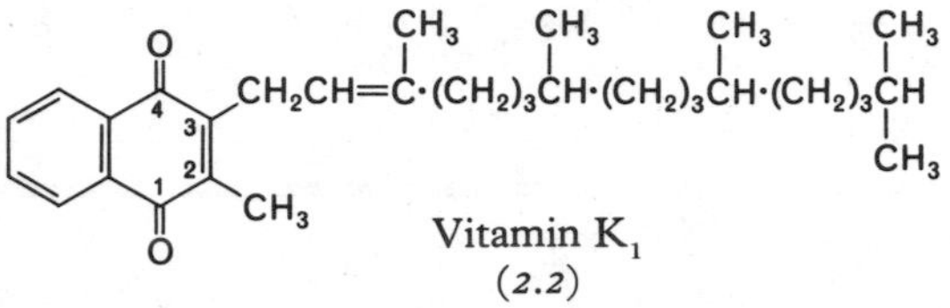

Vitamin K_1
(2.2)

Synthetic drugs show a similar dependence on minute detail. In benzene-sulphonamide (2.3), an amino-group can be inserted in three different positions: in two of these it gives rise to an inactive substance, in the other it becomes the highly antibacterial substance sulphanilamide. In acridine (2.4), an amino-group can be inserted in five different positions: in three of these it gives aminoacridines that are almost inactive, but in the other two it gives powerful antibacterials. In quinoline (2.5), a hydroxy-group can be inserted in seven different positions: in six of these, completely inert substances arise, but in the remaining position a strong antibacterial and antifungal substance is produced. What is more, the reasons why the active isomerides are active, and the inactive ones inactive, are well understood and will be described in what follows. The marked biological differences shown by optical isomers (Section 2.1) further illustrate this point. At this stage, before plunging into these details, it will help to stand back a little and take a broader view of how the ideas of structure-activity relationships arose.

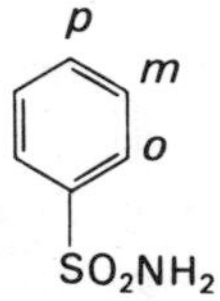

Benzenesulphonamide
(2.3)

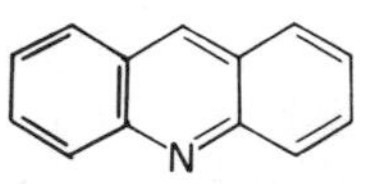

Acridine
(2.4)

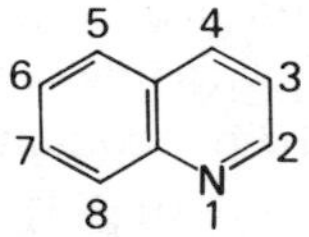

Quinoline
(2.5)

2.0 The earliest correlations

In Renaissance times, Paracelsus (1493–1541) taught: 'All substances are poisons; there is none which is not a poison. Only the right dose differentiates between a poison and a remedy'. This somewhat nihilistic view began to undergo modification, very slowly it is true, through scientific observation and reasoning in the 19th century. Thus in 1848, Blake, in the United States, published his opinion that the biological activity of a salt was due to its basic *or* its acidic component, and not to the whole salt. Thus the poisonous entity in lead acetate and lead nitrate was the lead moiety and not the acetate or nitrate part. Similarly, the toxicity of sodium, potassium, and calcium arsenites resided only in the arsenite portion of these salts. This was, for its time, a daring thought, because it was not until 1884 that Arrhenius introduced his theory of electrolytic dissociation (namely: salts dissolved in water are dissociated into oppositely charged ions).

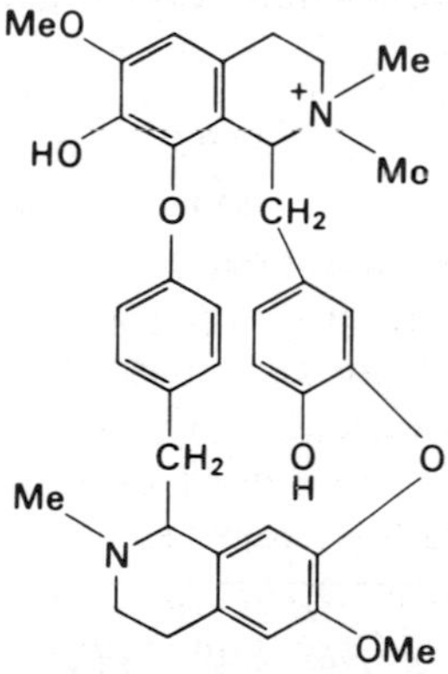

Tubocurarine
(revised formula, 1970)
(2.6)

The next correlation was found in Scotland where Crum Brown and Fraser (1869) made a major discovery. They showed that several alkaloids, when quaternized, lost their characteristic pharmacological properties (many of them spasmogenic or convulsant) and acquired the muscle-relaxing powers of tubocurarine (2.6) (itself a quaternary amine), whose site of action had been shown to lie at the junction between nerve and voluntary muscle, a few years earlier, by Claude Bernard (1856). Strychnine, bruceine, thebaine, codeine, morphine, nicotine, atropine, and coniine were quaternized into curarimimetic substances, by reaction with methyl iodide. The Scottish authors wrote: 'There can be no reasonable doubt that a relation exists between the physiclogical action of a substance and its chemical composition and constitution, understanding by the latter term the mutual relations of the atoms in the substance.'

These discoverers of the first structure-action relationship among organic substances entitled their paper 'On the Connection between Chemical Constitution and Physiological Action'. However, no other example came to light of a single chemical group being able to confer a single pharmacological action on a variety of complicated nuclei. A solution of this puzzling correlation came only in the present century, for it had to await development of the idea of drug receptors and the discovery of some analogous phenomena in enzyme chemistry.

Meanwhile attention was drawn to the overriding importance of a physical property when, at the turn of the present century, Overton and Meyer independently put forward a 'Lipoid Theory of Cellular Depression'* (Meyer, 1899; Overton, 1901). This stated that chemically inert substances, of widely different molecular structures, exert depressant properties on those cells (particularly those of the central nervous system) that are rich in lipids; and that the higher the partition coefficient (between any lipid solvent and water) the greater the depressant action. This statement requires only insertion of the words, 'up to the point where hydrophilic properties are almost extinguished' after 'partition coefficient' to outline the present day viewpoint. It is now appreciated that the relationship between lipophilicity and depression of nerve functioning is a parabolic one, because substances that are entirely lipophilic become trapped in other lipids and do not enter the cell (Hansch *et al.*, 1968). Table 2.1 offers

Table 2.1

CORRELATION OF LIPID/WATER PARTITION COEFFICIENTS WITH
BIOLOGICAL DEPRESSION
(SUPPRESSION OF MOTILITY OF TADPOLES)

Substance	Partition coefficient olive oil/water	Minimal immobilizing concentration. mol/l (water)
Trional	4.46	0.0018
Butylchloral hydrate	1.59	0.0020
Sulphonal	1.11	0.0060
Triacetin	0.30	0.010
Diacetin	0.23	0.015
Chloral hydrate	0.22	0.020
Ethyl urethane	0.14	0.040
Monacetin	0.06	0.050

(Meyer, H., 1899; Baum, F., 1899)

* 'Lipoidtheorie der Narkose' (Meyer, 1899).

an example of the original results (see Table 15.1 for more recent data).

Depressants may be hydrocarbons, halogenated hydrocarbons, alcohols, ethers, ketones, weak acids (like the barbiturates), weak bases, or simple sulphones. They are the selectively toxic agents used in medicine as hypnotics and general anaesthetics. This is the only kind of biological activity in which structure simply does not matter (there is much more about this in Chapter 15). See Section 3.2 for the general function of partition effects in securing selective distribution of drugs.

In the present century, the most valuable correlations have come from receptor theory and from a study of physical properties, and particularly from the reconciliation of these two approaches originally seen as rivals. These concepts will now be expanded, in turn.

2.1 The concept of 'receptors'. The receptor as an enzyme or other protein

Three striking characteristics of the action of drugs indicate very strongly that they are concentrated by cells on small, specific areas known as receptors. These three characteristics are, (i) the high dilution (often 10^{-9}M) at which solutions of many drugs retain their potency, (ii) the high chemical specificity of drugs, so discriminating that even the D- and L-isomers of a substance can have different pharmacological action, and (iii) the high biological specificity of drugs, e.g. adrenaline has a powerful effect on cardiac muscle, but very little on striated muscle.

The idea that drugs act upon receptors began with J. N. Langley in Cambridge who, after studying the opposing actions of atropine and pilocarpine on the flow of saliva in the cat, wrote: 'We may, I think, without much rashness, assume that there is some substance or substances in the nerve endings or gland cells with which both atropine and pilocarpine are capable of forming compounds. On this assumption, then, the atropine or pilocarpine compounds are formed according to some law of which their relative mass and chemical affinity for the substance are factors' (Langley, 1878).

However, the word 'receptor' was introduced later, by Paul Ehrlich. His experiences, first with immunochemistry and then in his new subject, chemotherapy, led him to visualize receptors as chemical groups that gave a biological response by uniting with chemically complementary groups either of tissue nutrients and chemical messengers, or of drugs (when medication was in progress). To Ehrlich, receptors were small, chemically defined areas on large molecules. Thus he wrote. 'That combining group of the protoplasmic molecule to which the introduced group is anchored will hereafter be termed *receptor*', and later a receptor is defined as: 'That combining group of the protoplasmic molecule to which a foreign group, when introduced, attaches itself' (Ehrlich and Morgenroth, 1910). Ehrlich's

Nobel lecture in 1908 discussed his concept of receptors (see Section 6.1 for a brief account of his development of this concept). Here it is sufficient to say, by way of example, that Ehrlich believed, as we still do, that the mercapto-group (-SH) is the arsenic receptor in trypanosomes and that the blockade of this receptor by arsenic causes the death of these organisms.

Early confirmation of the existence of drug receptors was provided by substances that form pairs of optically-active stereoisomers. Numerous drugs, including morphine, atropine, and adrenaline, can be obtained in two forms, namely as dextro- and laevo-rotatory isomers (see Section 13.1), which differ strikingly in biological potency. Because the two members of such pairs have identical chemical and physical properties, and differ only in that their molecules are built as mirror images of one another, it is evident that the *shape* of a drug molecule is crucial for its action and that a part of the molecule may have to fit a structure complementary to it (Cushny, 1926).

At first the receptor concept was received with scepticism because of repeated failure to isolate any such substance. However, the idea of receptors became more firmly established by the quantitative work of A. J. Clark (1937)*, who showed that (drug-receptor) combination obeyed the law of mass action. He also showed that a great deal of the most accurate quantitative data on drug action could be interpreted as the result of the formation of a bond (not necessarily covalent) between a drug and a receptor specific for this drug. This relationship is discussed further in Section 7.5. The high specificity of many drugs for their receptors seemed analogous to that of a substrate for its specific enzyme, and in 1929 (see below) the receptor for pilocarpine was found to be acetylcholinesterase. In the 1940s, the hydroxy-group of serine in this enzyme was pinpointed as the receptor site for organophosphate insecticides (see Section 12.3), and in the 1950s the antimalarial action of pyrimethamine was traced to its blocking the enzyme dihydrofolate hydrogenase (see Section 9.3c). Both of these enzymes have been obtained pure. Yet it was clear from the start that agonistic drugs were analogous not to the *substrates* of enzymes (because they were not changed by their receptors) but to *coenzymes* which assist the enzyme to function.

Reversibility of combination with receptors.   The majority of drugs and other selectively toxic agents combine very loosely with their receptors. They can usually be easily washed off the receptors, which then cease to register the adverse effects produced by the agent. It is comparatively rare for agents to form covalent bonds with their receptors (covalent bonds are defined in Section 8.0), but those that can do so inflict a change that is difficult to reverse.

Ehrlich, who discovered the firmness of the arsenic-sulphur bond in

---

* Work begun about 1920.

arsenic-medicated trypanosomes (Ehrlich, 1909), nevertheless knew that other, more easily reversible, bonds were concerned in the action of most drugs, because he wrote: 'If alkaloids, aromatic amines, antipyretics or aniline dyes be introduced into the animal body, it is a very easy matter, by means of water, alcohol or acetone, to remove all these substances quickly and easily from the tissues' (Ehrlich, 1900).

The chemotherapeutic worker, with the examples of arsenicals and penicillin in mind, may tend to think that agents generally act by forming covalent bonds. But the worker in pharmacodynamics, used to washing organ-preparations and using them over and over again, is better informed in this matter. Fig. 2.1 gives a typical example of the ease with which drugs can be removed from their receptors by washing.

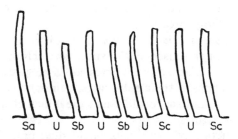

Sa U Sb U Sb U Sc U Sc

FIG. 2.1 Easy displacement of drug from receptors by washing. This example is the assay of histamine by immersing guinea-pig gut alternately in unknown and standard solutions, made up to 2 ml with isotonic saline.
  S. Standard solution (1 in 5 000 000)
      (a) 0.1 ml, (b) 0.07 ml, (c) 0.09 ml.
  U. Unknown solution (0.1 ml).
Between each reading, the tissue was washed with saline, which restored it to its original condition. (Result of assay: 0.1 ml of unknown has the potency of 0.09 ml of standard.) (Gaddum, 1936.)

The number of agents known to act by covalent-bond formation is quite small. It comprises mainly the arsenicals, mercurials, and antimonials which act on parasites by combination with mercapto-groups; penicillin, the phosphorus-containing anticholinesterases, and the nitrogen-mustards, all of which either acylate or alkylate certain receptors; and finally some altered purines and pyrimidines which become built into the structure of nucleosides, for example, 8-azaguanine. These covalent-bond forming agents are dealt with in detail in Chapter 12. Although new examples may be discovered, there is little doubt that most of the known drugs react with receptors by readily reversible bonds, namely ionic, hydrogen, and van der Waals bonds (see Section 8.0), and that combination with receptors by covalent bonds is a rarity.

Although covalent bonds are firmly maintained, they are not all of the same strength and some of the weaker ones can be exchanged for other covalent bonds. Thus although poisoning of a cell takes place when an arsenical agent combines with vital mercapto-groups, a swamping excess of an antidote which has a reactive mercapto-group, e.g. thioglycollic acid, can liberate the mercapto-group (Voegtlin, 1925). To overcome stronger arsenic-sulphur bonds in the cell, a stronger dimercapto reagent was devised, namely dimercaprol (Peters et al., 1945). Similarly, when the organic phosphorus agents injure a tissue by forming phosphorus-oxygen bonds with vital enzymes (see Section 12.3), the use of organic hydroxylamines can break all but the strongest of these bonds by offering the hydroxyl-group of the antidote for phosphorylation (Wilson and Meislich, 1953; Childs et al., 1955). In spite of these successes, most other covalent bonds between drugs and receptors are probably too tight to be broken by exchange processes.

Acetylcholine: agonists and antagonists. With this background in mind, the narrative of the discovery of drug correlations can be resumed. By 1910, it was known that many enzymes could be blocked by substances that structurally resembled their substrates. For example amylase, which hydrolyses starch to maltose, could easily be blocked by glucose (Wohl and Glimm, 1910). Although suspected, no close connexion between this discovery and the action of drugs was established until the Scottish bio-chemist Stedman (1926) showed *in vitro* that the alkaloid physostigmine (*2.7*) blocked the enzyme acetylcholinesterase whose normal function is to destroy acetylcholine (*2.8*) as soon as it has completed its task of carrying the nerve impulse across the nerve-muscle gap (this neurotransmitter function of ACh was suspected by Loewi in 1921 and confirmed by Loewi and Navratil in 1926).

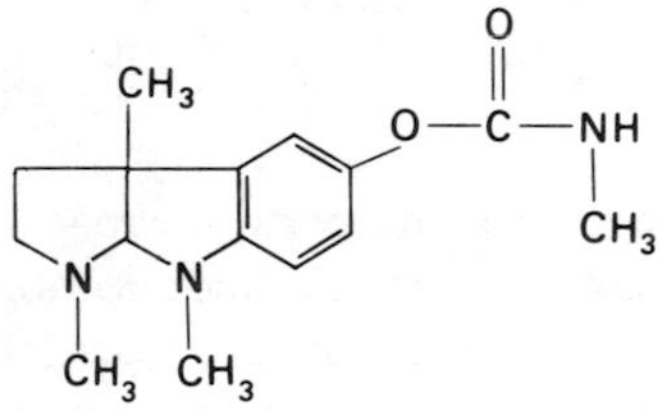

Physostigmine (eserine)
(2.7)

Acetylcholine (cation)
(2.8)

(2.9)

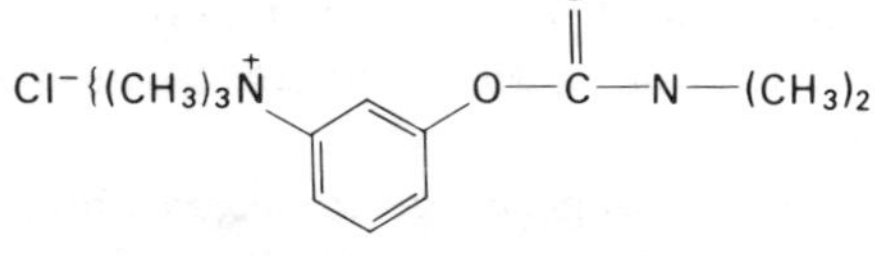

Neostigmine
(2.10)

Carbachol (cation)
(2.11)

Stedman went on to show that the reason that physostigmine contracts the pupil of the eye, in ophthalmic medicine, is that it is a strong inhibitor of acetylcholinesterase in the nerve-muscle synapse (gap), thus allowing the muscle to be contracted by the ACh that slowly leaks from the nerve ending between impulses (Stedman, 1929). This work established that an enzyme could be a drug receptor. Physostigmine, although it mimics the action of ACh, is not a true agonist because it does not act on the muscle ACh receptor; it is classed as a pseudo-agonist.

Synthesis of analogues soon showed that the two portions of the physo-stigmine molecule needed to inhibit the esterase were the basic group and the methylcarbamoyloxy group (2.9) (Stedman and Stedman, 1931). Neostigmine (2.10), synthesized as a simplified analogue of physostigmine (Aeschlimann and Reinert, 1931), was found to be a more powerful drug than the latter for treating myasthenia gravis, a muscle-wasting disease with symptoms similar to those of tubocurarine poisoning. Neostigmine, like physostigmine, carries a carbamoyloxy group, but the basic group of the latter is that of acetylcholine. These two groups together make neo-stigmine an excellent substitute for ACh at the active site of acetylcholine-sterase, but unlike physostigmine it also has a direct true agonistic effect on the ACh receptor of muscle.

These indications that the carbamoyloxy (or 'urethane') group could mimic the acetyl group of ACh, led to the introduction of carbachol (carba-mylcholine) (2.11) whose actions resemble those of acetylcholine but are much longer lasting (Molitor, 1936). Although its action is, in part, truly agonistic (replacing ACh on the muscle receptor) carbachol acts principally as a pseudo-agonist, yet in a way totally different from that of physostig-mine: namely, carbachol drives ACh from its stores in the nerve terminal. Carbachol neither blocks nor is hydrolysed by acetylcholinesterase. It is valuable for restoring tone to the bladder and intestines of patients recovering from surgery.

This accumulated evidence led Ing (1936) to conclude that tubocurarine (2.6), and other large-molecule quaternized amines, relax muscle by blocking the acetylcholine receptor there. This penetrating conclusion was to bring far-reaching benefits; in particular it was to indicate the source of simple synthetic compounds to act as muscle relaxants during surgical operation, thus permitting the introduction of lighter anaesthetics for major operations (see Section 7.3). Ing (1936) also indicated that the somewhat weak, but typically curariform, action of numerous quaternary phosphonium, arsonium and stibonium salts, and the analogously consti-tuted sulphonium and iodinium salts, arose from their competition with acetylcholine for the ACh receptor.

By this time it was clear that drugs with a given group (here, the tetra-methylammonium group) could impose two quite opposite actions, one action if they resembled a natural messenger (here, acetylcholine) sufficient-

ly well to take its place, at least in some situations, but the exact opposite
action if they differed from the messenger enough to interfere with its
working (see further, Section 9.2). For further information on the physiological functions of ACh, its receptors, agonists and antagonists, see Sections
7.5a, 7.6c, and 13.6.

This interpretation shed a new and unfavourable light on the 'one-
group one-action' hypothesis that had dominated the thoughts of many
workers in this field, especially in the drug industry (e.g. I. G. Farben,
1933–8; Dyson, 1928). This hypothesis had been born with the Crum
Brown and Fraser correlation and was nurtured by Ehrlich's successes in
the cure of trypanosomiasis and syphilis with the aromatic arsenicals, and
by the wide range of barbiturates (and other ureides) that had shown
hypnotic action.

Sulphanilamide and its derivatives.   The concept that a drug receptor
could be an enzyme was extended from pharmacodynamics to chemotherapy when Woods (1940) demonstrated the reversal of the antibacterial
action of sulphanilamide (*2.12*) by *p*-aminobenzoic acid (*2.13*) and pointed
out that this reversal depended on the structural similarity of these two
substances. Later, the receptor for sulphonamides was found to be the
enzyme dihydrofolate synthetase, which incorporates *p*-aminobenzoic
acid into the molecule of dihydrofolic acid (*2.14*), an essential coenzyme
for the biosynthesis of purines and thymine, and hence of DNA. This
enzyme was isolated and purified by G. Brown (1962), and these functions
confirmed.

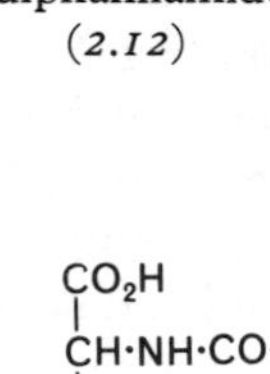

Sulphanilamide
(*2.12*)

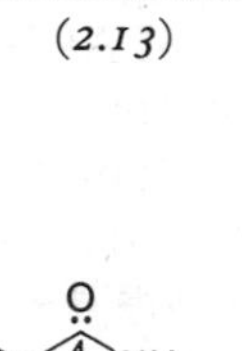

p-Aminobenzoic acid
(*2.13*)

Dihydrofolic acid
(*2.14*)

The sulphonamide antibacterials, which, soon after their discovery in the late 1930s, seemed to reinforce the 'one-group one-action' hypothesis, ended by dealing it a mortal blow. It soon became evident that the presence of a sulphonamide group would not introduce antibacterial properties unless the other conditions (such as *para* substitution) for fitting the enzyme-receptor were observed (see Section 9.3). If these conditions were met, the sulphonamide group could be replaced by a different group of similar polarity. Moreover many useful antidiabetic and diuretic drugs were launched, each with a sulphonamide group attached to a benzene, or other aromatic ring, but these drugs did not have the dimensions and charge-pattern suitable for becoming attached to dihydrofolate synthetase and hence had no antibacterial properties. The antibacterial enzyme-blockers, on the other hand can meet the enzyme specifications without even containing sulphur!

Other enzyme receptors.   Many other drugs have enzymes for receptors, including several antibiotics and synthetic agents which combine with DNA polymerase and RNA polymerase (see Section 4.0). Allopurinol (*9.30*) is particularly interesting case because it was carefully designed to fit (and block) its receptors, the two consecutive enzymes hypoxanthine oxidase, and xanthine oxidase (Elion *et al.*, 1966). It has provided the best of all treatment for gout, by preventing the formation of uric acid (see Section 9.4, p. 319). The receptor for cardiac glycosides in the heart is Na^+K^+-ATPase (Bonting, 1970; see also Section 14.1).

Non-enzyme proteins as receptors.   From about 1950, it began to be realized that the acetycholine receptor of muscle was a *permease*, namely a non-enzyme protein situated in the plasma membrane at the synapse. When coupled with ACh, it regulates the passage of sodium, potassium, and calcium ions (Karlin, 1974). Apparently, permeases provide the graded response needed at synapses. Initially, knowledge of permeases came from bacteria, where they were easier to isolate and study (see Section 3.1). Each molecule of ACh, by combining with its permease, allows 50 000 cations to cross the membrane (Katz and Miledi, 1972).

The homogeneity and richness in cholinergic synapses of the electric tissue (electroplax) of two fish species, *Torpedo* and *Electrophorus*, made it the ideal source of ACh receptor. Purification began with homogenization, differential centrifugation, and then sedimentation in sucrose density gradient solutions. The membrane fragments obtained in this way contained the receptor free from acetylcholinesterase (Cohen and Changeux, 1975; review). It was found that these fragments could be self-sealed to give vesicles whose permeability to $^{22}Na^+$, $^{42}K^+$, and $^{45}Ca^{++}$ was greatly increased by carbachol (Kasai and Changeux, 1971).

The receptor protein could be freed from the membrane by anionic and neutral detergents, and obtained apparently fairly pure, in milligram quantities (Karlin, 1974; O'Brien *et al.*, 1972, Miledi *et al.*, 1971). One

useful process for liberation was equilibrium dialysis in the presence
of ^{14}C-decamethonium bromide (7.20), with which it formed a complex.
It could be displaced from this complex by other ACh antagonists (tubocurarine, gallamine), and also by ACh agonists (carbachol, phenyltri-
methylammonium cation). Kinetic measurements were almost identical
with those obtained on the intact electroplax. The receptor protein was
stable for several days at 0° C (Changeux *et al.*, 1971).

The purified receptor, a glycoprotein of mol.wt. 250 000, spontaneously
dissociates into small proteins, at least one of which (mol.wt. 40 000) has
strong ACh-binding properties (Martinez-Carrion *et al.*, 1975). The isolated receptor, when mixed with lipid extracted from the vesicles (microsacs),
and calcium and magnesium ions, re-formed vesicles whose permeability
to ^{22}Na$^+$ was increased by carbachol and decreased by antagonists (Hazelbauer and Changeux, 1974).

The foregoing account is of the 'nicotinic' receptor from the neuromuscular junction. This work has been extended by isolation of a 'muscarinic' receptor from ox brain by simply extracting this organ with 2M-
sodium choloride ('nicotinic' and 'muscarinic' are defined in Section 13.6).
The brain receptor is recognizable by its intense power of binding an
ACh inhibitor, ^{3}H atropine, with an inhibitory constant (K_i) of 2×10^{-9}
This label can be displaced by unlabelled atropine and also by acetylcholine
and other agonists (Carson *et al.*, 1977).

Similar work on the isolation of catecholamine receptors is described
in Section 13.4; the receptors for the natural polypeptide anodynes (which
also bind morphine and other opioids) are discussed in Section 13.7.

In general, membrane-bound receptors are being located and purified
by incubation of a tissue homogenate with a radioactively-labelled agonist
or antagonist of the normal ligand (say, a neurotransmitter). If the marker
is chosen for the strength of its binding, it can guide the concentration
process. It can later be exchanged for weaker agonists or antagonists, or
removed by dialysis or affinity chromatography.

Molecular probes are also useful. These are small molecules with a
measurable physical property (such as fluorescence, visible absorption,
e.s.r., or n.m.r.) that is altered upon adsorption to the receptor. Fluorescent probes are sensitive to the polarity of the binding site; energy can be
transferred from the binding site to the probe, thus changing its fluorescence (Radda, 1971). For further reading on probes, see Chance *et al.*,
(1971). A fluorescent probe said to be specific for the ACh receptor
is 1-dimethylaminonaphthalene-5-sulphonamidoethyl trimethylammonium perchlorate. This can be competitively displaced by ACh, dimethyl-
tubocurarine, and decamethonium, thus providing a basis for identification and analysis (Weber *et al.*, 1971). For further reading on receptors,
see Rang (1973); for molecular aspects of hormone-receptor interaction,
see Levey (1976).

2.2 The receptor as a nucleic acid, or as a coenzyme or other small molecule. Other aspects of receptors

Nucleic acid receptors. The period of the Second World War (1939–1944) was a turning point in the study of structure-action relationships. Mere 'paper resemblances' between two formulae began to lose favour as a guide to biological action. Less often were groups (or nuclei) assumed to be the direct source of some pharmacological effect, and more attention was given to the physical properties which these groups (and nuclei) introduced and maintained. The chief physical properties studied were (a) electron distribution (e.g. ionization or dipole moment), which could facilitate or forbid the combination of a drug with its receptor, and (b) steric properties, which governed access to the correct receptor and a good fit upon arrival there. Both of these factors came to the fore in studies of the aminoacridines described briefly here, more fully in Section 10.3. First it was shown that the bacteriostatic action of these topical anti-bacterials was proportional to the fraction ionized as cation (Albert, Rubbo, and Goldacre, 1941). This was the first quantitative correlation of ionization with the biological properties of a chemotherapeutic drug. Acridine itself (*2.15*) is a weak base. With its pK_a of 5.3, it is only one per cent ionized at pH 7.3. However, two of the five monoaminoacridines are strong bases, and this strength (which secures a high degree of ionization) was traced to a resonance effect in their cations, which is not possible in the other three isomers. Formulae (*2.16*) and (*2.17*) represent the extreme or canoni-

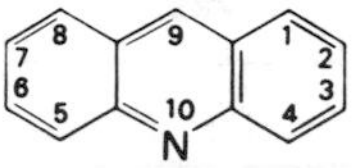

Acridine
(International Union of Chemistry numbering)
(*2.15*)

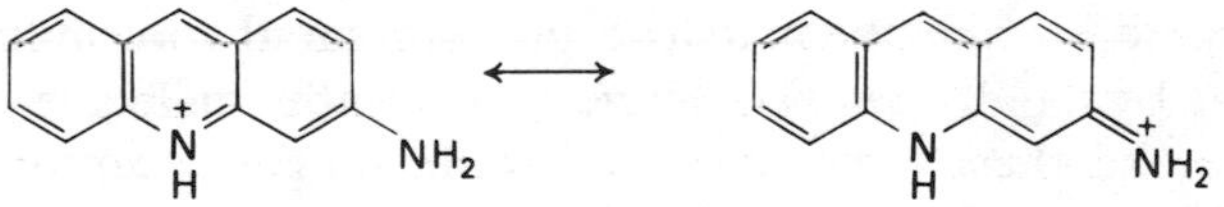

(*2.16*)   (*2.17*)

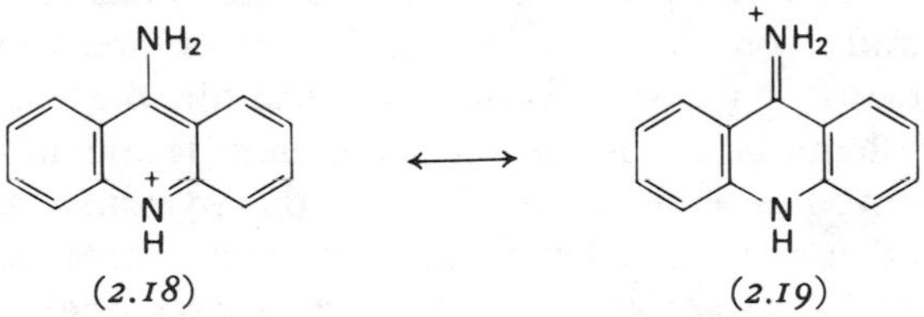

(*2.18*)   (*2.19*)

Cationic resonances which make 3- and
9-aminoacridines strong bases

cal forms which give rise to the high basic strength of 3-aminoacridine; similarly (*2.18*) and (*2.19*) are the canonical forms for 9-aminoacridine (Albert, Goldacre, and Phillips, 1948).

This positive correlation between ionization and bacteriostasis (illustrated in Table 2.2) was demonstrated over a wide range of bacterial species, anaerobes and aerobes, both Gram-positive and Gram-negative. Altogether over a hundred acridines were synthesized and tested, and it was always found that the substituents exerted no direct effect on the antibacterial action except in so far as they modified the ionization (Albert *et al.*, 1945). (For more on ionization, see Chapter 10.)

Table 2.2

DEPENDENCE OF ANTIBACTERIAL ACTION ON IONIZATION

-acridine	Minimal bacteriostatic concentration (Streptococcus pyogenes) 1 part in	Percentage ionized as cation pH 7.3; 37°C
1-Amino-	10 000	2
2-Amino-	10 000	2
3-Amino-	80 000	73
4-Amino-	5 000	< 1
9-Amino-	160 000	100
2,7-Diamino-	20 000	3
3,6-Diamino-	160 000	99
4,5-Diamino-	< 5 000	< 1

The antibacterial action of aminoacridines has these unusual characteristics: it takes place even at high dilution, is unchanged by the presence of serum proteins, and is without harm to mammalian tissues. Because no other cations known at that time had this combination of properties, it was tempting to ascribe them to the presence of the acridine nucleus. Nevertheless, by bold, stepwise alterations of the molecule, it proved possible to evoke these properties in a wide range of aromatic nuclei, even in non-heterocyclic ones! The important features for this kind of biological action were found to be: complete ionization as cation at the pH of the test, and a completely flat molecule with an area of not less than 0.39 nm^2 of flat surface (Albert, Rubbo, and Burvill, 1949). In this work, biological equivalents of the aminoacridines were found in the phenanthridine and benzoquinoline series, then in the pyridine and quinoline series provided that these smaller nuclei were given large, inert *coplanar* substituents. Finally these biological properties were coaxed out of the flat (but not heterocyclic) anthracene nucleus by providing a strong basic substituent (the guanidino group).

That aminoacridines were accumulated by the nucleic acids of cells was known through their use in vital staining (Strugger, 1940). The reason for the need for molecular flatness, as just described, became evident in 1961 when Lerman showed that aminoacridine molecules were intercalated into DNA by stacking between layers of base pairs, to which they were attached by van der Waals forces supplemented by stronger ionic bonds to phosphate anions (see Fig. 10.6). The resultant increase in 'melting temperature' showed that intercalation interfered with the unwinding of DNA strands, and hence with its normal functioning.

In the very next year, it was demonstrated that aminoacridines injure bacteria by blocking the DNA template required by the enzymes which synthesise DNA and RNA (Hurwitz *et al.*, 1962). These aspects are discussed more fully in Section 10.3.

These studies of structure-action relationships in the aminoacridines, and their physically-related analogues, have established that nucleic acids can be receptors. In fact, the drug-receptor interaction was observed here in unusual detail, much of it at the level of molecular biology.

Nucleic acids have been found to be the receptors for other classes of drugs. Furanocoumarins, particularly derivatives of psoralen (*2.20*), are given orally to repigment skin that has lost its natural colour. Methoxsalen, the 8-methoxy derivative, has a rapid action whereas trioxsalen, the 4,8,5'-trimethyl derivative gives a slower, more controllable response. These drugs add across the 5,6-double bond of the pyrimidine bases (thymine and cytosine) in DNA (Musajo and Rodighiero, 1970). This molecular change stimulates the melanocytes to active mitosis at doses that produce little change elsewhere (Africk and Fulton, 1971).

Psoralen
(*2.20*)

DNA is also the eventual receptor for steroid hormones, as shown by the antagonistic action of actinomycin D, a specific DNA inhibitor. *Sequential receptors* are concerned, the first of them a protein. The pioneering studies of Jensen and Jacobson (1962) revealed that a receptor protein, specific for oestrogens, existed in the cytosol of the uterus, vagina, and anterior pituitary gland. They had applied 17β-[³H] oestradiol to various tissues and found it was selectively bound to these few. Next, the receptor was isolated by ultracentrifugation (Toft and Gorski, 1966). Similarly the oviduct was shown to have specificity for progesterone (O'Malley and Means, 1974). These steroid-receptor complexes diffuse into the nucleus of the same cell where they bind to the chromatin (no steroid is bound in absence of its protein). In this way, a length of DNA (codon) is de-repressed and produces the required mRNA which, in turn, uses cytoplasmic ribosomes to make the characteristic protein. So rapid is this process that the physiological response characteristic of the hormone can sometimes be seen within an hour. These are very typical examples of the *induction of* a characteristic protein (for a review of induction, see Cohen, 1966).

Many other examples were then discovered. The principal androgenic steroid, dihydrotestosterone, was found to be quite specifically bound by an acidic protein in androgen-dependent tissues such as the prostate gland (Anderson and Liao, 1968). Corticosteroids, too, are bound by specific protein in the cytoplasm of liver and some other cells, and the complex enters the nucleus where it is bound by DNA. This leads to the appearance of a specific mRNA (its formation suppressable by actinomycin D) which, in turn, produces enzymes characteristic of the corticosteroid (Sekeris, 1971). A similar sequence governs the diuretic effect of aldosterone (Edelman et al., 1963). Steroid hormones, just like cholesterol, also exert a direct effect on membranes (Bangham et al., 1965), but this seems to be, relatively speaking, of only minor significance.

The importance of nucleic acids as receptors extends even more widely. Cholecalciferol (vitamin D_3), a seco-steroid, indirectly affects calcium absorption through its inductive action on DNA in the cells lining the intestine (Haussler and Norman, 1969). Ecdysone (*4.49*), the steroid insect hormone, induces DNA to make (through RNA) the enzyme synthesizing *N*-acetyl-3,4-dihydroxyphenylethylamine, which then interacts with cutaneous protein to bring about moulting (Karlson and Sekeris, 1962). Among plant hormones, the gibberellins induce DNA to yield amylase (Varner and Chandra, 1964), and both the cytokinins and auxins stimulate DNA to make specific RNA (Matthyse and and Abrams, 1970).

Small molecules as receptors. Another kind of drug-receptor relationship was brought to light through investigating the antibacterial and antifungal properties of 8-hydroxyquinoline (*2.21*), commonly known as oxine (Albert et al., 1947). Typical of early ways of thinking, Hata (1932) had supposed that oxine owed its antibacterial properties to a combination of those of quinoline and phenol in the one molecule. Yet neither quinoline nor phenol is at all antibacterial at dilution of 1:5000, whereas oxine is active at 2 parts/million. That the biological properties of two substances could be combined by introducing their individual groups into a single molecule strikes us today as absurd, because the favourable distribution of electrons in each of the constituent molecules (here, phenol and quinoline) must, far more often than not, be incompatible in the hybrid.

In the new study (Albert et al., 1947), it was found that the six isomers of oxine, obtained by moving the hydroxy group in (*2.21*) to each other possible position, were non-antibacterial. This suggested that the biological properties of oxine were linked to its ability to chelate, i.e. to bind metal cations tightly by two or more atoms so that a 5- or 6-membered ring (no other size is stable) is formed. When tested, the six inert isomers failed to chelate, whereas oxine chelated strongly to give complexes such as (*2.22*) (oxine has long been used in the analysis of metals because of this property).

8-Hydroxyquinoline (oxine)
(*2.21*)

The 1 : 1-ferrous complex of oxine
(*2.22*)

Thus both the outstanding chelating and antibacterial properties of oxine required the juxtaposition of the oxygen and nitrogen atoms which permits the tight binding of heavy metal cations in a five membered ring, as shown in (*2.22*). The remaining positive charge on the metal can be removed by further addition of oxine, and the complexes become more liposoluble due to removal of the charge.

The question was then posed: does oxine act on bacteria by removing metals essential to bacterial welfare, or does it cause traces of metals to become more toxic to the bacteria? The latter proved to be the case, as first indicated by the following example of 'concentration quenching'. Staphylococci were completely killed in an hour by 0.01 mM oxine but were unharmed by 0.70 mM oxine; in fact even a saturated (5.0 mM) solution would not kill them (Albert, Gibson, and Rubbo, 1953). Streptococci behaved similarly. The meaning of this phenomenon became clear when it was found to occur only in media containing traces of iron or copper. The viability of staphylococci for 24 hours in distilled water permitted the decisive experiments, summarized in Table 2.3, to be made.

It is easy to see from Table 2.3 that oxine (0.01 mM) is biologically inert, but becomes bactericidal in the presence of a similar quantity of iron. Clearly the toxic agent is neither oxine nor iron, but the oxine-iron complex. When broth replaced water, no added iron was necessary because it was present in the medium. When the concentration of oxine was increased to 1.25 mM, the bactericidal action disappeared. This was attributed to formation of a non-antibacterial 2:1-oxine-iron complex because, when sufficient extra iron was added to the broth so that the 1:1 complex was re-formed, full bactericidal properties were restored (Albert, Gibson, and Rubbo, 1953).

In the absence of external heavy metals, oxine has been found to enter the cells of bacteria and fungi without harming them (Beckett, Vahora, and Robinson, 1958). Yet if iron (the more potent for bacteria) or copper (for fungi) is present, the combination is rapidly lethal.

Table 2.3

THE INNOCUOUSNESS OF OXINE IN THE ABSENCE OF IRON
(Bactericidal test)
Staphylococcus aureus: pH 6–7 (20°C).

Oxine	FeSO$_4$	Growth on plating out after 1 h	
mM	mM	In glass-distilled water	In untreated meat broth
nil	nil	prolific	prolific
0.01	nil	prolific	nil
nil	0.01	prolific	prolific
0.01	0.01	nil	nil
1.25	nil		prolific
nil	1.25		prolific
1.25	1.25		nil

(Albert, Gibson, and Rubbo, 1953).

Other chelating antimicrobials have been found that, while having a totally different structure, mimic the action of oxine by being active only in the presence of a variable-valence metal, and hence show concentration quenching. Such a substance is 1-hydroxypyridine-2-thione (pyrithione), (*2.23*) (Albert, Rees, and Tomlinson, 1956), which is much used in the dermatology of the scalp. Another example is dimethyldithiocarbamic acid (*2.24*), whose salts are widely used as selective fungicides in agriculture.

All three types have a third property in common: their antimicrobial action is prevented by a small concentration of cobalt ions, even though the requisite iron or copper has been supplied (Sijpesteijn and Janssen, 1959). Cobalt is well known as an anti-oxidant, which can break an oxidatively destructive chain reaction catalysed by another metal (cf. Baur and Preis, 1936). This suggested to the Dutch workers that the iron and copper complexes of oxine, pyrithione, and dimethyldithiocarbamic acid were oxidatively destroying thioctic acid (lipoic acid) (*2.25*) which is the essential coenzyme for the oxidative decarboxylation of pyruvic acid. This was confirmed when they found pyruvic acid accumulating in the medium (Sijpesteijn and Janssen, 1959; also personal communication from these authors). Apparently the receptor in all three examples is the small molecule (*2.25*).

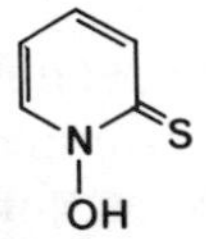

Pyrithione
(*2.23*)

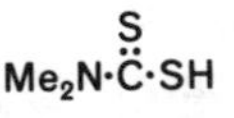

$Me_2N \cdot \overset{S}{\overset{..}{C}} \cdot SH$

Dimethyldithiocarbamic acid
(*2.24*)

$\overset{SH}{|} \quad \overset{SH}{|}$
$CH_2 \cdot CH_2 \cdot CH(CH_2)_4 \cdot CO_2H$

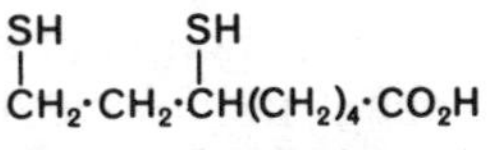

Thioctic acid
(*2.25*)

Both the aminoacridine and the oxine projects were begun at a time when interest was awakening in the possibilities of physical chemistry as a basis for drug action. Biological activity in both series was dependent on cation uptake, the acridines needing to have high affinity for the hydrogen cation, and the oxines for a heavy metal cation accidentally present in the environment. In both series, the likely efficacy of new analogues could be gauged quickly by a potentiometric titration. In both series, too, molecular structure was found to have little significance so long as it provided the essential physical properties, and in this there was great latitude. Nevertheless, at a more fundamental level, the two series differed greatly in the type of receptor on which their members acted. They both extended the current concept of a receptor in, at that time, unimagined directions. Lipoic acid is now considered the most likely receptor for arsenical drugs also (Section 12.0).

An earlier example of a coenzyme acting as a receptor is the porphyrin molecule of cytochrome oxidase. The lethal action of hydrogen cyanide, counter-selective for mammals, follows directly from the binding of this poison to the free valence of the chelated iron in the porphyrin. Many bacteria, lacking this enzyme, are not affected.

Other aspects of receptors.   When a receptor is one enzyme in a series of enzymatic reactions, it is most likely to be the one that is relatively unabundant and hence the *pacemaker* of the series (Krebs, 1957). The triosephosphate dehydrogenase system in glycolysis is an example.

Because substrates often change the *conformation* of enzymes and enzymes that of substrates (Koshland, 1964), it is likely that receptors and drugs can change one another's conformations. Of course some drugs have quite rigid structures, but others could be deformed by the receptor, and a protein receptor should be deformable by the drug, so that in some cases the drug may be acting in a cavity that its presence has created, a case of 'induced fit'. This concept is developed further in Section 7.5b. Stereochemical specificity (see earlier in this chapter) made people think, wrongly, that receptors must be quite rigid. For more data on conformation, see Section 13.3.

The introduction of penicillin into medical practice in 1941, and of streptomycin, chloramphenicol, and the tetracyclines in the following 8 years, opened up a new vista in chemotherapy. *Antibiotics* were at first regarded with much awe, and a completely new mode of action was predicted for them. In the course of time, though, they have been found to use the established types of receptor. Those antibiotics like penicillin and cephalosporin which prevent the synthesis of bacterial cell-wall have turned out to have an enzyme for receptor (Section 12.1), and this is true of the simpler oxamycin (Section 9.4). Many other antibiotics act on DNA, preventing its replication or transcription: such are adriamycin, actinomycin, mitomycin, and bleomycin (Section 4.0). Rifamycin, however, acts on the *protein* of DNA-primed RNA-polymerase.

Most of the other antibiotics inhibit protein synthesis on the ribosomes, where the receptor has to be either RNA or a protein: for example, chloramphenicol, the tetracyclines, gentamicin, streptomycin, and erythromycin (Section 4.1). The polyene antibiotics, such as amphoteracin, become attached alongside the sterol in fungal plasma membrane, thus making the cell porous, and the polypeptide antibiotics, which act on bacterial membrane, may be the only antibiotics to have found new types of receptor, namely organized lipids.

A property that sets many antibiotics apart from synthetic drugs is their complex stereochemistry which, being laid down in contact with living matter, often makes a remarkably effective fit in a therapeutic situation, but not always a selective one. For further reading on the mode of action of antibiotics, see Franklin and Snow (1975), and Gale *et al.* (1972).

In the past, there was much puzzlement as to why drugs of quite different chemical and physical properties could bring about the same physiological result. Surely they could not all act on the same receptor? Actually, there is often a *succession of receptors*, each of which can be controlled by a drug selective for it. For example, in treating high blood pressure, it is possible to medicate peripherally by relaxing the muscle of blood vessels with hydrallazine (*11.43*) or nitrites. However, one can proceed a little higher up the chain of command by blocking the sympathetic nerve-endings at their junction with these muscles, using a β-receptor blocker such as propranolol (*13.41*). It is possible to work at a still higher stage of organization by blocking the sympathetic ganglia with hexamethonium (*7.24*). Finally one can act on the highest level of all, the central nervous system, with clonidine (*9.34*). Naturally, these four kinds of drug do not share any physical or chemical properties, for they act on four chemically distinct receptors.

Just as there are analogous enzymes (Section 4.6), so there are *analogous receptors*. For instance, the acetylcholinesterase in sheep's gut combines more reversibly with organic phosphates than the analogous enzyme (the receptor) does in worms parasitizing the intestine. Highly selective de-worming can be accomplished thanks to this (Lee and Hodsden, 1963). The human body has at least three main types of receptor for catecholamines (Section 13.4), two for histamines (Section 9.4), and two (called nicotinic and muscarinic) for acetylcholine (Section 7.5a): selective drugs have been found for each of these.

Rarely, targets of drugs can be *non-receptors*. Several chelating agents are routinely used in hospitals as antidotes for poisoning by inorganic substances; examples are dimercaprol (dithioglycerol) (*11.19*), used to treat poisoning caused by compounds of arsenic, antimony, mercury, and gold; and calcium edetate (*11.22*), an effective remedy for lead poisoning (see Section 11.6). Because these metals are not normal body constituents, they are not receptors. However the metals involved in the action of the oxine family may be thought of as the first of two sequential receptors, following the pattern of steroids.

For further reading on receptors and mechanism of action of steroid hormones, see Pasquelini (1976).

2.3 How a small change in a molecule can lead to large changes in biological properties

It is quite common to find a pair of closely related molecules, of which the first has much biological action but the other has none. How can two such substances, which may differ in composition by only a single methyl-group, perform so differently in a biological test?

In this Section, a study of methyl- and methylene-groups will be made as examples of what are commonly classed as 'chemically inert' groups. If suitably placed, these groups can profoundly change the chemical behaviour of molecules, by well-understood steric and electronic effects. It can be shown that their altered biological properties are related to these changes.

(a) *Steric influences*

The steric effects introduced by small, inert groups are of two kinds. Some are evident even in aqueous solution; others require a suitable, partly complementary surface for manifestation, as in enzyme reactions.

Steric influences on solubility. It might be thought that the insertion into a given molecule of a methyl-group would always lower solubility in water. It is true that, because the methyl-group is water-repelling (see Appendix II), it usually does lower solubility, but there are interesting exceptions. Table 2.4 lists the aqueous solubilities of some aliphatic alcohols. It can be seen that the solubility of the isomeric pentanols increases

Table 2.4

SOLUBILITIES OF ALCOHOLS
(g per 100 g water at 20°C)

Pentanols	
$CH_3-CH_2-CH_2-CH_2-CH_2-OH$	2.4
$CH_3-CH_2-CH_2-\underset{\underset{OH}{\vert}}{CH}-CH_3$	4.9
$CH_3-\underset{\underset{OH}{\vert}}{\overset{\overset{CH_3}{\vert}}{C}}-CH_2-CH_3$	12.2
n-Butanol (for comparison)	8.2

(Ginnings and Baum, 1937.)

as the side-chain is broken up into smaller lengths. This is the expected behaviour, because of the strong hydrogen-bonding that exists between water molecules. In order that a substance may dissolve, these water molecules must be forced apart by breaking their hydrogen bonds. The lower alcohols, methanol and ethanol, readily do this because the hydroxyl-group forms such a large part of each molecule, and this group forms hydrogen-bonds to water. But in higher alcohols, the paraffinic side-chain becomes a more dominant feature: it cannot be accommodated in interstices, it cannot force the water molecules apart, and hence it tends to be squeezed out of the water, dragging the whole molecule with it. This effect is considerably lessened by shifting the hydroxyl-group to the centre of the molecule (as in tertiary amyl alcohol) which is consequently more soluble than its lower homologue n-butanol. No less surprising, the 2-amino-butyric acids are more soluble than 2-amino-propionic acid (alanine) because of chain folding (Cohn *et al.*, 1934).

The sulphonamidopyrimidine drugs are another series where the addition of methyl-groups strikingly increases solubility (see Table 2.5). At first sight this seems surprising, because these substances are acids and the addition of each methyl-group decreases the ionization of the acidic (SO_2NH-) group as would be predicted from the inductive effect of methyl-groups (see Appendix III). Thus it would not be expected that sulphadiazine would be less soluble than its methyl-derivatives, because sulphadiazine

Table 2.5

INCREASED SOLUBILITY IN WATER CAUSED BY
INSERTION OF METHYL-GROUPS

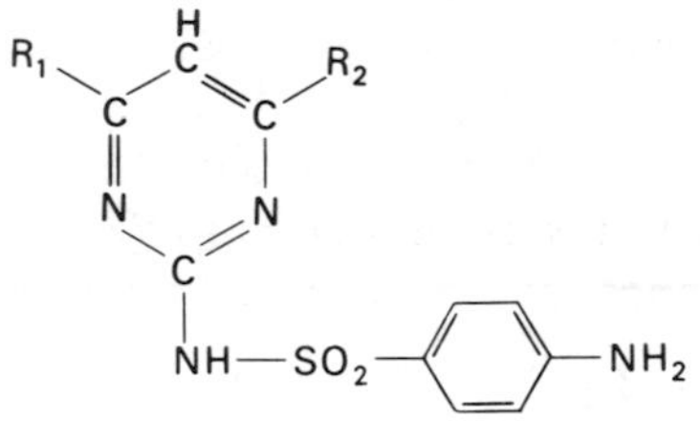

R_1	R_2	Drug	pK (acidic)	Per cent Ionized at pH 5.2	Solubility at pH 5.2 (g mol/litre) (37°C)
H	H	Sulphadiazine	6.5	3.9	0.0005
CH_3	H	Sulphamerazine	7.1	1.4	0.0013
CH_3	CH_3	Sulphadimidine	7.4	0.7	0.0024

(Gilligan and Plummer, 1943.)

is the most ionized member of the series and it is normal for an ion to be more soluble than the corresponding neutral species. This abnormal effect of methyl-groups, to be found also in other molecules having a similar degree of complexity and rigidity, is due to the protruding methyl-groups preventing the ready adsorption of dissolved solute on to the crystal-lattice of the solid phase, thus displacing the final equilibrium in the direction of increased solubility. The solubility measurements in Table 2.5 were made at pH 5.2 because this has practical significance in urinary disinfection and also in assessing the ease of clearance of the drug by the kidneys.* The same solubility sequences were found also at pH 6 and 7.

A further, and biologically very important, instance of methyl-groups increasing solubility is found in the triazine herbicide series. Non-symmetrical examples such as atrazine (*2.26*) are more soluble in water than symmetrical lower homologues such as simazine (*4.3*). These two examples have aqueous solubilities of 70 and 5 p.p.m. respectively, at 25°C, and as a consequence atrazine is much the more toxic to leaves.

Atrazine
(*2.26*)

One of the most striking cases where an inert substituent exerts a profound change in biological action is the homologous series. In such a series, each member is usually found to be more biologically active than the previous one until, suddenly, the addition of just one more $-CH_2$-group severely diminishes, or even abolishes, the biological effect. This 'cut-off' occurs at a different place in the series for different test-objects. Now, it is not surprising that toxicity should increase as a series is ascended, because the addition of each methylene-group makes possible the creation of another van der Waals bond, thus adding to the adsorptive factors which bind each substance to the organism's receptors. At the same time, there is no increase in the desorptive forces, because the kinetic energy of every molecule is identical, regardless of its size. The 'cut-off', however, was unexplained until Ferguson (1939) showed that, in a homologous series, the equitoxic concentrations for various members usually fall on a straight line, if plotted logarithmically: solubilities also fall on a straight line, but these two lines are not quite parallel and hence they intersect. It is at those points where the lines intersect that the sharp cut-off occurs (Fig. 2.2). A discussion of this effect, from the viewpoint of thermodynamic activities versus concentrations, is given in Section 15.0

* All three drugs are less soluble than their acetyl-derivatives, otherwise the solubility of the latter would be of more relevance.

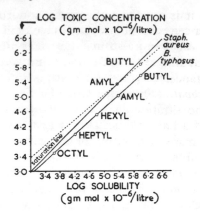

FIG. 2.2 Plot of bactericidal concentration versus solubility for normal primary alcohols.

In Fig. 2.2, where the toxic concentrations of primary alcohols have been plotted against their aqueous solubilities, it can be seen that the Gram-negative organism *B. typhosus* is very sensitive to these alcohols. Hence, even as high up in the series as octanol, the required lethal concentration is not in excess of the solubility. On the other hand, the Gram-positive organism *Staphylococcus aureus* is less sensitive to alcohols, so that a higher concentration is required for the killing. Consequently a sharp cut-off occurs at amyl alcohol because the predictable lethal concentration of hexanol is in excess of the solubility (see also Badger, 1946). In Fig. 2.2, the 'saturation line' is a diagonal, i.e. the plot of log solubility versus log solubility. It is the line on which all the points would fall for an imaginary series of substances that were optimally active in saturated solutions.

Sometimes the loss of biological activity in the upper part of a homologous series has a slightly different cause from that just discussed. The primary aliphatic amines, for example, have solubility and toxicity curves which are adequately spaced. Nevertheless, for most bacteria, a maximum in toxicity is reached somewhere about the C_{12} member (dodecylamine) and a rapid falling-off occurs when one or two more carbon atoms are added to the long paraffinic side-chain (see Fuller, 1942). It should be noted that this falling-off occurs in that part of the series where micelle-formation (Section 14.0) is beginning to increase rapidly with increase in chain-length. Thus, as the critical micelle concentration falls from 0.01 to 0.003 M in passing from the C_{12} to the C_{14} amine (Klevens, 1948), each higher homologue contributes fewer and fewer molecules of monomer, even in moderately dilute solutions. If we assume (and this is very likely) that bacterial receptors and micelles are in competition with one another for the unassociated molecules, it is easy to understand how this decreasing concentration of monomer can cause the decline in biological activity.

Steric influences on covalent hydration. A methyl-group prevents the addition of water to an adjacent double-bond, thus greatly increasing the lipophilicity of a substance. To place this remarkable effect in perspective, the phenomenon of *covalent hydration* will first be described. Discovery that the potentiometic titration of pteridin-6-one (6-hydroxypteridine) gave a loop instead of a line (Albert, Brown and Cheeseman, 1952a) led to the recognition that many nitrogenous heterocyclic substances add water, covalently across a double-bond, in at least one ionic species (for reviews, see Albert, 1967, 1976; Perrin, 1965). Thus the neutral species of quinazoline in aqueous solution consists largely of the anhydrous form (*2.27*), but its cation is the hydrate (*2.28*) (Albert, Armarego and Spinner, 1961).

Quinazoline
(*2.27*)

Hydrated quinazoline (cation)
(*2.28*)

Pteridine
(*2.29*)

There are three reliable methods for detecting covalent hydration, and each works by revealing deletion of a double bond by the addition across it of a water molecule. Thus ultraviolet spectra are displaced to lower wavelengths, determination of ionization constants reveal acids to be weaker, and bases stronger, than normal, and proton magnetic resonance spectra show the signals displaced upfield. The first and third of these methods can indicate, in addition, which ionic species is the hydrated one. For all these methods, normal values can be predicted from isomers, and from molecules with one fewer ring-nitrogen atom or one benzene ring less. Similarly, values for the hydrates are approximated by those for the corresponding dihydro-compounds.

An example: the spectrum of quinazoline is unexpectedly displaced to much shorter wavelengths when the solution is acidified (Fig. 2.3); also the pK_a is 3.51 (an equilibrium value) instead of 1.9, the pK_a for totally anhydrous species, determined in rapid-reaction apparatus (Bunting and Perrin, 1967). Covalent hydration is largely suppressed if a methyl-group is present on the carbon atom which is attacked by the OH-group of water. This effect has been shown to be due to a steric effect reinforced by induction (Albert *et al.*, 1961). Thanks to this, 4-methylquinazoline shows a normal spectral shift on acidification (Fig. 2.4), and has a pK_a of 2.52 in agreement with calculations.

Pteridine (*2.29*) has a higher tendency to hydrate than quinazoline, hence even the neutral molecule is 22 per cent hydrated (in aqueous solu-

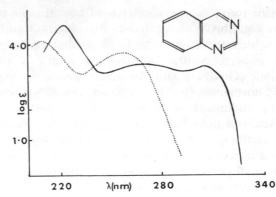

FIG. 2.3 Ultraviolet spectra of quinazoline in water. The solid line shows the neutral species, the dotted line the cation.

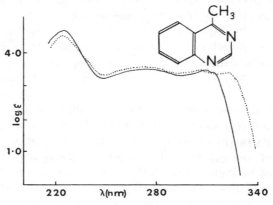

FIG. 2.4 Ultraviolet spectra of 4-methylquinazoline in water. The solid line shows the neutral species, the dotted line the cation.

tion, at 20°). Here again a methyl-group in the 4-position substantially prevents hydration of this substance (Perrin, 1962); it also prevents hydration of 2-aminopteridine (Albert, Howell and Spinner, 1962), and of pteridin-2-one (Albert and Howell, 1962). The hydration of pteridin-6-one, which occurs in the 7, 8-position (Brown and Mason, 1956), is similarly hindered by a methyl-group in the 7-position (Albert and Reich, 1961).

The extra hydroxyl-group furnished by covalent hydration, as in (2.28), reduces lipid/water partition coefficients and hence membrane-permeability. It is thus easy to visualize how the presence of a favourably situated methyl-group could increase permeability by diminishing hydration (see Appendix II) and thus completely change physiological properties.

Several naturally occurring pteridines, such as xanthopterin, are hydrated, whereas 7-methyl-xanthopterin (also naturally occurring) is not

(Albert and Reich, 1961; Inoue and Perrin, 1962). Several other natural products are in equilibrium with covalently hydrated forms, e.g. the aflatoxins with which the fungus *Aspergillus flavus* contaminates food (Patterson and Roberts, 1972); anthramycin (*4.26*), a pyrrolobenzo-diazepine antibiotic (Goldberg and Freidman, 1971); the blood-pressure lowering alkaloid hortiamine (Pachter, Raffauf, Ullyot and Ribiero, 1960); tetrodotoxin, the sodium-channel blocker from Japanese puffer fish (Goto, Kishi, Takahishi and Hirata, 1965); and the ergot alkaloids if expos-ed to sunlight (Hellberg, 1959). The oxidation of purines by xanthine oxidase is thought to require prior covalent hydration of these substances, although only a small percentage may be hydrated at equilibrium (Berg-mann, Kwietny, Levin, and Brown, 1960).

Steric influences on chelation. The antibacterial action of 8-hydroxy-quinoline (discussed in Section 11.7a) is seriously decreased by a methyl-group in the 2-position (Albert, Rubbo, Goldacre and Balfour, 1947). This deactivating effect of the methyl-group is most likely exerted through a steric effect at a biological surface. Even in solution, this substance (2-methyl-8-hydroxyquinoline) has lost affinity for Al^{3+} (while retaining it for Fe^{3+}) because of the steric effect of the methyl-group. Other examples of steric hindrance by a methyl-group are described in Section 11.4.

Steric influences on receptors and enzymes. Most molecules that fit the receptor of acetylcholine (and thus imitate the muscarinic action of this neurotransmitter) have a quaternary nitrogen atom of which one substituent is a straight chain of five atoms in length (see Section 13.6). The addition of just one more methylene-group to this chain causes a dramatic loss of biological effect. Two of the other substituents on the nitrogen atom must be methyl-groups to achieve maximal action; if one of these is substituted by either hydrogen on ethyl, a sharp drop in action takes place.

Enzymes, also, are often so specific that the addition or elimination of a single methyl-group in a substrate or coenzyme can cause a large, or even complete, loss of reactivity. How the biological action of thiamine is affected by the addition or loss of a single methyl-group was recounted at the begin-ning of this Chapter.

Indoleacetic acid (*4.52*), one of the natural growth-regulators of plants, is an example of a substance whose powerful action is abolished by the insertion of a methyl-group in the 2-position. On the other hand, in the K family of vitamins, e.g. menaphthone (*2.30*), the presence of a methyl-group in the 2-position is absolutely essential for biological activity (see also below).

Sometimes a methyl-group increases the biological effect of a drug by making it a poorer fit for a *destructive enzyme*. Thus amphetamine (*7.42*) (1-methyl-2-phenylethylamine) has a much more prolonged hypertensive effect than 2-phenylethylamine. This has been traced to the resistance of amphetamine to monoamine oxidase which rapidly destroys the lower homologue (Blaschko, 1952). Similarly the action of corticosteroids and the steroid sex hormones can be intensified by inserting a methyl- or fluorine-substituent, a device which has produced many clinically valuable drugs. Such seemingly inert substituents probably turn the steroids into poorly-fitting substrates for their natural destructive enzymes (Ringold, 1961).

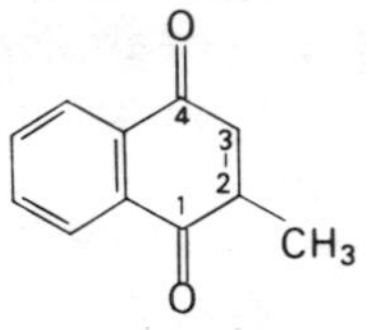

Menaphthone	Barbituric acid
(2.30)	(2.31)

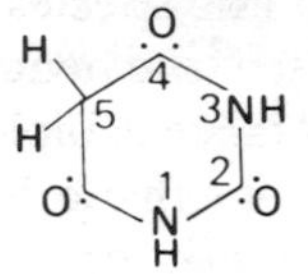

(b) *Electronic influences*

The methyl-group is the commonest example of those few substituents which release electrons in any environment, no matter whether inductive or mesomeric mechanisms are operating (see Appendix III).

Electronic influences on ionization. Because of its electron-releasing nature, a methyl-group, if attached to a carbon atom, strengthens a base and

Table 2.6

CONNECTION BETWEEN IONIZATION AND
ANTIBACTERIAL ACTIVITY IN A SET OF
TRIPHENYLMETHANE COMPOUNDS

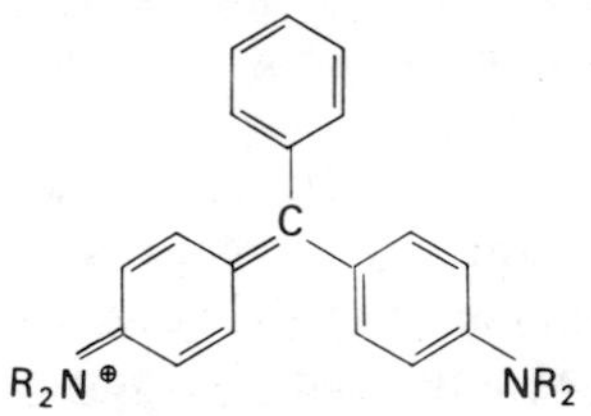

Substance	R (all four)	pK (equil.)	Per cent Ionized at pH 7.3	Min. bacteriostatic conc'n for Staph. aureus (24 h at 37°C and pH 7.3)
Doebner's Violet	H	5.38	2	1 in 20 000
Malachite Green	CH_3	6.90	28	1 in 80 000
Brilliant Green	C_2H_5	7.90	80	1 in 1 280 000

(Goldacre and Phillips, 1949.)

weakens an acid. Also, a methyl-group attached to a nitrogen, so as to make a secondary amine, is base-strengthening, but most tertiary amines are weaker than secondary amines. Such changes in strength are usually less than one pK unit, but can influence biological results if the pK falls within one unit of the pH at which the biological test is made (see Section 10.0). Under these circumstances, a difference of one pK unit between two drugs can cause a tenfold increase in the ionization of one of them. When, as so often happens, one ionic species (say, the cation) is far more biologically active than another (say, the neutral species), this change in ionization can decide whether a substance is biologically active or not (see Section 10.3).

The triphenylmethane dyestuffs, whose somewhat complicated chemistry is discussed in Section 10.2, show a very remarkable increase in basic strength on N-alkylation. It can be seen from Table 2.6 that antibacterial activity is strongly correlated with ionization for the substances examined, and that the antibacterial activity thus depends on the presence of 'chemically inert groups'.

It is obvious enough that methylation of an acidic $-OH$ or $-NH$ group must abolish its ability to ionize. The consequences of this in the barbituric acid series are particularly interesting. In aqueous solution, barbituric acid exists in the trioxo-form (*2.31*), and forms the mono-anion by loss of a proton from C-5. It is a fairly strong acid (pK_a 3.9). The insertion of one alkyl-group into the 5-position decreases the acidic strength only slightly, but two such groups remove any possibility of an anion being formed in the 5-position. In the latter case the anion is formed from N-3, but is much weaker. Thus barbitone (5,5-diethylbarbituric acid) has a pK_a of 7.9 and hence is 10^4 times weaker than barbituric acid. The consequences of the insertion of these inert ethyl groups, for structure-activity relationships, is momentous. A substance with a pK_a of 3.9 is completely ionized at pH 7.3 (see Appendix I) and hence quite unlikely to pass the blood-brain barrier. But when the pK_a is 7.9, as in barbitone, the substance is 80 per cent non-ionized (as anion) at pH 7.3, and hence should pass without any difficulty. So essential is lipophilicity for hypnotic action that no less than four carbon atoms (altogether) must be present in the substituents of the 5-position (see further Chapter 15).

Electronic influences on reduction-oxidation (redox) *potentials.* The electrons released to the rest of a molecule by a C-methyl substituent lower the redox potential (E_o). As a result, the affected substance becomes a more active reducing agent and a less active oxidizing agent (i.e. it is more resistant to becoming reduced) than is the unmethylated homologue. Redox potentials are defined in Section 11.4 and refer to the equilibrium between oxidized and reduced forms (all values in this book are versus the normal hydrogen electrode).

To give an example of this lowering of E_o, a methyl-group inserted into the 2-position of 1,4-naphthoquinone, to give (*2.30*), depresses the potential (by 76 mV) to + 408 mV (Fieser and Fieser, 1935). This 408 mV is a very workable potential for an oxidizing agent in the living cell. On the other hand, the reduction potential of NAD (nicotinamide adenine dinucleotide) is − 280 mV, a value so low that a substituted NAD of slightly lower potential can probably not become reduced to its NADH. If it could not be reduced in the living cell, it could not act as an important hydrogen carrier. It is probably for this reason that 2-methylnicotinamide has no biological activity, although the effect of the methyl-group may also be partly steric.

Electronic influences on reactions where a covalent bond is broken. The electron-releasing effects of a methyl-group described above were of a virtually instantaneous character. Some time-dependent (i.e. kinetically controlled) effects will now be mentioned. Methyl-groups, because of their electron-releasing properties, promote electrophilic substitution, e.g. they make neighbouring amino-groups readier to be acylated, or to form an azomethine (Schiff-base) with an aldehyde. A methyl-group also constitutes a side-chain that is often bio-degraded. Thus the metabolic oxidation of a methyl-group to a carboxylic acid in an aromatic hydrocarbon completely changes the distribution of the substance and leads to its rapid excretion (cf. Schultzen and Naunyn, 1867).

Methyl-groups can stabilize a molecule by replacing a hydrogen atom that would otherwise be split out in conjunction with a neighbouring atom. Thus dithiocarbamates split out hydrogen sulphide if at least one alkyl-group is replaced by hydrogen. In this way they produce *iso*thiocyanates. For example, the agricultural fungicide nabam breaks down in this way, and the *iso*thiocyanate that is produced on the plant seems to be the true active agent. However, fully alkylated dithiocarbamates, e.g. (*2.24*), are stable, and act as such (mode of action was described in Section 2.2).

Solubility.   In an aromatic nitrogen heterocycle, replacement by methyl of the hydrogen in an − OH, − NH$_2$ or − C(: O)-NH group can increase solubility in water dramatically, even in the pyridine series. Substituents with a bondable hydrogen atom (e.g. − NH$_2$) decrease the solubility in water through hydrogen-bonding of the substituent to the highly polar ring-nitrogen atom; in short, the attraction of one molecule for another is greater than its attraction for water molecules. As a result, the crystal lattice energy is increased, and the substance falls out of solution. Such an effect is rarely observed among non-heterocyclic compounds. This is not strictly an electronic effect of a methyl-group, but rather the consequence of the ability of a methyl-group to prevent the strong, electron-mediated self-polymerization by hydrogen bonds.

Some examples will be given from the pteridine (*2.29*) series (all in water at 20°). 4-Aminopteridine is soluble only 1 in 1400, but 4-dimethyl-aminopteridine 1 in 2 (Albert, Brown and Cheeseman, 1952b). Similarly, 7-hydroxypteridine is soluble only 1 in 900, but both its *O*- and *N*-methyl-derivatives are soluble 1 in 50. Again, 6-aminopurine (*4.3*) (adenine) is only soluble 1 in 1100 but 6-dimethylaminopurine 1 in 120 (Albert and Brown, 1954).

2.4 Correlations today

Each* early discovery of a structure-activity relationship seemed, to its contemporaries, to be a universal explanation of drug action, and it was not clearly seen that, had this been true, drugs could evoke only one kind of biological effect. Nowadays, more correctly, we accept different explanations for different biological actions, but are still troubled by our nomenclature. Thus when we say 'structure', we mean 'constitution', namely all the information on physical and chemical properties that is stored in the chemical formula, or that can be discovered by measurement and experimentation. Also when we say 'activity' we mean the action on the drug-receptor, but this effect, we know, is often connected to the desired physiological result only through a long chain of other reactions. It is only with reference to the action at the receptor that the constitution of the drug has any relevance.

A rich harvest of chemical and physical properties can now be gleaned from a chemical formula. Students of medicinal chemistry are taught to 'read out' properties when confronted by structures. For example, the formula of phenol shows it to be a weak acid of pK_a about 10; moreover, if it were a substituted phenol, the rise or fall in acidic properties could be read out at once by subtracting the Hammett σ-constant for that substituent (see Appendix III) from the pK_a of phenol. It is clear that the molecule can be readily attacked at the electron-rich 2, 4, and 6-positions by electrophilic reagents. In addition, the hydroxy-group is available for esterification and ether-formation. The ease with which all these reactions can take place in a substituted phenol is governed by the sign and magnitude of Hammett σ-constants for the substituents, electron-attracting groups disfavouring and electron-releasing groups aiding the reaction. Nucleophilic attack and reactions of addition are clearly unlikely, reduction difficult, and oxidation likely to produce quinones and hence self-condensation. Powerful, electron-attracting substituents ($-CN$, $-NO_2$, $-CONH_2$) will favour nucleophilic attack, addition reactions, and reduction; but will disfavour oxidation. The distribution of a phenol between an aqueous and a lipoid solvent can be approximately calculated by use of the π-constants for each substituent, as derived by Hansch and Rekker (see Appendix II).

Similarly the formula of pyridine reveals that it is a weak base, with a pK_a about 5, and the basic strength of substituted pyridines can quickly be calculated by the procedure of Clark and Perrin (1964). Further, the formula shows that there is a large deficiency of electrons in the 2, 4, and 6-positions, which are therefore liable to nucleophilic attack; only the nitrogen atom is open to addition reactions; electrophilic reactions are extremely unlikely; reduction, although not easy, is possible and oxidation unlikely. The rules, allowing these categories of information to be read out of the formulae of various kinds of heterocycles, are easy to memorize and have been set out in convenient form for this purpose (Albert, 1968).

There are some kinds of drug action where the structure itself plays an outstanding part, namely in the use of metabolite analogues. In many other kinds of action, a physical property is its main source, and this property could be provided by many kinds of structure.

In seeking correlations today, the outstanding interest lies in the nature of the receptor, whether this is in the isolated state or merely gleaned by inference. The key physical properties sought for correlations are: ionization and other equilibrium properties, electron-distribution, partition between phases, and stereochemistry.

For information on the chemistry of drugs, see Wade (1977), Burger (1970), and Wilson, Gisvold, and Doerge (1977).

3 Differences in distribution: the first principle of selectivity

Of the various principles that govern selectivity, that concerned with distribution is (even when its contribution is relatively small) never completely absent. At the other extreme, it can be the principal source of the whole selective gain.

It is remarkable that selectivity through distribution can take place even when the agent is toxic to both economic and uneconomic cells, provided that it is accumulated only by the latter. An example where the economic and uneconomic cells are in different species is illustrated in Plate 1. Some years ago a Frenchman discovered that an aqueous solution of sulphuric acid could safely be sprayed on cereal crops to destroy the weeds (Rabaté, 1927). The unsprayed strip at the right shows wild radish in full bloom among the wheat, but the crop is seen uncontaminated on the sprayed side of the field (Ball and French, 1935; Robbins, Crafts and Raynor, 1952). The strength used was 10 per cent (w/w) H_2SO_4 at about 120 gallons per acre. Sulphuric acid is, of course, injurious to the cytoplasm of both wheat and weed, but it never reaches that of the former for two reasons. The exterior of cereal grasses is smooth and waxy, whereas that of dicotyledonous weeds is rough and wax-free; the acid runs off the former but is accumulated by the latter. Moreover the tender new shoots of cereals arise from the base of the plant and are protected by leaf-sheaths, whereas the growing point of the dicotyledons is exposed and vulnerable because it is the apex of the shoot (Fig. 3.1). Hence the weeds die, and the economic crop persists, because of a selective action that depends entirely on distribution (Blackman, 1946).

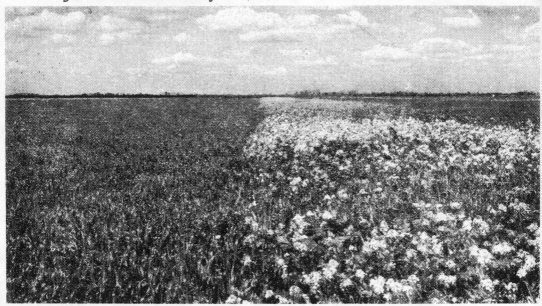

PLATE I   Elimination, by early spraying with 10 per cent sulphuric acid, of wild radish from a wheat crop. The strip on left was sprayed at emergence. (Ball and French, 1935.)

The selectivity of the tetracyclines, so much used in treating bacterial infections in mammals, depends on a similarly favourable distribution: the bacteria concentrate these antibiotics whereas mammalian cells do not. Concentration of tetracyclines by bacteria (both Gram-positive and -negative types) was found to be a function of the cytoplasmic membrane (Franklin, 1971). Because of the difference, tetracyclines inhibit ribosomal protein synthesis in bacteria at doses which do not affect it in higher organisms (Franklin, 1963b, 1966). This selectivity depends on the intact-

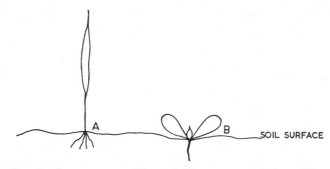

FIG. 3.1   Sketch of emergent seedlings of (A) a monocotyledon; (B) a dicotyledon.

ness of the mammalian cell membrane, because isolated ribosomes (rat liver was used) were found to be as subject to inhibition of protein synthesis as bacterial ones were (Franklin, 1963a; Section 11.8).

Other cases are known where an invading organism concentrates a poison which selectively injures it. A remarkable feature of trypanosomes is the speed and extent of their concentration of organic arsenicals. Within ten minutes of first contact, these drugs may reach a level several hundred times greater than in the surrounding fluid. This is thought to be due to the relatively greater number of mercapto-groups on the organisms' cell surface: in one calculation, it was estimated that every fifth atom forming the surface has a -SH group (Eagle, 1945).

Similarly phenothiazine, a highly effective oral anthelmintic in sheep, is accumulated by intestinal worms but not by the cells lining the sheep's gut: yet, when given intravenously, it is toxic for both species (Lazarus and Rogers, 1951).

Examples will now be given of selective partitioning between the tissues of a single organism.

After oral administration, griseofulvin is specifically localized in a patient's keratinized cells, namely the epidermis, hair, and nails, and is used to injure fungi parasitizing these tissues. Griseofulvin blocks fungal mitosis, causing multinucleate cells to be formed (Gull and Trinci, 1973): mammalian (and plant) cells suffer similarly, so the selectivity depends on the initial distribution.

Cyanocobalamin (vitamin B_{12}), injected into a muscle, travels to the bone-marrow and is accumulated there after a dilution of 10^{10}-fold in the body fluids. Even a microgram, injected in this way, is enough to cause new reticulocytes to form in the marrow of a patient suffering from pernicious anaemia. The process of distribution has been followed with ^{57}Co.

Iodine, which is selectively accumulated by the thyroid gland, provides another good example of selective action through specific distribution. This process is easily followed with radioactive iodine (^{131}I, half-life 8 days), which is used for the treatment of thyrotoxicosis. Depending on the dosage, the radioactive chemical can merely inhibit the excessive metabolism of the gland or actually attack a tumour in it. The usual oral dose is only 10^{-12}g, yet 80 per cent of this can be demonstrated in the gland soon after administration.

Inorganic phosphates are accumulated specifically by the trabecular bone-tissue which lies close to the haemopoietic red bone marrow. The overproduction of red cells in polycythaemia is treated clinically with ^{32}P (half-life 14 days).

The safe and accurate diagnosis of diseases by using radiopharmaceuticals represents an important contribution of atomic energy to human health. Mercury, as ^{197}Hg (half-life 64 h), is much used for kidney screening as it is selectively concentrated in the renal tubules. Leucocytes labelled with indium (^{111}In, half-life 67 h) are now injected intravenously to locate all forms of abscess, making use of the natural swarming of leucocytes to diseased areas (Segal, Arnot, Thakur, and Lavender, 1976). A different isotope (^{113}In, half-life 99 min) is used to scan the lungs by first adsorbing it on to particles of 30–60 µm, a size that the lung selectively retains. Technetium (as ^{99}Tc, half-life 6 h), a powerful but safe emitter of soft gamma rays, is also used in this way, and also (in simple solution) to localize brain tumours which selectively accumulate it. Similarly thallium (^{201}Tl) is used to locate damaged cells in a patient's heart. For more details on radiopharmaceuticals, see Wade (1977).

The daring but successful therapy of brain tumours with boron rests on the isotope ^{10}B which is not radioactive, but has an extraordinary ability to capture neutrons. These are converted to alpha particles which have 100 million times the energy of the neutrons. Normal brain tissue is little affected by neutrons, and the alpha particle has a range of only 10 µm in tissues. Normally boron compounds penetrate the blood-brain barrier quite poorly, but the tumours have large gaps in this membrane: hence the boron-containing agent accumulates in the malignant tissue, as was first shown by Kruger (1955) using mouse brain.

The boron is injected into the patient usually as a carborane (e.g. the ring-compound $C_2H_{12}B_{10}$) which is furnished with two mercapto-groups to give affinity for protein. Although there is 19 per cent of ^{10}B in natural boric acid (the rest is mainly ^{11}B), the therapeutic material is further enriched. One hour after the injection, a neutron beam from a thermonuclear reactor is lined up with an appropriately localized hole made in the patient's skull. The pioneer clinical work was done in Tokyo (Hatanaka and Sano, 1973; cf. Wong, Tolpin, and Lipscomb, 1974).

Many organic compounds containing normal iodine (^{127}I) are used as radiopaques (X-ray contrast agents) in the radiography of the area where each is selectively accumulated. For delineating the gall-bladder and biliary ducts, sodium ipodate or iopanic acid (*3.1*) are given orally. Similarly the urinary tract is selected by intravenous diatrizoic acid (*3.2*) or its isomer iothalamic acid.

Iopanic acid
(*3.1*)

Diatrizoic acid
(*3.2*)

N-substituted phenothiazines with basic side chains (e.g. the antihistamine promethazine, and the tranquillizer chlorpromazine) are accumulated in the eyes of all mammals. A concentration 50 times as great as in other tissues is often reached (Potts, 1962).

Each naturally occurring steroid has a specific protein to transport it to the nuclear DNA in the cells which it selectively influences (see Section 2.1, p. 33).

The next example of selectivity through favourable distribution is culled from anticancer therapy. Heidelberger, knowing that many malignant cells take up uracil more readily than normal cells, synthesized 5-fluorouracil (*3.3*) and introduced it into the clinic (Heidelberger, Griesbach, Cruz, Schnitzer and Grunberg, 1958). Today it is used by dermatologists to cure skin cancers (both squamous and basal cell carcinomas). So selective is this substance that the 5 per cent cream is usually rubbed in with the bare hand without harmful effect, and there is no objection to covering the whole face or even trunk with it when the growths are widely distributed. The malignant tissue, only, becomes inflamed and finally disintegrates being replaced by healthy granulation tissue followed by new skin (Williams and Klein, 1970; Belisario, 1970). Surgery and diathermy act more quickly but produce scarring. The biochemistry of 5-fluorouracil action is discussed in Section 12.5.

5-Fluorouracil
(*3.3*)

Particles, injected into the human circulation, are distributed according to size, whether they are radiopharmaceuticals (see the foregoing) or inert material such as glass microspheres. Thus particles of 30 μm diameter lodge in the Kupffer cells of the liver, whereas those 1000 times this width are retained by lung capillaries. When particles are inhaled, those above 5 μm diameter remain in the nasal passages, those of about 2 μm lodge in the larger bronchial areas, whilst particles must be narrower than 1 μm to reach the smallest bronchi and alveolar sacs, as is necessary for effective medication by aerosols (nasal sprays).

The processes by which distribution achieves selectivity will now be outlined in the following Sections.

3.0 Absorption, distribution, and excretion of drugs

Whether an agent is given by mouth or injected, it must usually traverse one or several semi-permeable membranes before the required receptor is encountered. For example, an antimalarial, such as chloroquine (*10.28*), given by mouth, must penetrate the barrier that lies between the gastro-intestinal tract and the blood-stream, then the erythrocyte membrane, and finally that of the malarial parasite. On both sides of each membrane the concentration of a drug continually decreases through storage, excretion, and inactivation. Examples of storage are (i) in lipoids for liposoluble substances such as thiopentone, (ii) on nucleic acids or chondroitin for cationic substances such as chloroquine, and (iii) on serum albumin for anionic substances such as suramin and sulphonamides (Brodie and Hogben, 1957). Storage is usually freely reversible and can be beneficial, e.g. when it tends to keep the blood-level of a drug constant in septicaemia; but it can be disadvantageous, e.g. when, after a bedtime dose of a hypnotic, the patient cannot keep awake at his work next day.

Excretion may be through the kidneys, the bile-duct (and hence into the gut), or through the lungs (as with general anaesthetics). Ether and strychnine are examples of drugs which are rapidly excreted (in the urine) without storage or chemical change. For many other drugs, excretion is preceded by inactivation, a process which involves the making or breaking of covalent bonds and hence is not freely reversible. When the drug has penetrated into the tissues through membranes of the blood-vessels, it is subject again to loss by storage and inactivation, but in many situations it cannot be excreted until it penetrates back into the blood-stream. Finally, when the drug penetrates the last membrane surrounding the relevant receptor, combination occurs with the receptor, a signal is generated, and the physiological effect characteristic of the drug begins. This effect usually continues as long as the concentration is high enough to keep a significant number of receptors activated (see further, Sections 2.2 and 7.5). However, as the concentration is falling all the time, the receptors will not stay activated unless more of the drug is administered.

These competing effects are shown diagrammatically in Fig. 3.2, which shows how the frequency and size of the dose depend on all these factors, each arrow representing an equilibrium or a steady state (see Section 3.6, below). Sometimes there is an additional complication: the drug which

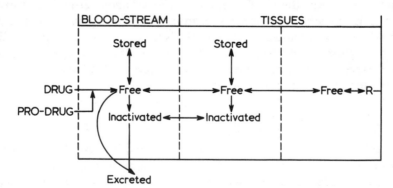

FIG. 3.2 Distribution of a drug or other biologically active substance. The broken vertical lines indicate selective membranes and R stands for a receptor.

acts on the receptor is not administered as such, put as a 'pro-drug' which is turned into the drug by metabolism (see Section 3.5).

In this picture of distribution (Fig. 3.2), the reversibility of most of the steps should be noted.

The useful concept of *apparent volume of distribution* (V_D) of a drug is defined:

$$V_D = \frac{\text{Weight of drug in the body}}{\text{Plasma concentration of the free drug at equilibrium}}$$

Thus V_D is the apparent fluid volume in which the drug is dissolved. Values of V_D compatible with the known volume of a body compartment may suggest that the drug is confined to that compartment. Values of V_D greater than the total body volume indicate that the drug is deposited in a tissue (Goldstein, Aronow and Kalman, 1974). Some relevant volumes of body compartments are (in litres): circulating plasma of blood (3), erythrocytes (3), extracellular water other than blood (11), intracellular water (24); the total is 41 litres or 58 per cent of body weight (average values) (Goldstein *et al.*, 1974).

The picture of distribution would not be complete without mentioning some recycling mechanisms. Drugs in circulation enter the liver by the hepatic artery and portal vein. From the liver's two lobes, the drugs emerge (as such, or in a degraded state) with the bile which passes down the 'common duct' into the gall-bladder, which exists for bile storage. At intervals, bile leaves the gall-bladder by the bile-duct which discharges into the second part of the duodenum; this is a slender tube about 30 cm long which connects the stomach to the rest of the small intestine. Some drugs are absorbed from the small intestine by the portal vein and pass by the bloodstream to the liver, which secretes them into the small intestine again, through the bile. Phenolphthalein and biallylamicol ('Camoform') are examples, and the last-named is also recycled by the following pathway: intestine-lungs-bronchi-trachea-pharynx-intestine. Both circuits involve a gradual decrement via the faeces, and the latter circuit also involves loss through expectoration (Dill, Fisken, Reutner, Weston and Glazko, 1957).

Redistribution in plants is a similar phenomenon. When a field is sprayed, much of the plant surface is shadowed by other parts of the plant and hence does not receive the spray. However, redistribution of the sprayed agent is effected by wind and by moisture. Because the surface of plants is negatively charged, redistribution is efficient mainly for positively charged substances (such as Bordeaux Mixture, or streptomycin) (Dimond and Horsfall, 1959).

From the above it will be apparent that the physicochemical properties of a potential agent must be very finely adjusted if it is to avoid the many casualties of storage, excretion, and degradation. In many cases, by accident or by design, substances have been obtained with properties favourable for their *accumulation* near one or other kind of receptor; then, if their chemical structure is complementary to that of the receptor, the desired biological action takes place.

Apart from concentration at effector sites, high concentrations of drugs are commonly found in the liver and kidneys, arising from the functioning of these organs as centres of detoxication and excretion.

'Compartmentalization', a word coined by A. Zaffaroni, is the restriction of agents to the target tissue by mechanical means. In its commoner form, a small piece of plastic, impregnated with the drug, is inserted at the desired site of action. The uses of this type of sustained release (see Section 3.6) range from controlling glaucoma to birth control. In another field of use, rubber sheets impregnated with organic tin compounds are fixed on ships' keels to prevent fouling by barnacles. Copper compounds are similarly being compartmentalized and anchored in tropical streams to kill schistosome-infected snails. In a different approach, artificial sweeteners have been covalently bonded to polymers which impart a sweet taste to food, but are not absorbed from the gastrointestinal tract.

For further general reading on the distribution of drugs, see La Du, Mandel and Way (1971) and Saunders (1974).

The structure of water.   The role of water in all distribution phenomena is dominant. Because water is so familiar to us, we are not inclined to think of it as one of the most complex of all liquids. Its irreplaceable role in all living processes calls for deeper understanding: water is not just an inert medium, accidentally present, of little more relevance than a reaction vessel. In fact, water has unique physiocochemical properties: it has a broad domain of thermodynamic stability and can participate in acid-base equilibria over a wide range (actually over 16 pH units); and it can sustain redox equilibria over a potential range of more than 2 V (Section 11.4). The curious fact of a maximal density at $4°C$, and the ability of water to absorb or release calories without much change in temperature, have profoundly influenced the distribution of life on earth. All these properties point to a structure immensely more complex than the common symbol H_2O would indicate, because water is, from the melting temperature of ice to the condensation temperature of steam, a large and complex polymer.

In the molecule of steam (Fig. 3.3a), two protons and two lone-pairs of electrons occupy tetrahedrally disposed, hybridized orbitals. In ice, hydrogen bonding between molecules leads to the formation of a five-molecule structural unit, which is approximately tetrahedral (Fig. 3.3b). Each oxygen atom is surrounded by four others at a distance of 2.75 Å; three of them are in the same layer (forming, with other water molecules, puckered six-membered rings) and the fourth is in an adjacent layer. Large polyhedral cavities lie between these layers.

Liquid water is unique in its ability to promote three-dimensional order, for it is the only molecule which, from a single atomic centre, can give rise to *four* hydrogen bonds (two as a donor, and two as an acceptor). The

(a)   (b)

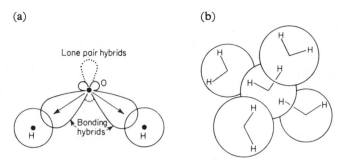

FIG. 3.3 (a) The water molecule, as in steam; (b) primary unit of water association, as in ice. (Ives and Lemon, 1968.)

hydrides most closely related to it (NH_3 and HF) can form only two hydrogen bonds (by acting once as a donor and once as an acceptor). As a rule, only *equal* numbers of donor and acceptor bonds are energetically stable in liquids.

Of the many hypotheses of the structure of liquid water that have been proposed, that of Pople (1951) agrees very well with all experimentally determined properties. In this, water is formulated as a continuous polymer in which H_2O units are united by a network of hydrogen bonds that extend throughout the whole liquid, which is, in this sense, one large molecule. This formulation is compatible not only with the evidence from density, dielectric constants, spectroscopy, and X-ray diffraction, but also with the extraordinarily large heat capacity of water which arises from the ability of H-bonds to absorb thermal energy (confirmed by Weres and Rice, 1972). No support remains for older ideas of 'flickering clusters', monomeric inclusions, or other types of discontinuity.

When water molecules are in close contact with a paraffin, the hydrocarbon side-chain of a molecule, or an inert gas, they obviously cannot use their normal quota of four hydrogen bonds. This limitation leads to a measurable loss of entropy, and a gain in density of structure. Some authors interpret this as the formation of 'icebergs' at the non-bonding boundaries. However, ice is a little less dense than water! Careful measurements have shown that the loss of entropy is proportional to a change at the boundary only (Miller and Hildebrand, 1968).

Chaotropic agents are those used to open up the structure of water. The best-known are urea, guanidine, and inorganic ions. They are much used to change the conformation of enzymes and other macromolecules in contact with water by removing the structure which is extending them. Some enzymes are inactivated by this treatment, others activated.

For further reading on the structure and properties of liquid water, see Eisenberg and Kauzmann (1969), Franks (1972), and Lewin (1974).

3.1 The permeability of natural membranes

It is evident that the distribution of an agent is highly dependent on its ability to penetrate semi-permeable membranes. The plasma membrane is discussed in Section 5.2. In the classical conception of this membrane, its behaviour was static, something like a dialysis sac. More recent work discovered its latent dynamic properties, such as phase-reversal and processes akin to enzymic activity (e.g. permease activity, and transport in response to the metabolism of glucose). In the following pages, membranes will be discussed according to their observed functions and classified as four main types.

'*Type 1' membrane.*   This seems to be the most common; it hinders the passage of ions, and permits that of neutral molecules. Through this type of membrane, those molecules that have high oil/water partition coefficients (and hence are quite lipophilic) diffuse fastest. The time for half-equilibrium can vary from about 1 min to 30 days. The action of this membrane is exemplified in Table 3.1.

The influence of chemical constitution on partition coefficients is discussed in Section 3.2, and also the effects of varying the organic phase.

Table 3.1 illustrates a general trend: the higher the lipid/water coefficient of a substance, the greater the proportion of it found inside the cell after equilibration has taken place. For example, the insertion of another hydroxyl-group into 1,2-dihydroxypropane, giving glycerol, causes a large

Table 3.1

THE PERMEABILITY OF NATURAL MEMBRANES

Non-electrolytes	*Partition coefficient (olive oil/ water)* $\times 10^5$	*Permeability of living cells* (Mol/s/μm²/molar conc. difference) $\times 10^{20}$				
		A	*B*	*C*	*D*	*E*
1,2-Dihydroxypropane	570	—	13 200	13 000	4000	24 000
Propionamide	360	2200	—	23 000	—	36 000
Acetamide	83	800	—	10 000	—	15 000
Glycol	50	1100	6700	7300	2100	12 000
N-Methyl-urea	44	90	—	—	—	1900
Urea	15	15	2500	—	78 000	1000
Glycerol	7	18	180	50	17	210
Erythritol	3	3.1	—	—	—	13
Sucrose	3	0.8	—	—	—	8

A, Curcuma (flowering plant) (Collander, 1937); *B, Gregarina* (protozoon) (Adcock, 1940); *C, Arabacia* eggs (marine animal) (Stewart and Jacobs, 1936); *D,* Ox erythrocytes (Jacobs *et al.* 1935); *E, Chara* (green alga) (Collander, 1937).

—signifies 'not determined'.

fall in partition coefficient, and it can be seen that there is a corresponding decrease in penetration. In fact, few molecules penetrate readily that have more than three water-attracting groups and a molecular weight over 150 (Davson and Danielli, 1952). The size of the molecule and the nature of the groups also exert an effect (usually only secondary). The outstanding exception in Table 3.1 is the easy penetration of urea into ox erythrocytes. This facilitated uptake of urea occurs in all mammalian red cells, but not in those of birds.

The Type 1 membrane appears to be about 5 nm thick and to consist mainly of lipoidal material mixed with some protein. The presence of this type is diagnosed if substances of similar molecular weight and molecular diameter are found to penetrate at a rate proportional to their partition coefficients. It is interesting to note that if the partition coefficient is too high, the substance enters the membrane freely but cannot leave it (it would take 60 kcal/mol to release a lipophile from the membrane into water).

For a discussion on membrane permeability and equilibria see Wilbrandt (1959), for the kinetics of diffusion see Laidler and Shuler (1949), and Zwolinski, Eyring and Reese (1949).

A useful *permeability constant* (K) can be calculated, for a particular substance and membrane, by the following equation (Lueck, Wurster, Higuchi, Lemberger and Busse, 1957). This equation describes a diffusion process under quasi steady-state conditions in which two agitated liquids are separated by a membrane permeable to a solute:

$$\log\left(C_\mathrm{o} - 2C_\mathrm{b}\right) = -\frac{2K}{2.303}t + \log C_\mathrm{o}$$

where C_o is the initial concentration of the solute, C_b is the concentration beyond the membrane, and t is the time of sampling. A plot of $\log\left(C_\mathrm{o} - 2C_\mathrm{b}\right)$ against time gives a straight line of slope equal to $-2K/2.3$ from which K can readily be found. K (the permeability constant) also equals ADD_c/VL, where A is the cross-sectional area of the membrane, L is its thickness, V is the volume of each of the two chambers (fore and aft of the membrane), D is the diffusion coefficient, and D_c is the distribution coefficient between solution and membrane. This relationship enables other interesting data to be calculated.

The cardiac glycosides afford clinically important examples of the effect of partition coefficients on permeability. Digitoxin, the most readily accumulated of these glycosides, is the most lipophilic. It is excreted only slowly into the bile and is largely reabsorbed from this fluid. Related glycosides which are more hydrophilic because of the presence of extra sugar groups, or extra hydroxyl- or carboxyl-groups in the steroid nucleus, are more rapidly excreted into the bile. Digoxin and lanatoside C are examples of glycosides which have less clinical activity for this reason (Wright, 1960). For the mode of action of cardiac glycosides, see Section 14.1.

A simple apparatus has been designed for measuring the passive diffusion of drugs through an artificial lecithin membrane. It is claimed that this model system gives results similar to those obtained with natural Type 1 membranes (Misra, Hunger and Keberle, 1966). Other work with artificial membranes is in Chapter 14.

'*Type 2*' *membranes* differ by requiring a carrier in the membrane. This gives *facilitated diffusion* (sometimes called mediated transport). The transported molecule combines reversibly with a carrier which is thought to oscillate between the inner and outer surfaces to release, or pick up, this molecule. Because of the thinness of the membrane, this conformational motion may be very small; a mere shift of charge in a suitable receptor could suffice to shed the transported molecule. The tests for this type of membrane are (a) that the carrier can become saturated, whereupon little of the substance is transported for a while, even though the gradient is favourable, and (b) metabolic energy is not consumed by the act of transportation, e.g. no increase in respiration can be detected. The Type 2 facility usually occurs as isolated patches in a normal Type 1 membrane. It seldom leads to concentration of the substance against a gradient.

Examples of facilitated diffusion: (a) choline, a permanently ionized cation unable from its nature to penetrate by simple diffusion, is easily transported into erythrocytes and some other cells by carriers in the membranes; (b) tetramethylammonium cations, which can enter cells on the choline carrier, a facility which is unavailable to tetraalkylammonium homologues which can, however, block the physiological uptake of choline (Martin, 1969).

The transport of glucose in human erythrocytes is the best-known example of facilitated diffusion (Wilbrandt and Rosenberg, 1961). In general, the hydroxyl-group at C-2 of a hexose is essential for active transport through the intestinal membrane. It is thought that the carrier esterifies this group. A hydrogen-bonding substituent is essential at the C-3 position also (e.g. – OH, or even – Cl or – F) (Barnett, Ralph and Munday, 1970).

At least seven carriers control entry through the mitochondrial membrane. One carrier facilitates entry of succinate, D- and L-malate, malonate, and *meso*-tartrate anions, but not tartrate, maleate, or fumarate. Another mediates the entry of citrate, *cis*-aconitate, *iso*citrate, and D- or L-tartrate, but not furmarate or maleate. A third carrier transports adenosine nucleotides. Also phosphate anions can enter mitochondria whereas other inorganic anions cannot (Chappell, 1966). Apart from these processes, many substances (e.g. ammonia) enter by simple diffusion as non-ionized substances, and many anions flow in and out of mitochondria if cations are present (Pressman, 1970).

'*Type 3*' *membranes*, most complex of all, operate an energy-consuming process, and can concentrate substances against a gradient if necessary. In this *active carrier transport*, as it is called, the penetrating molecule is believed to combine with the carrier, as in Type 2. The metabolic energy is consumed in modifying the carrier structure.

Examples of permeability through a Type 3 membrane are: (a) the transport of Na^+ and K^+ in mammalian cells (see Section 14.1), (b) the absorption and secretion of wide range of ionized and non-ionized substances by the kidney tubules and, to a less extent, by the gastrointestinal membrane, (c) the uptake of inorganic ions, aminoacids, and sugars by bacteria, (d) accumulation of the iodide anion by the thyroid gland, and (e) accumulation of K^+, Na^+, Ca^{2+}, and Mg^{2+} against a concentration gradient in mitochondria (Margoliash, *et al.*, 1970).

For each 18 sodium ions transported through the frog's skin, one extra molecule of oxygen is consumed (Zerahn, 1956). Toad bladder and guinea-pig intestine behave similarly. Many cathartics (e.g. cascara, phenolphthalein, podophyllin) inhibit absorption of sodium by the membrane of the intestinal lumen (from experiments in living rabbits), thus causing accumulation of sodium salts in the colon, and hence retention of water (Phillips, Love, Mitchell and Neptune, 1965).

Activated processes also exist for some anions and for the more hydrophilic non-electrolytes. As with cations, these processes are highly specific. For example, the kidney tubules which resorb glucose from the glomerular filtrates cannot take up mannose or arabinose. The responsible enzyme can be inhibited by phlorizin whereupon the uptake of glucose ceases (Wilbrandt, 1950). For more information on the passage of inorganic cations through membranes, see Section 14.1.

The Type 3 membrane, which seems to occur in scattered spots on a membrane that is otherwise normal Type 1, can be recognized by (a) the ease of saturation of the carrier (as in Type 2), and (b) the increased metabolic activity during transport (absent from Type 2).

It is not yet clear how the carriers in Types 2 and 3 membranes operate (Le Fevre, 1975). Many examples isolated from eukaryotic membranes were found to be dimeric glycoproteins of mol.wt. about 100 000. Most think that they are transmembrane proteins (see Section 5.2) which effect transport by undergoing small conformational changes. Examples are (a), the Na^+ and K^+ ATPase which transports sodium and potassium ions across membranes of all eukaryotic cells (Skou, 1964); (b), the Ca^{2+} and Mg^{2+} ATPase which transports calcium ions into muscle cells; (c), the anion-exchange protein that regulates the passage of CO_2 through the red blood-cell membrane; (d), rhodopsin, the retinal-binding visual pigment which governs permeability within the retinal rods; and (e), the acetylcholine receptors which change the ionic permeability of nerve and muscle cells after combination with acetylcholine (Section 2.1). More complex is the protein (mol. wt. 50 000) which actively transports both glucose and histidine from the jejunum across the brush border into the blood stream (Faust and Shearin, 1974) (see Section 14.1 for recent examples).

In bacteria, the active carriers (permeases) are specific sugar-free proteins of molecular weight about 30 000 (Rickenberg, Cohen, Butlin and Monod, 1956). Permeases for galactose and other carbohydrates, arginine, leucine, and several anions have been isolated from *E. coli*. Each molecule of sulphate permease binds, with a dissociation constant of $10^{-7}M$, one sulphate ion (Pardee, 1967). Type 3 membranes are also active in the higher plants. Carrot roots, for example, can take up sodium chloride only while extra glucose is being consumed (Lundegårdh, 1937).

When new drugs are being designed, the requisite permeability has usually been obtained by stepwise increases in liposolubility, a strategy aimed at Type 1 membranes. A different and more selective approach makes use of Types 2 and 3 membranes by designing a part of the drug to resemble a natural substance for which a specific transport mechanism exists in particular cells. That this approach can be highly successful was exemplified by a project for increasing the penetration of nitrogen-mustard anticancer drugs into cells (Bergel and Stock, 1954). Of the various amino-acids attached, the phenylalanine analogue, melphalan (12.34), penetrated best and has given excellent results in the clinic. As would be expected, the D-alanine isomer was inactive. Other workers have obtained promising results with sugars (cf. Barnett, *et al.*, 1970), and yet others with uracil (cf. Schanker and Jeffrey, 1961). The idea is capable of tremendous expansion, and the rewards should be considerable.

For a review of permeability through Types 2 and 3 membranes, see Wilbrandt and Rosenberg (1961).

'*Type 4*' *membranes* are distinguished from Type 1 by the presence of pores, the size of which can be gauged from the size of the largest molecule which can penetrate them. As a homologous series is ascended, substances are obtained which penetrate Type 4 membranes less (and Type 1 membranes more) readily. One of the best-known examples of a Type 4 membrane is the glomerular tuft in Bowman's capsule of the kidney (see later). This tuft is permeable to all molecules smaller than albumin (mol. wt. 70 000). The pore size is estimated as 3 nm, and inulin (mol. wt. 5000) passes through easily. Small anions, such as chloride, often pass into cells through aqueous channels lined with positively charged groups. These channels exclude cations by coulombic repulsion.

Pinocytosis is a process in which a membrane (usually Type 1) develops invaginations that are then pinched off to form vesicles. It is a device for passing through a membrane those molecules which are too large to diffuse in the normal way, especially proteins. In this way material formerly outside the cell appears inside it, and also vice versa. For example, the proximal tubules of the kidney resorb protein in some such way while engaged in discriminating between many kinds of smaller molecules (Woodin, 1963).

Phagocytosis, a somewhat similar process, allows the passage of still larger particles. Thus the electron microscope clearly shows solid particles passing across the cell membranes of mammalian capillaries, the entire surface of which seems to be available for this purpose. Enzymes and hormones are often extruded from cells as vesicles enclosed in a lipid membrane. The five hydrolytic proenzymes of the pancreas are thus extruded together as 'zymogen granules' (Palade, 1959). The vesicles in which acetylcholine is secreted by nerve-endings (Whittaker, 1963), and the granules in which noradrenaline leaves the medulla of the adrenal gland (Blaschko, 1959), seem to have a similar origin.

★   ★   ★   ★

The permeability of various mammalian tissues. In recent years, a great deal of work has been done on the comparative permeability of mammalian tissues. It has been found that the mechanism of absorption and distribution of foreign organic substances is much simpler than those of natural cell substrates and constituents. The following structures offer a Type I lipid barrier to the passage of many foreign molecules: the gastro-intestinal epithelium, the renal tubular epithelium, the blood-brain barrier, and the blood-cerebrospinal fluid barrier (Schanker, 1961).

In the *stomach* (rat), it was found that drugs were absorbed well only if non-ionized. Thus, when the pH of the stomach contents was raised, basic drugs were better absorbed, because more of their molecules became non-ionized; but this pH change decreased the absorption of acidic drugs, because less of the non-ionized form remained (see Section 10.0 for an outline of the chemistry of ionization). The value of lipophilic properties in assisting absorption was demonstrated with three barbiturates of similar pK_a but different lipid/water partition coefficients (see Table 3.2): absorption rose proportionally as the coefficient rose (Schanker, Shore, Brodie and Hogben, 1957; Brodie, Kurz and Schanker, 1960). The pattern

Table 3.2

CORRELATION OF GASTRIC ABSORPTION WITH LIPOSOLUBILITY

	pK	A	P_c
Barbital	7.8	4	< 0.001
Quinalbarbital (secobarbital)	7.9	30	0.10
Thiopental	7.6	46	3.30

Where A is the per cent absorption from rat stomach when fed a solution (pH 1) orally, and P_c is the partition coefficient between heptane and water (pH 1): the higher values of P_c are the more lipophilic. (Schanker, *et al.*, 1957.)

of absorption from human stomach contents (pH 1) was very similar. Weakly acidic drugs, such as salicylic acid, aspirin, thiopental and many other lipophilic barbiturates, were readily absorbed because they were not ionized at pH 1, whereas basic substances such as quinine, ephedrine, and amidopyrine were not absorbed because they were totally ionized at this pH (Hogben, Schanker, Tocco and Brodie, 1957).

It is in the *small intestine* that the main absorption of all drugs takes place. The epithelial lining of the small intestine (rat) was found to permit the penetration of non-ionized drugs and impede the passage of the corresponding ions (Hogben, Tocco, Brodie and Schanker, 1959). Three permeability barriers have to be passed, in this order: the lumen-facing membrane of intestinal cells, the capillary-facing membrane of the same cells, and the basement membrane of a capillary. Two experimental methods are available: a length of intestine can be removed, the lower end tied, and the whole placed in an organ bath (Smyth and Taylor, 1957). Alternatively a sac of the intestine can be everted from the living rat and surrounded by Ringer's solution in a glass jacket (Crane and Wilson, 1958). Both methods gave similar results (Misra, *et al.*, 1966). The kinetic and physiochemical factors underlying these absorption processes have been described by Nogami and Matsuzawa (1963). The average pH (6.6) of the small intestine membrane is higher than that of the stomach, and hence it permits the passage of aromatic amines but not of the stronger aliphatic amines (see Section 10.0 for the chemistry of ionization). Absorption of drugs from the small intestine must be through the lipid-rich areas rather than through the aqueous channels, because liposoluble drugs of high molecular weight were absorbed more rapidly than lipid-insoluble substances such as urea or deuterium oxide. Raising the pH increased the absorption of bases and decreased that of acids, just as in the stomach. Moreover, substances whose degree of ionization was not changed by such alterations in pH showed no change in the rate of absorption.

The absorption of foreign ions from the small intestine (rat) was found to be very slow, and declined with time. It would be valuable to discover how ions are absorbed from this organ, because some highly ionized drugs are given orally, e.g. quaternary ammonium salts, and the tetracyclines which are zwitterions (see Section 11.8) (Schanker, Tocco, Brodie and Hogben, 1958; Hogben *et al.*, 1959). The absorption from the small intestine of natural substrates, e.g. L-aminoacids, glucose, and uracil, uses specific activated transport systems which can work against a concentration gradient, and can be saturated.

The absorption of drugs from the *colon* (rat) is similar to that from the small intestine (Schanker, 1959). All absorption in the gastro-intestinal tract can be slowed by atropine which decreases mobility of the muscular lining.

The distribution of drugs between *blood-plasma and the tissues* is essentially the same as between the gastro-intestinal tract and the blood-plasma, as described above (Waddell and Butler, 1959). Only the fraction *not* strongly bound by plasma albumin is free to diffuse in this way. A weakly-bound drug can be displaced from blood proteins by another drug for which they have a higher affinity.

The epidermis is the permeability barrier of the *skin*. Various neutral organic substances diffuse across the skin proportionally to their lipid/water partition coefficients (Treherne, 1956).

The permeability of vertebrate *erythrocytes* has been extensively studied, and has already been referred to in Table 3.1 and associated text. In general the membrane is Type 1, but the entry of particular substances is facilitated in certain species, e.g. glucose in humans and primates (Le Fèvre, 1961). A special peculiarity of red blood cells is the ease with which they admit inorganic anions, by exchanging them for bicarbonate ion, which is then dehydrated to (non-ionic) carbon dioxide.

The tissues discussed above are examples of cellular permeability, but capillary permeability must now be discussed. The *capillaries* of the blood-system, like those of the kidney glomerulus (see below), have porous Type 4 membranes and allow the passage of ions and proteins. However the capillaries of the brain are differently structured: see 'blood-brain' barrier, in the following.

The fundamental unit of the *kidney* is the nephron, of which about 1.2 million are present in each human being. If uncoiled and placed end to end, one individual's nephrons would stretch about 50 miles. Structurally each nephron consists of a porous tube within a non-porous tube and is U-shaped (see Fig. 3.4). At the beginning of each nephron is a little tuft of blood capillaries called the glomerulus. Blood flows into this tuft which has a Type 4 (porous) membrane that retains all the particles and most of the protein: it feeds the rest into the nephron. The tubule cleanses the blood, exudes most of it back into the circulation, and sends the waste (urine) down the ureters into the bladder. The human kidney produces about 185 litres of glomerular filtrate each day, but the tubules resorb all but 1.5 litres of water, and also many dissolved substances, some of them of great value in the body's economy. The renal tubules, which effect this resorption, have a normal Type 1 membrane, which permits the passage of liposoluble substances in either direction (i.e. to or from the blood-stream), depending upon the concentration gradient (Orloff and Berliner, 1956; Waddell and Butler, 1957). The tubules and accompanying cells also have specialized patches of activated transport for secreting many kinds of organic ions, even against a gradient. For cations, see Peters (1960), and for anions, Sperber (1959). There is no corresponding process for the resorption of these organic ions. The most important physiological role of the tubules is the resorption of water, bicarbonate, chloride, and other inorganic ions.

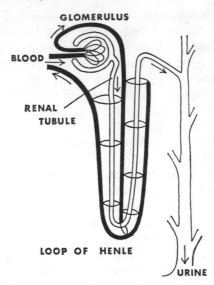

FIG. 3.4 Unit structure of the human kidney.

Of two similar drugs, the one that is more strongly bound to blood-albumin is excreted by the glomerulus with more difficulty. This means that porosity is of little avail against the forces (electrostatic, van der Waals, or hydrogen-bonding) which tie the drug to a blood-protein. On the other hand, protein-binding is of little avail when the constitution of the drug makes it eligible for one of the activated transport mechanisms in the kidney tubule. These principles can be borne in mind when re-designing a drug so as to reduce the dose.

The mechanism of *biliary excretion* of drugs is still insufficiently known. The pathway is blood → liver interstitial fluid → hepatic parenchyma cells → bile → small intestine. Active transport is provided for anions and cations whereas liposoluble neutral molecules diffuse through a Type 1 membrane. Molecules heavier than 250 daltons, even inulin (mol. wt. 5000), pass readily from blood into the bile. This facility seems designed to allow the passage of bilirubin glucuronide (Schanker, 1961). For substances in the molecular weight range of 350–500, strong species differences were found, and substances of lower mol. wt. were poorly excreted in bile, seemingly because they were more quickly excreted by the kidney. The overall picture of biliary excretion of drugs is one in which foreign substances whose molecular weight is too high for excretion by the kidneys can be returned to the bowel. Unfortunately such substances are likely to be resorbed from the bowel and recycled as above, so that little loss from the body can take place (phenolphthalein is an example). Drugs that are enterohepatically circulated, especially if they are metabolized with difficulty, can build up dangerously large blood levels. The liver has large pores (which have no parallel in other animal cells) in the membranes of the hepatic parenchymal cells (Schanker, 1961).

For further reading on biliary excretion, see Hirom, Millburn, and Smith (1976), also Smith (1973).

Many drugs were found to penetrate from the blood into the *cerebrospinal fluid* (dog, rabbit) by simple diffusion at rates roughly parallel to their lipid/water partition coefficients at pH 7.4 (Brodie *et al.*, 1960; Mayer, Maickel and Brodie, 1959; Mark *et al.*, 1958). When the pH gradient between blood and cerebrospinal fluid (CSF) was altered by changing the pH of plasma, those drugs which underwent no ionization change (e.g. sulphanilamide) retained their normal distribution ratio, whereas those drugs which became more highly ionized achieved a poorer CSF/plasma concentration ratio than before (Rall and Zubrod, 1960). Cations and anions penetrate the CSF and the brain exceedingly slowly; among the few exceptions are the phenylarsonic acids used in trypanosomiasis (Section 6.2) which may be taken up by the phosphate transport mechanism. Regardless of their rate of entry into the CSF, drugs often disappear quite rapidly from this fluid, a poorly explained phenomenon (Pappenheimer, Heissey and Jordan, 1961).

Towards the end of the last century, Ehrlich injected the dye trypan blue intravenously and found that it entered all tissue except the central nervous system. Conversely, when he injected this dye into the cerebrospinal fluid, the brain was stained rapidly, but none of the dye entered the bloodstream. Diffusion of drugs from the blood to the brain is more restrictive than elsewhere. This barrier (known as the blood-brain barrier) is capillary endothelium in which intercellular clefts are more tightly sealed and the cell overlap is tighter than in other parts of the body (Rapoport, 1976). This barrier is unusually permeable to lipids, but particularly impermeable to ions. When the barrier membranes are inflamed, however, a wider range of substances can pass through.

After passing this barrier, a drug still has to penetrate the membranes of the brain. Transfer of drugs occurs between various regions of the brain. Highly lipophilic substances (such as thiopental, chlorpromazine, and DDT) were found in the grey regions (of high vascularity) soon after oral administration; but a few hours later they were seen to be localized in the white regions which are richer in lipids.

Barriers to *permeability within cells* largely consist of the membranes of mitochondria and of the endoplasmic reticulum, both of which appear to be Type 1 with patches of Types 2 and 3, also the nuclear membrane which appears to be the porous Type 4.

Penetrability of other types of cell.   Bacteria whether intact or freed from cell walls have, on the exterior of the cytoplasm, a membrane which appears to be mainly Type 1 and is their sole permeability barrier. This has been studied in, for example, *Staph. aureus*, *Micrococcus lysodeikticus*, and *Sarcina lutea* (Mitchell and Moyle, 1959). Organic substances with more than four hydrogen-bonding groups (e.g. – OH groups), or ions that transport more than four water molecules, cannot penetrate the membrane at a significant rate (see Section 4.1). Whereas lysine can penetrate this membrane by diffusion, the more hydrophilic aminoacids, such as glutamic acid and histidine, penetrate only by activated transport (Gale, 1947) as glucose does.

The membranes of diatoms, and the chitin-impregnated membranes of arthropods, are Type 4.

The common belief that the integument of *insects* is penetrated faster by chlorinated insecticides than is mammalian skin has been disproved (O'Brien, 1967). It has been found that, when grain-weevils were exposed to deposits of BHC and its three isomers, the γ-isomer penetrated about fifty times more rapidly than α- β-, or δ -isomers. Hence the γ-isomer was accumulated in far greater quantity, and only it was toxic (Armstrong, Bradbury and Standen, 1951).

The membranes of *plant cells* are remarkably like those of animals. The plasma membrane of plants seems not to offer so great a barrier as that of the mitochondria, or of the cytoplasmic reticulum, or of the vacuole (a feature absent in animals). Most, if not all, movement into plant roots is physical diffusion unaided by biochemical processes. The plasma membrane of roots seems to have a special structure with unusual selectivity.

Maleic hydrazide causes chromosome breakages in plant cells, but not in mammalian cells. As mammalian and plant chromosomes have the same chemical composition, a difference in permeability is indicated (Barnes *et al.*, 1957).

For more on the nature of membranes, see Section 5.2. For further reading on the movement of molecules across membranes, see Bittar (1970), and Stein (1967).

3.2   The significance of the partition coefficient

Chemists and pharmacologists began to take an interest in partition coefficients at the turn of the present century, as outlined in Section 2.0. Their stimulus was the positive correlation that Overton and H. Meyer had demonstrated between the bio-depressant (e.g. hypnotic) action of many chemically unrelated substances, and their preference for the lipoid layer when partitioned between olive oil and water. This work was continued by K. Meyer and Hemmi (1935) who obtained more precise correlations by refinement of the technique.

Interest in partition coefficients then waned, but was renewed in the early 1960s when a group in Pomona College, California, under the leadership of Corwin Hansch, showed that this relationship is parabolic and hence, after an optimal degree of lipophilicity had been built into the molecule, further increases diminish the biological action *pro rata* (Hansch and Fujita, 1964; expressed more clearly in Hansch, 1971). The Pomona school widened drug scientists' interest in partition coefficients by pointing out that, no matter what electronic or stereochemical factor was chiefly responsible for the action of a class of drugs, the partition coefficient usually played *some* part in the delivery of the drug to its site of action. For this reason, a favourable balance between lipophilic and hydrophilic properties should help any type of agent to reach its receptor. Even when partitioning is only a secondary property, they concluded, it cannot be neglected.

Recalculating the published data on bio-depressants, Hansch and his colleagues found that the following regression equation made a good fit (the squared term ensured a parabolic relationship):

$$\log(1/C) = k(\log P) - k'(\log P)^2 + k''$$

where C is the concentration that produces a standard biological response, P is the partition coefficient, and k, k', and k'' are constants to be selected by computer (using the method of least squares) to make a 'best fit' of the experimental results (Hansch, Steward, Anderson and Bentley, 1968; Hansch and Anderson, 1967). Because this equation describes an equilibrium, a *linear free-energy relationship* is said to exist between the logarithms of the two sets of data (dosage and liposolubility). It will be noted that the provision of no less than three kinds of k, allows of much adjustment in fitting the data to the equation.

This, and other statistical work, is reported with the following information:

n, the number of data points used,
s, the standard deviation for the regression, and
r, the correlation coefficient, which should be, ideally, 1.00.

For drugs which are not simple bio-depressants, it is necessary to insert one or more further terms into the above equation to convert it to *multiple* regression analysis. This modification is developed in Chapter 16 (see also Hansch, 1968, 1971).

The practical details of measurement of partition coefficients are described in Appendix II. In seeking the ideal non-aqueous solvent for determinations, Meyer and Hemmi (1935) replaced the traditional olive oil by oleyl alcohol, thinking it nearer in properties to actual membrane components. In current terms, it had a better ratio of hydrophilic to lipophilic properties than oil, and the hydroxyl group also provided hydrogen-bonding properties. Collander experimented with a large number of non-aqueous phases (Collander, 1933, 1937, 1947, 1954). He found that the logarithm of the partition coefficient in a pair of solvents is *linearly* related to the logarithm of the partition coefficient in a second pair of solvents, one solvent being water in each case, thus:

$$\log P' = a \log P + b$$

where P and P' are partition coefficients of one substance in two different solvent pairs, and a and b are constants. The less the lipoidal solvent was capable of dissolving water, the more 'discriminatory' it was, spreading the values further apart but usually without altering their ratios (Collander, 1954). This work was extended by Leo and Hansch (1971), who compiled a list of a and b values.

Setting a at 1 for octanol, both chloroform and ether become 1.13, and butanol 0.70, and most other a values lie between these extremes. However, b varies more widely. Setting it at 0 for octanol, it ranges from $- 2.85$ for heptane, through $- 1.34$ for chloroform, $- 0.58$ for oleyl alcohol, $- 0.17$ for ether, right up to $+ 0.87$ for cyclohexanol. A substrate with P of 2.0 in octanol has $P - 0.14$ in cyclohexane.

Some exceptions have been encountered where partition coefficients, between water and two non-aqueous solvents, do not run parallel. A common example is the solute that forms a hydrogen bond with one non-aqueous solvent but not with the other, e.g. phenol with oleyl alcohol but not with dodecane (Burton, Clarke and Gray, 1964). Similarly, carboxylic acids form dimers in hydrocarbons, but not in moist alcohols (Biagi, Barbaro, Guerra, Forti, and Fracasso, 1974).

In selecting octan-1-ol as their standard non-aqueous solvent, the Pomona school were influenced by its ease of handling, comparative freedom from anomalous results, and closeness of discriminatory power to at least some natural membranes. Typical P_{octanol} values are: benzene 2.13 (± 0.01), nitrobenzene 1.85, aniline, 0.90, phenol 1.46, and benzyl alcohol 1.10. A table of 5806 experimentally-determined partition coefficients, by many authors and from various non-aqueous phases, has been compiled (Leo, Hansch, and Elkins, 1971).

Lipophilicity falls by a factor of about 10 000 when ionization occurs (Hansch, Leo et al., 1973). The Pomona school showed how $P_{\text{obs.}}$ is liberated from its ionic contribution (treated as being entirely in the aqueous phase) by the equation:

$$P_{\text{true}} = C_{\text{octanol}} \, / C_{\text{water}} \, (1 - \alpha)$$

where α is the fraction ionized (Fujita, Iwasa, and Hansch, 1964). See Scherrer and Howard (1977) for several biological correlations discovered by separating ionized and non-ionized contributions to the partition coefficient.

Small changes in temperature, such as $\pm 5°$, have little effect on partition coefficients.

A liquid becomes partitioned between itself and water just as it would between a foreign solvent and water. Hence the partition coefficients of neutral liquids run parallel to their solubility in water. This general observation does not apply to saturated hydrocarbons (Hansch, Quinlan, and Lawrence, 1968).

The π values.   Hansch and colleagues formulated a substituent constant (π) that was intended to be proportional to the free energy of transfer of the substituent from one phase to another. This constant was defined as $\pi = \log P_X - \log P_H$, where P_X is the partition coefficient of a derivative and P_H of the parent (Fujita, Iwasa, and Hansch, 1964). A table of 128 aromatic π values was published by Hansch, Leo *et al.* (1973), and their additivity was stressed. It was pointed out that when a partition coefficient could not be determined experimentally, it could be calculated by adding the π values of the substituents to the P of the nucleus (Hansch, 1971). Although enjoying great popularity among the more theoretical of contemporary drug designers, the concept of π values was adversely criticized by Davis (1973) and Nys and Rekker (1973).

Hansch and his colleagues obtained these π values by a process analogous to the derivation of Hammett's sigma constants, which the Pomona school was already applying to their investigation of plant growth-factors. Unfortunately, the analogy was not close enough, and this derivation robbed π values of thermodynamic significance. The fault in the derivation is evident in the following example:

$$\pi_{methyl} = \log P_{toluene} - \log P_{benzene}$$

because this calculation really furnishes only $\pi_{methylene}$. Arising, apparently unconsciously, from their earliest publications on π, the Pomona school have always taken π_{methyl} and $\pi_{methylene}$ to be identical (about 0.5). Similarly they assumed that $\log P_{benzene}$ is identical with π_{phenyl}, and (hence) that π_H is 0.

Rekker's f values.   Rekker, wishing to overcome this error, introduced f, the hydrophobic fragmental *constant*, to replace π which is the hydrophobic fragmental *substituent*. Thus:

$$f_{methyl} = \log P_{toluene} - f_{phenyl}$$

The calculations were performed on a computer using a multiple regression analysis programme, into which 128 published values of $\log P$, directly determined in octanol, were processed statistically (Nys and Rekker, 1973; Rekker, 1977). Inspection of these f values shows that they tend to be about 0.2–0.3 higher than π values. The f value for methyl is 0.17 higher than that for methylene, and a hydrogen atom is now seen to contribute about 0.2 to lipophilicity. The Pomona school, conceding the merits of the f system, published their own experimentally-determined f values (Leo, Jow, Silipo, and Hansch, 1975). Given P (experimentally determined) for hydrogen gas (0.45), they assigned half of this (0.225) to fH, and this value, when subtracted from $P_{methane}$ (1.09) gave 0.865 for

fCH$_3$, a value later refined to 0.89; similarly 0.66 for fCH$_2$. See Appendix II for a selection of these f values.

One immediate gain from adopting f values was the disappearance of former abnormalities in the values for omega-substituted phenylpropanes, which have erroneously been supposed to have *folded* molecules because of the seeming irregularities. Unfortunately other abnormalities remain, and some of these will now be mentioned.

Aromatic π or f values derived from *meta* and *para* substituents tend to be identical, but *ortho* substituents often give outlying values, e.g., when they permit internal hydrogen bonding, lipophilicity is increased. Apart from this, these π and f values are very sensitive to polar environments. For example, π for chlorine substituted in benzene is 0.71, but this becomes (insertion is in all cases, *meta*) 0.61 in nitrobenzene, 0.68 in phenylacetic acid, 0.83 in benzoic acid (all ionizable substances are corrected for ionization), 0.98 in aniline, and 1.04 in phenol. This difference of 0.43 between extremes is increased to 0.90 when nitro-group replaces chlorine in the same nuclei (Hansch, Leo *et al.*, 1973). Two highly polar substituents, particularly if both are nucleophilic, show enhanced lipophilicity (often 0.8) if separated by only one carbon atom, and about half this enhancement if separated by two carbons (Leo, Hansch, and Elkins, 1971; Rekker, 1977, pp. 49, 98, 293).

Continuing with anomalies of the values: small molecules like ethane are highly irregular (Leo *et al.*, 1975). Then there is the strangely enhanced hydrophilicity of pyridinium salts after alkylation on the nitrogen atom (Leo, Hansch, and Elkins, 1971; Rekker, 1977, p. 150). Covalent hydration (described in Section 2.3) introduces an alcoholic group, not allowed for in the usual calculations. The formation of micelles in the aqueous phase, by compounds bearing a long hydrocarbon chain, presents a further difficulty.

The Pomona school recommends drug designers to calculate, from a table of f values, the P value of a molecule which they are thinking of preparing to make sure that it lies within the range where the desired biological activity has already been found (Leo *et al.*, 1975).

Chromatography can provide R_M values, similar in nature to π or f values. They were first obtained by using reverse-phase paper and the following equation (Bate-Smith and Westall, 1950):

$$R_M = \log(1/R_F - 1)$$

A stationary phase of octanol and silica on a glass plate, developed by an aqueous buffer, can be used instead, and corrections for ionization have been developed (Biagi *et al.*, 1974). Not only are ΔR_M values both constitutive and additive, but there is a linear relationship between ΔR_M and π (Iwasa, Fujita, and Hansch, 1965). Similar values can also be obtained by high-pressure liquid chromatography (Mirrlees, Moulton, Murphy and Taylor, 1976).

Biological implications of partition coefficients. Thanks to the initial stimulus of the Pomona school, experimental modification of the P values of common drugs was soon under way. The sulphonamide antibacterials were recognized as slightly hydrophilic substances whose performance improved slightly when they were made a little more lipophilic, but declined with further increases. The penicillins and cephalosporins, on the other hand, improved slightly in performance when made a little more hydrophilic (Biagi *et al.*, 1974), but declined when this quality was accentuated. These results seem to be typical of what can be accomplished when lipophilicity (or its converse) is *not* the principal factor in the action of a class of drugs.

Partition coefficients can have directional significance, particularly in the more rigid molecules. For example, benzamides that carry a large hydrocarbon group in the 4-position are strong inhibitors of alcohol dehydrogenase, but the same group in the 3-position does not make the molecules inhibitory (Hansch, Kim, and Sarma, 1973). This example suggests that it may be futile to quote P values without further qualifying information.

The principal biological interest of P values is as models for the penetration of drugs through membranes, but to obtain this type of information presents great experimental difficulties. At least we know that the partition coefficients of a series of alcohols between red cell ghosts and water shows a free energy of about $- 690$ cal/mol for the transfer of each methylene group, approximately the same result as between octanol and water (Seeman, Roth, and Schneider, 1971).

The buccal membrane is, so far, the best investigated of all living membranes. Healthy volunteers are asked to retain a drug in the mouth while its appearance in the blood-stream is measured at intervals (Beckett, Boyes, and Triggs, 1968). These authors thought that their results were typical of a highly discriminating system, like heptane/water. However, rigorous statistical analysis by Rekker (1977) showed that it was less discriminating than octanol/water and more like the system butanol/water. Rekker thought that the gastrointestinal membrane behaved more like octanol/water, whereas the blood-brain barrier, most discriminating of all, had a resemblance to the heptane/water system (Rekker, 1977). It is to be hoped that the next decade will reveal what differences in the lipoid and protein content of various kinds of membranes are responsible for these differences in partitioning.

3.3 Mechanisms of loss. Storage and elimination

Three principal mechanisms whereby an active substance can be lost before it reaches the effective receptor are: storage, elimination, and chemical inactivation (Fig. 3.2). Veldstra referred to the loci where these processes occur as 'sites of loss' and suggested that the well-known synergistic action of biologically inert substances is actually a blocking of such sites, which allows a higher concentration of the drug to reach the receptor (Veldstra, 1956).

Storage.   Three important storage sites of loss are lipids (for neutral substances), ribonucleic acid (for cations), and albumin (for anions). Body-fat is such a lipid, and it stores drugs of high liposolubility, e.g. thiobarbiturates [such as thiopental ('Pentothal') (*3.4*)], and dibenamine. This appears to be a simple lipid/water partition effect (Brodie and Hogben, 1957). Plant-growth accelerators, such as α-naphthylacetic acid, are taken up by the fatty reserves of pea shoots; these sites of loss can be blocked with a biologically inactive, but more liposoluble, analogue such as decahydro-naphthylacetic acid (Veldstra, 1956).

Thiopental
(*3.4*)

Ribonucleic acid combines with the cations of highly basic substances. Thus the principal storage of mepacrine (*6.9*) after intravenous injection is in the nuclei of capillaries where this antimalarial does no harm and is available for replenishing the blood-level (Hecht, 1936). Chondroitin and other anionic biopolyers also store cations.

Several proteins in the mammalian blood-stream are capable of binding drugs, but albumin is by far the most effective of these. Neither fibrinogen nor the γ-globulins combine with drugs; and α- and β-globulins are usually enzymes whose affinity is almost confined to their substrates (although β_1-globulin combines with iron, zinc, and copper). Lipoproteins, related to the globulins, combine with steroid hormones (lipid-lipid attraction). However, the substances enumerated are natural metabolites, and suramin seems to be the only drug that is bound by a globulin.

Serum albumin, on the other hand, is a storage site for many drugs, most of which are weak acids. Table 3.3 shows how this affinity varies not only from species to species, but also among two series of chemically related substances. Man, who binds drugs by serum albumin more strongly than other mammals do, usually metabolizes drugs less readily than other mammals.

Human serum albumin, of which blood contains about 4 per cent, has a mol. wt. of 69 000, and possesses 109 cationic and 120 anionic groups. Although, at pH 7.3, it contains a net negative charge, one of the cationic groups must be particularly accessible because this albumin binds mainly

Table 3.3

BINDING OF DRUGS BY SERUM ALBUMIN

Animal species	Percentage unbound			
	Benzylpenicillin	Cloxacillin	Sulphadiazine	Sulphisoxazole
Man	49	7	67	16
Horse	59	30	—	—
Rabbit	65	22	45	18
Rat	—	—	55	16
Mouse	—	—	93	69

(Penicillins: Rolinson and Sutherland, 1965; sulphonamides: Anton, 1960.)

anions, and in a 1:1 ratio. This binding site seems to be on arginine (Jonas and Weber, 1971). Binding of anions to serum albumin increases with the drug bound; the presumed mode is by van der Waals bonding between the benzenoid rings of aromatic molecules and the flat ring of the solitary tryptophan residue in serum albumin, the fluorescence of which is quenched on binding by, for example, warfarin and dicoumarol (Chignell, 1970). The increase in binding to serum albumin with rising partition coefficient has been strikingly demonstrated in a series of penicillins (Bird and Marshall, 1967).

Examples of anionic drugs that have been shown to be bound at a single site of high affinity on serum albumin are: sulphonamides (Wood and Stewart, 1971), thiazide diuretics (Ågren and Bäck, 1973), pyrazolone analgesics (Rosen, 1970), and penicillins (Phillips, Power, Robinson and Davies, 1970).

This binding follows the law of mass action (Krüger-Thiemer and Bünger, 1965). Hence C^1 (concentration of drug in plasma) and C (concentration of drug in the water of plasma) are related thus:

$$C^1 = C \left(w + \frac{\beta \cdot p}{K + C} \right)$$

where w is the water content of blood-plasma (ml/ml),
      β (the saturation capacity factor) is the maximal specific binding capacity of the plasma albumin (μmol per g),
      p is the albumin content of plasma (g per litre),
      K is the dissociation constant of the drug-protein complex (μmol per litre).

The terms w and p vary slightly from patient to patient and are not influenced by the drug. The constant K varies from 900 for sulphadiazine, which is poorly bound, to 11 for sulphadimethoxine ('Madribon', see Section 9.3), which is almost too well bound to be a useful drug. Unless more than 95 per cent of a drug is bound by albumin, renal clearance is not slowed, and the serum protein acts as a depot and not a site of loss.

This dissociation constant (K) is the reciprocal of the affinity constant, calculated as $[DP]/[P][D]$, where $[D]$ is the molar concentration of the free drug, $[P]$ that of the free protein, and $[DP]$ that of the drug-protein complex. In practice, the concentration of the free drug $[D_f]$ is obtained by ultra-filtration, equilibrium dialysis, or measuring the displacement of the absorption maximum in the ultraviolet spectrum. From this is calculated the value of $\bar{v}$ (called 'nu-bar') which is the average number of moles of drug bound per mole of protein. When $\bar{v}/[D_f]$ is plotted against $\bar{v}$, a Scatchard plot is usually obtained in the form of a straight line. If the line is curved, the presence of two sites, binding independently, is disclosed. This treatment follows from general experience that the binding of drugs to serum albumin is reversible and obeys the law of mass action.

The clinical effect of a drug is increased, sometimes dangerously, if a second drug displaces the first one from serum albumin (Oliver *et al.*, 1963). Thus aspirin chases phenylindanedione (a frequently prescribed anticoagulant) out of its store in serum albumin and often precipitates a crisis of bleeding.

The percentage (of a drug) bound to serum albumin decreases as the concentration in the plasma is increased; i.e., as the albumin store becomes progressively more saturated, there is difficulty in loading it further. For this reason it is desirable, when quoting the percentage bound, to give the total drug concentration (bound and unbound).

The drugs most readily bound by serum albumin are aliphatic acids, aromatic acids (including salicylic acid, and related anti-inflammatory agents), sulphonamides, and barbiturates. The iodinated anions used as X-ray contrast agents (e.g. diodone) are also well bound. Neutral substances with a strong, localized, negative polar charge combine with serum albumin: naphthaquinones, coumarins [e.g. warfarin (6.53)], indanediones, lactones including the cardiac glycosides, and porphyrins. Among the many simple drugs and metabolites *not* bound by albumin are ether, glucose, and urea.

The triterpenoid drug carbenoxolone (glycyrrhetic acid hydrogen succinate) (3.5) has a very high affinity for human serum albumin (K 10^{-7} mol/l), apparently through the binding of the unsaturated ketone to the tryptophan residue, also a highly lipophilic nature. It is suggested that the remarkable ability of this substance to heal gastric ulcers depends on this affinity (Parke and Lindup, 1973).

For further reading on the binding of agents to the proteins of blood, see Goldstein, Aronow, and Kalman (1974); Meyer and Guttman (1968).

In a great many cases the level of free drug in the tissue fluids eventually becomes the same as that in the plasma. This relationship is convenient because the plasma is more accessible for analysis. Among examples investigated are the antibacterial sulphonamide sulfadoxine ('Fanasil')

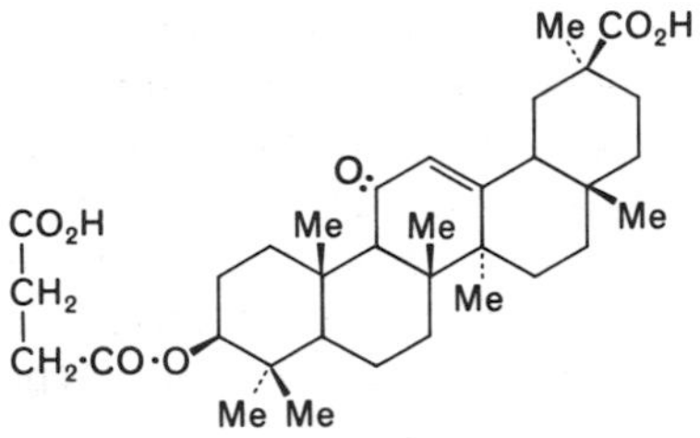

Me CO_2H

O.

CO_2H Me   Me   Me

CH_2

$CH_2 \cdot CO \cdot O$ Me

Me Me

Carbenoxolone

(3.5)

in the intraperitoneal cavity of rats after oral injection (McQueen, 1968), also various penicillins in lymph of dogs. The literature of this correlation has been reviewed by Robinson (1966).

Many hydrophilic drugs are excreted unchanged by the human body (see under kidney and bile in Section 3.1), but much excretion occurs only after metabolic alteration, as discussed in the next Section.

Radioisotope labelling is the perferred method for locating and measuring drugs after administration, and for following their fate in the test animal or human subject. The products are usually isolated by chromatography, sometimes on paper, in other cases by gas chromatography followed by mass spectroscopy; the electrophoresis of urine is also useful. After isolation, they can be measured by scintillation-counting, or by scanning, or autoradiography. The most used label is carbon-14, next comes the less expensive tritium, and sometimes 'double labelling' with both isotopes is practised. In planning a radiochemical synthesis, the first consideration is to choose the most useful labelling position in the molecule. Then the specific activity must be decided, according to the experimental dose levels planned.

For further reading on the storage and elimination of drugs, *see* Brodie, Gillette, and Ackerman (1971).

3.4 Metabolic change as an early step in excretion. Synergism and antagonism.

Metabolic alteration of drugs involves the making or breaking of covalent bonds (defined in Section 8.0) and hence is seldom reversible. Although many hydrophilic drugs are excreted unchanged by the mammalian body, others are 'conjugated', i.e. they are joined to small metabolites to assist excretion. For example, organic acids that are too weak to be ionized at the low pH of urine, and which would therefore be difficult to eliminate, are conjugated with glycine in the mitochondria of liver, and are then readily excreted by the kidney. Some amines become acetylated by acetyl coenzyme A in the liver cytosol (cell sap), but most of them are conjugated with glucuronic or sulphuric acid. Thus *p*-acetamidophenol (paracetamol, acetaminophen) (*3.6*), the much-used headache remedy, is changed partly to the glucuronide (*3.7*), and partly to the sulphate ester (*3.8*). Glucuronides are formed in the endoplasmic reticulum (*e.r.*) of liver, kidney, and gut. Provided that they are liposoluble enough to get into the *e.r.*, amines, alcohols, phenols, amides and carboxylic acids can be converted to glycosides. Sulphation takes place in the liver cytosol (for sterols), and also in that of the kidney and gut cells (for hydrophilic alcohols and phenols).

p-Acetamidophenol (*3.6*)

Glucuronide of (*3.6*) (*3.7*)

Sulphate ester of (*3.6*) (*3.8*)

The glucuronides of amines and phenols are easily hydrolysed by the β-glucuronidase of the gut and bladder. Hence to a certain extent, the formation of glucuronides can become a step in a recycling mechanism. Thus *o*-aminophenols, which are carcinogenic, are converted by the liver into innocuous glucuronides; but if β-glucuronidase activity is high in the bladder, the aminophenol will be re-formed and the risk of cancer is increased (Boyland, Wallace and Williams, 1955).

Drugs which are more lipophilic than the above examples are resorbed by the renal tubules. If they were not submitted to metabolic degradation, a single dose could remain in the body for many weeks. However, they are usually concentrated in a membranous organelle in the liver. This organelle, the *endoplasmic reticulum*, contains many kinds of scavenging enzymes, which alter them chemically so that they become more hydrophilic. Each altered drug is then excreted, either as such or (if it acquired a hydroxy-, carboxy-, or primary amino-group) in one of the conjugated forms favoured by hydrophilic drugs. For example toluene is oxidized by the *e.r.* to benzyl alcohol, the oxidation of which is continued in the cytoplasm to give benzoic acid, which is then conjugated with glycine in the mitochondria, and the resultant benzoylglycine (hippuric acid) is rapidly eliminated in the urine.

Although this example shows that *e.r.* is not the sole site of metabolic degradation, this organelle is by far the most versatile. It can be separated from liver by differential ultracentrifugation and is similarly freed (Rothschild, 1961) from the neighbouring ribosomes which are sites of protein synthesis. During the course of much purification, the *e.r.* is broken up into spherules ('microsomes') without loss of enzyme activity. These enzymes, which are numerous, are mainly oxidative, but a few of them perform reductions, hydrolyses, and at least one synthesis (Fouts, 1962;

Gillette, 1966). The following typical oxidative processes are performed by these enzymes (at least one enzyme for each process).

(i) Aliphatic C-hydroxylation ($R \cdot CH_3 \rightarrow R \cdot CH_2OH$), for which the side-chains of barbiturates are common substrates.

(ii) Aromatic C-hydroxylation, e.g. the conversion of acetanilide to p-hydroxyacetanilide. This aryl-hydrocarbon hydroxylase detoxifies some hydrocarbons by oxidation to phenols, but converts others to carcinogenic epoxides.

(iii) N-Oxidation ($R_3N \rightarrow R_3NO$), for which both aliphatic and aromatic tertiary amines are good substrates.

(iv) S-Oxidation ($R_2S \rightarrow R_2SO$), as in the oxidation of chlorpromazine.

(v) O- and S-Dealkylations (e.g. $ROC_2H_5 \rightarrow ROH + CH_3 \cdot CHO$), for which phenacetin and codeine are well-known substrates.

(vi) N-Dealkylation ($RNH \cdot CH_3 \rightarrow R \cdot NH_2 + H \cdot CHO$), as in the conversion of methylaniline to aniline.

(vii) Deamination ($R \cdot CH(NH_2) \cdot CH_3 \rightarrow R \cdot CO \cdot CH_3 + NH_3$), as in the metabolism of the side-chain of amphetamine.

Moreover, at least two reducing enzymes are present: a nitro-reductase ($-NO_2 \rightarrow NH_2$), for which chloramphenicol is a substrate, and an azoreductase.

Brodie (1956) has convincingly argued that the enzymes of the *e.r.* exist for the degradation of toxic substances normally occurring in food or produced by bacterial decomposition in the gut. In addition, they have a normal role to play in steroid metabolism, particularly in the hydroxylative destruction of such hormones as oestradiol, testosterone, progesterone, and the corticoids (Conney *et al.*, 1968). The *e.r.* enzymes are not very demanding about the structure of their substrates and hence are capable of attacking drugs not previously encountered.

Apart from N-oxidation, most of the above reactions require a special cytochrome coenzyme known as p_{450} (because it absorbs visible light intensely at 450 nm), also the coenzyme NADP, and a flavoprotein enzyme (cytochrome c reductase) which utilizes the oxygen of air (Gillette, 1966). These *e.r.* enzymes, by their requirement for NADP, stand apart from the many NAD-requiring enzymes that the body's intermediary metabolism uses in its stepwise conversions of nutriment into energy. Conversely, the *e.r.* enzymes attack neither the raw materials nor the products of inter-mediary metabolism, partly because such substances are too hydrophilic to penetrate into the *e.r.*

The *e.r.* enzymes can be selectively inhibited, e.g. 6-aminochrysene inhibits the N-demethylation enzyme while increasing the activity of the hydroxylating and O-demethylating enzymes (Russo *et al.*, 1976). The *e.r.* drug-metabolizing enzymes are largely, but not entirely, confined to the liver. At least the *e.r.* of lung tissue similarly degrades inhaled foreign substances (Matsubara, Nakamura, and Tochino, 1975). The destructive effects of *e.r.* enzymes can be avoided by inserting a group that makes the drug a poor substrate. Thus, insertion of ethinyl $(-C\ \vdots CH)$–into the 17-position of oestradiol prolongs the contraceptive action from a minute to a day.

Metabolic alteration of foreign substances has often been called 'detoxification', but many examples are known where the product of an *e.r.* enzyme is more toxic than the substrate. The example of oxidizing hydrocarbons to carcinogens has just been cited. Also, the *e.r.* converts dimethylnitrosamine to a substance which methylates the guanine of RNA to 7-methylguanine, a reaction which leads to acute liver necrosis (Magee, 1964). For related examples see under alkylation and lethal synthesis in Sections 12.4 and 12.5 respectively. The toxic action of methanol, including eventual blindness, is caused by its transformation by the body into formaldehyde (Kini and Cooper, 1962).

For a review of microsomal oxidation and reduction, see Gillette, *et al.* (1969); Boyd and Smellie (1972).

For most experiments on the enzymes of the *e.r.*, the source has been rat liver. However, it has been shown that human *e.r.* enzymes are qualitatively similar to those of the rat, but act at different rates, some faster and some slower (Kuntzman *et al.*, 1966). It has been suggested that the large differences in effective dosage that exist between man and laboratory animals depend more on such species differences in the rate of destruction than on any species differences in the sensitivity of target organs. Hence a given pharmacological effect should appear at a similar blood-level in all mammals, even though the doses required to produce this level are known to vary greatly from one species to another (Brodie, 1964). Table 3.4 supports this argument; it shows some quantitative data on carisoprodol (*3.9*), a muscle relaxant. However, too little information is available to say how widely the above hypothesis is valid.

Exceptions to the hypothesis obviously exist in those cases, possibly rare, when the major pathway of metabolism is not the same in two species. Thus the mouse simply hydrolyses 6-propylthiopurine (*3.11*) to 6-mercaptopurine (*3.12*), and hence it has excellent carcinostatic properties in this animal. Man, on the contrary, oxidizes the drug in two places, without hydrolysis, and the product (*3.10*) is not carcinostatic (Elion, Callahan, Rundles and Hitchings, 1963).

The possibility of species variations is recognized also in the narrower field of conjugation. Phenylacetic acid, the classic example of divergent paths, is conjugated with glutamine in man and chimpanzee (only), with glycine and with glucuronic acids in most other mammals, and with ornithine in the hen (Williams, 1959). Again, amphetamine is metabolized in the rat by *para*-hydroxylation, but by deamination in man, monkey, and guinea-pig (Dring, Smith and Williams, 1970). Interestingly, rabbits

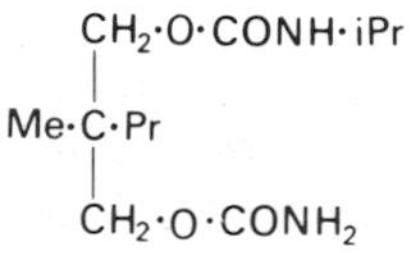

$$CH_2 \cdot O \cdot CONH \cdot iPr$$
$$|$$
$$Me \cdot C \cdot Pr$$
$$|$$
$$CH_2 \cdot O \cdot CONH_2$$

Carisoprodol
(3.9)

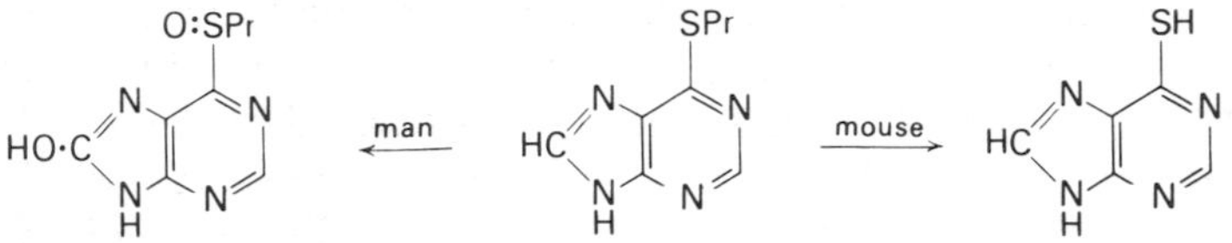

8-Hydroxy-6-propyl-   6-Propylthiopurine   6-Mercaptopurine
sulphinylpurine   (3.11)   (3.12)
(3.10)

$$\overset{Ph}{\underset{Ph}{Pr \cdot \overset{\bullet}{C} \cdot CO \cdot OCH_2CH_2 \cdot NEt_2}}$$

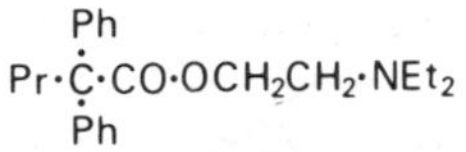

SKF 525-A
(3.13)

Table 3.4

SPECIES DIFFERENCES AND SIMILARITIES IN
THE ACTION OF A DRUG, CARISOPRODOL (3.7),
GIVEN INTRAPERITONEALLY
(0.2 g/kg)

Species	Duration of action (loss of righting reflex) h	Plasma level on recovery µg/ml
Cat	10	125
Rabbit	5	100
Rat	1.5	125
Mouse	0.2	130

(Brodie, 1964.)

can eat belladonna leaves with impunity because they have an esterase in the blood-serum able to hydrolyse the tropine alkaloids, but other mammals lack such an enzyme.

Other drug changes that take place in the liver cytosol (not the *e.r.*) include mercapturic acid formation from a few aromatic hydrocarbons, the oxidation of cyclohexanes to benzenes, of alcohols to aldehydes, and both oxidation and reduction of aldehydes. Esters and anides are rapidly hydrolysed in the bloodstream and many other tissues. An important

O-methylating enzyme, catechol-*O*-methyl transferase, is found in many tissues.

For further reading on the metabolic alteration of drugs, a specialized subject with an enormous literature, see Williams (1959), Goodwin (1976), Fishman (1970–1973), La Du, Mandel, and Way (1971) Testa and Jenner (1976) and Jenner and Testa (1978); also the journal *Xenobiotica* (London) which began publication in 1971.

Synergism. Much light has been thrown on the synergism of drugs by the use of the substance SKF 525-A (*3.13*). This substance, the di-phenylpropylacetic ester of diethylaminoethanol, can synergize the action of a wide variety of drugs by preventing their metabolism in the *e.r.* It seems to exert this effect, not by making the membrane of the *e.r.* imperme-able to lipophilic drugs, but by non-competitive inhibition of all hydroxyla-tion reactions and by competitive inhibition of hydrolytic reactions (Gillette, 1966). These actions of SKF 525-A are examples of a very common type of synergism, namely, blocking sites of loss (Veldstra, 1956). It is not used medicinally.

Metabolic inactivation, whether taking place in the *e.r.* or at other sites, is often accidentally inhibited by other drugs. Thus many patients have died as a result of the simultaneous administration of an inhibitor of monamine oxidase (an enzyme present in mitochondria) and an amine drug which is not toxic on its own. Thus the inhibitor phenelzine (*9.36*) (phenylethyl-hydrazine) has caused deaths after usually safe doses of amphetamine, pethidine, nortriptyline, or amitriptyline, or after the patient has consumed amine-rich food such as cheese, red wine, meat-extract, yeast-extract, or broad beans. These are examples of unfortunate synergism, but many favourable examples are known, examples of which will now be given.

Loss by elimination can sometimes be blocked by an analogue of similar charge type. Thus the penicillins belong to the class of moderately lipo-soluble acids which get facilitated transport through the proximal tubules of the kidney. This elimination can be largely blocked by physiologically inert substances of similar physical properties, such as probenecid (*3.14*) ['Benemid', *p*-(dipropylsulphamoyl) benzoic acid]. This substance is used clinically to increase the action of penicillins when a highly resistant bacterium is encountered.

$$HO_2C - \bigcirc - SO_2 \cdot NPr_2$$

(*3.14*)

Piperonyl butoxide

(*3.15*)

Loss by enzymic destruction can be overcome through use of a synergist. Thus pyrethrins in fly sprays are commonly formulated with a methylene-dioxybenzene synergist, often derived from piperic acid. One of the most used synergists of this class is piperonyl butoxide (*3.15*), but even quite simple methylenedioxy-derivatives of benzene show the effect. Metabolites of these compounds bind to cytochrome P_{450} (the terminal oxidase of the microsomal electron transport system) which is thus hindered in its usual oxidative destruction of pyrethrins, carbamates, and organic phosphates (Franklin, 1972). Use of a synergist can be avoided by inserting a blocking group into the agent to prevent oxidative degradation, as has been much used by designers of new steroid drugs (cf. Ringold, 1961).

Apart from the synergism that arises from blocking sites of loss, some other types are known. The first of these is sequential blocking (the inhibition of two or more consecutive metabolic processes) which is dealt with in Section 9.5. The other type of synergism is the attempt to retard the growth of bacterial mutants, based on observations that a mutant resistant to one drug does not easily undergo further mutation to give a strain resistant to two or more drugs. It is for this reason that the weakly antitubercular substance *p*-aminosalicylic acid is included in the isoniazid therapy of tuberculosis (see Section 6.5 for discussion of drug-resistance).

Resembling synergism in its effects is the genetically determined lack (in an individual or a race) of a detoxifying enzyme, as a result of which a patient reacts to a small dose of a drug as though it were a large one (see Section 9.8). This phenomenon differs from gradual sensitization to a particular drug, which is an immune response.

Antagonism by the induction of drug-destroying enzymes. Examples of unintentional overdosage were described above; in these a drug blocks an enzyme that normally detoxifies a second drug taken at the same time (e.g. phenelzine taken with the opioid pethidine). In contrast to this type of mishap a patient may be subjected to underdosage through a drug-induced induction of *e.r.* enzymes (Conney and Burns, 1962). The anti-rheumatic drug phenylbutazone (*10.32a*) is one of several drugs known to induce the excessive production of these enzymes, so that a fixed daily dose eventually produces an ever-decreasing effect; this is a consequence of the faster rate of destruction. Thus, 25 hours after a dose of 0.1 g/kg of phenylbutazone, the plasma of a dog showed a concentration of 100 µg/ml; but after five consecutive daily doses, the level of the drug had fallen to 15 µg/ml. If medication is suspended for a week or more, the patient can regain good use of the drug.

Similarly, successive doses of various barbiturates in mice and rats produced shorter and shorter periods of sleep. A similar induction of the barbiturate-destroying enzyme occurs in man, usually within a week of the patient's beginning to take a small, nightly dose. If the patient increases the dose, the accustomed sedation will return, but only for a few nights, because the induction of the barbiturate-destroying enzyme in the *e.r.* will have escalated. If he continues to increase the dose, habituation and withdrawal symptoms are to be expected. On the other hand, the patient may discontinue the drug as soon as he felt the first decrease in action. After one or two weeks, the excess of enzyme will have disappeared and the original potency of the drug will be available. During the period of abstinence, the patient is at no disadvantage because withdrawal symptoms do not occur at low doses of barbiturates.

That an inducing drug actually increases the amount of destructive enzyme in the *e.r.* has often been shown, e.g. by administering an azo-dye to laboratory animals for several days; then, when excretion of the dye was sharply diminished, hepatic *e.r.* was isolated, and the relevant enzyme found, by assay, to have increased greatly (Porter and Bruni, 1959). In one experiment in dogs, the amount of enzyme did not return to normal until 10 weeks had elapsed.

Examples of other substances which stimulate their own metabolic destruction are chlorcyclizine, probenecid, tolbutamide, aminopyrine, meprobamate, glutethimide, chlorpromazine, chlordiazepoxide, methoxyflurane, 3,4-benzpyrene, and DDT.

Moreover, heavy dosage with a drug can induce increased production of an enzyme capable of destroying a different drug introduced into the dosage scheme simultaneously, or many days later (Remmer, 1962). For example phenylbutazone, also barbiturates, speed up the metabolism of the coumarin anticoagulants in man. Hence a patient on anticoagulant therapy may be worse off if (as often happens) a barbiturate is also prescribed. For example a patient, who was taking 75 mg daily of bishydroxycoumarin and was later given 60 mg daily of phenobarbitone as well, showed a large decrease in plasma level of the coumarin drug, and the anticoagulant power fell. Yet soon after the phenobarbitone was discontinued, the coumarin drug regained its former level and so did the prothrombin time (Cucinell, *et al.*, 1965; cf. Robinson and MacDonald, 1966). Examples of pairs of drugs, the first of which can accelerate the metabolic destruction of the other *in man*, are: phenobarbitone and diphenylhydantoin, phenobarbitone and griseofulvin, phenylbutazone and aminopyrine, and phenobarbitone and digitoxin. Similarly, administration of the following drugs has been found to accelerate destruction of steroid hormones by the *e.r.*: phenobarbitone, chlorcyclizine, and phenylbutazone (Conney, 1967).

Some of the most powerful inducers of these drug-destroying enzymes are found among the chlorinated insecticides. A small dose of DDT or benzene hexachloride can make laboratory animals highly resistant to the effects of other agents. Hence such insecticides must not be used on animals when drug tests are to be carried out on them. Moreover chlorinated insecticides increase the metabolism of progesterone, oestradiol, and testosterone.

The primary site of action of these inductive antagonists, such as phenobarbitone and 3-methylcholanthrene, is on the DNA core of RNA-polymerase. By increasing the activity of this enzyme, more RNA is synthesized, and finally more of the metabolizing enzymes (Gelboin, Wortham and Wilson, 1967).

For further reading on the induction of *e.r.* enzymes, see Swidler (1971); Parke and Rahman (1970). For general reading on the topics discussed in this Section, see La Du, Mandel, and Way (1971); Brodie *et al.*, (1971); Gillette and Mitchell (1975). For an encyclopaedic listing of drug bio-transformations, see Pfeifer (1975).

In concluding this Section, it is worth noting that an organism's normal reaction to a foreign substance is simply to burn it up for food. In general, heterocyclic nuclei have proved the most resistant to these destructive processes, and hence are being used more and more in designing new agents.

3.5 Metabolic changes as an early step in activation

As indicated in Fig. 3.2, it has sometimes happened that a substance thought to be a drug is really a pro-drug* which is converted to the actual agent *after administration.* Thus 'Prontosil' (*3.16*), the first of the antibacterial sulphonamides, was thought to be the true drug when it was introduced into medicine in 1935. But workers in the Institut Pasteur were able to show, in the same year, that this substance was inactive, and suggested that the true drug was *p*-aminobenzenesulphonamide (sulphanilamide) (*3.17*) which was formed by reductive fission in the body (Tréfoüel, *et al.*, 1935). Accordingly, sulphanilamide replaced 'Prontosil' in the clinic because it acted more promptly and directly. The reductive fission is effected by intestinal flora and by cells of the intestinal wall (Gingell and Bridges, 1973).

'Prontosil'
(*3.16*)

Sulphanilamide
(*3.17*)

Much earlier, it had been shown that phenylarsonic acids, of which the parent is (*3.18*), were inactive until converted in the body to the corresponding arsenoxides, e.g. (*3.19*) (Ehrlich, 1909). In treating trypanosomiasis, it was found useful to let phenylarsonic acids diffuse into the site of infection in the central nervous system and there become reduced to the true drug. In this example, the latentiation of the arsenoxide was advantageous, but the reverse was the case for arsenobenzenes [trimers of (*3.20*)], which act only after oxidation to arsenoxides (*3.19*) (Voegtlin, 1925). In the U.S.A. this knowledge led to arsenoxides such as oxophenar-

* I must apologize for having invented this term, now too widely used to alter, for purists tell me they would have preferred 'pre-drug'.

sine ('Mapharsen') being preferred to arsenobenzenes such as arsphenamine ('Salvarsan') in the treatment of syphilis, because the patient could be cured with a much smaller dose, thus increasing the margin of safety (Tatum and Cooper, 1934; see Section 12.0).

The first pro-drug to be designed as such was hexamine (urotropin, methenamine), which was introduced in 1899 as a source of formaldehyde, liberated from it by the acidity of urine. However, most of the early pro-drugs were discovered accidentally. The anthracene glycoside purgatives had been used for centuries (in crude forms, as cascara, senna, rhubarb, etc.) before recognition that their aglycones (e.g. emodin) were the true active forms (Straub and Triendl, 1937). Castor oil, which acts on the bowel as ricinoleic acid, and sodium citrate, which, after partial combustion in the body to sodium bicarbonate, basifies the urine, are other early examples of pro-drugs.

OH
|
⬡—As:O
|
OH

(3.18)

⬡—As:O

(3.19)

⬡—As:As—⬡

(3.20)

Among drugs introduced in the nineteenth century, chloral hydrate (*3.21*) is reduced in the body to trichloroethanol (*3.22*) which is also hypnotic (Butler, 1948); and acetanilide (*3.23*) and phenacetin (*3.24*) acts as analgesics after metabolism to *p*-acetamidophenol (*3.6*) which has now replaced these pro-drugs (Brodie and Axelrod, 1948, 1949). An old suggestion that codeine exerts some of its analgesic effect after demethylation to morphine has been confirmed (Adler, 1963).

Aspirin, one of the most heavily prescribed drugs of our day (4 to 10 g daily for arthritis) has a pro-drug background. The antifebrile properties of willow tree bark (*Salix alba*), well-known to the ancients, were due to a glucoside called salicin. The patient's gastrointestinal tract hydrolysed this to glucose and salicyl alcohol; the latter underwent cytoplasmic oxidation to salicylic acid, the true drug. Following this train of thought, Buss (1875) introduced oral sodium salicylate, but this was found to be an irritant and became slowly superseded by aspirin (acetylsalicylic acid) put forward by Dreser in 1899. For the mode of action of aspirin, see Section 12.5.

$CCl_3 \cdot CH(OH)_2$

Chloral hydrate
(*3.21*)

$CCl_3 \cdot CH_2OH$

Trichloroethanol
(*3.22*)

⬡
|
NH·COCH₃

Acetanilide
(*3.23*)

OC_2H_5
|
⬡
|
NH·COCH₃

Phenacetin
(*3.24*)

Whenever it is found that there is no correlation between mean plasma concentration and therapeutic effect, the 'drug' must be suspected to be a pro-drug. From such a clue it was established that the antimalarial proguanil (*3.25*) acted only after cyclization in the body to the dihydro-triazine (cycloguanil) (*3.26*) (Crowther and Levi, 1953). The pro-drug is almost inactive against cultures of malarial parasites *in vitro*, whereas (*3.26*) is highly active.

By similar means, it was found that the gametocidal antimalarials derived from 8-amino-6-methoxyquinoline, such as primaquine (*3.27*), act only after demethylation and oxidation to the corresponding 5,6-quinone (*3.28*) (cf. Smith, 1956).

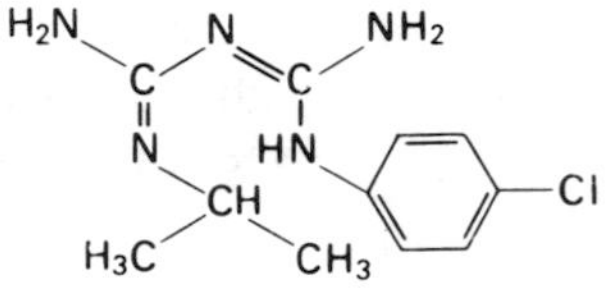

Proguanil
(*3.25*)

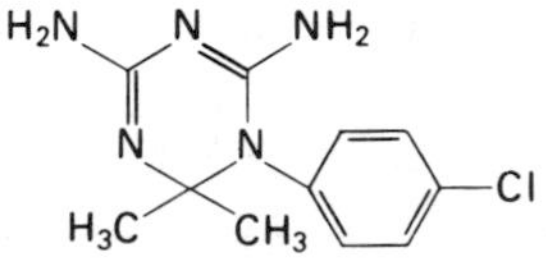

Cycloguanil
(*3.26*)

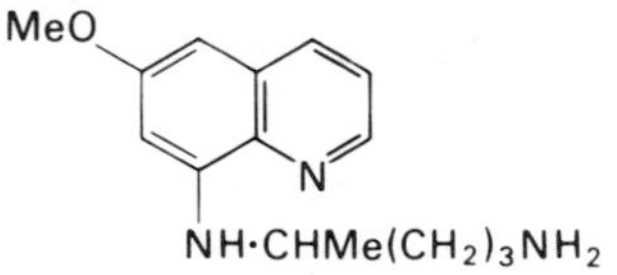

Primaquine
(*3.27*)

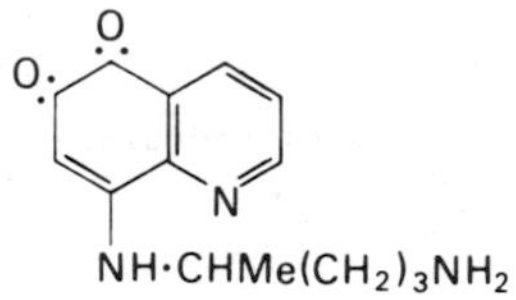

(*3.28*)

N-Demethylation of drugs takes place very readily in the *e.r.* of liver: thus 1-methylphenobarbitone (mephobarbital) becomes phenobarbitone; hexobarbitone (5-cyclohex-1′-enyl-1,5-dimethylbarbituric acid) similarly loses the 1-methyl-group; methoin (*3.29*) (5-ethyl-3-methyl-5-phenyl-hydantoin, 'Mesantoin') loses the 3-methyl-group, giving ethotoin; 3,5,5-trimethyl-2,4-oxazolidinedione (troxidone, trimethadione), and 5-ethyl-3,5-dimethyl-2,4-oxazolidinedione (paramethadione) both lose a 3-methyl-group. The original methylation was not wasted, because it increased the liposolubility of the drug, leading to faster acting sedatives with (usually) improved anti-epileptic properties (Butler, 1955). The antidepressive drug imipramine ('Tofranil') (*3.30*) loses one of the terminal methyl-groups to give the corresponding secondary amine desipramine ('Pertofran'), which is often preferred because it has a more immediate clinical effect (Sulser, Watts and Brodie, 1962).

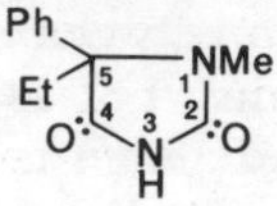

Ph
Et —NMe
5   1
4   3   2
O   N   O
H

Methoin
(3.29)

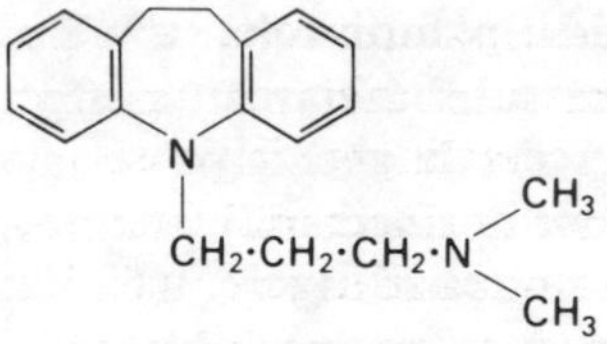

CH₃
CH₂·CH₂·CH₂·N
CH₃

Imipramine
(3.30)

N-Demethyl-diazepam, a metabolite of diazepam (*13.77*) has a quicker onset and more prolonged hypnotic action than diazepam, and may be responsible for the latter's therapeutic benefits (Nicholson *et al.*, 1976).

The much used anticancer drug, cyclophosphamide (*3.31*), is inert until converted to the active agent by hepatic *e.r.* Some workers think that this active agent is the 4-hydroxy-derivative formed by metabolism (Takamizawa *et al.*, 1975), but metabolism continues right down to the acyclic derivative (*3.32*), and this, or something in between, may be the true drug (Connors *et al.*, 1974).

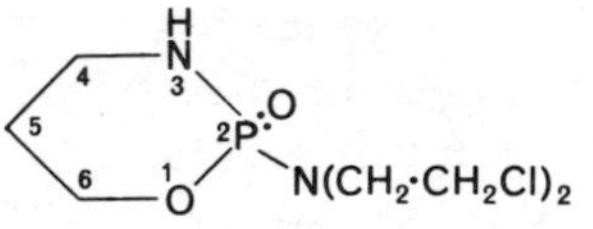

H
N
4   3
5   2P   O
6   1
O   N(CH₂·CH₂Cl)₂

Cyclophosphamide
(3.31)

O   OH
H₂N·P
N(CH₂·CH₂Cl)₂

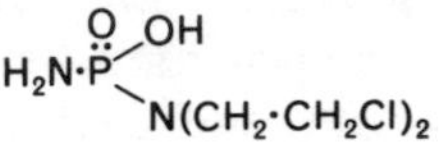

Metabolite of (*3.31*)
(3.32)

Ftorafur (*3.33*), the Russian-discovered anticancer drug, which is also made and used in Japan, is an *N*-tetrahydrofuryl derivative of 5-fluorouracil (*3.3*) to which it is slowly broken down in muscle and liver. Given intravenously, it has the same spectrum of clinical usefulness as 5-fluorouracil (cancer of the breast, rectum, and colon) but is much better tolerated (Blokhina, Vozny, and Garin, 1972).

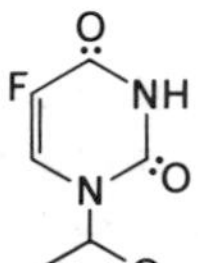

O
F   NH
N   O
O

Ftorafur
(3.33)

O₂N
N
S
N
Me
N
N
N   N
H

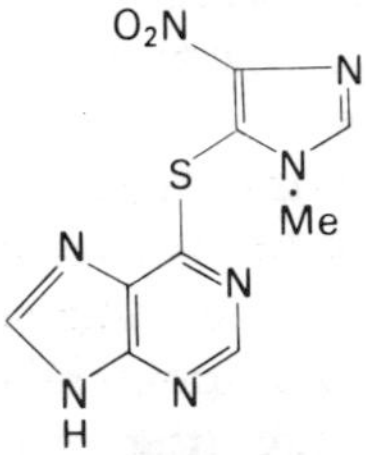

Azathioprine
(3.34)

Succinyl-sulphathiazole, a valuable remedy in bacterial dysentery, differs from sulphathiazole in that it is poorly absorbed from the small intestine. Accordingly, it passes on to the colon in high concentrations. Although not antibacterial *in vitro*, it is hydrolysed by benign bacteria in the colon to sulphathiazole, which sterilizes the bowel. Cycloguanil (*3.26*), re-introduced as an insoluble salt under the name cycloguanil pamoate ('Camolar'), is used as a depot antimalarial; a single intramuscular dose can protect a man against malaria for five months (Elslager and Worth, 1965).

6-Mercaptopurine (*3.12*) strongly suppresses the immune reaction in the human body and hence could be useful to secure survival donor grafts, but it is eliminated too fast for a sustained effect. Hence less easily eliminated derivatives were sought. The best of these was found to be azathioprine (6-1′-methyl-4′-nitroimidazol-5′-ylthiopurine, 'Imuran') (*3.34*), which is slowly cleaved (non-enzymatically) in the body to 6-mercaptopurine and hence serves as a depot. The electron-attracting properties of the nitro-group give the desired lability to the C–S bond (Elion, 1967).

An ingenious use of masking to overcome a problem in transport is the administration of 6-azauridine (see Section 4.0, p. 119) as its liposoluble 2′,3′,5′-triacetyl derivative, for oral medication in psoriasis. Whereas 6-azauridine was not taken up from the intestines, the triacetyl-derivative was absorbed, and then deacetylated to the true drug in the bloodstream (Welch, 1961).

Somewhat similarly, 5-hydroxytryptophan (which, like most amino-acids, passes the blood-brain barrier by a Type 3 mechanism) is decarboxy-lated in the brain to 5-hydroxytryptamine (serotonin), a substance which could not enter directly. This device is used to get amines such as dopamine (*3.35a*) into the brain by giving laevodopa (*3.35b*), orally, in the treatment of parkinsonism. This form of replacement therapy was developed after finding that the concentration of dopamine was much below normal in the basal ganglia of the brain in this disease (Ehringer and Hornykiewicz, 1960). The initial clinical work was done by Cotzias, Van Woert, and Schiffer (1967). Many thousands of patients have benefited from this therapy, but about 95% of the dopa is wasted by decarboxylation before absorption into the central nervous system. More of the drug is spoilt by O-methylation. To conserve the drug, it is often given along with specific enzyme inhibitors.

Methimazole, 2-mercapto-1-methyl-imidazole ('Mercazole'), a useful agent in thyrotoxicosis, is usually given as the 2-ethoxycarbonyl-derivative (*3.36*) (carbimazole, 'Neo-Mercazole') which forms a depot.

Experiments are in progress with anticancer pro-drugs which hydrolyse and liberate the true drug only at the lower pH (often about 6) which obtains in tumour cells (see Section 4.6). In a completely different approach, nitrogen-mustard anticancer drugs were coupled to an antiserum against

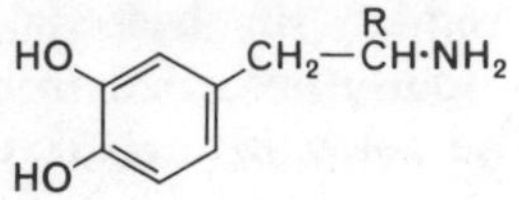

(a) Dopamine (R = H)
(b) Laevodopa (R = CO₂H)
(3.35)

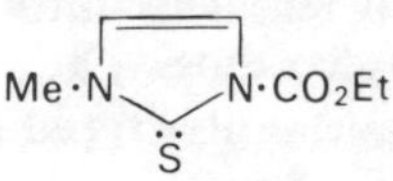

Carbimazole
(3.36)

lymphoma cells. Powerful anticancer properties were evinced in the mice and it was suggested that the antibody operated a homing mechanism for the drug so that it could act at shorter range and in higher local concentration (Rowland, O'Neill, and Davies, 1975).

The administration of pro-drugs is an artifice that is most used when the true drug is excreted or metabolized too fast for effective medication. In most cases, medical practitioners prefer to give the true drug in order to control the dosage according to the patient's response. Sustained release is discussed in Section 3.6: for more on the use of pro-drugs as controllable delivery systems of this kind, see Higuchi and Stella (1975).

Agricultural examples. Many highly successful organophosphorus insecticides have been designed to be degraded to a more toxic product by the insect, and simultaneously degraded to a less toxic product by the host (see Section 12.3).

DDT (chlorophenothane, or dicophane) (3.37) has been made selective against those cellulose-digesting insects which bite plants, by forming it into granules coated with cellulose or hemicellulose (Ripper *et al.*, 1948). Three decades ago it was much discussed whether DDT could be a pro-agent which broke down to hydrogen chloride and dichlorodiphenyl-dichloroethylene. However, it is now known that many insect strains are resistant to DDT just because they can accomplish this reaction, which turns out to be a detoxification (Winteringham, Loveday and Harrison, 1951). Actually, many chlorine-free analogues of DDT, such as 1,1-dianisyl*neo*pentane (3.38), have strong, typical DDT activity (Brown and Rogers, 1950).

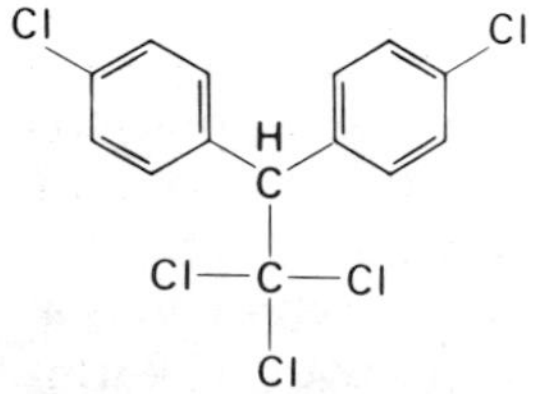

DDT
(3.37)

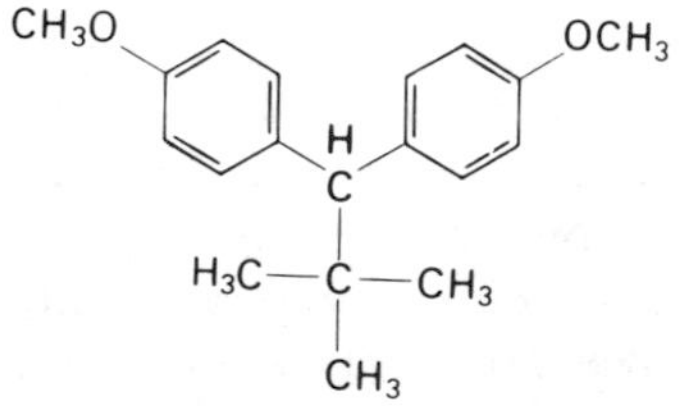

(3.38)

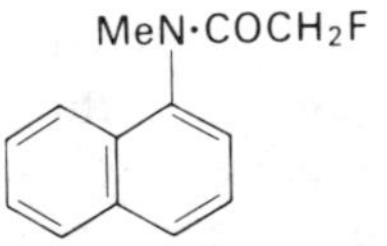

(3.39)

The highly selective N-methyl-N-(1-naphthyl) fluoroacetamide (*3.39*) ('Nissol'), is lethal to mites because they liberate fluoroacetic acid from it (see Section 12.5), but has little toxicity to mammals because they do not degrade it in this way (Hashimoto *et al.*, 1968).

Tetramethylthiuram disulphide (*3.40*), which is used to check the growth of fungi in seeds and turf, acts by reduction to dimethyldithiocarbamic acid (*3.41*), which is a widely used chelating fungicide (see Section 11.7c).

$$(CH_3)_2N \cdot C \cdot SS \cdot C \cdot N(CH_3)_2$$
$$\overset{..}{S} \quad \overset{..}{S}$$

$$(3.40)$$

$$(CH_3)_2 \cdot N \cdot C \cdot SH$$
$$\overset{..}{S}$$

$$(3.41)$$

When the fungicide benomyl (*3.42a*) was introduced in 1966, it proved to be more active than any known agent by several powers of ten. This substance (methly 1-butylcarbamoyl-2-benzimidazolecarbamate) easily loses the butylcarbamyl-group (which may assist penetration into the plant) to give methyl 2-benzimidazolecarbamate (BCM) (*3.42b*) which has the same degree and range of activity (Clemons and Sisler, 1969). It has been quite clearly established that BCM is the only fungitoxic substance in plants treated with benomyl (Peterson and Edgington, 1969). Moreover another commercial fungicide, methyl thiophanate (1,2-*bis*-3′-methoxy-carbonylthioureidobenzene) (*3.43*), similarly generates BCM when wet, and this seems to be the sole form in which it is active (Vonk and Sijpesteijn, 1971).

(a) R = −C(O) · NHBu (benomyl)
(b) R = −H   (BCM)

(*3.42*)

Methyl thiophanate
(*3.43*)

A most ingenious way has been found to increase the selectivity of herbicides in the phenoxyacetic acid series. Many weeds can degrade the side-chain of the intrinsically harmless ω-2,4-dichlorophenoxy-aliphatic acids until the lethal 2,4-dichlorophenoxyacetic acid is produced, whereas many economic crops lack the β-aliphatic oxidase necessary for this degradation (Wain, 1955, 1964) (see Plate 2). The following observation led to this ingenious masking. In a homologous series of seven ω-2,4-dichlorophenoxyalkylcarboxylic acids, an alternation of growth-accelerating activity was found to occur as the series was ascended; but only the members with an *odd* number of methylene-groups had any activity and this led to

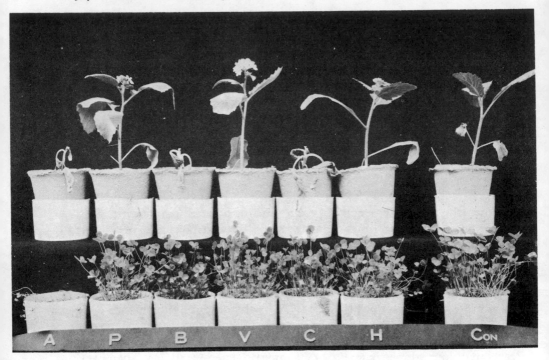

PLATE 2 Selective latency in herbicides. Effect of spraying 0.2 per cent
solutions of ω-(2,4-dichlorophenoxy) (−)acetic (A), (−)propionic
(P), (−)butyric (B), (−)valeric (V), (−)caproic (C), and heptanoic
(H) acids on charlock (top row) and clover (bottom). Control plants
are on right. Photographed after 2 weeks (Wain, 1964.)

the suggestion of β-aliphatic oxidation (first demonstrated in mammals
by Knoop in 1904). Wain's masked herbicides are used commercially,
e.g. MCP (γ-2-methyl-4-chlorophenoxybutyric acid), which efficiently
kills the weeds in a legume crop, or flax in a field of clover.

2-Chloroethanephosphonic acid is used as a masked source of ethylene
(a natural growth inducer in plants) to force flowering, and the ripening
and abscission of fruit (Edgerton and Blanpied, 1968).

       ★   ★   ★   ★

Although several substances originally thought to be agents have turned
out to be only pro-agents, there is abundant evidence that the *majority*
of agents act on their receptors in the same chemical form as that in which
they are administered or applied. A detailed knowledge of permeability
and enzymes can assist a skilful designer in finding useful pro-agents,
but he must bear in mind that he is adding more complications to the long

list of distribution problems that lie between administration and arrival at the receptor. For further reading on metabolic activation, see La Du, Mandel, and Way (1971); Higuchi and Stella (1975).

3.6 Quantitative aspects of distribution. Pharmacokinetics. Sustained release

The earlier parts of this Chapter showed that selectively-permeable membranes regulate the access of a drug to its receptor. This was indicated qualitatively in Fig. 3.2. To transfer this thinking to the quantitative level, it is necessary to perform experiments to find the constants which govern each unit of the total process. Two quite distinct types of constant are relevant, (a) kinetic constant (also called rate constants, or velocity constants), and (b) equilibrium constants. The former give information on the speed of a process, the latter on the percentage composition of the mixture remaining when the process is completed and equilibrium has been reached. Of the two, the kinetic constants are usually easier to measure in the living organism and are sufficient to provide a scientific basis for formulating dosage schedules. This concept of affixing constants to units of drug distribution is shown, in barest outline, in Fig. 3.5. Each pair of constants (one for each forward, and one for each backward direction) is usually determined first as a single overall constant, and then split into microscopic (i.e. constituent) constants only if the nature of the work calls for it.

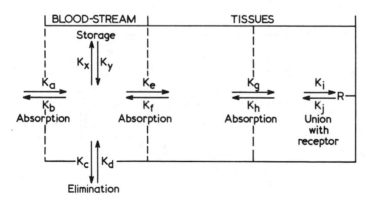

FIG. 3.5 Quantitative aspects of distribution.

The subject of pharmacokinetics, i.e. the kinetics of drug absorption, distribution, metabolism, and excretion (all of which are rate-controlled), was initiated by Widmark (1920) and Dominguez (1933), then extended greatly by Krüger-Thiemer (1960) and Nelson (1961). The term pharmacokinetics was proposed by Dost in 1953. Much of the stimulus for the vigorous development of this topic in the 1940s and 1950s came from Bernard Brodie, founder of the Laboratory of Clinical Pharmacology in the U.S. National Institutes of Health.

Even between substances that are chemically closely related, large kinetic differences operate at the various stages of distribution shown in Fig. 3.2, and these differences contribute very much to the selectivity of drugs. Thus the fate of each drug is ordained by the sum of the constants with which its chemical constitution has endowed it. (It should be borne in mind that these figures are constant only for the animal species in which they were determined.)

Without guidance from calculations based on experimentally determined constants, the physician finds himself perched on a tight-rope stretched between two extremes: ineffectiveness if the dose is too low, and poisoning the patient if it is too high. He needs to be given a dosage schedule which he can use to control two factors, (a) the degree of the drug's action and (b) the duration of this action. The rates of absorption and distribution govern the time of onset of the drug's action; the rates of metabolism and excretion govern the duration; the size of the dose, in combination with these effects, governs the intensity. This information is no more than vaguely indicated by animal experiments, and so the help of human volunteers is needed.

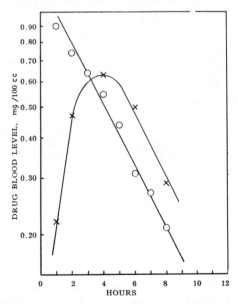

FIG. 3.6 Average blood levels of theophylline for human subjects given the same dose intravenously (circles) or orally (crosses). (Swintosky, 1956.)

The usual difference in times of onset which occur when a dose is given intravenously or orally is shown in Fig. 3.6. It is evident that injection instantly gives the highest attainable blood concentration, whereas oral dosage gives a more delayed and less intense effect; however, the intensity of both effects declines at about the same rate.

The rate of transfer of a drug across a membrane can be best described by the differential dD/dt, where dD is the microscopic amount transferred in dt (the very short time taken to transfer it). The amount (D) of drug on the outside of the membrane determines the rate of transfer across the membrane, as follows,

$$- dD/dt = kD$$

where k is the absorption constant. The rate of transfer will be faster the greater D is, in fact doubling the dose will double the rate. Similar differential equations govern distribution (which tends to be faster than absorption and elimination). D_o, the amount of unabsorbed drug at zero time is, of course, the dose.

The apparent volume of distribution (V_D) (see Section 3.0), discloses whether the drug remains in one compartment (usually the blood stream) or is shared with a second compartment (usually the tissues). Chemotherapeutic agents work best if shared, because infection is commoner in the tissues than in blood. A two-compartment distribution can be confirmed by the biphasic character of the first-order plot of concentration against time. The symbol k_{12} relates to any transfer from compartment 1 to compartment 2, whereas k_{21} reverses the direction (examples of microscopic constants). Kinetics for two-compartment absorption were worked out by Loo and Riegelman (1968). The cardiac glycoside digoxin is typical of a two-compartment drug. With barbiturates, the second compartment is the tissue lipoid and not the tissue water.

Unlike the absorption constant, which is linked to the dose, all other constants must be linked to concentrations. This does not require any great change in the foregoing equation, which now becomes

$$- dC/dt = \beta C$$

where C is the concentration in the compartment in front of the relevant membrane, β is the elimination constant, and $- dC/dt$ is the 'disappearance rate'. The elimination constant is usually taken as the sum of the metabolism and the excretion constants. Although first-order constants are most often encountered, a few of 'zero order' have been found. Zero-order constants are independent of the amount (or concentration) of drug present (Nelson and O'Reilly, 1960, 1961).

To obtain blood levels as constant as possible during therapy, the best interval between doses is derived from the half-life of the drug in the blood-

Table 3.5

HALF-LIVES OF VARIOUS DRUGS
IN THE HUMAN BODY

Tubocurarine	13 minutes
Penicillin	28
Erythromycin	1.6 hours
p-Aminosalicylic acid	1.9 ”
Streptomycin	2.3 ”
Chlorotetracycline	3.5 ”
Imipramine	3.5 ”
Aspirin	5.8 ”
Glutethimide	10.0 ”
Sulphaphenazole ('Orisul')	10.3 ”
Sulphamethoxypyridazine ('Lederkyn')	21.4 ”
Pentobarbital	42.0 ”
Phenylbutazone	45.0 ”
Bromide ion	7.5 days

(Wilbrandt, 1964.)

stream. This half-life $(t_{0.5})$ is calculated from the elimination constant by the equation

$$t_{0.5} = 0.693/K_e$$

and it represents the time taken for half of the drug to disappear from the blood. Table 3.5 lists the half-lives of several common drugs. For a large table of $t_{0.5}$ values, see van Rossum (1971).

The ideal dose interval (τ) is $3.32\, t_{0.5}.\log(1 + C_o/C_{min})$ where C_o is the initial blood concentration and C_{min} is the lowest blood concentration that is therapeutically effective. Unfortunately, this equation often produces dose intervals that are too difficult to observe, such as 19 hours. It has become more usual to decide on a convenient dose interval (4, 8, 24, or 48 hours) and substitute it, as τ, into the following equation to find the best dose (D) (Wagner, 1967):

$$D = \tau \cdot V_D \cdot C_{av} / 1.44\, t_{0.5} F$$

where C_{av} is the average required blood level, F is the fraction absorbed (ideally 1.0), and the other symbols have their previous significance.

The ideal dosing intervals can also be determined by drawing a line parallel to the base line of curves, constructed as in Fig. 3.6, at the minimal effective blood level of the drug, i.e. the level below which no beneficial effect on the patient can be observed.

In oral therapy, a *priming dose* may be needed for the drug to reach an effective blood level as quickly as possible. If the drug is one with a long half-life, a priming dose is essential, because it takes five half-lives for a drug to reach its plateau. Further doses are determined as in the foregoing.

Ideally, the size of doses should be determined for each patient by blood analyses performed at the beginning of treatment. This procedure builds the patient's idiosyncrasies (of distribution or metabolism) into the dose. When it is not possible to do this, it is usual to take published average figures, derived from a group of patients.

The pioneer studies of Krüger-Thiemer have established dose intervals and ratios of initial to maintenance doses for a large number of sulphonamide antibacterial drugs of which Table 3.6 presents a selection (Krüger-Thiemer and Bünger, 1961, 1965). In the early days of treatment with sulphonamide drugs, the wide span of their half-lives was not realized, and examples with long half-lives were often discredited because unwitting overdosage harmed the patients.

Table 3.6

RECOMMENDED DOSE INTERVALS. RECOMMENDED RATIOS OF PRIMING DOSE $(D^\star)$ TO MAINTENANCE DOSE (D) FOR OBTAINING STEADY BLOOD LEVELS OF DRUG

	Average half-life (hours)	Dose interval (hours)	$D^\star/D$
Sulphathiazole	3.5	4	1.8
Sulphisoxazole	6.1	6	2.0
Sulphanilamide	8.8	8	2.1
Acetylsulphisoxazole	13.1	12	2.1
Sulphadiazine	23.5	24	3.0
Sulphamerazine	23.5	24	3.0
Sulphadimethoxine	41.0	24	3.0

(Krüger-Thiemer and Bünger, 1961.)

One sometimes reads that a drug is 'cumulative' but accumulation in the body is often a function of the dosage pattern and not of the drug. Any drug, given too often or in too large a dose, will accumulate; the problem is most evident with drugs that have a long $t_{0.5}$.

Once the principles of these studies have been grasped, the distribution of a drug can be investigated in more detail. The dose schedules for sulphonamides in Table 3.6 were obtained as follows. The drug was given orally to healthy human volunteers, and specimens of blood and urine were taken at frequent intervals and analysed. The rate constants for the metabolism of various sulphonamides were obtained; also those for their excretion (see Fig. 3.7). Further work enabled the composite excretion constant β_1 to be split into two microscopic constants describing respectively the secretion of the drug by the kidney glomerulus, and the resorption from the kidney tubules into the blood stream.

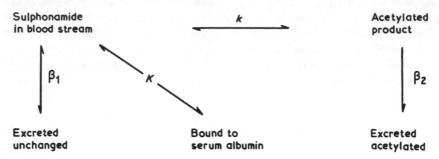

FIG. 3.7 Kinetics of the metabolism and excretion of sulphonamide drugs in the human body. (Nelson and O'Reilly, 1960.)

Studies such as these have made valuable contributions to selectivity, for they showed that drugs had many unsuspected *independently variable* constants; hence the pattern of drug distribution could be varied at will by making minute changes in the molecular structure. Two decades ago, this knowledge opened a new door for the drug designer to improve selectivity by controlling distribution, and at once led to improved antibacterial sulphonamides, many with specialized uses in therapy (see further Section 9.3).

The use of pro-drug in place of a drug requires a complete set of constants to be determined for each (Martin, 1967). When the elimination rate of the precursor is less than that of the drug, a blood level (of the drug) is obtained which declines more slowly than that obtained when the drug is given as such. The rate of conversion of precursor to drug also governs this result. When the drug-designer perseveres until he finds a precursor with favourable values for both these rates, he has on hand a substance capable of extending the dosage interval and maintaining a more uniform level of the drug between doses.

The absorption of orally administered *solids* is slow, and exponential. The solution rate is proportional to the drug's surface area, and the availability for absorption decreases in the order: solutions, suspensions, capsules, compressed tablets, coated tablets. Sodium salts of poorly soluble weak acids usually produce higher blood-levels than the free acids, because the hydrochloric acid of the gastric juice liberates the weak acid from its salt in a much finer form than any in which it can be marketed. The kinetics of dissolving drugs is reviewed by Wagner (1961).

The *bioavailability* of different specimens of a poorly soluble drug, when given orally and measured by the rate of the rise of plasma levels, varies enormously because of differing particle sizes. This test has revealed important differences between different brands of aspirin, diphenylhydantoin, cardiac glycosides (especially digoxin), tetracyclines, chloramphenicol, and bishydroxycoumarin. 'Micronization' of the powder often provides the remedy.

Sustained release. For some therapeutic uses, slow absorption of drugs is a nuisance, but in other cases it may represent the ideal state, so long as it is regular. At first this effect was achieved by enteric coatings of shellac, waxes, or cellulose esters to protect the drug from gastric fluid but liberate it in the small intestine. Later, concentric coating was developed to provide an initial dose followed by one or more delayed doses. Alternatively, tiny pellets, with different coatings timed to dissolve after a series of intervals, were incorporated in a single capsule. Although these devices work well for some patients, much evidence of individual variability has been met. The kinetics of slow dissolution of pellets of steroids, implanted under the skin, have been worked out (Ballard and Nelson, 1962). Other examples of slow release from a depot are provided by the intramuscular injection of insoluble hormones dispersed in wax or oil, and of penicillin as its insoluble procaine salt.

Remarkable new developments are advancing the subject of delayed action. The use of microencapsulation, an idea derived from modern copying papers, provides capsules as small as a few μm in diameter filled with micronized drug particles or ultrafine droplets. A coacervate of gelatin and gum acacia has been much used to form these microcapsules (Luzzi, 1970). Alternatively, liposomes which are oil drops of radius about 20 nm, are filled with hydrophilic or lipophilic drugs and injected into the blood stream. They have special affinity for the spleen and liver into whose cells they discharge their contents by endocytosis or by fusion with the plasma membrane. Insertion of organic antimonials into liposomes increases potency 300-fold in treatment of visceral leishmaniasis, because both parasite and drug become concentrated in the same liver cells (Alving *et al.*, 1978). Attempts are being made to label the surface of liposomes with 'homing substances' to dispatch them to other organs (Gregoriadis, 1977).

The advent of silicone rubber ('Silastic Polymer') has further widened the possibilities for ensuring sustained release (Zaffaroni, 1974). When this substance is prepared by polymerization in the presence of the drug, the latter can be relied upon to diffuse from it at a slow, steady rate, in any moist situation (for equations of diffusion, see Roseman and Higuchi, 1970). Thus a silicone rubber membrane, impregnated with pilocarpine, is used successfully in the treatment of glaucoma when implanted in the conjunctival sac (Goodman and Gilman, 1975, p. 474). A sealed tube of the polymer, filled with progesterone, has been found to act efficiently as a contraceptive when implanted in the uterus, and a vaginal silicone-rubber ring charged with medroxyprogesterone is also reliable (Mishell, *et al.*, 1970).

Research is now proceeding into micro-instruments, sensitive to feedback from high levels of a hormone or other blood constituent, to be implanted in the body and control the release of a drug with which they have been charged.

For further reading on the modification of a drug's structure to improve the pharmacokinetics, see Notari (1973). For theory and calculations of kinetic studies, see Krüger-Thiemer (1966); for the design of dose schedules, see Goldstein, Aronow, and Kalman (1974), also van Rossum (1971); for books on pharmacokinetics, see Gibaldi and Perrier (1975), and Notari (1975).

4 Comparative biochemistry: the second principle of selectivity

Of the three approaches to selectivity outlined in Section 1.2, Comparative Biochemistry has so far proved the most successful. In retrospect, it is surprising how slowly this subject developed, but the widespread misunderstanding among biochemists that all living cells had a common ground-plan of metabolism (see Section 1.2) hardly left the subject room to exist. Baldwin's book *An Introduction to Comparative Biochemistry* first appeared in 1937 and opened many people's eyes to the interest and possibilities of the subject, but it is only in the last two decades that comparative biochemistry has supported a substantial number of senior research workers. Today, however, it is a thriving and successful subject. In fact comparative biochemistry has undergone such a rapid growth in recent years that even the seven volumes of Florkin and Mason (1960–4) do not hold more than the outline of it. The following account of selectivity through comparative biochemistry will begin with the nucleic acids, because of their dominant position in the life of the cell.

4.0 Nucleic acids

The biological importance of nucleic acids began to emerge with the discovery by Oswald Avery, and his colleagues at the Rockefeller Institute, that the deoxyribonucleic acid of pneumococci carried heritable information, so that a specimen from one strain of this bacterium could confer its properties on a different strain, a process called transformation (Avery, MacLeod, and McCarty, 1944).

Deoxyribonucleic acid (DNA), the most important of the nucleic acids, occurs in mitochondria and chloroplasts, but most of it is in the nucleus. It is the carrier of all the cell's genetic information, the appropriate portion of which is placed in service instantly to meet changing circumstances in the cell. The information stored in DNA is encoded by the nature and order of the pyrimidine bases, thymine (*4.1b*) and cytosine (*4.2*), and the purine bases adenine (*4.3*) and guanine (*4.4*). Each strand of DNA has a deoxyribose-phosphoric acid backbone to which these bases are attached. Usually DNA has two such strands wound around one another in a double helix and held together by H-bonds between each opposing pair of bases (Watson and Crick, 1953; for bond lengths and angles, see Donohue, 1968).

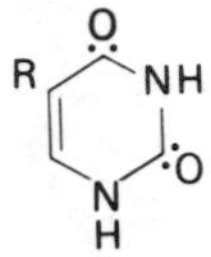

(a) R = H (uracil)
(b) R = Me (thymine)
(*4.1*)

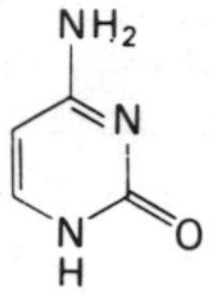

Cytosine
(*4.2*)

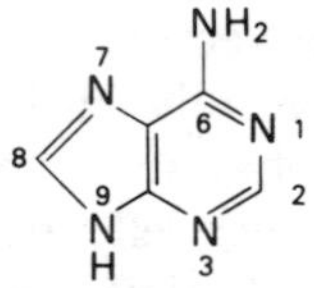

Adenine
(*4.3*)

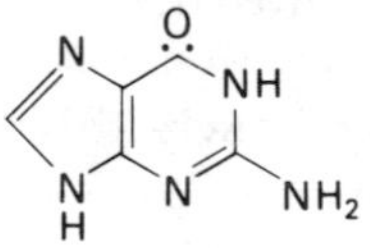

Guanine
(*4.4*)

DNA, from many sources including mammalian and bacterial, has a molecular weight between 10 and 100 million. In the vertebrate nucleus, the spirals usually form rods of about 3 μm in length, and 18 Å diameter. [However, non-nuclear DNA (as in mitochondria and bacteria) is often circular and in the latter, single-stranded.] The vertical distance between the layers of bases is about 3.3 Å (measured from centre to centre of the molecules) so that there is no free space between these layers (Jordan, 1968). The purine and pyrimidine bases are planar, and the paired bases are in the same plane with one another and with the C-1′ and C-4′ atoms of the sugars to which they are attached. However, the planes of the sugars are nearly at right angles to those of the bases.

The structure of the DNA molecule is intimately related to its two primary roles: replication (gene duplication by synthesis of more DNA) and transcription (gene expression by synthesis of RNA) (see Fig. 4.1).

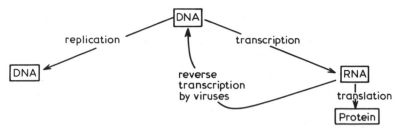

FIG. 4.1 Roles of nucleic acids in the living cell.

In the nucleus, DNA is synthesized from mononucleotides (such as deoxyadenosine triphosphate) by a polymerase. Some preformed DNA is required as a template. Several substances are known which inhibit this synthesis by combining with the template and making it unavailable (see, for example, the acridines, below). Many tumour-producing viruses, which have RNA as their sole nucleic acid, contain reverse transcriptase, i.e. a polymerase that forms new DNA as a copy of viral RNA (Temin and Mizutani, 1970). Agents to inhibit this enzyme selectively are being sought.

The four bases mentioned account for most of those found in the DNA of higher forms of life. 5-methylcytosine forms the principal exception; 25 per cent of the cytosine in the DNA of plants is in this form, but animals have much less, and bacteria have only 0–2 per cent (Vanyushin *et al.*, 1968). Bacterial and viral DNAs sometimes contain other methylated bases, such as 6′-methyladenine, 2-methyladenine, or 5-hydroxymethyl-uracil. In some phages, all cytosine is replaced by 5-hydroxymethyl-cytosine, made by a virus-induced enzyme in the bacterial host (Cohen, 1963).

The ratio of bases in bacterial DNA differs greatly from one bacterial species to another. This is evident from Table 4.1 where the last column gives the sum of the two amphoteric bases divided by that of the two mono-functional bases (Belozersky and Spirin, 1958). This figure ranges from 0.45 to 2.80, whereas in higher animals and plants it varies only between 0.6 and 0.9. In spite of the variable GC/AT ratio in bacteria, the purine/pyrimidine ratio remains at 1.0. Ratios of GC to AT have also been determined for protozoa (flagellates, 0.85 to 1.56; ciliates, 0.28 to 0.54), fungi (0.56 to 1.17), algae (0.56 to 2.00), and invertebrate animals (0.50 to 0.78) (Schildkraut, *et al.*, 1962; Sueoka, 1961). Because some DNA antagonists prefer to attack a particular kind of base-pair, the above data can be used to assist selectivity.

Chromatin. DNA does not exist free in the nucleus, but is organized into a continuous rope of flat, wedge-shaped *nucleosomes.* Each nuclesome contains a double-helix of 200 base-pairs, superwound around a core of 9 molecules of basic proteins (histones). Apparently the outside of each

Table 4.1

BASE RATIOS IN DNA OF BACTERIA

Species	$\dfrac{\text{Guanine + Cytosine}}{\text{Adenine + Thymine}}$
Clostridium perfringens	0.45
Staphylococcus aureus	0.53
Pasteurella tularensis	0.53
Proteus vulgaris	0.68
Escherichia coli	1.09
Shigella dysenteriae	1.14
Salmonella typhosa	1.14
Corynebacterium diphtheriae	1.20
Azotobacter spp.	1.28
Brucella abortus	1.37
Pseudomonas aeruginosa	2.03
Mycobacterium tuberculosis	2.08
Actinomyces spp.	2.80

(Belozersky and Spirin, 1958; Hill, 1966.)

nucleosome is available for union with RNA-polymerase and the information-masking acidic proteins. During mitosis, this 'rope' can be folded into chromosomes. This example is from rat liver, typical for eukaryotes. The rather different structure of bacterial chromatin is also described (Finch, et al., 1977).

Ribonucleic acids (RNAs). Besides reproducing itself, DNA acts as a template for the synthesis of ribonucleic acids, of which the three principal kinds are messenger RNA (mRNA), transfer RNA (tRNA) sometimes called 'soluble RNA', and ribosomal RNA (rRNA). The RNAs closely resemble DNA in general structure, but only a portion of each molecule is in the helical form, and they have ribose in place of deoxyribose, and uracil in place of thymine. All three kinds of RNA have some methylated bases. All types of RNA have their part to play in the synthesis of proteins. The details of protein synthesis differ little, whether taking place in bacteria or in the most highly evolved organisms. The molecular weights of all RNAs are lower than that of the parent DNA; that of a typical mRNA is often about one million, and of a tRNA about 25 000.

Messenger RNA (mRNA) is actually a whole family of RNAs, upon each member of which the DNA has transcribed a message which the mRNA has to translate into synthesis of a protein that is chosen according to the needs of the cell at that time (see Fig. 4.1). Each mRNA travels rapidly to the ribosomes, selects the tRNA-bound aminoacids (see below) in the order required to make the needed protein, leaves the ribosome, and is destroyed. Each triplet 'codon' of consecutive mRNA bases specifies a particular aminoacid, as listed by Nirenberg *et al.* (1963), and Khorana, *et al.* (1966). This genetic code is identical for all forms of life.

Transfer RNAs (tRNA) occur in many varieties, each of them specific for one aminoacid to which they become esterified. These esters are attracted to the ribosomes in an order predetermined by the messenger RNA that is passing through the ribosome at that time (see Fig. 5.7). The ribosome is able, by expending the energy of guanosine triphosphate, to add each new aminoacid residue to the $-CO_2H$ terminal of the growing polypeptide chain, at the same time casting the tRNAs back into the cytoplasm to make a new supply of aminoacid esters.

In detail, the 3'-hydroxy-group of the ribose (in the terminal adenosine residue of each tRNA molecule) is acylated, enzymatically, by an activated form of that aminoacid for which this tRNA is specific. Amide-ester exchange of these esters with peptidyl-tRNA on the ribosomes then occurs under the direction of mRNAs. In the latter step, the growing peptide is transferred from the tRNA bond on the 'donor' site of the ribosomes to an aminoacyl-tRNA bond on the 'acceptor' site of the same ribosome. This reaction is catalysed by the enzyme peptidyl transferse. The peptide, lengthened in this way, is then entirely shifted to the donor site with the help of a translocation enzyme. The next aminoacyl-tRNA then becomes bound to the vacant acceptor site, and the process repeated. The terminal groups of the tRNAs are always – XCCA, where C is a cytidylic, and A an adenylic, acid residue.

Several of the nucleotides in tRNAs have bases unusual for RNA. For example, the alanine-specifying tRNA has hypoxanthine, 1-methyl-hypoxanthine, 1-methylguanine, 2-dimethylguanine, thymine (ribose-bound), dihydrouracil (three times), and pseudouracil (ψ), i.e. uracil with ribose attached to C-5 instead of to nitrogen (twice). Other unusual bases often found in tRNAs include: 5-methylcytosine, 7-methylguanine, 2-methylguanine, and 1-methyl-, 2-methyl-, and 6-methyl-adenine. The precursors of all tRNAs have the usual purine and pyrimidine bases which are changed *in situ* by a methylase that transfers the methyl-group from methionine. This methylation increases specificity. In mammals, methylation occurs only in the nucleus, and is quite specific in pattern for each tissue. Malignant tumours perform such methylations at an abnormally high rate, producing some tRNAs different from those of the tissue of origin (Kuchino and Borek, 1978).

Ribosomal RNA (rRNA) is associated with about 50 different proteins in the ribosomal sub-units (see Section 5.3). A precursor of the rRNA is synthesized in the nucleoli and is then partly methylated there.

For further reading on the chemistry of nucleic acids, see Davidson (1977).

Substances which inhibit the synthesis of DNA. A large number of the most successful antibacterial, antiprotozoal, antiviral, and anticancer drugs act by inhibiting the synthesis of DNA, whether directly or indirectly. Understandably enough, many of these substances became established clinically before it was realized that their mode of action was interference with the cell's genetic material, the prime governor of its present health and future inheritance. To interfere deliberately in this way with the un-economic cell has long been a cherished dream, but one that we held back by fear of damage to the genes of the economic cell. Consensus has now been reached that a drug is acceptable even if it interferes slightly with the synthesis of DNA in the host, provided that it does not damage (or even covalently combine with) the DNA of the host. The application of this rule safeguards the host's cells from the possibility of any mutation, while retaining many of the most selective drugs that Man has yet discovered.

It will be convenient to divide these drugs into classes, such as (a) those that exert their effect on DNA somewhat remotely, namely by influencing a biochemical process that normally produces the components from which DNA is synthesized, and (b) those which directly affect the replication of existing DNA.

Outstanding among drugs which inhibit the production of DNA from several stages back in the biosynthetic pathway are the sulphonamides and the 2,4-diaminopyrimidines used so much as antibacterials and anti-malarials. All of the chemotherapeutic sulphonamides, whether simple sulphanilamide (4.5a) or its more complex heterocyclic derivatives (4.5b) including sulphadiazine, competitively inhibit the enzymes dihydrofolate synthetase which produces dihydrofolic acid (2.14) (see p. 28). The basis of this inhibition, as outlined in Section 2.1 (p. 28), is the similarity in the steric and electronic properties of p-aminobenzoic acid (2.13) (which the enzyme is ready to build into new molecules of dihydrofolic acid) and the sulphonamides (4.5) which, when taken up by the enzyme, merely block it. The basis of the *selectivity* of these antibacterial sulphonamides depends on two factors, which reinforce one another: (i) mammals lack the enzymes necessary for the synthesis of dihydrofolic acid, and hence they tolerate these sulphonamides very well; (ii) pathogenic bacteria lack the permease with the aid of which mammals absorb dihydrofolic acid from the diet. Further relevant data will be found in Section 9.3. Dihy-drofolic acid is only two steps away from the coenzyme required for bio-synthesis of thymine and all the purine bases. Deprived of the substrates, especially thymine, bacteria soon die because they can make no new DNA.

Another class of much used drugs, interfering with the synthesis of DNA, acts by inhibiting dihydrofolate hydrogenase. This is the enzyme that reduces dihydrofolic acid to 5,6,7,8-tetrahydrofolic acid, a substance only one step short of the coenzymes for synthesis of the purine bases and thymine. Analogues of folic acid, based on 2,6-diaminopteridine, such as methotrexate (4.6), are useful anticancer drugs (see Section 9.3c) but

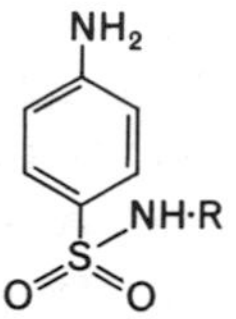

Sulphanilamide, and
derivatives
(a) R = H
(b) R = heterocyclic ring
(4.5)

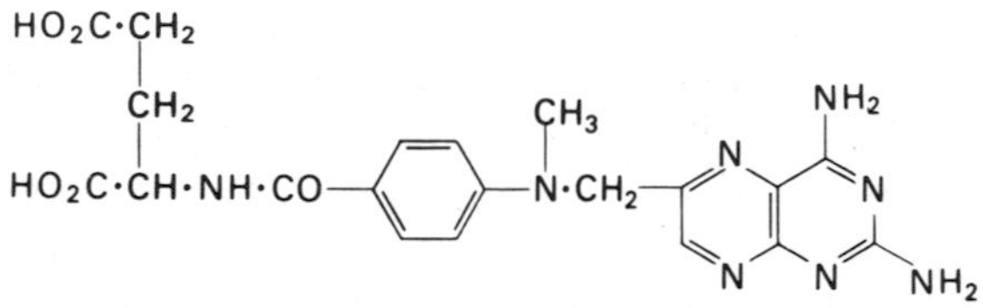

Methotrexate; amethopterin
(4.6)

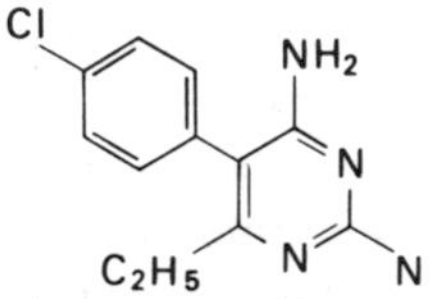

Pyrimethamine
(4.7)

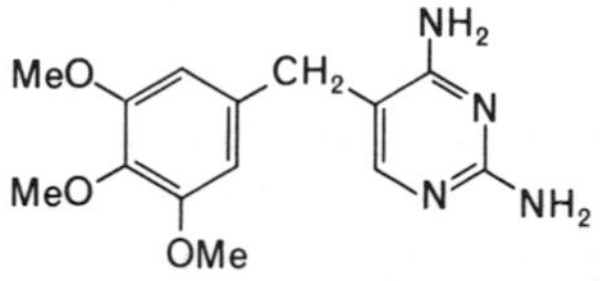

Trimethoprim
(4.8)

are not absorbable by micro-organisms. To overcome this defect, Hitchings pared away at the molecule of methotrexate until he found that the power to inhibit dihydrofolate hydrogenase resided in 2,4-diaminopyrimidine. The addition of some lipoidal groups furnished the powerful antimalarial drug, pyrimethamine ('Daraprim') (4.7) (Falco, et al., 1951). Pyrimethamine (2,4-diamino-6-ethyl-5,p-chlorophenylpyrimidine) has become the most widely used of all prophylactics against malaria. The lipoidal groups in the molecule favour its uptake by the tissues and the malarial parasite (Hitchings, 1952), and these groups also increase the adsorption of the drug to the reductase by van der Waals forces (Baker and Shapiro, 1966).

The selectivity of this class of drugs depends on the existence of *analogous enzymes*, namely dissimilar enzymes carrying out apparently identical functions in dissimilar organisms (more about these in Section 4.6). Dihydrofolate reductase, isolated from the malarial parasite *Plasmodium berghei*, was found to have a molecular weight of 200 000, which is 10 times as large as those of analogous enzymes purified from mammals and bacteria.

As can be seen from Table 4.2, the plasmodial enzyme is inhibited by pyrimethamine at a concentration about 2000 times lower than that inhibiting the analogous mammalian enzymes. The concentration that inhibited the plasmodial enzyme corresponded to that achieved in the tissues after the usual prophylactic dose. These data established that the selective action of pyrimethamine in malaria is due to the extraordinary sensitivity of the enzyme in the parasite compared to the analogous enzyme in the host (Burchall and Hitchings, 1965).

Cycloguanil (*3.26*), the triazine antimalarial formed in the human body from the inert pro-drug proguanil, also acts by inhibiting dihydrofolate hydrogenase (Wood and Hitchings, 1959).

The degree of inhibition of dihydrofolate hydrogenase by pyrimethamine was decreased very little when the chlorophenyl-group was changed to a butyl-group (Baker and Shapiro, 1966). However, quite a different substitution pattern was required to persuade the 2,4-diaminopyrimidine series to show effective antibacterial action. Eventually excellent results were obtained by providing the lipophilic substituent with a somewhat hydrophilic periphery, as in trimethoprim (*4.8*), a very successful oral antibacterial (Roth, Falco, and Hitchings, 1962). Table 4.2 shows that, whereas pyrimethamine is the most selective (of representatives of the three classes of anti-dihydrofolate hydrogenase) against the malarial parasite enzyme, trimethoprim is most selective against the bacterial enzyme. It will be observed that methotrexate, although no longer kept apart from the target enzyme by a permeability barrier, remains a poorly selective drug against micro-organisms.

Table 4.3 demonstrates the high selectivity that trimethoprim exerts

Table 4.2

CONCENTRATIONS (× 10^8 M) OF ANTIFOLIC DRUGS NEEDED
FOR 50 PER CENT INHIBITION OF DIHYDROFOLATE
HYDROGENASE, ISOLATED FROM SIX SOURCES

Substance	Human liver	Rat liver	Mouse erythrocyte	Pl. berghei	Tryp. equiperdum	E. coli
Pyrimethamine (*4.7*)	180	70	100	0.05	20	2500
Trimethoprim (*4.8*)	30 000	26 000	100 000	7.0	100	0.5
Methotrexate (*4.6*)	9	0.2	(not done)	0.07	0.02	0.1

(Burchall and Hitchings, 1965; Ferone, *et al.*, 1969; Jaffe and McCormack, 1967.)

Table 4.3

EFFECT OF TRIMETHOPRIM (*8.25*a) ON
ISOLATED DIHYDROFOLATE HYDROGENASE
Concentration (× 10^8 M) causing 50% inhibition

SOURCE: Mammalian liver		Bacteria	
Man	30 000	E. coli	0.5
Rat	26 000	S. aureus	1.5
Rabbit	37 000	P. vulgaris	0.4

(Burchall and Hitchings, 1965.)

against the dihydrofolate reductase of bacteria, both Gram-positive and Gram-negative types, while leaving the analogous mammalian enzyme unharmed. For clinical uses of this drug see Section 9.5.

A third class of drugs, one that inhibits a much later stage in DNA synthesis, consist of analogues of pyrimidine and purine bases. Several members of this class have earned a valued place in the treatment of cancer, and others are the mainstay of such antiviral therapy as has yet been achieved. Many of these analogues are metabolically changed to deoxyribosides and deoxyribotides which compete with normal nucleosides and nucleotides (Langen, 1975). Thus 5-fluorouracil (3.3), whose outstanding selectivity in treating various skin cancers has already been referred to (see Introduction to Chapter 3), exerts its major effect on the enzyme thymidylate synthetase. As has already been explained, much of the selectivity of this drug rests on its pattern of distribution, but there is some evidence of additional selectivity through the existence of analogous enzymes, as will now be outlined.

5-fluorouracil becomes an active cytostatic drug only after conversion to its nucleotide (5-fluorodeoxyuridylic acid) by the enzyme phosphoribosyl transferase. This nucleotide has an affinity for thymidylate synthetase that is several thousand times greater than that of the enzyme's natural substrate, deoxyuridylic acid. Thus it is able to keep the substrate off the enzyme, and no more DNA is synthesized (Reyes and Heidelberger, 1965). (This is the enzyme that normally transfers a methyl-group from methylene-tetrahydrofolic acid to deoxyuridylic acid, which is the key step in passing from the uracil series to the thymine series.) Further selectivity was found in leukaemia cells (mouse) which had an analogous enzyme in place of normal phosphoribosyl transferase. This analogous enzyme had almost no affinity for uracil, but a very strong one for 5-fluorouracil (Kessel, Hall, and Reyes, 1969).

Apart from its topical use in curing skin cancers, 5-fluorouracil (usually as the ribotide, 5FUdR) is given intravenously to increase the postoperative survival rate in cancer of the colon and rectum (Li and Ross, 1976) and in adenocarcinoma of the breast or colon, and in metastases of the liver (once thought to be inevitably fatal). However, it has yet to be shown that systemic use of this drug can prolong the survival rate beyond 5 years.

Idoxuridine
(4.9)

Cytosine arabinoside
(4.10)

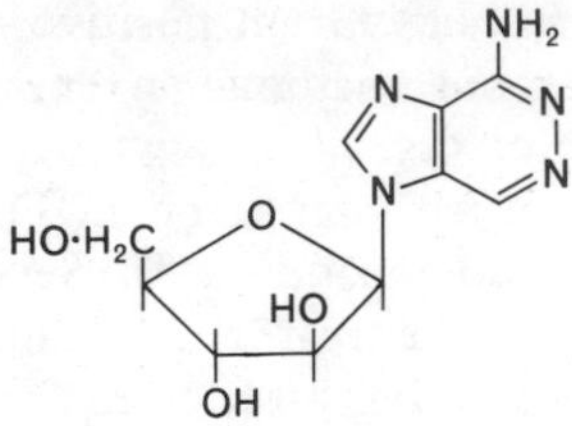

Adenine arabinoside
(4.11)

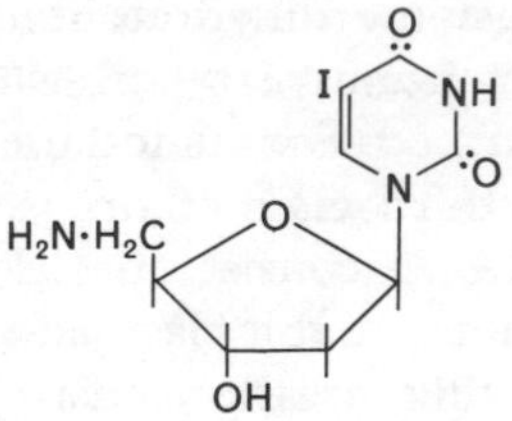

'Ald Urd'
(4.12)

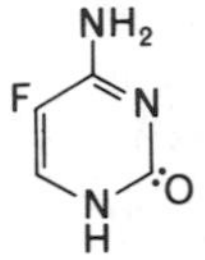

Flucytosine
(4.13)

Turning now from anticancer to antiviral drugs, the narrative must begin with 5-iododeoxyuridine (4.9) (IUdR), which made history by actually curing a virus-caused disease, herpetic keratitis (Kaufman, 1962; Perkins, et al., 1962). Such treatment is now much used to terminate, quickly, what was usually a long-lasting and painful illness. It interferes with the utilization of thymidine in cells by becoming converted to the 5′-monophosphate, which interferes with the use of thymidine. Unfortunately, it is also incorporated into DNA (in place of thymine), not only in typical DNA-containing viruses such as vaccinia and herpes simplex (Welch and Prusoff, 1966), but also into the DNA of mammals. Therefore care is taken not to use it systemically, for fear of mutagenesis. In the conjunctival sac, sealed off from the tissues and not easily absorbed, it has proved to be completely safe.

An insight into the mode of action of this drug is possibly given by the following work. When pseudo-rabies virus was exposed to IUdR, most of the thymine in the viral DNA was replaced by 5-iodouracil. The virus, when allowed to infect cultured mammalian kidney cells, continued to produce DNA, but this did not become protein-coated and hence did not generate new virus particles. That the new DNA was potentially infective was then shown by exposing it to thymidine: when much of the iodouracil had been replaced by thymine, infectivity was restored (Kaplan and Ben-Porat, 1966).

Cytarabine (4.10) is a more selective drug, never incorporated into DNA. It is also known as Ara-C, cytosine arabinoside, and 1,β-D-arabinofurano-sylcytosine. It cures herpetic keratitis, also severe generalized herpes in man. During treatment of the latter (2 to 6 days of continuous intravenous infusion), no serious injury to the bone-marrow occurred (Chow, Foerster, and Hryniuk, 1970; Juel-Jensen, 1970). It is also used in cancer therapy and many consider it the treatment of choice for acute myelocytic leukaemia, alone or with methotrexate. The unfortunate need for intravenous infusion stems from the rapid deamination of this drug in the body. Its valued medical action follows from selective inhibition of (a) nucleoside reductase (blocking biosynthesis of deoxycytosine) and (b) DNA polymerase, in herpes infected cells (Chu and Fischer, 1965) and in cancer cells (Burgoyne, 1974).

The related drug vidarabine (4.11) (Ara-A, 9,β-D-arabinofuranosyl-adenine) has shown impressive antiviral activity with no serious side-effects in man (including children). Useful in viral pneumonia, its most spectacular effect was achieved in herpes virus encephalitis (Whitley, et al., 1977), several thousand cases of which break out in the U.S.A. every year, killing 70% of the victims. Although the drug does not appear to enter Man's DNA, it is teratogenic in mice and its mutagenic possibilities are being assessed.

An amino-analogue of idoxuridine known as Ald Urd (4.12) may have clinical potential, because of its very unusual biochemistry. This substance (5-iodo-5'-amino-2',5'-dideoxyuridine) is activated to its cytostatic tri-phosphate by the kinase of herpes virus, but not by kinases in uninfected human, murine, or simian cells. It inhibited herpes simplex infection with no sign of toxicity to the host. However, when a mammalian cell was infected with herpes virus, the drug was incorporated into the DNA of both host and virus (Chen, Ward, and Prusoff, 1976). This incorporation will not matter, provided that all infected cells die, and the replication of the virus is halted. Acycloguanosine, recently developed, is 3000 times more toxic to herpes simplex virus than to mammalian cells. This substance, 9-(2-hydroxyethoxymethyl)guanine, 'zovirax', is phosphorylated by virus-specified thymidine kinase and the product is highly lethal to the virus (only). Healthy human cells carry out little of this phosphorylation, and are unharmed by the product, hence the phenomenal selectivity (Elion et al., 1977) and its clinical usefulness.

6-Mercaptopurine (3.12), first made by Elion, Burgi, and Hitchings (1952), has an established place in the treatment of the acute leukaemias (Hitchings et al., 1950; Burchenal et al., 1953; Brulé et al., 1973). Resistance studies suggest that it acts after conversion, in the cell, to its nucleotide 6-thioinosine-5'-phosphate (Brockman, 1963). Although this affects several stages of the cell's metabolism, the therapeutic benefit of 6-mercaptopurine seems to be due mainly to its inhibition of (a) the conversion of inosine-5'-phosphate to adenosine-5'-phosphate (Salser and Balis, 1965), and (b) (surprisingly) the amination of phosphoribosyl pyrophosphate to phosphoribosylamine, the latter being one of the earliest steps in purine biosynthesis (Bennett, et al., 1963). It does not become incorporated into the nucleic acids, but brings their synthesis to a stop. The 2-amino-derivative of 6-mercaptopurine, known as thioguanine, has special value in treating granulocytic leukaemia (Clarkson, 1972). Azothioprine (*3.34*, p. 90), the *S*-(1-methyl-4-nitroimidazol-5-yl) derivative of 6-mercaptopurine (which it slowly releases in the body) is much used as an immunosuppressant to prevent the rejection of organ grafts, particularly of the kidney (Elion, 1967; Elion, *et al.*, 1963).

Flucytosine (*4.13*) (5-fluorocytosine, 'Ancobon') has proved clinically successful as an oral fungicide for treating such systemic diseases as candidosis and cryptococcal meningitis. It has turned out to be remarkably non-toxic to the patient, even after 3 months of continuous therapy (Casemore, 1970; Bennett, 1977). Its selectivity depends on the fact that mammals secrete it unchanged (just as they do cytosine), whereas fungi convert it to 5-fluorouracil and then elaborate this to its cytostatic nucleotide.

For further reading on the metabolic basis of the medicinal use of purines and pyrimidine analogues, see Langen (1975).

A fourth class of agents which interfere with DNA does so by intercalating into the DNA molecule by stacking between the layers of base pairs. Section 2.2 (p. 33) describes how simple aminoacridines, such as 9-aminoacridine (*2.18*) act in this way, and hence injure bacteria by blocking the DNA template in DNA- and RNA- polymerases (Hurwitz *et al.*, 1962). These substances, strongly antibacterial against both Gram-positive and Gram-negative species, are highly selective when used topically, on mucous membranes and in deep wounds. Their selectivity seems to depend on (a), the vulnerability of the bacterial chromatin, exposed as it is in the plasma membrane (a subject expanded in Chapter 5) and (b), an apparent preference for circular DNA. As it is not certain that their selectivity is related to comparative biochemistry, these, and all other basic intercalating drugs are dealt with under 'ionization' in Section 10.3. Such drugs include the antimalarials mepacrine ('Atebrin') and quinacrine, the aminophenanthridines used for the prophylaxis of trypanosomiasis in cattle, several other trypanocides, and the valuable anticancer drug adriamycin (*10.23*).

Several useful drugs will now be mentioned which affect the synthesis or use of DNA in yet other ways.

A urinary antiseptic with high selectivity, nalidixic acid (*4.14*) ('Negram', 1-ethyl-7-methyl-4-oxo-1,8-naphthyridine-3-carboxylic acid), has high potency against Gram-negative, and inertness toward Gram-positive, bacteria (a reversal of the usual trend in antibacterials). It has proved very successful in the clinic for curing urinary infections caused by rod-shaped bacteria which are usually difficult to treat. Nalidixic acid inhibits the synthesis of DNA in bacteria (but not in man) without affecting either the use of existing DNA or the synthesis of RNA and protein (Goss, Deitz and Cook, 1965). The presence of an ionizing carboxylic acid group guarantees elimination of this drug in the urine (Section 3.4). The antibacterial properties of nalidixic acid are shared by the simpler 1-alkyl-4-oxoquinoline-3-carboxylic acid which, however, causes optical damage, lacking in (4.14). For speculation on the molecular basis of its selectivity, see Franklin and Snow (1975); Chao (1978).

The bleomycins, a family of copper bonded antibiotics isolated in Japan from *Streptomyces verticillus*, decrease the melting temperature of DNA by breaking a single strand of DNA and preventing its repair, but they have no effect on RNA (Nagai *et al.*, 1969). They have a mol. wt. of about 1550, and the molecule includes one imidazole, one pyrimidine, and two thiazole rings strung along a polypeptide chain (Umezawa, 1973). The virtues of the bleomycins are that they give a prompt response in treating cancers (squamous cell carcinomas, lymphomas), and they do not depress the bone marrow, a rare feature in anticancer drugs. Unfortunately, they are highly toxic to the human lung, which they fibrose. Their principal use is in synergism with other anticancer drugs, such as adriamycin (Carter and Blum, 1976).

The phleomycins are a family of copper-containing antibiotics, isolated from the same *Streptomyces* (Takita, Maeda, and Umezawa, 1959). They differ from the bleomycins only in the presence of two extra hydrogen atoms in the thiazole rings, and they give the corresponding bleomycins on oxidation (Umezawa, 1973). They cause breakdown of DNA in bacteria provided that the excision-endonuclease is present) by attacking at the thymine residue (Pietsch, 1966). This action is strongly potentiated by otherwise inert purines, which are thought to unwind the DNA helix partly, thus allowing the antibiotic better access (Grigg, Edwards, and Brown, 1971). Delayed renal toxicity in mammals makes the future of these otherwise selective antibiotics doubtful (Umezawa, 1973).

Camptothecin, an alkaloid from the Tibetan shrub *Camptotheca acuminata*, cleaves DNA in a way that the cell ligases can repair (Horowitz and Brayton, 1972). It has some selective anticancer (Kessel, 1971), and antiviral properties (Kelly, 1974). The molecule has five fused rings (Meyers *et al.*, 1973), of which the active portion is a pyridine lactone (4.15). It is principally used as a biochemical reagent for inhibiting biosynthesis of ribosomal and messenger RNAs while permitting formation of mitochondrial RNA (Abelson and Penman, 1972).

Nalidixic acid
(4.14)

Active portion of camptothecin
(4.15)

Hydroxyurea (*4.16*) is a derivative of hydroxylamine that is well tolerated by the patient in the large doses required for the management of chronic granulocytic leukaemia resistant to busulphan (*12.31*) (Kennedy and Yabro, 1966). The molecular basis for its selectivity lies in its sequestering the iron required by the iron-dependent enzyme *ribonucleoside diphosphate reductase*, essential for the conversion of ribo- to deoxyribo-nucleosides, and hence a vital stage in DNA synthesis (Krakoff, Brown, and Reichard, 1968). It does not affect RNA synthesis. The same enzyme is inhibited by two other drugs that show clinical promise: guanazole (*4.17*), 3,5-diamino-1,2,4-triazole (Brockman *et al.*, 1970), and 5-hydroxypicolinic aldehyde thiosemicarbazone (*4.18*) (Agrawal and Sartorelli, 1975). All these substances are specific for the S phase of the cell cycle (see Section 5.0).

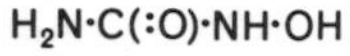

$$H_2N \cdot C(:O) \cdot NH \cdot OH$$

Hydroxyurea
(*4.16*)

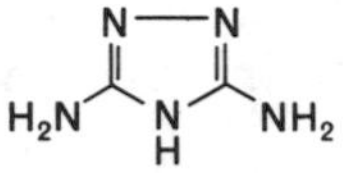

Guanazole
(*4.17*)

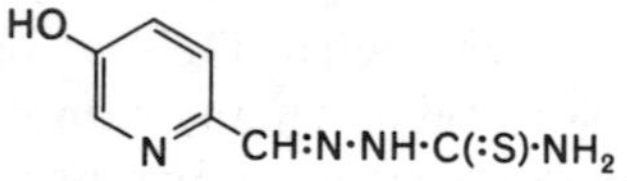

5-Hydroxypicolinic aldehyde
thiosemicarbazone
(*4.18*)

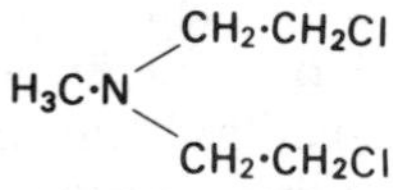

Chlormethinum
(*4.19*)

Chlormethinum (*4.19*) (mustine, mechlorethamine), the parent of the nitrogen-mustard class of cytostatic drugs, was the first substance to win clinical approval for the treatment of cancer (Gilman and Philips, 1946; Goodman *et al.*, 1946). These 'mustards', which have a very unusual chemistry (discussed in Section 12.4), act by locking together two strands of DNA by their guanine residues (Goldacre, Loveless, and Ross, 1949; Lawley and Brookes, 1967). The selectivity of the early nitrogen-mustard drugs was only moderate, but was enhanced by physical localization, such as injection directly into the tumour, or the use of tourniquets, or temperature gradients.

Caffeine, which is consumed daily in vast quantities by millions of people without harm, increases the rate of spontaneous breakdown of DNA in *E. coli* and it is highly mutagenic in this bacterium (Grigg, 1970). It is a sobering thought that, under legislation current in many advanced countries, these adverse effects of caffeine on DNA could hold up the introduction of tea and coffee were they not already in common use. In assessing this, and other possible mutagens, it has to be borne in mind that

most mutated cells are not viable, and a (very small) percentage of muta-
tions are actually beneficial.

In concluding this section, two precautions necessary for responsible
use of newly introduced anti-DNA drugs will be emphasized. Regular
blood counts should be made, and the drugs should be withheld from women
in the critical months of pregnancy.

(a) Rifamycin SV, R = H   CH$_2$ ——————— CH$_2$

(b) Rifampin,   R = $-$CH$\,$:$\,$N$\cdot$N$\cdot$CH$_2\cdot$CH$_2$NMe

(4.20)

Substances that inhibit the synthesis of RNA.   The rifamycins are antibiotics isolated in Italy from *Streptomyces mediterranei*, and then chemically
altered in the laboratory to give more useful products. Of these, rifamycin
SV (*4.20a*) provided early clinical experience, but rifampin (rifampicin)
(*4.20b*) has become the standard medication. Among the most selective
of all known drugs, the rifamycins are used early in tuberculosis, and also
for curing drug-resistant tuberculosis; also for resistant staphylococcal
infections. Were they less expensive, they would be used a great deal
more.

Chemically, the rifamycins belong to a group of natural products known
as ansamycins, from the Latin *ansa*, a handle. The name ansa-compound
was coined by Lüttringhaus and Gralheer for substances containing
an aromatic nucleus (naphthalene in the present case) around which is
wrapped the 'handle' in the form of an aliphatic chain, joined in two places
(Maggi *et al.*, 1966, 1968). At least three of the hydroxyl-groups are necessary for their action. The structure, which has not been synthesized,
lends itself to chemical alteration, but principally only in the 3-position.
A whole wealth of products altered in this position have been made and
tested.

Rifamycins act on the β-subunit of the protein in bacterial DNA-dependent RNA-polymerase. Combination is tight, though not covalent, and
occurs in a 1 : 1 molecular ratio (this union does not take place in rifampin-
resistant organisms). As a result, no more RNA is synthesized, but

neither DNA nor protein syntheses are affected. There is no action whatsoever on the RNA-synthesizing mechanism of mammals, which lacks a
β-subunit, and hence the selectivity experienced by the patient is of the
very highest degree (Tocchini-Valenti, Marino, and Colvill, 1968). Rifamycin SV also inhibits reverse transcriptase, the RNA-dependent synthesizer of DNA, e.g. in murine leukaemia virus (Brockman *et al.*, 1971).
A substance with this property could be an outstanding antiviral drug,
but it has not proved to be so. Rifampicin (*4.20b*), on the other hand,
inhibits the replication of poxviruses and adenoviruses in mouse cells;
yet this is accomplished by inhibiting the DNA-primed, and not the
RNA-primed, enzyme (Heller *et al.*, 1969).

Other ansamycins are found in Nature, e.g. streptovaricin (from another
Streptomyces) which acts in the same way as rifamycin but is not so selective;
amanitin (from the fungus *Amanita phalloides*) which is counter-selective,
inhibiting eukaryotic but not prokaryotic DNA-dependent RNA-polymerase; and maytansine (from the bark of an African flowering plant) which
has anticancer properties, but is not yet established in the clinic (Kupchan
et al., 1974).

Actinomycin D (*4.21*); a bright red antibiotic isolated by Waksman and
Woodruff in 1940, has an aminophenoxazine nucleus which bears two
identical cyclic side-chains, each of which has one ester and five peptide
linkages (*4.22*). The residues in each side-chain are: *N*-methyl-valine,
sarcosine, proline, valine, and threonine (Brockmann, 1960). Evidence from
n.m.r. indicates that the −NH of valine is strongly hydrogen bonded to the
CO of sarcosine.

Actinomycin D is remarkably specific in inhibiting the synthesis of
ribosomal RNA (DNA-primed) without any effect on the synthesis of DNA
(Reich *et al.*, 1962). Use of radioactive actinomycin showed that it was
covalently bound to the guanine of the DNA starter, and did not combine
with any other cell component at concentrations that block RNA synthesis.
The phenoxazine nucleus intercalates into DNA near to a G-C pair, and the
peptide portions project into the minor groove (Müller and Crothers,
1968) (for more on intercalation see Section 10.3b). Whereas the action of
the aminoacridines is sensitive to magnesium ions and insensitive to urea,
precisely the reverse is true of actinomycin. Again, proflavine prevents the
enzymatic synthesis of guanine-free polynycleotides, but actinomycin
does not.

Actinomycin D (under the name dactinomycin) has shown its most
striking anti-cancer properties in postoperative treatment of Wilms's
tumour of the kidney which forms a high proportion of all malignant
tumours in children. Under its influence, pulmonary metastases caused by
this tumour regress (Farber and Mitus, 1968). Forms of cancer requiring
longer treatment are not suitable for this drug, which has only moderate
selectivity.

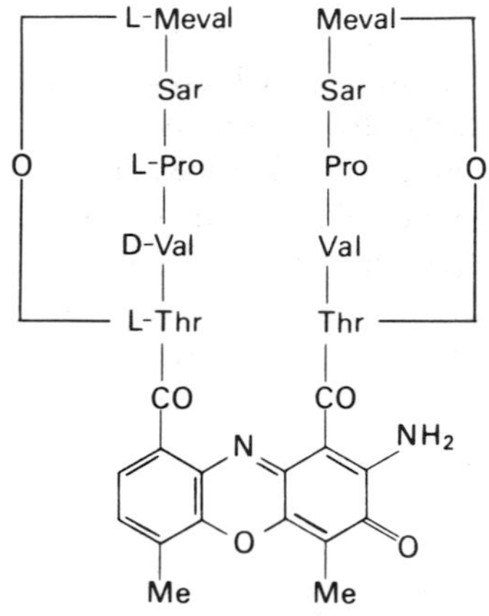
L-Meval
Meval
Sar
Sar
O
L-Pro
Pro
O
D-Val
Val
L-Thr
Thr
CO
CO
N
NH2
O
O
Me
Me
Actinomycin D
(*4.21*)

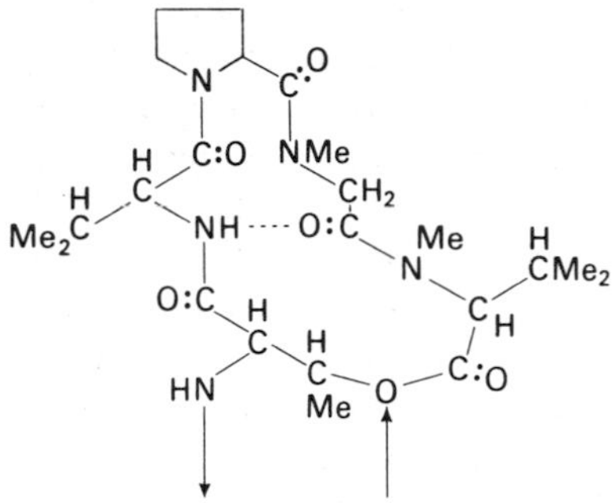
N
C:O
H
C:O
NMe
H
C
CH2
Me2C
NH····O:C
Me
H
N
CMe2
O:C
H
C
H
C
H
H
C
HN
C
O
C:O
Me
Side-chain of actinomycin D
↓ indicates point of attachment to nucleus
↑ indicates ester linkage
(*4.22*)

8-azaguanine (*4.23*) was first prepared by synthesis (Roblin *et al.*, 1945), but the antibiotic, pathocidin, isolated later from *Streptomyces albus* (Anzai and Suzuki, 1961), is identical. 8-azaguanine is used to treat cancer of the brain, kidney, and liver because these organs are rich in guanase which deaminates it to harmless 8-azaxanthine, whereas tumours common in these organs lack this enzyme (Levine, Hall, and Harris, 1963). A strong inhibitor of protein synthesis, 8-azaguanine is not incorporated into DNA in *E. coli*, T_2 bacteriophage (Smith and Matthews, 1957), cancer cells in culture or in the intact mouse (Nelson *et al.*, 1975). Instead, it is converted by guanosine-5′-phosphate pyrophosphorylase into the nucleotide which is incorporated into messenger RNA, causing polysomes to break down into monomeric ribosomes: this puts a stop to protein synthesis (Kwan and Webb, 1967). In addition, 8-azaguanosine-5′-phosphate inhibits phosphoribosylpyrophosphate amidotransferase at an early step in purine biosynthesis (McCollister *et al.*, 1964).

Mithramycin, which has a tetrahydroanthracene nucleus with two chains of pyranose rings attached, is obtained from several species of *Streptomyces*. It inhibits synthesis of RNA while that of DNA continues. It can cause hypocalcaemia and, in general, is not very selective, but has proved useful in treating testicular tumours (Northrup, Taylor, and Northrup, 1969).

6-azauracil (*4.24*) is used in agriculture as a fungicide to inhibit powdery mildew (e.g. in cucumbers). It is converted in the fungal cell to the ribotide which, being an analogue of orotidylic acid, blocks orotidylic decarboxylase (Dekker, 1968; Pasternak and Handschumacher, 1959). Although a side-effect on the central nervous system precluded its use in man, the triacetyl-derivative, azaribine (see Section 3.5, p. 91), has proved valuable in the oral treatment of psoriasis (Calabresi and Turner, 1966).

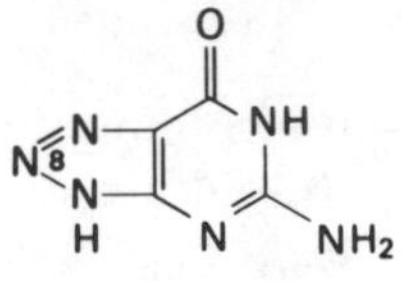

8-Azaguanine
(4.23)

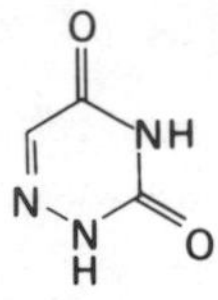

6-Azauracil
(4.24)

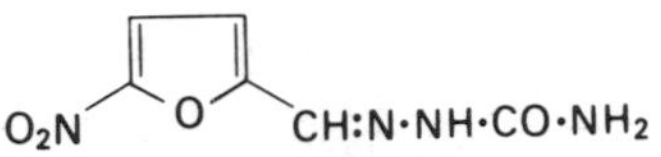

Nitrofurazone
(4.25)

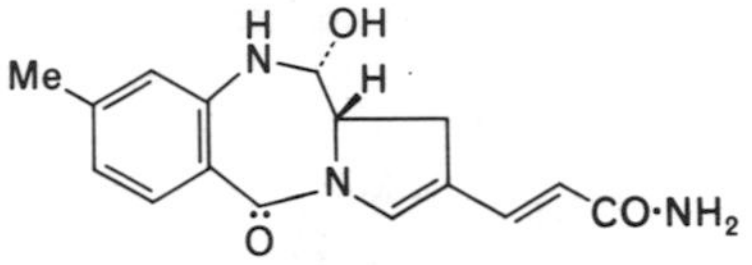

Anthramycin
(covalently hydrated form)
(4.26)

Nitrofurazone (*4.25*) (5-nitrofurfural semicarbazone, 'Furacin') is used topically with great success as a broad-spectrum antibacterial. It is also kept in reserve for arsenic-resistant late stages of trypanosomiasis. In dilute solution, nitrofurazone inhibits the formation of all types of RNA in *E. coli* (Tu and McCalla, 1976). Mutants that lacked 'nitrofuran reductase' are not attacked, and hence reduction must precede activity of this drug. The active form is either the hydroxylamino analogue of this nitro-compound, or one differing from this by one electron. Nitrofurazone, with its reduction potential of − 0.425 volts (versus the standard calomel electrode at pH 7) is an electron acceptor at a highly negative potential, just on the lower border of the biological range. The corresponding derivative of benzene, *p*-nitro-benzaldehyde semicarbazone, has a reduction potential of −0.580 V, considered to render it biologically unreducible (Sasaki, 1954). Of the nitro-furans, those with a conjugated side-chain are most easily reduced because the radical anion thus formed is stabilized by resonance (Lindberg, 1970).

Related drugs include nitrofurantoin (*6.14*, p. 200) (a urinary antiseptic) and metronidazole (*6.19*, p. 205) (a nitroimidazole much used in amoebiasis and trichomoniasis). Clearly, there is much to be discovered before it can be said how any of these drugs act so selectively, but the recent link of nitrofurazone with inhibition of RNA synthesis seems an important clue.

Anthramycin (*4.26*), which readily undergoes covalent hydration (Section 2.3, p. 45), inhibits the synthesis of RNA by binding to the DNA primer in RNA polymerase, which could account for its antitumour and antimicrobial action (Horwitz and Grollman, 1968; Kohn and Spears, 1970).

4.1 Proteins

In every living cell, proteins are assembled on ribosomes by the co-poly-merization of about 20 kinds of aminoacids, all with the same L-optical configuration (see Fig. 5.7). The molecular weight of proteins varies from about 6000 to well over a million daltons, but all have the common structure shown in Fig. 4.2, where R represents the familiar side-chains, such as methyl (for alanine) and *p*-hydroxybenzyl (for tyrosine). The *Atlas of Protein Sequence and Structure* (National Biomedical Research Foundation, Georgetown University, Washington, D.C), published at intervals, contains the aminoacid sequences of many hundreds of proteins.

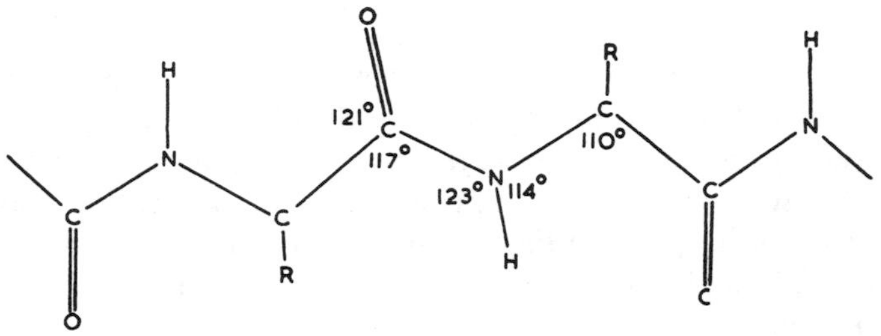

FIG. 4.2 Portion of primary polypeptide chain.

The sequence of the aminoacid residues is determined by the genetic information in the cell's DNA, and expressed through the combined operation of mRNA and tRNA. This sequence is known as 'primary structure'. Such a polypeptide chain is always folded into a secondary struc-ture which is retained by multiple hydrogen bonding between the – CO groups in one strand and the NH – groups in the next (the reversal of the chain's direction, to give strands, is forced wherever proline residues occur in it). This sheet has a repeat distance of 7.2 Å between *alternate* aminoacid residues. As it occurs in nature, the sheet is slightly pleated to make room for small-to-medium side-chains, and the repeat distance is about 7.0 Å, as in fibroin, the protein of silk.

When the average size of the side-chain is large, a helix is formed instead of a pleated sheet. These helices (also called α-helices, but the α is un-necessary) are all right-handed and have 3.7 aminoacid residues in each turn, shown in Fig. 3.8. As Pauling and Corey showed, this is the structure of a wool fibre. These spirals have a repeat distance of 1.5 Å between amino-acid residues measured along the *axis*; neighbouring aminoacids unite the loops of the spiral by CO . . . HN bonding. Apart from X-ray crystal-lography at a resolution of 2 or 3 Å, knowledge of this secondary structure has been acquired by investigating the optical rotatory dispersion, and by measuring the number of hydrogen atoms which exchange *slowly* with the deuterium of D_2O (i.e. those forming interhelical bonds).

These helices are long strands which, in globular (i.e. non-fibrous) proteins, including enzymes, are folded back on themselves to give the irregular loops characteristic of tertiary structure. These loops are usually set in a form pre-determined by the order of the aminoacids (Perutz, Kendrew and Watson, 1965). The setting is effected by covalent (disulphide), ionic, van der Waals, or hydrogen bonds. The molecule is compact but with a few water molecules inside. Almost all the polar groups (e.g. $-OH$, $-NH_2$, $-CO_2H$) are on the outside of the molecule. Because of this, globular proteins dissolve in water. The $S-S$ bonds, which give ribonuclease (for example) the conformation on which its enzymatic action is dependent, unite the following pairs of aminoacid residues, counting from the NH_2 end of the chain: 28–84, 65–72, 40–95, 58–110 (there are 124 residues in this protein).

Globular proteins have been found (by X-ray diffraction examination of their crystals) to be partly helical, partly pleated, and partly random. Randomness seems to be encouraged by residues of asparagine, aspartic acid, and phenylalanine; it also appears that threonine, and aspartic and glutamic acids occur preferentially near the NH_2 end of the chain, whereas lysine, arginine, and histidine are found more often towards the CO_2H end (Cook, 1967).

For a discussion of enzymes, see Section 9.0. For further information on the structure of proteins, see Neurath and Hill (1975), and the periodical, *Advances in Protein Chemistry*. Models of proteins may be visualized in three dimensions by using the Stereo Supplement to the book *Structure and Action of Proteins* (Dickerson and Geis, 1969).

Substances that inhibit the synthesis of proteins. The considerable structural differences between bacterial ($70S$) and mammalian ($80S$) ribosomes may suggest that the discussion of the inhibitors of protein synthesis should be deferred to Section 5.3, where the different kinds of ribosomes are compared. However, several relevant details of comparative biochemistry are emerging, and this indicates that the protein-synthesis inhibiting drugs should first be presented in this Chapter.

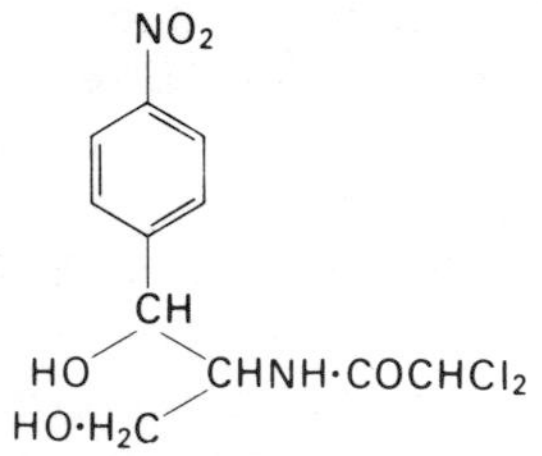

Chloramphenicol
(4.27)

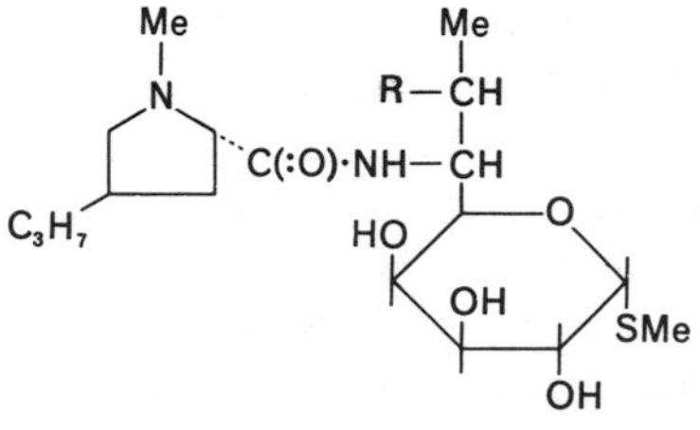

(a) Lincomycin (R = OH)
(b) Clindamycin (R = Cl)
(4.28)

Chloramphenicol (*4.27*), isolated from *Streptomyces venezuelae* in 1947 but now obtained entirely by synthesis, is the D-(-)*threo* isomer of 2,2-dichloro-*N*-[2-hydroxy-1-(hydroxymethyl)-2-(4-nitrophenyl) ethyl] acetamide. Its selective antibacterial effect, when given orally, depends on its inhibition of protein synthesis on the ribosomes of bacteria without affecting that taking place on mammalian ribosomes, even when it has free access to the latter (Rendi and Ochoa, 1962; Gale and Folkes, 1953). The other three stereoisomers have no effect on protein synthesis.

X-ray crystallography shows that the two hydroxy-groups lie close together (the amide-group points away from these), and the whole aliphatic portion is in a plane roughly at right angles to the benzene ring (Dunitz, 1952). The n.m.r. spectrum indicates that the two hydroxyl groups are hydrogen-bonded mutually (Jardetzky, 1963), and this confers a steric resemblance to uridine-5-phosphoric acid. On the other hand Das, Goldstein, and Kanner (1966) thought that the amide-group of chloramphenicol made it a stereospecific metabolite analogue of a natural amino-acid, and other authors have deemed chloramphenicol to be a structural analogue of yet other molecules engaged in protein biosynthesis. So far, none of these suggestions has helped to elucidate details of its action at the biochemical level, and what little is known has been inferred from the following facts.

The antibacterial properties of chloramphenicol are unimpaired when the nitro-group is replaced by another strongly electron-attracting group, such as methylthio- (MeS-), sulphamoyl- ($H_2N.SO_2$-), or methylsulphonyl ($MeSO_2$-), hence the role of the nitro-group is simply electron-attracting (Cammarata, 1967). Of these analogues, the methylsulphonyl-compound, known as thiamphenicol, is used clinically in Italy and Japan (unlike chloramphenicol, it is excreted through the kidneys, thus extending the usefulness of this series). The D-*threo* configuration has proved as essential for these altered molecules as it is for chloramphenicol itself (Freeman, 1970).

The aliphatic portion of the molecule is more sensitive to change, e.g. the substitution of any hydrogen atom by a methyl-group leads to complete inactivation; however, an increase in activity was seen when the dichloro-group was replaced by a trifluoromethyl-group (Nagawa, 1960).

Bacteria at once absorb chloroamphenicol which is rapidly accumulated on the 50*S* subunit of the 70*S* ribosomes typical of bacteria, and protein synthesis is rapidly halted (learnt from studies with ^{14}C-chloramphenicol followed by ultrasonic rupture of cell walls; Wolfe and Hahn, 1965). On the ribosome, chloramphenicol prevents formation of the peptide bonds by inhibiting peptidyltransferase at the A site (Jacoby and Gorini, 1967), presumably by blocking interaction between this enzyme and the aminoacyl end of aminoacyl-tRNA (Pestka, 1970). Work with ribosome cores that have been depleted of specific proteins, has indicated that it is protein L 16 which binds chloramphenicol most specifically (Nierhaus and Nierhaus, 1973; Roth and Nierhaus, 1975).

Chloramphenicol was the first of the broad-spectrum antibiotics to be used in medicine, but it came under a cloud when long-continued administration produced many cases of aplastic anaemia, which can be life endangering. Its use is now restricted to diseases where it is the most active known remedy, and which are likely to be cured quickly, within the safe period of the drug. Hence it is used to cure typhoid fever, cholera, bacterial meningitis, rickettsioses (including Rocky Mountain spotted fever), and intra-ocular infections; also, as a single dose, to terminate rapidly the acute symptoms of a dysentery that is being treated with the safe, but slower-acting derivatives of sulphathiazole.

Lincomycin (4.28a), from *Streptomyces lincolnensis*, and its derivative clindamycin (4.28b), are given orally for resistant strains of Gram-positive cocci, and also for intestinal anaerobes, such as *Bacteroides* which builds up in postoperative blind-loops. It inhibits peptidyl transferase on the 50S ribosomal subunit, much as chloramphenicol does (Smithers, Bennett, and Struck, 1969). The principal side-effects are diarrhoea, and even colitis.

Erythromycin
(4.29)

Erythromycin (4.29) is a much-used orally-active macrolide antibiotic isolated in 1952, from *Streptomyces erythreus* in soil from the Philippines. Studies with ^{14}C-erythromycin show that it inhibits protein synthesis in 70S (but not in mammalian 80S) ribosomes. In detail, it prevents peptidyl-tRNA trasferring from the A to the D site on the 50S ribosomal subunit during translocation (Mao, Putterman, and Wiegand, 1970).

Erythromycin has much the same spectrum of antibacterial activity as penicillin, and is specially valued for penicillin-sensitive patients. It has almost no side-effects and is well tolerated by children. Because it is acid-labile, it is often prescribed as an insoluble salt (especially the stearate) from which it is liberated in the small intestine, or as an ester (e.g. the propionate). Both erythromycin and lincomycin inhibit the uptake of ^{14}D-chloramphenicol by ribosomes, which points to similar sites for attack by all three antibiotics (Wolfe and Hahn, 1964).

Tetracycline
(4.30)

Tetracycline (4.30) and its derivatives are the most used of all 'broad-spectrum antibiotics'. Their selectivity depends on their preferential accumulation by bacteria, as was outlined in the introduction to Chapter 3. Chelation of magnesium also plays an important part in their action, and this is discussed in Section 11.8. Tetracycline is prepared by the dechlorination of its 7-chloro-derivative ('Aureomycin'), the first medicinal tetracycline, isolated in 1947 from *Streptomyces aureofaciens*. It is a dimethyl-aminopentahydroxydioxo-octahydro*napthacene*carboxamide.

By using ^{3}H-tetracyclines it was shown that these antibiotics were bound to the $30S$ ribosome subunit (e.g. Connemacher and Mandel, 1965), where they inhibited the *m*RNA-directed binding of aminoacyl-tRNA (Sarkar and Thach, 1968). In this way they efficiently inhibit bacterial protein synthesis. Orally administered, tetracyclines cure infections caused by many species of Gram-positive and -negative bacteria, spirochaetes, and rickettsiae, with very few side effects, none of them serious. The earlier types, which needed large and frequent doses, have been supplemented by (a) two long-acting examples: demeclocycline [as (4.30) but with Cl in 7-position, and no Me in 6] and methacycline [gain of OH in 5-position, and dehydration of 6 to $= CH_2$], and (b) two much longer-acting examples which have the further advantage of being better absorbed: doxycycline [OH moved from 6 to 5 position], and minocycline [loss of Me and OH from 6-position, gain of NMe$_2$ in 7].

Fusidic acid resembles the tetracyclines in being almost equally inhibitory to both bacterial and mammalian ribosomes while normally leaving the latter unharmed through inability to penetrate the mammalian cytoplasmic membrane (Franklin and Snow, 1975). However, there is no chemical resemblance, for fusidic acid is a steroid. Although liable to produce mild diarrhoea, fusidic acid is well tolerated orally, even by children. It is usually reserved for pneumonia, or other coccal infection, resistant to the commoner antibiotics.

Spectinomycin (4.31) (decahydro-4a,7,9-trihydroxy-2-methyl-6,8-*bis*-methylaminopyrano[2,3-*b*]benzodioxin-4-one, 'Trobicin') inhibits protein

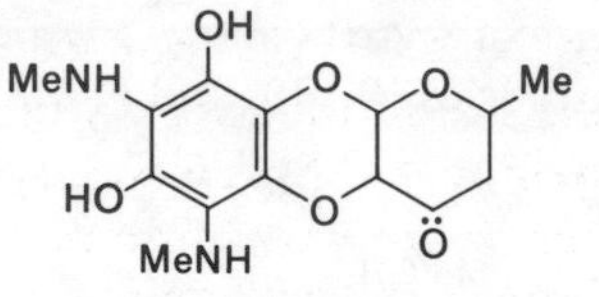

OH

MeNH

HO

MeNH

Me

O   O

O

Ö

Spectinomycin
(4.31)

synthesis by binding to the 30S ribosomes. It is selective, but weak, and is reserved for treating, intramuscularly, cases of gonorrhoea resistant to penicillin and the tetracyclines (Reyn *et al.*, 1973).

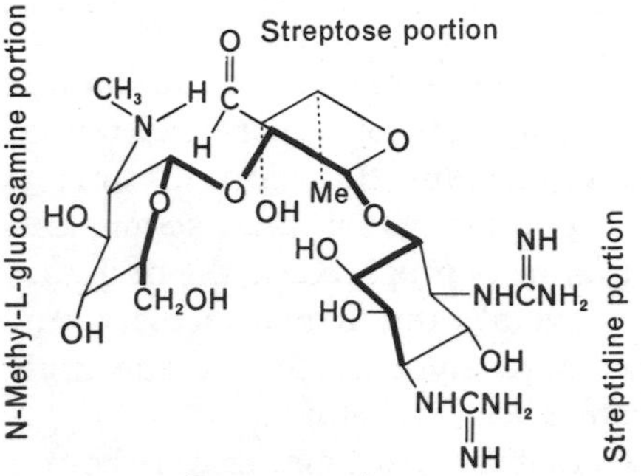

N-Methyl-L-glucosamine portion

Streptose portion

CH₃   H   C
    N
   H

HO

CH₂OH

OH

O

OH   Me

HO

HO

O

—NHCNH₂

OH

NHCNH₂

NH

NH

Streptidine portion

Streptomycin
(4.32)

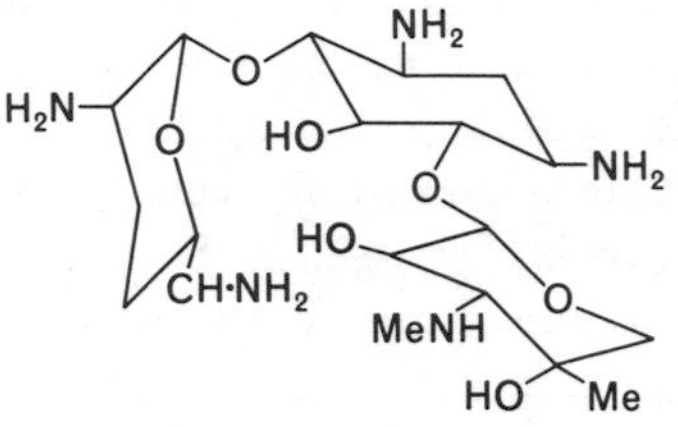

H₂N

NH₂

O

HO

—NH₂

O

HO

CH·NH₂

MeNH

HO   Me

O

Gentamicin-1a
(4.33)

Streptomycin (4.32), the first of the aminoglycoside antibiotics, was discovered in *Streptomyces griseus* by Waksman and colleagues in 1944 during their systematic quest for an antibiotic which, unlike penicillin, would be sensitive to Gram-negative as well as Gram-positive bacteria. Chemically it is an *N*-methyl-1-glucosamido-streptosido-streptidine in which the guanidine base (streptidine) is linked to a disaccharide. Streptomycin penetrates through the bacterial plasma membrane in a rather complex way, described in Section 14.2 It does not harm the mammalian (80S) ribosome, but binds to the ribosomal protein S12 on the 30S sub-unit of the bacterial (70S) ribosomes. This protein, in streptomycin-resistant bacteria, has a single aminoacid replacement for one or other of its two lysine moieties (Ozaki, Mizushima, and Nomura, 1969). The binding of streptomycin to the bacterial ribosome seems to cause some distortion of the site, and a loss of magnesium ions (see Section 11.9).

The ability of streptomycin, under certain conditions, to induce mis-reading of the genetic code and to produce nonsense polypeptides, may be phenomena of the laboratory unrelated to the clinical use of this drug (Luzzatto, Apirion, and Schlessinger, 1968). Streptomycin is lethal to cells only when they are vigorously engaged in protein synthesis. For this reason, some other inhibitors of protein synthesis, notably chloramphenicol and tetracycline, interfere with the antibacterial action of streptomycin.

Streptomycin-dependent bacteria do not owe this genetically-based oddity to contact with the drug, but have an inbuilt metabolic error that the drug corrects (Goldstein, 1954; Mitchison, 1962).

Streptomycin, being unabsorbable from the bowel, is injected intra-muscularly. It leapt to fame as the first drug that could cure tuberculosis, but its toxic effect on the eighth cranial nerve often led to permanent deafness. It is now used mainly as an auxiliary to other drugs, notably isoniazid, to prevent the emergence of resistant strains in tuberculosis. Another current use of streptomycin is with either penicillin or tetracycline for treating chronic bacterial infections.

Gentamicin, a mixture of (4.33) with two of its methyl homologues, is the most important of all aminoglycosides in current clinical use. It was isolated in 1964 from an actinomycete (prokaryote) named *Micromonospora purpurea*. Its mode of action is similar to that of streptomycin, but it is more selective (Milanesi and Ciferri, 1966). Highly active against all common Gram-positive and -negative bacteria, gentamicin is injected intramuscularly to combat infections of the respiratory and urinary tracts, being specially valued for Gram-negative infections of the latter. Un-fortunately about 3% of the patients receiving it develop (reversible) kidney damage and sometimes irreversible deafness has occurred.

Kanamycin, tobramycin, neomycin and viomycin are aminoglycosides chemically similar to gentamicin and with similar clinical properties. Of these, neomycin and viomycin have proved to be too little selective, and are now used only in ointments. Kanamycin is more selective, but apparently not so much as gentamicin. Tobramycin has recently been introduced because of its intense activity against that very individualistic and difficult bacterium, *Pseudomonas*. All three drugs can cause nephro-and oto- toxicity, although to different degrees. Finally, the aminoglycoside paromomycin provides the shortest course yet discovered for treating amoebiasis (Woolfe, 1965).

The alkaloid emetine (4.34), the first of all drugs against amoebiasis (see Section 6.0), is now losing ground against such non-nauseating but highly effective remedies as metronidazole and chloroquine. However it is still considered a useful adjuvant to have on hand. Emetine acts on both parasite and host by suppressing protein synthesis namely by preventing the translocation of peptidyl-tRNA from the acceptor site to the donor site in the ribosomes (Huang and Grollman, 1970). The likely basis of its selectivity is that the amoebae, unlike mammalian liver cells, cannot quickly enter into a recovery phase between courses of the drug (Grollman, 1966).

Cycloheximide (4.35), (obtained from *Streptomyces griseus* along with streptomycin) is counter-selective, for it inhibits protein synthesis in mammalian, but not in bacterial, cells. It is widely used by biochemists to inhibit protein synthesis whenever it is desired to establish if a given biochemical effect depends on the synthesis of new protein. It also has limited use as an agricultural fungicide.

There are configurational and conformational similarities between emetine and cycloheximide. In emetine, the R (rectus) configuration at C-1′ and the secondary nitrogen atom at N-2′ are essential for activity, as inspection of a series of analogues, active and inactive, showed. Cycloheximide, which has a hydrogen-bonded nucleus (Siegel, Sisler, and Johnson, 1966), shares much of emetine's essential structure (Grollman, 1966, 1968).

For a review on the design of drugs intended to inhibit protein synthesis, see Grollman (1971).

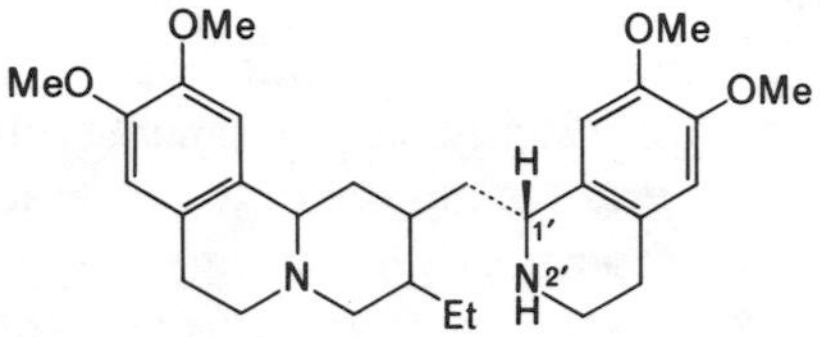

Emetine
(4.34)

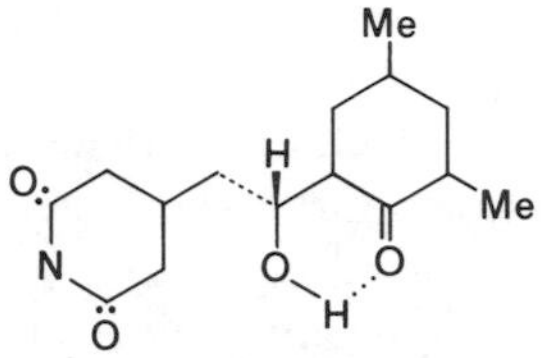

Cycloheximide
(4.35)

4.2 Nitrogen and phosphorus metabolism

This Section and the next deal with catabolic processes. Because these are known to follow fairly uniform patterns in most living cells, the expectation of variations that could be exploited selectively may not seem very high. In spite of that, some variations do exist, and a selection of them is recorded here together with indications of their use.

Nitrogen metabolism has end-products more varied than those of fat or carbohydrate metabolisms, ranging in complexity from ammonia to the alkaloids. What is still more surprising, the end-products of nitrogen metabolism can vary within a single species, depending on the stage of development. For example, Fig. 4.3 shows that a chicken, in the egg, passes in turn through the stages of excreting ammonia (as though it were a fish), urea (as though it were a frog), and uric acid (typical of birds), all within a few days. This sequence may shed light on the well-known necessity for using different selectively toxic agents to deal with parasites at different stages. For example, the sexual form of the parasite of malignant tertian malaria can be attacked only by 8-aminoquinolines, e.g. primaquine (3.27); whereas the asexual form, although coexisting with the other in human erythrocytes, is injured by drugs of quite different molecular structure such as chloroquine (10.28) and mepacrin (6.9).

Some unusual aminoacids occur in the cell walls of bacteria (Section

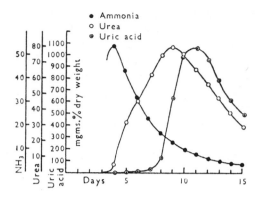

FIG. 4.3 Nitrogen excretion of chick embryo (after Needham).

Maximum of	Days after fertilization
Ammonia	4
Urea	9
Uric acid	11

(Baldwin, 1948a.)

5.1). Several unusual biosyntheses of common aminoacids have been recorded. Thus plants and bacteria make lysine only by decarboxylating diaminopimelic acid, but the lysine of fungi and mammals is made from 2-aminoadipic acid (Vogel, 1959). No aminoacid of the D-series has been found in an active cell constituent of any creature higher on the evolutionary scale than the earthworm (*Lumbricus terrestris*), which contains the phosphagen lombricine (*O*-phosphodiester of guanidinoethanol and D-serine) (Ennor *et al.*, 1960).

The aromatic aminoacids, phenylalanine and tryptophan, are made in bacteria and plants from shikimic acid (*4.36*) (3,4,5-trihydroxy*cyclo*hex- Δ^1-ene-1-carboxylic acid); but mammals cannot form the benzene ring and hence have to obtain these two aminoacids from the diet (Gibson, 1964). From shikimic acid, plants elaborate gallotannins, and insects harbour bacteria which make protocatechuic acid (3,4-dihydroxybenzoic acid) which tans the proteins of their integument. Because shikimic acid does not enter into mammalian metabolism, its synthesis and use are clear targets at which to aim selective toxicity. In bacteria, shikimic acid arises by cyclization of the carbohydrate 3-deoxy-2-oxo-D-*arabino*-heptulosonic acid 7-phosphate, which is formed by the condensation of erythrose-4-phosphate and phosphoenolpyruvic acid. Shikimic acid undergoes biosynthesis to chorismic acid (4-hydroxy-3-pyruvylenoloxy*cyclo*hex- Δ^1-ene-1-carboxylic acid), which leads in turn to phenylalanine (and hence tyrosine), anthranilic acid (and hence tryptophan), ubiquinone, vitamin K, and *p*-aminobenzoic acid (and hence folic acid). Inhibition of shikimic acid metabolism is a field worthy of intense study.

Shikimic acid
(4.36)

Stibophen
(4.37)

Adenosine triphosphate (ATP) is employed by all multicellular organisms for energy storage and transfer, but some bacteria (e.g. *Rhodospirillum rubrum* and *Proprionibacterium shermanii*) use inorganic pyrophosphate, and so does the dysentery-causing protozoon *Entamoeba histolytica*. The work of ATP is assisted by phosphagens which differ, interestingly, among the different forms of animal life. Phosphocreatine, which is the sole phosphagen for vertebrates, occurs in a few invertebrate species, but phosphoarginine is more common, and a few invertebrate species have both. Within any given phylum, the distribution of these two phosphagens often differs between closely related species, and even between the tissues of a single animal (Florkin and Mason, 1960). Some rarer phosphagens, which have a distribution restricted to a few invertebrates, are phospho-guanidoacetic acid, phosphoguanidotaurine, and lombricine (see above).

4.3 Carbohydrate and lipid metabolism

Carbohydrate metabolism has at its core the chemical sequence known as glycolysis, i.e. the conversion of glucose (or glycogen) to lactic acid. This takes place, in all living cells, by the pathway uncovered by Meyerhof, Embden, Parnas, and Cori. Oxygen is not utilized, but nicotinamide adenine dinucleotide (NAD) is reduced in proportion as glyceraldehyde-3-phosphate (anion) is oxidized to phosphoenol-pyruvate. The NADH produced in this way is then used to reduce pyruvate to lactate. Glycolysis takes at least 11 steps, each with its own enzyme. The net balance of energy storage is that two (and three) molecules of adenosine triphosphate (ATP) are made for each molecule of glucose (and glycogen, respectively) utilized.

Such anaerobic metabolism can sustain life in animal cells only for short periods. However, if there is free access of oxygen, pyruvic acid passes from the above Meyerhof sequence to the tricarboxylic acid cycle (see Section 4.4), where it is completely oxidized to carbon dioxide and water. An alternative pathway exists for degrading glucose, through pentose phosphate as in bacteria (see below). The relative importance of the two pathways has not yet been assessed in vertebrates, but clearly varies from organ to organ.

Investigation of the comparative biochemistry of normal and cancerous cells has revealed few significant differences in glycolysis (Greenstein, 1954). Moreover, the enzymes used seem identical, even immunologically. However, Warburg (1927) showed that cancer cells have less oxidative phosphorylation than normal cells and hence more anaerobic glycolysis leading to enhanced production of lactic acid. In fact, rapidly dividing cancer cells have been found to lack glycerol-3-phosphate dehydrogenase (NAD-linked type) in the cytoplasm, an important difference from normal cells (Criss, 1973; Fondy, Ghangas, and Reza, 1970). Malignant tumours usually have a core of hypoxic (almost anaerobic) cells, resistant to both chemotherapy and radiation. Such cells are selectively attacked by miso-nidazole, particularly if irradiated. This drug, 1-(2-nitroimidazol-1-yl)-3-methoxy-2-propanol, is undergoing clinical trials (Flockhart et al., 1978). Selective avoidance of other hypoxic tissues (e.g. nerves, skin, cartilage) is being monitored (Josephy, Palcic, and Skarsgard, 1978).

Several instances are known where enzymes performing similar functions in two species are chemically distinct. Examples of such 'analogous enzymes' are mentioned below under 'helminths', and several more will be found in Section 4.6. The following paragraphs summarize variations of glycolysis in invertebrates.

Insect muscle utilizes the Meyerhof sequence only as far as pyruvate, and the NADH produced during triosephosphate oxidation seems to be reoxidized by the reduction of dihydroxyacetone phosphate to glycero-phosphate (Chance and Sacktor, 1958). The major sugar in the plasma is α,α-trehalose, a disaccharide of glucose, and it plays a major part in the glucose transport system of insects (Wyatt and Kalf, 1957). For a review of insect biochemistry, see Goodwin (1965).

Helminths are characterized by a high rate of carbohydrate metabolism associated with incomplete substrate oxidation. This is the case whether they live anaerobically (as intestinal worms do) or aerobically (like schisto-somes). The Meyerhof sequence is the major metabolic pathway in worms for the utilization of carbohydrate. Trehalose (see above) plays an important part in helminth carbohydrate metabolism. For a review of helminth biochemistry, see von Brand (1974).

Kinetic studies of the lactic dehydrogenase of schistosome worms and of rabbit muscle showed a large rate difference (Mansour and Bueding, 1953), also the pH optimum for the schistosome enzyme was significantly lower. The dissociation constant for the enzyme-pyruvate complex was 6–12 times higher for the worm enzyme than for the mammalian. An even more strikingly different pair of analogous enzymes in these worms is displayed in Table 4.4. In short, the phosphofructokinase of schistosome worms (the enzyme which converts fructose-6-phosphate to the diphosphate) is much more sensitive to the inhibitory effect of antimonials than is mammalian phosphofructokinase. The therapeutic success of antimonials in treating bilharziasis depends on blocking this enzyme selectively (see Section 12.0 for more on antimonials). Because glycolysis is the main source of energy for the parasite, and this enzyme is a pacemaker (as defined in Section 2.2, p. 37), its substrate (fructose-6-phosphate) accumulates (Mansour and Bueding, 1954; Bueding and Fisher, 1966).

Table 4.4

PERCENTAGE INHIBITION OF PHOSPHOFRUCTOKINASE
ACTIVITY BY ANTIMONIALS

Concn. of antimonial M	Antimony potassium tartrate (12.5)		Stibophen (4.37)	
	(A) Enzyme from Schistosoma Mansoni	(B) Enzyme from rat brain	as (A)	as (B)
1×10^{-3}	100	32	100	0
5×10^{-4}	100	4	100	0
3×10^{-4}	100	0	85	0
1×10^{-4}	70	0	44	0
3×10^{-5}	32	0	0	0
1×10^{-5}	2	0	0	0

(Mansour and Bueding, 1954.)

Protozoa, in general, can utilize exogenous acids but not carbohydrates for energy. They lack hexokinase, and accumulate starch as an energy reserve. However, the bloodstream form of African trypanosomes are completely dependent on glycolysis (of the host's glucose) for their energy supply. They excrete pyruvic acid into the host's blood-stream because they lack both lactic dehydrogenase and the citric acid cycle. The NAD which they produce is reoxidized by a cyanide-insensitive glycerol-3-phosphate oxidase that is not present in the vertebrate host. If this enzyme is blocked, glycerol accumulates from the enforced anaerobic pathway. Following up this clue, it was found that an injection of salicylhydroxamic acid (to block glycerol-3-phosphate oxidase) with glycerol (for its mass-action effect) could destroy all trypanosomes (*T. brucei*) in the mammalian host (rat) in a few minutes (Clarkson and Brohn, 1976). It is hoped that this will lead to a new clinical treatment for trypanosomiasis.

The schizont stage of the malarial parasite utilizes the Mayerhof sequence efficiently to convert glucose to lactic acid. In *Entamoeba histolytica*, the major pathway of glucose utilization is the formation of pyruvate from phosphogluconate and from 2-keto-3-deoxy-6-phosphogluconate (Florkin and Mason, 1960).

Plants follow the Meyerhof pattern, but no less than three different glyceraldehyde-3-phosphate dehydrogenases exist: one reacts with NAD, two with NADP, processes linked to photosynthesis. In older plant tissues, the pentose phosphate pathway is also utilized and up to 50 per cent of all carbohydrate may be metabolized by this route.

Bacteria often use the Meyerhof sequence, but at least two alternative pathways have been found. In one of these (the pentose phosphate pathway) glucose-6-phosphate is oxidized to ribulose-5-phosphate, two molecules of which are quickly changed to one molecule each of glyceraldehyde-3-phosphate and sedoheptulose-7-phosphate. These phosphates then yield fructose-6-phosphate and a tetrose phosphate. In the other (the 2-keto-3-deoxy-6-phosphogluconate pathway), glucose is oxidized to gluconate by a primitive route without prior phosphorylation. The non-Meyerhof routes are favoured by those bacteria, such as the pseudomonads and aerobacters, which cannot utilize glucose-6-phosphate.

When nutrients are present in excess, many bacteria accumulate special energy reserves such as glycogen or β-hydroxybutyric acid (Wilkinson, 1966). Yeasts, and some bacteria, convert pyruvic acid to ethanol (instead of lactic acid), an idiosyncrasy which man has carefully exploited.

CH$_2$O·OC·R
|
R'·CO·OCH
| O
CH$_2$O·PO·CH$_2$CH$_2$·N$^+$Me$_3$
|
O$^-$

Phosphatidylcholine (lecithin)
(*4.38*)

HO
HO   HO
HO   3   1   O·PO$_3$H$_2$
OH   2

OH

Myoinositol phosphate
(*4.39*)

Lipid metabolism. Lipids are divided broadly into fats (triglycerides, esters of glycerol with three moles of fatty acids), sterols, and phospholipids such as phosphatidylcholine (lecithin) (*4.38*). All natural phospholipids have the L-3-glycerophosphoric structure. Each phospholipid is a family rather than a pure substance. The 2-position of lecithin is usually esterified by an unsaturated, and the 1-position by a saturated, fatty acid of the C$_{16}$ or C$_{18}$ series. Double unsaturation in the 2-position is common (esterification by linoleic acid). Phosphatidylethanolamine and phosphatidylserine (both found in the 'cephalin' of brain) are variations on the lecithin structure. Inositol phosphates, e.g. (*4.39*), occur in fungi, higher plants and animals. About 35 per cent of the phospholipids of mammalian brain and nerves is in the form of plasmalogens; these resemble phosphatidylethanolamine, but the 1-chain is not an ester but an α,β-unsaturated ester, a structure which yields an aldehyde on hydrolysis. Many bacteria have phospholipids which are esterified by aminoacids (CO of acid to OH of glycerol) (Macfarlane, 1962). Branched chains and the cyclopropane ring are often found in the fatty side-chains of bacterial phospholipids.

Phospholipids in mammals are synthesized (from smaller molecules supplied by the blood-stream) mainly in the tissues which use them, and they are broken down by a series of phospholipases secreted by the pancreas and gut. Flatworms cannot synthesize the fatty acids required to make their triglycerides and phospholipids, but they can alter their host's lipids to suit their requirements. Cholesterol, their only sterol, comes directly from the host (Meyer *et al.*, 1970). For further reading on phospholipids, see Schettler (1973); and Slotboom and Bonsen (1970).

In the oxidation of fats, the classical β-oxidation to acetyl coenzyme A occurs in the mitochondria of all kinds of cells. Some cells have one or two subsidiary mechanisms as well. Because the metabolism of fat produces twice as much water as that of either carbohydrate or protein, cells which have to encounter sudden dehydrating conditions usually have a high fat metabolism. Parasitic nematode worms are a striking example of this (Baldwin, 1948b).

4.4 The tricarboxylic acid cycle, and electron transport

After the glycolysis of carbohydrates and the β-oxidation of fats has taken place, the greater part of the energy of these nutrients still remains to be liberated, but only well-aerated cells can do this. These aerobic cells utilize acetyl coenzyme A for this purpose. They obtain it not only from lipid metabolism but from the pyruvic acid which is the final product of glycolysis if conditions are aerobic. This acetyl coenzyme A is utilized as fuel by being passed through the tricarboxylic acid cycle (synonyms: citric acid cycle, Krebs cycle), which converts it to carbon dioxide, water, and energy (see Fig. 4.4). Bacteria convert the pyruvic acid to acetyl coenzyme A through acetyl phosphate, whereas vertebrate animals use adenyl acetate as the intermediate and a different set of enzymes.

Contrary to what was formerly believed, all bacteria and yeasts use the tricarboxylic acid cycle as the major pathway for terminal oxidation. A small shunt in the cycle is made by some bacteria (e.g. *E. coli* and *Pseudomonas aeruginosa*) and fungi (e.g. *Aspergillus* and yeasts) as follows. Isocitrate is dismutated to succinate and glyoxylate; the latter is then dimerized to malate which, like succinate, is a normal constituent of the cycle. The blood-stream form of many parasitic trypanosomes, which lack mitochondria, have no tricarboxylic acid cycle (Grant and Fulton, 1957).

The operation of the cycle produces large quantities of the reduced forms of the nucleotides of adenine with nicotinamide (NAD and NADP) and riboflavine (FP). The regeneration of these coenzymes is effected

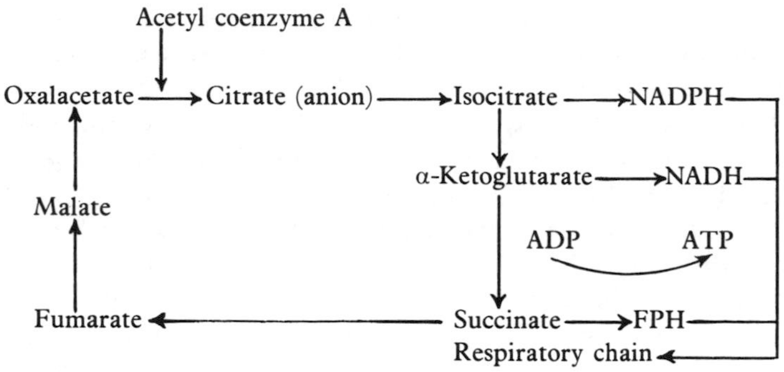

Acetyl coenzyme A

Oxalacetate ——→ Citrate (anion) ——→ Isocitrate ——→ NADPH—

α-Ketoglutarate ——→ NADH—

Malate   ADP   ATP

Fumarate ←——————— Succinate ——→ FPH—
                                  Respiratory chain ←

Overall: $(CH_3CO) + 2O_2 \longrightarrow 2CO_2 + 2H_2O + energy$

FIG. 4.4 The tricarboxylic acid cycle (abridged)

by a transfer of electrons from the reduced forms to the oxygen of the atmosphere. In almost every kind of living cell, this transfer is mediated by some or all of the cytochrome respiratory chain (Section 5.3). Most of the organisms that lack all cytochromes have insignificant aerobic metabolism. Few enzymatic differences in the cycle have been demonstrated in mammals, but in the rat there is six times more aconitate hydratase in the heart than in skeletal muscle (Dixon and Webb, 1964).

Inhibitors of the respiratory chain. This chain terminates in cytochrome oxidase for which the cyanide ion is a powerful and specific inhibitor. Antimycin A, obtained from a *Streptomyces*, specifically inhibits the chain between cytochromes-b and -c_1. Its iron-chelating properties are mentioned under salicylic acid in Section 11.9.

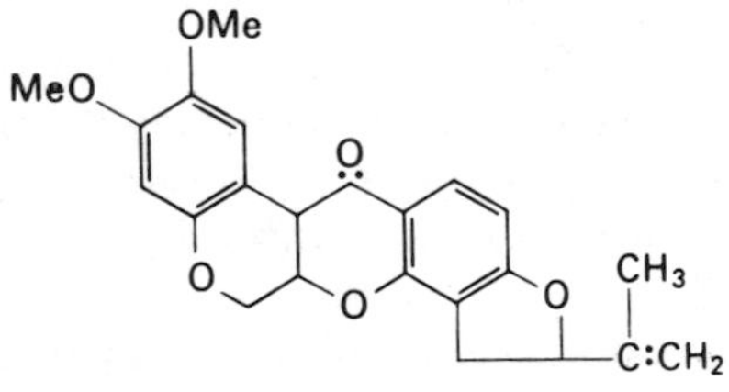

OMe

MeO

CH₃

$C:CH_2$

Rotenone
(4.40)

Rotenone (4.40), an insecticide of vegetable origin, blocks the dehydrogenation of NADH in the respiratory chain, at a dilution of 10^{-8} M, by displacing ubiquinone from NADH dehydrogenase (Gutman *et al.*, 1971). It thus prevents the oxidation of pyruvate and glutamate (but not succinate). Fish, but not mammals, are highly susceptible to rotenone: mammals are selectively protected by rapid metabolic oxidation, but their *isolated* mitochondria are very susceptible (Ernster *et al.*, 1963). For a review on rotenone, see Yamamoto (1970).

Good selectivity is shown by a soil fungicide, sodium *p*-dimethyl-aminobenzenediazosulphonate ('Dexon'), which inhibits mitochondrial oxidation of NADH in the fungus *Pythium ultimum*. Sugar beets, which this fungus infects, have an enzyme in the mitochondria which decomposes this fungicide (Tolmsoff, 1962).

Many simpler molecules can uncouple oxidation from phosphorylation, so that the energy obtained by the combustion of nutrients ceases to be stored as ATP. Three classes of uncoupling agents are recognized: liposoluble weak acids, alkylating agents, and liposoluble strong bases (Skulachev *et al.*, 1969). Phenols and other weak acids, by far the most numerous of the uncouplers, act by transporting hydrogen ions across the inner mitochondrial membrane until its resting potential is discharged (Hemker, 1962; Stockdale and Selwyn, 1971; Scherrer and Howard, 1977). Artificial membranes made from mitochondrial lipoprotein similarly lose their potential (Büchel and Schäfer, 1970; Skulachev, *et al.*, 1969). The following examples of the selective use of uncoupling agents could be supplemented by the antifungal substances in Section 10.5, especially 2,4-dinitrophenol, a well-known uncoupler.

The point of attack of trialkyltin salts (R_3Sn^+), which are highly active fungicides, is believed to lie in the oxidative phosphorylation of mitochondria (Aldridge, 1958). The tributyl homologue is the most used because it is the least toxic for mammals (Barnes and Stoner, 1958).

Because many anti-inflammatory drugs, such as salicylates, are strong uncouplers of oxidative phosphorylation in the mitochondria, it had been thought that the anti-inflammatory action might be the result of such uncoupling (Smith and Smith, 1966). However 2,4-dinitrophenol, a strong uncoupler, is not anti-inflammatory, and the anti-inflammatory action of salicylates is an anti-prostaglandin effect (see Section 4.7).

The terminal respiratory systems of some bacteria (Dolin, 1961), protozoa (trypanosomes) (Grant, Sargent and Ryley, 1961), and helminths (*Ascaris*) (Kmetec and Bueding, 1961) are insensitive to concentrations of cyanides and antimycin A that are lethal to mammalian cells. It is evident that they can dispense with the whole respiratory chain after cytochrome-b. However, they are particularly sensitive to vitamin K analogues, e.g. 2-hydroxy-3-2′-methyloctyl-1,4-naphthoquinone.

4.5 Photosynthesis

All green plants and a very few bacteria (non-pathogens) can utilize sunlight to split water into hydrogen and oxygen. The plant releases this oxygen to the atmosphere, thus helping to reconstitute the air that we breathe. More important for the plant's nutrition is its ability to combine the hydrogen with carbon dioxide from the air to produce carbohydrates, proteins, and even fats, by an exceedingly complex cycle of reactions. Photosynthesis commences with the absorption of visible light by quantasomes (aggregates of about 200 molecules of chlorophyll) in the chloroplasts described in Section 5.3. This brings about the photolysis of water, which provides hydrogen radicals for reductive processes and electrons for replenishment of the chlorophyll. This part of the process is called the Hill reaction.

At the same time the light-excited chlorophyll molecules reduce the ferredoxin in the chloroplast to an unusually low potential (about -400 mV). This electron-transfer from water is used to reduce NADP and to phosphorylate ADP to ATP. These co-factors then carry the sun's energy to an elaborate synthetic cycle, in which ribulose and sedoheptulose are important intermediates, and most paths lead to glyceraldehyde-3-phosphate (and hence to starch or pyruvic acid). For further reading on photosynthesis, see Rabinowitch and Govindjee (1969). In the red algae (and the 'blue-green algae' now classified with bacteria) the primary absorbers of light are not chlorophyll but phyco-erythrin and -cyanin (respectively). These pyrrole pigments seem to be the evolutionary precursors of phytochrome (see Section 4.6).

Herbicides. In recent years, many herbicides have been found that attack only the Hill reaction and hence are harmless to all animals. The most used of these herbicides are triazines such as simazine (*4.41*), which is non-toxic to mammals, no matter how great the dose. The action of the triazines can be demonstrated on isolated chloroplasts at the same concentration (10^{-7}M) at which the substances exhibit herbicidal action. Cereal crops absorb simazine, but detoxify it by hydrolysing the chloro-substituent to a hydroxy-group (Exer, 1958; Gysin, 1962). One of the largest uses of simazine is to kill weeds in maize crops. Although most vegetables are adversely affected by the triazine herbicides, the berry fruits are resistant, also rose bushes and garden shrubs; it has now become a common sight to see plants chemically weeded by triazines. These herbicides (also monuron, see below) are not destroyed by bacteria but remain in the soil for many years.

Simazine
(2-chloro-4,6-*bis*ethylamino-
1,3,5-triazine)
(*4.41*)

Diuron
(3,4-dichlorophenyl-dimethylurea)
(*4.42*)

3,4-Dichlorophenyl-2'-
methylbutyramide
(4.43)

Other much-used herbicides which depend on inhibition of the Hill reaction are phenylureas, acylanilides, and uracils such as bromacil. The most potent member of the urea family is diuron, 3-(3,4-dichlorophenyl)-1,1-dimethylurea (4.42), but monuron (the earlier and slightly less active 4-monochloro analogue) is still in use. The most potent amide is 3,4-dichlorophenyl-2-methyl-pentanamide (4.43). For activity, these substances require a free imino-group, a carbonyl-group, a side-chain of rather critical length, and 4- (Preferably 3,4-) substitution in the benzene ring. The best substituents are halogens, or methoxy- or methyl-groups (Good, 1961).

The bipyridylium herbicides, used as a substitute for ploughing in erosion-prone country, are transformed to stable free radicals in the process of exerting their herbicidal action. They are contact herbicides, and because they are not appreciably translocated, weeding with them produces a razor-sharp boundary. The most potent of these is paraquat (4.44), 1,1'-dimethyl-4-,4'-bipyridylium cation (used as the dichloride). This substance has long been in use in another connection, namely as an indicator for low reduction potentials. This colourless substance, known as methyl viologen, functions by forming a violet-coloured stable free radical (4.45) when the potential falls to -446 mV (Michaelis and Hill, 1933).

It was quickly noted that the 3,3'-bipyridyl analogue of paraquat was not herbicidal; what was needed was a structure that permitted formation and stabilization of a free radical upon reduction. Stabilization requires a coplanar molecule, so that in (4.45) the unpaired electron (shown as a large dot) can exchange rings with the positive charge and so obtain stabilization by the resonance of similar canonical forms (Brian, 1965).

It was next found that substances with too low a reduction potential formed too little of the free radical form in the plant; and when the results were recalculated on the basis of the amount of free radical formed, all members of the series were equitoxic (Homer, Mees and Tomlinson, 1960). High herbicidal activity is confined to analogues with E_0 between -300 and -500 mV. This makes it likely that they are reduced to free radicals by ferredoxin.

After application of these herbicides, rapid uptake into the chloroplast

$$\text{MeN}^{+}\text{—}\langle\text{—}\rangle\text{—}\langle\text{—}\rangle\text{—}\text{N}^{+}\text{Me} \quad \overset{+\epsilon}{\rightleftharpoons} \quad \text{MeN}\text{—}\langle\text{—}\rangle\text{·}\langle\text{—}\rangle\text{—}\text{N}^{+}\text{Me}$$

Paraquat (cation)   (4.45)
(4.44)

$$\text{H}_2\text{N}\text{—}\langle\overset{\text{N}}{\underset{\text{N}—\text{N}}{}}\rangle$$
                         H

3-Aminotriazole
(4.46)

follows, and death occurs when the ratio of one molecule of paraquat to 100 molecules of chlorophyll is reached (Baldwin, Clarke and Wilson, 1968). Plants kept in the dark are unaffected by this concentration, but they rapidly die when light is admitted. Also there is no injury if oxygen is excluded or the amount of chlorophyll is deficient.

The bipyridyl free radicals are not a direct cause of death, but just a stage in a rapid cycle of reduction and re-oxidation. In the course of this cycle much hydrogen peroxide is formed, and some superoxide free radical (O_2-), which is considered to be the true toxic agent (Davenport, 1963; Fridovich, 1975). When monuron (see above) is used to inhibit photosynthesis, diquat loses most of its effect (Mees, 1960). Although paraquat is completely safe in normal usage, large oral doses cause fibrosis of the lungs, and death may follow.

3-amino-1,2,4-triazole (4.46) (amitrole) is a selective herbicide that acts by inhibiting the synthesis of chlorophyll (see also Section 9.4).

4.6 Analogous enzymes. Coenzymes

Enzymes. Many examples are known where the enzymes carrying out apparently identical catabolic functions in two dissimilar genera are themselves dissimilar. These are known as analogous enzymes (sometimes, as homologous enzymes). This has been demonstrated in many ways: by differences in immunology, kinetics, electrophoresis, or specificity (of coenzymes, substrates, or inhibitors). Examples of analogous enzymes are being found even for *cata*bolic steps in metabolism which are often assumed to be identical in almost all forms of life. In carbohydrate catabolism, it is quite usual for analogous enzymes to be immunologically distinct. For example, crystalline glyceraldehyde-3-phosphate dehydrogenase of yeast is immunologically distinct from that of rabbit muscle (Krebs and Najjar, 1948). Even different organs in the one species can show this effect; thus, the phosphorylase of dog heart is serologically different from that of dog liver.

Some chemical differences exist between analogous enzymes. Numerous hexokinases have a high specificity for a single hexose, whereas others catalyse the phosphorylation of several carbohydrates. Differences in requirements for coenzymes, particularly metals, can be found. Thus, crystalline aldolases from yeasts and moulds require iron (Warburg and Christian, 1943), and so does that from the bacterium *Clostridium perfringens* (Bard and Gunsalus, 1950), whereas those from mammals, plants, and trypanosomes do not (Taylor, Green and Cori, 1948). Again, the enzyme superoxide-dismutase occurs as a copper + zinc requiring form in eukaryotes, whereas in prokaryotes it needs either manganese or iron to function (Lumsden and Hall, 1975). There are two distinct classes of the enzymes known as FDP (fructose-1,6-diphosphate) aldolases, which carry out an important and early stage in glycolysis: (a), the varieties found in animals and higher plants cleave FDP by way of a Schiff base, whereas (b), those which occur in bacteria and fungi require a metal (usually Zn^{2+}) bound to the carbonyl group in the enzyme-substrate complex; special inhibitors exist for the second variety (Lewis and Lowe, 1973). More examples of differing metal requirements will be found in Section 11.1: see under *Helminths* in Section 4.3 for some other differences in analogous enzymes. Table 4.4 clearly shows how antimonial drugs can distinguish between a pair of analogous enzymes, one in a parasitic worm, the other in its mammalian host. This is the selectively toxic basis of the classical treatment of schistosomiasis.

The ability of various diaminopyrimidines to distinguish between analogous forms of the enzyme dihydrofolate hydrogenase is the basis of some of the best contemporary antimalarial and antibacterial therapy (see Section 4.0, p.108, Tables 4.2 and 4.3, and Section 9.3c and 9.5). A new form of treating leprosy has been proposed depending on the ease of inhibiting tyrosinase in *Mycobacterium leprae* with sodium diethyl-dithiocarbamate, cf. (*2.24*), whereas the host's enzyme withstands this drug (Prabhakaran, 1973). The acetylcholinesterase in the worm *Haemonchus contortus*, which parasitizes the sheep's gut, is irreversibly inhibited by the organophosphorus drug, haloxon (*12.25*), a much-used vermifuge. Yet the acetylcholinesterase of the sheep's gut is only temporarily affected and rapidly recovers. Worms not affected by haloxon have been shown not to have this *Haemonchus* variant of the enzyme (Lee and Hodsden, 1963). Pure glutamate dehydrogenase from *Trypanosoma cruzi* has a structure very different from that of the mammalian enzyme (Juan *et al.*, 1978).

Parallel enzymes in two mammalian species can be analogous instead of (as expected) identical. For instance, rabbit muscle adenylate kinase is inactivated by 0.8 mM N^6-iodoacetamidohexyl-adenosine-5′-phosphate, whereas the corresponding enzyme in pig muscle was quite unaffected even by a 2.8 mM solution (Hampton, 1976).

Table 4.5

PROPORTIONS OF ENZYMES
IN MUSCLE
(RAT)

	Heart	Skeletal
Aconitase	6	1
Aldolase	1	16

Apart from such inter-species differences, many differences have been found in the proportions of enzymes in the different tissues of a *single organism*. Thus aconitase and oxaloacetate transacetase are much more abundant in heart than in skeletal muscle, but the reverse is true of aldolase (Dixon and Webb, 1964; cf. Table 4.5). Similarly, in mouse tumour cells (Ehrlich ascites), the specific activity of purine phosphoribosyltransferase was found to be between 15 and 60 times the activity of that in liver, brain, spleen, heart, or kidneys of the same animal (Murray, 1966).

The following three characteristic mammalian liver and kidney enzymes are absent from muscle: catalase, xanthine oxidase, and D-amino oxidase. The distribution of many other enzymes in mammals is limited to particular organs. Thus arginase occurs only in the liver, alkaline phosphatase in the intestinal mucosa, acid phosphatase in kidney, spleen, and prostate, 5-nucleotidase in the testis, and α-mannosidase in the epididymis (see Table 4.6). The blood is disproportionately rich in carbonic anhydrase, and the pancreas in ribonuclease. Glutamine synthetase, which condenses

Table 4.6

ENZYMES THAT OCCUR MAINLY IN SPECIAL ORGANS
OF MAMMALS

Enzyme	Organ	Enzyme	Organ
Arginase	liver	α-Mannosidase	epididymis
Alkaline phosphatase	intestines	Carbonic anhydrase	blood
	⎧ kidney	Ribonuclease	pancreas
Acid phosphatase	⎨ spleen	Glutamine synthetase	⎧ brain
	⎩ prostate		⎩ liver
5-Nucleotidase	testis		

(Dixon and Webb, 1964.)

glutamic acid with ammonia, is abundant in brain and liver, but almost absent from all other human tissues (Dixon and Webb, 1964). Thus the more specialized the mammalian tissue, the more individual its enzymes.

The organ-specific character of so many enzymes suggests possibilities for devising selective pro-drugs, masked with a group that the target tissue can specifically remove. An example is fosfestrol USP (diethyl-stilboestrol diphosphate), which remains biologically inert until hydrolysed by the acid phosphatase which is abundantly present in the prostate gland when carcinoma is present there. The liberated diethylstilboestrol brings about regression of the growth and this treatment is considered life-saving (Lambley and Ware, 1967).

An enzyme that is present in two communicating tissues may be active in only one of them because of a difference in pH. For example, the pH of cancer cells, provided glucose is available, tends to be lower (often pH 6) than that of the surrounding healthy cells (pH 7.3) (Rauen, 1964; Schloerb et al., 1965). As a result of this difference, the enzyme β-glucuronidase (which has a pH optimum of 5.2) is much more active in tumours than in normal cells (Bicker, 1974). The glucuronide of 8-hydroxyquinoline, cf. (3.7), injected into the peritoneum of a sarcoma-bearing rat, remained as such in the healthy muscle cells, but was hydrolysed to 8-hydroxyquinoline in the tumour. Bicker suggested that glucuronides of cytostatic phenols and amines could be highly selective in cancer therapy.

A different kind of enzymatic individuality in cancer cells is shown by three liver tumours (from mouse, rat, and human) which had lost feedback control of cholesterol synthesis while the surrounding healthy liver tissue was exercising normal restraint on this synthesis. The site of this failure of control was traced to HMG-reductase, the enzyme that converts β-hydroxy-β-methylglutaric acid to mevalonic acid, on the way to squalene (Siperstein and Fagan, 1964).

For more information on enzymes, see Section 8.0.

Coenzymes.   Many remarkable species differences have been found among the coenzymes. Most plants and animals synthesize their own ascorbic acid which is (among other tasks) essential for the hydroxylation of proline and lysine in the biosynthesis of collagen. However, man, other primates, and the guinea pig are notable exceptions, so that for them, and for them alone, it is a vitamin, and must be taken in with food.

Differences between bacteria and man in the absorption and the biosynthesis of dihydrofolic acid (2.14) and its derivatives are so great that the whole system of sulphonamide chemotherapy rests on it (Section 9.3a). In brief, pathogenic bacteria can synthesize their requirements of folic acid, but cannot absorb preformed folic acid in their nutriment. Man, on the other hand, cannot synthesize this coenzyme, but has no difficulty in absorbing it from food.

Tumour cells (ascites hepatoma) of the rat liver can take up (i) pyridoxine phosphate and (ii) pyridoxal phosphate without eliminating the phosphate group, but the liver cells of normal rats always completely dephosphorylate these forms of vitamin B_6 (Ito, Nakahara, and Sakamoto, 1964).

Early work on members of the cytochrome family established that the pattern of distribution varied more widely among bacteria than among eukaryotes. The extreme position is occupied by the anaerobic genus *Clostridium*, members of which have no cytochromes whatsoever (Keilin, 1933). The parasitic worms *Ascaris lumbricoides* var. *suum* (a nematode) and *Moniezia expansa* (a cestode) lack cytochrome P-450. This suggests that helminthicidal drugs can be designed which will persist in these parasites but be destroyed by the P-450 linked oxidases of their hosts (Douch, 1976).

The sideramines, iron-containing substances found only in bacteria, and thought to be bacterial equivalents of the cytochromes, are dealt with in Section 11.1, along with the ferredoxins, non-haem iron-containing proteins confined to bacteria and plants.

In plants, many aspects of morphogenesis are regulated by light, e.g. control of budding and flowering, leaf and stem expansion, seed germination, and the biosynthesis of many pigments. The chief mediator of these changes are the phytochromes, blue metal-free complexes of a tetra-pyrrolemethine (similar to a bile pigment in structure) with proteins. Confined to green plants, phytochromes absorbs at 660 nm, but the red rays of sunlight transform them to another active form absorbing at 730 nm. Located in semipermeable membranes, the phytochromes are thought to react to illumination by regulating membrane potential (Roux and Yguerabide, 1973). Like everything else that has specialized biochemistry, they offer the opportunity for selectively toxic interference.

4.7 Hormones and pheromones

Animal hormones. It is known that vetebrate hormones influence invertebrates, and vice versa. Substance that show the pharmacological action of adrenaline on the frog's heart have been extracted from protozoa, annelid worms, molluscs, and arthropods (cf. Wense, 1939). Conversely, pure adrenaline causes increased muscle-tone in annelida, molluscs, and arthropods. Again, substances with oestrogenic action on vertebrates have been extracted from protozoa, coelenterates, annelid worms, molluscs, and echinoderms (Steidle, 1930). It seems to be Nature's way, to use chemicals already present in the environment (arising by degradation of nutrients, for example) as messengers that become more and more specialized as the evolutionary tree is ascended. Thus glycine has no hormonal function in plants, and may have none in worms, but in Man it is an important transmitter in the central nervous system. *Schistosoma mansoni* adults contain a high concentration of 5-hydroxytryptamine which they use as a neuro-transmitter after obtaining it from their hosts (Bennett and Bueding, 1973).

Currently, much interest is being taken in selective possibilities of the prostaglandins, a family of secondary messengers discovered by von Euler in 1934. They have since been found to be widespread in Nature, and in mammals their task is usually to translate a flux of a hormone or neuro-transmitter into the appropriate physiological result. Their action, which can be violent, is usually short-lived; specific dehydrogenases exist to degrade them rapidly after release. Some are stimulant, even irritant, whereas others have healing properties.

The starting point of their biosynthesis is linoleic acid, an essential dietary constituent for man. This is converted, through arachidonic acid (a 20-carbon aliphatic acid with four double bonds) to a partly cyclic structure, the endoperoxide (4.47). From this key intermediate, the working prostaglandins are formed by simple chemical changes, for instance, pro-staglandin E_2 (4.48) arises by simple isomerization. Until required, the prostaglandins are stored as phospholipoid derivatives. The E series is distinguished by a hydroxyl-group at C-11 and an oxo-group at C-9; the F series has two hydroxyl-groups, at C-9 and C-11, and both series have in addition a hydroxyl-group on C-15. The subscript '2' signifies an extra double-bond, between C-5 and C-6. The prostaglandins are thought to exert their action on lipoid membranes.

Endoperoxide PGG$_2$
(4.47)

Prostaglandin E$_2$
(4.48)

The only prostaglandins yet used clinically are E_2 (for inducing labour) and F_2 (for terminating pregnancy). Their specificity is not high and use is accompanied by violent spasms in various organs of the body. Research is in hand to discover analogues with increased specificity and longer life. It has been found that by the substitution of a methyl-group into the 15-position, the allylic hydroxy-group in that position is protected from the destructive enzyme 15-hydroxyprostaglandin dehydrogenase. It is hoped to obtain use-ful analogues for treating asthma, gastric ulcer, and thrombosis.

Prostaglandins E_1, E_2, and apparently F, cause erythrema, oedema, and pain and, in addition, they sensitize pain receptors to other hyperalgesic substances such as histamine, bradykinin, and SRS (slowly reacting sub-stance) (Collier, 1971, Ferreira and Vane, 1974). The anti-inflammatory action of aspirin, which is still the most used drug for the treatment of arthritis and rheumatism, is due to its inhibition of the biosynthesis of

PGE_2 (4.48) (Vane, 1971; Roth, Standord and Majerus, 1975). This inhibition takes place at a concentration far below that which causes uncoupling of phosphorylation. Other non-steroidal, anti-inflammatory drugs act similarly, e.g. indomethacin, ibuprofen, and mefenamic acid (Ferreira and Vane, 1974). The site of action seems to be 'prostaglandin synthetase' a complex of enzymes which converts arachidonic acid, in several stages, to the endoperoxide (4.47) (Flower, Cheung, and Cushman, 1973; Flower, 1974). The action of these inhibitors is irreversible. The influence of ionization on activity in these drugs is mentioned in Section 10.3f. For the mode of action of aspirin, see Section 12.5.

The corticosteroids inhibit the synthesis of prostaglandins by a different, though unknown, mechanism (Tashjian et al., 1975).

Insect hormones.   In insects a high degree of control of physiological action is exerted by insect-specific hormones. These are being studied with two goals of interest for selective toxicity. One goal is to learn the nature of the hormones, to synthesize them inexpensively, and then to apply them in excessive amounts to confuse insect metabolism. The other goal is to synthesize antagonistic analogues (see Section 9.1) for use as insecticides.

The main types of insect-specific hormone are: α-ecdysone, from the prothoracic glands, which causes moulting; the brain hormone that stimulates the prothoracic glands; and the juvenile hormone, in the corpora allata, which causes metamorphosis. Further, the corpus cardiacum releases a hormone that increases the amplitude of the muscles of heart and gut (Davey, 1964), and also an adipokinetic hormone which regulates the use of lipids as a source of energy in flight (Stone et al., 1976).

Ecdysone (4.49) has the following features not found in mammalian steroid hormones: rings A and B are *cis*-fused, there is a hydrophilic substituent at C-2, the α-edge (which runs from C-3 to C-15) has hydrophilic substituents, and the side-chain on C-17 is very long (see Section 13.2 for more on steroids). The keto-group at C-6 is essential for action. This hormone was synthesized by Siddall, Cross and Fried (1966). Crustecdysone, the moulting hormone of crustacea (also present in some insects), is 20-hydroxyecdysone. Members of the ecdysone family can be prepared in quantity from plant products; but although many ecydsone analogues are insecticidal when injected, they are not absorbed through the insect cuticle and no practical use has yet been found. Because insects cannot synthesize this, or any other steroid, they have to absorb steroid intermediates from the diet (Lasser, 1966), a good point for selective attack.

Juvenile hormone (4.50) is a simple aliphatic substance: methyl 10-epoxy-7-ethyl-3, 11-dimethyl-2, 6-tridecadienoate in which both double bonds are *trans* (Röller et al., 1967). Activity is largely determined by the configuration at the C-1 end of the molecule.

Most of the active mimics have a terminal ester group that is conjugated with a double-bond held *trans* to a long alkyl chain. A typical mimic is

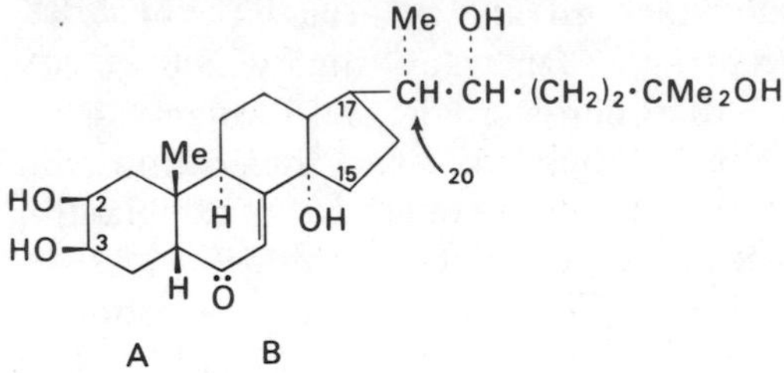

α-Ecdysone
(4.49)

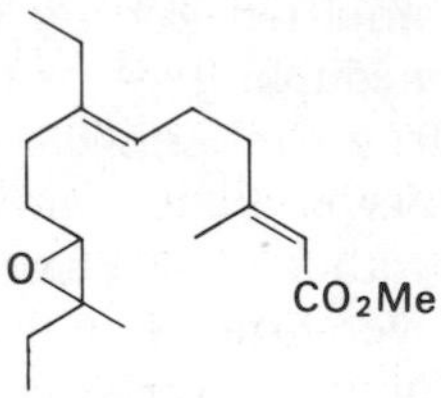

Juvenile hormone
(4.50)

methoprene ('Altosid') which is isopropyl (2E, 4E)-11-methoxy-3, 7, 11-trimethyl-2, 4-dodecadienoate. This has given good results in tests for floodwater mosquito control, when incorporated into slow-release polyamide micro-spheres. It is also successful in eliminating the manure-breeding flies that bother cattle and egg-laying hens; these animals are induced to swallow it in their feed. Methoprene has little toxicity to man, birds or fish, and it is active against resistant strains. For more on juvenile hormones see Section 6.4, also Gilbert (1976). The main problem with juvenile hormone *agonists* is that they keep the insect in the larval stage, where it usually does the most harm. Hence these mimics are most used against those few categories of insect, such as mosquitos and flies, where the adults do the most harm.

Juvenile hormone *antagonists* look more promising. The first of these were the precocenes, e.g. (4.51), chromanes occurring in the garden plant *Ageratum*. Even in low concentrations, they cause precocious moulting to give a sterile adult (Bowers *et al.*, 1976). Their site of action is the gland which synthesizes juvenile hormone.

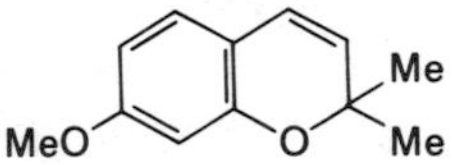

Precocene I
(4.51)

For an account of the physiology of insect hormones, see Novak (1966), and for insect biochemistry, see Goodwin (1965).

Insect pheromones, which serve to convey messages between insects, have been isolated from many species and found to be both highly specific, and effective in mere traces. They are usually aliphatic compounds, such as the termites' trail-following substance, dodecatrien-1-ol, but that secreted by the town ant is methyl 4-methylpyrrole-2-carboxylate.

Other, sex-attractant, pheromones are secreted by the female. That from the silkworm moth is hexadeca-10-*trans*-12-*cis*-dien-1-ol, that from the gipsy moth (*Porthetria dispar*) is *cis*-7,8-epoxy-2-methyloctadecane; and the attractant released by the female bollworm moth is 10-propyl-5, 9-tridecadienol. Field trials, where they are used as lures to poisoned bait, have shown promise, but they are not yet in general use. For further reading on insect sex pheromones, see Jacobson (1972).

The slow maturation of desert locusts (males) is accelerated when they are crowded together, which suggests that a volatile stimulant is emitted.

The 'queen substance', which inhibits conversion of larvae to queens, and is secreted by the mandibular gland in the queen bee's head, is 9-oxodec-*trans*-2-enoic acid:

$$CH_3CO(CH_2)_5CH:CH \cdot CO_2H$$

The oriental hornet, *Vespa orientalis*, uses δ-hexadecalactone to promote the production of queens.

Plant pheromones and hormones.   The ova of the common brown sea-weeds (*Fucus* spp.) release into sea water small amounts of *n*-hexane which attracts motile spermatazoa and so favours fertilization (Hlubucek *et al.*, 1970). Hexane is active at a dilution of 1 part in 10 million and exemplifies the principle that, no matter how commonplace a chemical may be, as soon as it gives an advantageous signal in a biological system, its specificity as a messenger can be perpetuated by natural selection. The female gametes of another marine brown alga *Ectocarpus siliculosus* produce a more complex sperm-attracting hydrocarbon, 1-*cyclo*heptadienylbutene (Müller *et al.*, 1971).

The fungus *Achlya* (male strain) secretes a hormone oogoniol which causes the female strain to form egg-bearing branches. This hormone is a steroid, with oxygen atoms attached to the 7- and 15-positions, (McMorris *et al.*, 1975).

Higher plants have numerous hormones which, being confined to the vegetable kingdom, offer us special opportunities for the exercise of selective toxicity. The most important of these hormones is usually considered to be indolyl-3-acetic acid (*4.52*), discovered in 1934. It, and some related substances, known collectively as 'auxins', bring about the lengthening of plant cells, the setting of fruit, and other expressions of growth. For stereochemical data on auxins, see Section 13.2.

The phenoxyacetic acids, which are cheaper to synthesize and have a more intense and prolonged action, are much used in agriculture to mimic the effect of the auxins. They were introduced (Zimmerman, 1942), and are still much used, for the rooting of cuttings, to prevent premature dropping of fruit, and to promote setting of fruit in the absence of pollination. When they were being used in high concentrations for this purpose, they were found to act as herbicides (Sexton, Slade, and Templeman, 1941;

Templeman and Sexton, 1946). At these higher concentrations, they are super-agonists, causing unrestrained growth which brings about death by exhaustion of reserves. This effect is highly selective, leading to the universal employment of phenoxyacetic acids for killing weeds in crops, and particularly in cereal crops.

The two most used herbicides in this class are 2-methyl-4-chlorophenoxyacetic acid (4.53) (MCPA or 'Methoxone'), and 2,4-dichlorophenoxyacetic acid (2,4-D, or 'Chloroxone'). The use of 2,4,5-trichlorophenoxyacetic acid has been suspended, because the usual process of manufacture contaminates it with a teratogenic dioxin (6.51). Tests carried out on 30 annual weeds that normally impoverish cereal crops showed that, by choosing the right compound and applying it at the right time, almost all the weeds can be killed. It is not known why cereals are relatively unaffected. In some experiments cereals were made to absorb as much of the phenoxyacetic acids as the weeds do (normally they absorb less), but the cereals remained unharmed (Wood, Wolfe and Irving, 1947). On the whole, dicotyledons are killed and monocotyledons survive, but there are striking exceptions. Thus onions (monocotyledons) are susceptible to the phenoxyacetic acids, whereas chickweed and cleavers (dicotyledons) are resistant because they have an enzyme that removes the side-chain.

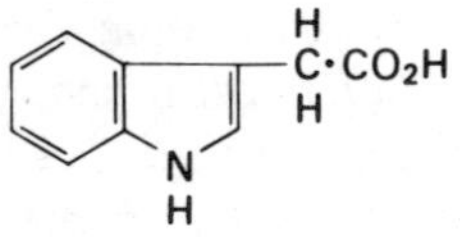

Indoleacetic acid
(4.52)

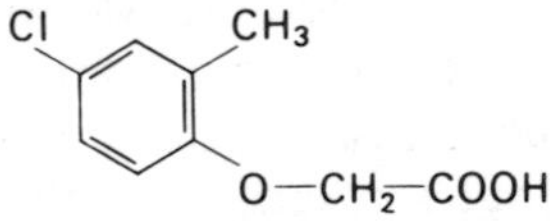

MCPA
(4.53)

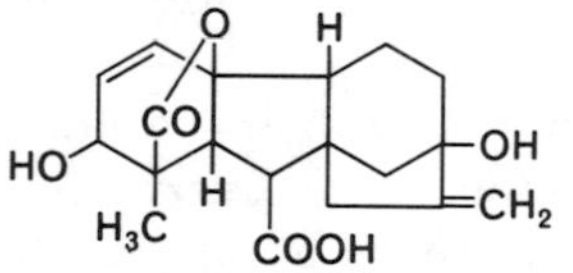

Gibberellic acid, GA$_3$
(4.54)

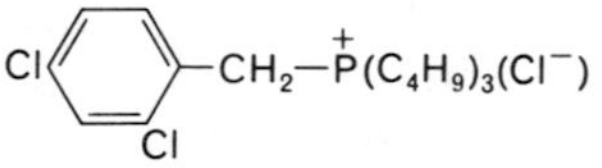

Phosphon-D
(4.55)

The gibberellins, e.g. (4.54) discovered in 1926, are a family of about 30 related diterpene acids which, like the auxins, are synthesized in the growing tips of plants. In nature, they work in conjunction with the auxins. In agriculture they are used to break the dormancy of seeds, delay the ripening of citrus fruits, increase the height of sugar cane (and hence increase yield per acre), and improve the malting properties of barley. They seem to function by inducing the biosynthesis of carbohydrate processing enzymes, such as amylase (Varner and Chandra, 1964).

Many simple synthetic compounds are used in agriculture to retard the action of gibberellins, for example chlormequat (2-chloroethyltrimethyl-ammonium chloride) which is used to dwarf cereal plants, N, N-dimethyl-aminosuccinamic acid, and phosphon D (4.55). These inhibit the bio-synthesis of gibberellic acid by fungi, and some of their effects on plants can be reversed by gibberellins (Lang, 1970; Cathey, 1964). These inhi-bitors are also used to coax fruit trees into a more compact growth, leading to a higher yield of fruit in a given area.

The process of cell division is managed by purine-based hormones known as 'kinins', which are formed in plant roots. Zeatin (4.56), isolated from maize (Letham, Shannon, and McDonald, 1964) is typical. Kinins are used to prolong the life of vegetables after harvesting.

Abscisins, e.g. (4.57), are sesquiterpenes widely distributed among plants and chemically related to vitamin A. They cause dormant phenomena such as the suspension of growth and the fall of leaves and fruit. The first of them was synthesized by Cornforth, Milborrow and Ryback (1965).

Ethylene is a very simple plant hormone, widespread in occurrence, which promotes or retards growth according to circumstances. It is much used in commerce to force the ripening of cold-stored fruit. For the use of chloroethanephosphonic acid, as a masked source of ethylene, see Section 3.5 (p. 94).

The related substance xanthoxin (4.58) clearly plays a fundamental part in normal plant regulation by antagonizing indoleacetic acid, gibberellic acid, and kinetin. It is readily oxidized to abscisic acid, of which it is prob-ably the natural precursor and with which it shares the *trans,trans* con-figuration (Taylor and Burden, 1972).

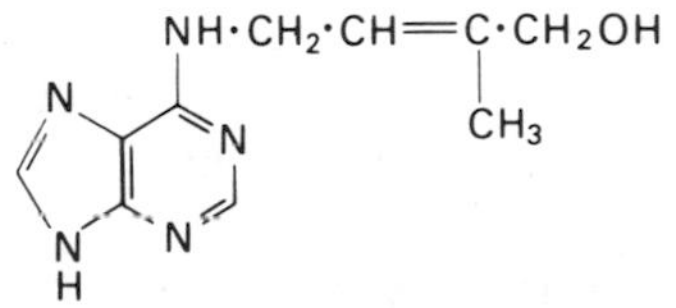

Zeatin
(4.56)

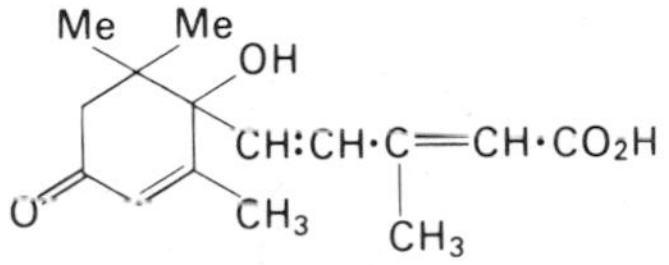

Abscisin II
(4.57)

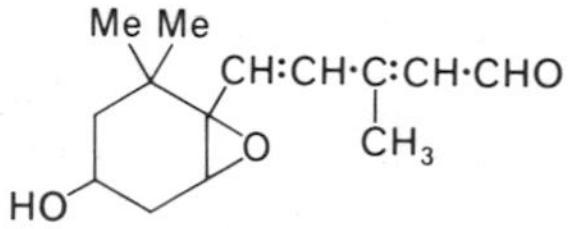

Xanthoxin
(4.58)

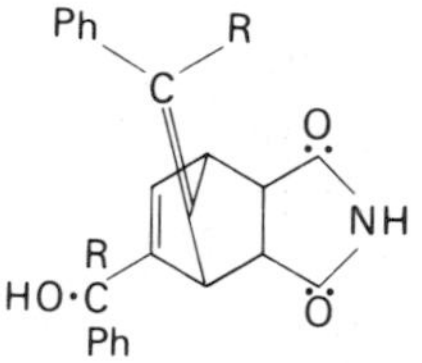

Norbormide
(R = 2-pyridyl)
(4.59)

4.8 Metabolism of foreign substances

Closely related genera often handle foreign substances in surprisingly different ways. The highly selective nature of many of the most useful of the organic phosphorus insecticides is due to two metabolic changes. The first of these (in the insect) makes the substance more toxic for insects, the second change (in the mammal) makes the substance less toxic for mammals. A large sector of the contemporary use of insecticides depends on this. For details see Section 12.3.

Some other examples of selective alteration will now be given. Whereas vertebrates convert phenols to β-glucuronides, most insects form phenyl-β-glucosides instead.

The aminoacid tryptophan is degraded by the higher plants to indole-3-acetic acid which is an important growth hormone for them, whereas bacteria usually degrade it to tryptamine, and mammals to 3-hydroxy-anthranilic acid and thence to nicotinic acid which is an indispensable metabolite.

The most cautionary examples of selective metabolisms are those in which man behaves differently from most other mammals, for herein lies one of the dangers in transferring results from laboratory animals to man. Here are some examples. The only animals that dehydrogenate quinic acid to benzoic acid are man and the Old World primates, for not even the New World primates do so. The antibacterial sulphonamide sulpha-dimethoxine is excreted by man and the primates as the N'-glucuronide, whereas the common laboratory animals excrete it as the N-acetyl-derivative (Adamson, Bridges and Williams, 1966). Other aromatic amines such as aniline and sulphanilamide are acetylated in man, and many other mammals, as well as in most species of birds, amphibia, reptiles, and fish; nevertheless dogs, frogs and turtles do not perform acetylation. Further examples of different metabolic paths followed by man on the one hand and mammals on the other have been traced for amphetamine, phenylacetic acid, and 6-propylthiopurine in Section 3.4 (p. 82).

The most selective known poison for mammals is norbormide (4.59), used as a rat-killer under the names 'Shoxin' and 'Raticate'. It is 5(α-hydroxy-α-2-pyridylbenzyl)-7(α-2-pyridylbenzylidene)-5-norbornene-2,3-dicarboximide. Only the genus *Rattus* is affected, and death follows its powerful and irritant local vasoconstrictor action; this leads to ischaemia of most of the vital organs which then cease to function. It is non-lethal to over 30 species of other mammals (including mice and other rodents), birds, and fish. It is suggested that all animals other than rats can detoxify norbomide (Roszkowski, 1965). Norbormide has not proved very successful in rat extermination because the vermin soon recognize its odour and learn to avoid it. More interest is being taken in another substance that is absolutely specific for *Rattus norvegicus*, 5-N-piperidino-10,11-dihydro-5H-dibenzocycloheptene (Savarie *et al.*, 1973).

4.9 Quantitative aspects of comparative biochemistry

So far, the differences discussed in the biochemistry of species have been mainly qualitative. But even where similar metabolic pathways are used by two species, *quantitative* differences become apparent. There are quantitative differences of accumulation (see Section 3.6), and quantitative differences in metabolism. An example of the latter is afforded by pathogenic trypanosomes which can be shown to utilize glucose two thousand times faster than their hosts, as follows. One million specimens of *T. rhodesiense*, weighing 0.0078 mg and consuming 0.031 mg of glucose in five hours, would consume 20 times their weight in 24 hours; but a man consumes only one-hundredth of his weight in that period. This intense carbohydrate metabolism of parasites is all the more vulnerable because usually so little energy is stored.

These quantitative differences do not always tell in favour of the larger creature. Man, for example, is 15 times more sensitive to atropine than the rabbit. However, he can safely take a dose of strychnine which would kill more than his own weight of rabbits, and he is unaffected by a concentration of hydrocyanic acid that is instantly fatal to dogs.

Remarkable differences can also be found within a single species. For example, the glutamine synthetase from rat kidney acts on its substrate ten times faster then does the analogous enzyme from rat muscle (Iqbal and Ottaway, 1970).

For further reading on biochemistry as the molecular basis of cell function, see Lehninger (1975). For more on plant biochemistry, see Bonner and Varner (1976). For a simple book, revising the basic facts of biochemistry, Campbell and Kilby (1975), available in paperback form, can be recommended.

5 Comparative cytology: the third principle of selectivity

It is an everyday observation that the various forms of life differ greatly in size. The frontispiece of this book shows pictorially how mammals, insects, and bacteria form a series in which the size of average members decreases a thousandfold, then a thousandfold again, whereas molecules (of the size of drugs, vitamins, and coenzymes) are a thousandfold smaller still.

However, the sizes of cells do not differ so greatly. The average diameter of bacteria ($1-4\,\mu$m) may be compared with that of a roughly spherical parenchymatous cell ($15-70\,\mu$m) of which the largest part of plant tissues is composed. A few kinds of plant cells are much larger, notably the pulp cells of fleshy fruits (up to 1 mm), and the fibre cells [usually $1-2$ mm (occasionally 100 mm) in length but of normal thickness]. Plant cells tend to remain small until the final division, after which they increase greatly in size as the vacuole fills with water.

Animal cells, which have no large vacuole, do not usually grow after division and tend to be slightly smaller than plant cells. Thus a typical epithelial cell may be $10 \times 10 \times 50\,\mu$m, and an erythrocyte $8\,\mu$m wide. A few kinds of animal cells are much larger, notably nerve cells [in mammals $1-20\,\mu$m in diameter (i.e. the long axon, but the body of the cell may be $100\,\mu$m), and from 20 mm to 1 m long]; the fertilized ovum is also unusually large.

5.0 The variations of cell architecture. Differentiation, de-differentiation, and cancer

Plants differ from animals in many ways: absence of a nervous system, of muscles (and hence of locomotion), and of an efficient circulatory system;

presence (except in fungi) of a photosynthetic mechanism. Animals, on the other hand lack two features very characteristic of plants, namely chloroplasts, and cell walls. Organophosphorus compounds, which kill insects by preventing transmission of the nervous impulse, cause no harm in a plant's sap because of the complete absence of a nervous system. On this basis rests the very successful practice of plant chemotherapy against insects (Section 12.3). The unique structure of chloroplasts (Section 5.3) offers the reverse opportunity, for example, to kill weeds without harming bees. In the structure of viruses, quite extraordinary features may lend themselves to selective interference (Section 5.4).

The organization of plant and animal cells into a variety of tissues makes a valuable division of labour possible in *multi*cellular creatures. But, apart from this, a further division of labour occurs at the cellular level by differentiation into nerve cell, muscle cell, epithelial cell, and so on.

The width of synapses. Many differences found by pharmacologists in the response of various adrenergically-innervated smooth muscles has been traced to the width of the synaptic gap (Burnstock and Costa, 1975). Across the wide gaps (80–400 nm) characteristic of blood vessels, nerve stimulation releases a concentration of noradrenaline which, even at its peak value, tends to be close to the threshold concentration. In such tissues, decreasing the amount of transmitter, either by depleting the vesicles (e.g. with reserpine) or by interfering with its release (using, e.g., bretylium), can easily inhibit neurotransmission to the involuntary muscle. On the other hand, these two types of drug have little effect on tissues in which this gap is small because the peak concentration of noradrenaline may normally be 100 times the threshold concentration. Examples of such tissues are the nictitating membrane, the vas deferens, and the sphincter papillae, all of which have a gap of about 20 nm only. The lack of inhibitory action of α-blocking agents in the 'narrow gap' tissues, follows from this: the usual blood levels of antagonists are not high enough to compete with the high concentrations of transmitter. The ability of cocaine to potentiate sympathetic postganglionic neurotransmission in some tissues but not in others can also be traced back to the gap size.

Cancer. Much of the most effective treatment of cancer with drugs depends on comparative cytology. Cancer cells are normally highly-specialized cells which have lost some or all of their differentiation. In short, they have regressed to a much simpler, more primitive type of cell* which (unlike the normal parent) divides continuously though inefficiently. Because a much higher proportion of cancer cells are actively

---

* They can even be viewed as cells which have devolved from a metazoan life (with its genetic instructions for mutual adhesion and shared growth-information) to a protozoan life (with complete independence for each cell (Goldacre, 1977).

dividing, they are more vulnerable than normal cells to drugs that are DNA antimetabolites. By giving the patient well-spaced courses of those anti-metabolites that interfere with the synthesis (or incorporation into DNA) of purines or pyrimidines, a selective action against the cancer cells can be obtained. (Normal cells divide more quickly than most cancer cells, although fewer are in a state of division at any one moment, and hence make a good recovery in the unmedicated intervals.) For examples of these drugs, see Sections 4.0 and 12.5. For the theory and practice of applying them, see Brulé *et al.*, 1973.

This leads to a discussion of what is known as the 'cell cycle'. All proliferating cells go through a series of phases when synthesizing new DNA. After mitosis (M phase), there is a resting phase (G_1) followed by the DNA synthesizing period (S), then a second resting phase (G_2) occurs before the cell enters mitosis. A third resting phase (G_0) is seen when the cell cycle is dormant, and this is so refractory to drugs that only the nitrosoureas can attack it.

The success of chemotherapy depends on (a) the tumour cells' susceptibility to the drug, and (b) the drug's reaching the tumour in an effective concentration (C) and remaining there long enough (T) to kill the cancer cells. The optimal product ($C \times T$) has to be related to the ruling phase of the cancer cell's cycle. Generally, with appropriate suspensions of therapy to allow all normal cells to catch up with their mitoses, chemotherapy must be continued for many weeks, or even months. For more information on the cell cycle, see Shall (1977).

Another form of cancer treatment makes use of hormones (especially androgens and oestrogens) to induce the cancer cells to re-acquire some differentiation, and hence behave more like the healthy cells of the tissue in which the malignancy occurs.

Post-menopausal breast cancers yield splendidly to treatment with oestrogens, whereas a common type of pre-menopausal breast cancer is actually stimulated by them and, in addition, can convert androgens to oestrogens (Brulé *et al.*, 1973). However, about one third of pre-menopausal breast cancers are dependent on a pituitary hormone, prolactin.

A new class of re-differentiating agents exists in relatives of Vitamin A, known as the retinoids. Vitamin A, itself, is too unselective in the required doses, but retinoic acid is more selective and prevents established epithelial tumours from developing (in mice), and it can sometimes even cause their retrogression (Bollag, 1972); again, retinyl acetate, given orally, abolishes carcinogen-induced mammary cancer (in mice) (Moon *et al.*, 1977). The epitheliomas include the most intractable tumours of all, namely cancer of the lungs, bladder, colon, rectum, breast, pancreas, and oesophagus, which collectively are responsible for half of all deaths from cancer. Clinical trials are at present being made with 13-*cis*-retinoic acid (*4.1*) in patients with early cancer of the bladder. A conservative prediction is that the tumour will cease to develop as long as medication continues, but it will not necessarily regress with any dose that is non-toxic to the patient. Although more than 100 retinoids have been tested in mice, an analogue with a really high therapeutic index has yet to be found; however, the patient seems injured by a retinoid-induced synthesis of prostaglandins which aspirin may control (Harrison *et al.*, 1977). Some retinoids are carcinogenic (Levine and Ohuchi, 1978).

For further reading on cell differentiation in malignant disease, see Sherbert (1973); for the growth kinetics of tumours, see Steel (1977). For general reading on cell differentiation, see Maclean (1977).

MeMe

—CH:CH·CMe:CH·CH:CH·CMe:CH·CO$_2$H

Me

Retinoic acid
(*5.1*)

Transformation, and lectins. In experimental cytology, viruses are used to convert normal cells, e.g. fibroblasts in culture, to what are known as 'transformed cells'. Although not malignant, these are partly de-differentiated and have, *inter alia*, the following properties: decreased self-cohesion, altered appearance due to surface changes, increased rate of growth, loss of the enzyme cyclic AMP phosphodiesterase, and decreased synthesis of sulphated mucopolysaccharides. All these trends can be reversed by adding dibutyryl cyclic adenosine monophosphate to the culture medium (Goggins, Johnson, and Pastan, 1972).

Lectins, of which concanavalin A (obtained from jack beans) is an example, are carbohydrate-binding proteins of vegetable origin. They agglutinate malignant cells, although normal cells are unaffected. Agglutin-ability tends to increase as malignancy increases (Inbar, Ben-Bassat, and Sachs, 1972). Usually agglutination leads to cell death without harm to normal cells present (Culp and Black, 1972), but a trypsin digest of con-canvalian A restores malignant cells to the growth pattern of normal cells (Burger and Noonan, 1970). Just how to adapt these very striking results to clinical use has, so far, proved elusive.

Sub-cellular structure. Apart from the division of labour brought about by cell differentiation, and the grouping of similar cells into organs, a further division exists at the sub-cellular level. In this way, the many conflicting chemical reactions that take place simultaneously inside cells, achieve the required isolation in specialized compartments formed of selectively permeable membranes. [These membranes can comprise 80% of the dry weight of an animal cell (O'Brien, 1967).] Knowledge of this ultrastructure was immensely furthered by the work of the Belgian Albert

Claude who, working in the Rockefeller Institute in New York City, diverted the electron microscope to this task in 1940, and used differential centrifugation to separate the various kinds of organelles.

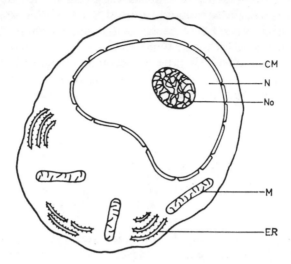

FIG. 5.1 Ultrastructure of a typical cell. CM, plasma membrane; N, nucleus; No, nucleolus; M, mitochondrion; ER, endoplasmic reticulum to which ribosomes are attached.

Figure 5.1 is a diagram of a typical cell showing the principal features seen under an electron microscope. Surrounding the whole cell is the plasma membrane, very thin, and highly selective of what it permits to enter. If a cell wall is present, it is external to this and is far thicker and more porous. Within the plasma membrane lies the cytoplasm, which is an ever-moving suspension of functional structures (called organelles) in the aqueous cytosol. The largest organelle inside the cell is the nucleus with its characteristic perforated membrane, and in the nuclear sap a nucleolus is shown. Also depicted in the cytosol (but in far fewer than their natural numbers, to assist clarity) are some of the other organelles that fill the cell: mitochondria, endoplasmic reticula, and ribosomes. These organelles provide compartments, interfaces, and membranes in which the chemical reactions of living matter take place in a specific order and facilitated by enzymes.

Such differences in comparative cytology can provide a basis for the exercise of selectivity in drugs and other agents. Nowhere is this more evident than in bacteria whose small size, compared to eukaryotic cells, leaves no space for a nucleus or even one mitochondrion. In place of a nucleus, the DNA is gathered into a single chromosome, laced through the plasma membrane; in place of mitochondria, the whole plasma membrane has to function as a mitochondrion, breaking down nutrients and storing the energy. Thus the exposed position of nuclear and mitochondrial functions in bacteria stands in contrast to the membrane-protected situation of these functions in the cells of higher organisms. But the most characteristic difference of bacteria is their need for a cell wall, of a construction found nowhere else in living matter. These cytological peculiarities of bacteria, particularly the last-named, have provided the basis for some of the most selective and successful drugs used in chemotherapy, and undoubtedly many more will follow. Figure 5.2, drawn to scale, allows comparison of the relative sizes of a typical bacterium, mitochondrion, and nucleus.

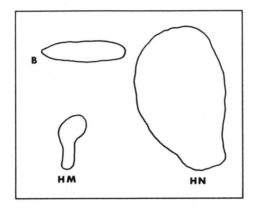

FIG. 5.2 Relative size of bacterium (B), host's nucleus (HN), and one of the host's mitochondria (HM) in mouse spleen infected with *B. anthracis*. Width of the bacterium is 0.5 µm. (Roth *et al.*, 1960.)

Even in mammals, selectivity between the various tissues is possible because of the great specialization in shape and structure of the cells, and this is true also of the cells' ultrastructure. Nuclei from the various human tissues differ so much in appearance that forensic pathologists have long based on entire system of tissue identification on these differences. Mammalian mitochondria, too, differ from organ to organ (Section 5.3). Such cytological differences (i.e. between two tissues in the one organism) could be used in therapy.

The remainder of this Chapter outlines the comparative morphology and function of organelles. Clearly, this is the youngest branch of our subject, and the least investigated of the three principles of selectivity. Some new workers are being recruited to the subject by the postdoctoral fellowships (two years in length) for correlations between morphology and pharmacology. These have been offered annually since 1964 by the Pharmaceutical Manufacturers Association in Washington, D.C.

For further reading on cytology and the division of labour inside cells, see Bourne (1970). For a descriptive atlas of the structure of cells and tissues, see Porter and Bonneville (1973).

5.1 The cell wall

A cell wall, when present, provides external support. It is highly porous and so does not regulate permeability which is a function of the plasma membrane (see next Section).

Animals. The cells of multicellular animals usually have no walls. Many protozoa (e.g. *Amoeba* and *Trypanosoma*) lack cell walls, whereas some others have walls of cellulose about 230 Å thick (e.g. *Chlamydomonas*), or of protein (e.g. *Eimeria*) or calcium carbonate (the *Foraminifera*).

Plants. Multicellular plants have cell walls formed from microfibrils of cellulose (10–20 nm wide and of variable length) embedded in an amorphous matrix of hemicelluloses and pectins. (Cellulose is the β-1,4-linked polymer of D-glucose.) The hemicelluloses are a family of polymerized anhydro-sugars of which xylan and arabogalactan are the commonest in higher plants. The pectins are straight-chain polymers of α-1,4-linked D-galacturonic acid residues, partly esterified with methyl-groups and partly present as calcium salts; the molecular weight ranges from 25 000 to 360 000. Primary cell wall is first laid down, and then thickened, and in some tissues finally impregnated with lignin. For further reading on the plant cell wall, see Siegel (1962). The cell wall is largely synthesized by enzymes present in the plasma membrane, and the various inhibitors of cell wall formation usually act on this membrane.

Fungi. The cell wall of fungi is a mosaic of various carbohydrates with a little lipid and protein. The principal carbohydrate is chitin* (poly-*N*-acetylglucosamine), although this is absent from some families of fungi, especially the yeasts.

Yeasts are single-cell fungi with cell walls consisting of two interlocking structures, either of which is sufficient to keep the characteristic shape. One structure is made entirely of glucan (a poly-anhydride of glucose), and the other is a mannan-protein complex bound to disulphide linkages (Nickerson, Falcone and Kessler, 1961). Only when both structures are broken is the cytoplasm extruded (Bacon *et al.*, 1965).

Unlike higher organisms, fungi are under high internal pressure and they burst if the cell-wall chitin is removed (e.g. with chitinase, obtainable from snails), unless the osmotic pressure of the medium is increased. Pentachloronitrobenzene (quintozene), a commercial agricultural fungicide, produces mycelial walls deficient in chitin (Macris and Georgopoulis, 1969).

Bacteria also are under a high internal turgor pressure, estimated as about

---

* Chitin also makes up a large proportion of the exoskeleton of insects and crustacea.

20 atmospheres for Gram-positive (and 5 for Gram-negative) types (Mitchell and Moyle, 1956b, 1957). Bursting is prevented by a thick cell wall which often constitutes 25 per cent of the dry weight. When the protoplast (i.e. all of the cell inside the wall) grows, additional quantities of cell wall must be synthesized. Several antibiotics owe their place in therapeutics to their ability to prevent this synthesis (see the following). In every case the bacterium ruptures under its own osmotic pressure, but only if it is growing and therefore in need of new cell wall. Lederberg (1957), who first reported this phenomenon (actually for penicillin), noticed that lysis can be prevented by making the culture medium hypertonic (see also Guze, 1967).

Bacterial cell walls have an effective pore diameter of about 1 nm (Mitchell and Moyle, 1956a). For an electron micrograph of bacteria, showing the thick cell wall external to the thin plasma membrane, see Roth, Lewis and Williams, 1960. The wall of Gram*-positive bacteria is only 15 to 50 nm in thickness and about half of it consists of murein*, a polysaccharide-polypeptide polymer which gives it its strength. Most of the rest of the wall consists of teichoic acids (to be described later). Murein is the specific substrate of lysozyme, an antibacterial enzyme found in tears and other body secretions, and in egg white; it is also used by phage viruses to gain access to bacteria.

The wall of Gram-negative bacteria is more complicated. Freeze etching, in combination with electron microscopy, reveals 5 or even 6 concentric layers of which murein (only 2 nm thick) is the innermost (murein forms only 5–20% of the wall mass). The surrounding layers are lipoprotein and lipo-polysaccharide, but teichoic acid is absent. The integrity of these layers depends on the presence of magnesium and calcium.

The structure of murein (also known as peptidoglycan) will be briefly described; then its biosynthesis will be outlined step-by-step. It is a cross-linked polymer of no fixed size, and it seems that one single molecule of it forms a sack around each bacterium. The latter can supply hydrolytic enzymes from the cytoplasm to help reshape this bag of murein when it is being enlarged during growth. In one direction, the molecule of murein consists of linear chains of disaccharides which are cross-linked, in the other direction, by side-chains of aminoacid residues (shown diagrammatically in Fig. 5.3). Not all of the aminoacid side-chains are used for cross-linking.

The biosynthesis of murein. The first stage is biosynthesis of the characteristic monosaccharide. To begin with, N-acetylglycosamine-1-phosphate and uridine triphosphate are united, in the cytoplasm, to give

* In 1884, the Danish bacteriologist Christian Gram published his method for selective staining with crystal violet and iodine followed by rinsing in ethanol. Many bacterial species, like *Staphylococcus*, and *Mycobacterium*, retained the stain and have come to be known as Gram-positive; other species remained unstained, e.g. *Escherichia* and *Salmonella*, and these are said to be Gram-negative. The name 'murein' was bestowed by J. T. Park (1966), the first chemical investigator of the mode of action of penicillin.

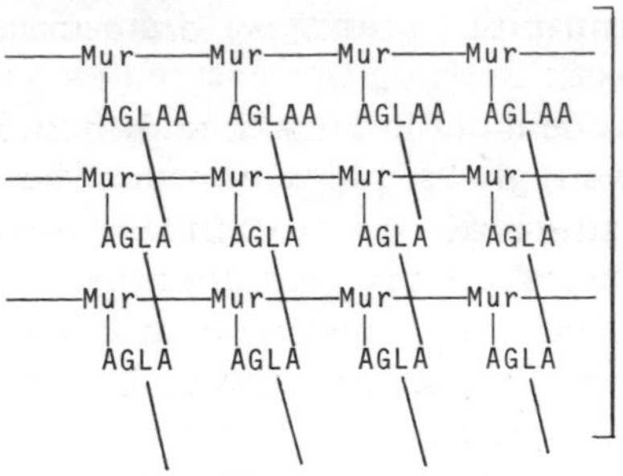

```
    ─Mur────Mur───Mur───Mur──
       │       │      │      │
     AGLAA   AGLAA  AGLAA  AGLAA

    ─Mur┐  ─Mur┐  ─Mur┐ ─Mur┐
       │  \    │ \    │ \    │ \
     AGLA   AGLA   AGLA   AGLA

    ─Mur┐  ─Mur┐  ─Mur┐ ─Mur┐
       │  \    │ \    │ \    │ \
     AGLA   AGLA   AGLA   AGLA
         \       \      \      \
```

FIG. 5.3 Fragment of murein showing cross-linking of muropeptide units through their aminoacids. Mur: the disaccharide. AGLAA: the five aminoacids.

N-acetylglycosamine-1-phosphate. This nucleotide then forms the 3-lactyl ether (in two steps), giving uridine diphospho-N-acetylmuramic acid [acetylmuramic acid is 3-O-D-lactyl-N-acetyl-glucosamine (5.2), a sugar found nowhere else than in prokaryote cell walls]. Five aminoacid residues are then added, the terminal two going on as the pair: D-alanyl-D-alanine. The composition of this pentapeptide varies slightly with the species; that for *Staphylococcus aureus* is shown here (5.3).

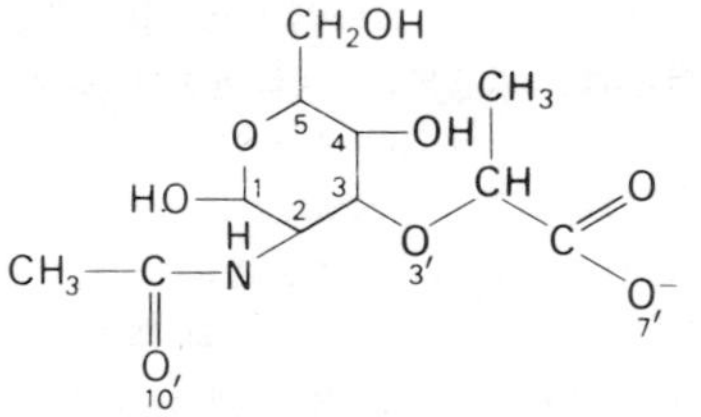

Acetylmuramic acid (anion)
(5.2)

(D-lactyl)-L-ala-D-*iso*glu-L-lys-D-ala-D-ala
(5.3)

This monosaccharide is transformed to the characteristic disaccharide as follows. It is first covalently united to a C_{55} isoprenoid alcohol in the plasma membrane, releasing uridine monophosphate (Higashi, Strominger and Sweeley, 1967). A molecule of N-acetylglucosamine is then incorporated, and five glycine residues are added to the lysine residue (this is done in the reverse direction to normal peptide synthesis, and without recourse to ribosomes). The product is usually referred to as the 'disaccharide decapeptide'.

The next stage is the polymerization. Breaking loose from the C_{55} group in the membrane, the disaccharide decapeptide forms a bond *from* the 1-position of the N-acetylmuramic residue *to* to 4-hydroxy-group of a terminal N-acetylglucosamine residue of another disaccharide unit. By repetition of this step (something like 50 times), the polysaccharide chain grows (Strominger et al., 1967).

The final stage is the cross-linking. This is a transpeptidation reaction, needing no external supply of energy, between the terminal amino-group in the pentaglycine side-chain and the carbonyl moiety of the penultimate D-alanine residue of another pentapeptide chain. In this way, one molecule of D-alanine is eliminated and a new peptide bond is formed (Wise and Park, 1965; Tipper and Strominger, 1965). By repetition of this process, the murein layer is completed.

The murein of Gram-negative organisms is constructed a little differently. No pentaglycine chain is present, and cross-linking takes place between the terminal amino-group of meso-diaminopimelic acid (which takes the place of lysine) and the penultimate D-alanine. The diaminopimelic acid is also linked covalently to the lipoprotein (Hofschneider and Martin, 1968). In spite of their lower content of murein, Gram-negative bacteria depend for their rigidity on murein, and burst if it is removed (Mandelstam, 1962).

Teichoic acids are polymers found on the C_{55}-site of the plasma membrane in Gram-positive bacterial species. They are composed of (polymerized) glycerol phosphate or ribitol phosphate; this polymer backbone carries species-variable substituents such as D-alanine, glucose, galactose, or amino-sugars. Teichoic acids take part in ion-exchange in the region between cell-wall and plasma membrane and they concentrate magnesium ions. They also confer group-antigenic properties on the cell walls. Teichoic acids are not found elsewhere in nature (Baddiley, Hancock, and Sherwood, 1973).

Bacterial spore walls are like cell walls, but surrounded by a calcium dipicolinate complex, exterior to which is a protein shell, rich in disulphide bonds (Gould and Hitchins, 1963).

For further reading on bacterial cell walls, see Gale, et al., (1972), and Franklin and Snow, (1975).

Several antibiotics are known which act through injuring different stages of the biosynthesis of bacterial cell wall. Cycloserine (5.4), from Streptomyces garyphalus, a structural analogue of D-alanine, has been found to inhibit two relevant enzymes, (a) the one that recemizes L-alanine to D-alanine (5.5), and (b) the enzyme that synthesizes D-alanyl-D-alanine from D-alanine (Strominger, Threnn, and Scott, 1959). Cycloserine is held about 100 times more tightly by the latter enzyme than is its normal substrate, although each is in free equilibrium. Cycloserine is used in resistant cases of tuberculosis (see, further, Section 9.4).

Benzylpenicillin (5.6), the first, and still the most used, member of the penicillin family, kills bacteria by combining covalently with a 'peptidoglycan transpeptidase', which normally brings about cross-linking, the final stage in murein biosynthesis (Izaki, Matsuhashi, and Strominger, 1968). Deprived of the opportunity to make new cell wall during a period of growth, the bacteria burst and die. This action of penicillin, which is discussed more fully in Section 12.1, is due to the acylating action of the 4-membered lactam ring. The action of the cephalosporin family (which is essentially similar) is described in Section 12.2. Some less used antibiotics that attack quite different stages in cell wall synthesis are mentioned in the latter Section.

Cycloserine
(5.4)

D-Alanine
(5.5)

Benzylpenicillin
(5.6)

3-Fluoro-D-alanine is a highly selective analogue of D-alanine with strong antibacterial properties (Kollonitsch *et al.*, 1973). In clinical trials, it was eventually given as the 2-deutero-derivative, to minimize metabolic loss. It was found to be rapidly absorbed through the small intestine, so that useful flora in the colon were undisturbed. An unexpected pheno-menon was encountered: in prolonged therapy, bacteria learnt to incorpo-rate the drug into the D-alanine position of cell wall precursor, whereupon it ceased to block the biosynthesis of new wall. This difficulty was overcome by simultaneous administration of cycloserine (Anon., 1975).

5.2 The plasma membrane

All cells have a thin, frangible, lipoprotein membrane which regulates permeability between the cytoplasm and the outer environment. It is usually 50–100 Å thick, and the electron microscope shows three parallel layers (after fixation with permanganate): dense lines, each 20–30 Å wide, separated by 25–40 Å (Robertson, 1959). A similar structure surrounds the organelles present in the cytoplasm, except that the membranes of nucleus, mitochondria, and chloroplasts are double. The originally accepted structure for such a membrane is shown in Fig. 5.4. This model was based on the high content of lipids and high electrical impedance of the plasma membrane, and its optical properties (all evidence for the lipid being present as a sheet), and the low surface tension towards water, which suggested that the lipid was covered by protein (Danielli and Davson, 1934; Davson and Danielli, 1952).

The application of other techniques, however, led to a rather different conception of the plasma membrane, as in Fig. 5.5. Freeze-etching sharpen-ed the image of the outer surface of the membrane, and freeze-fracture revealed planes of fracture within the membrane (both techniques used

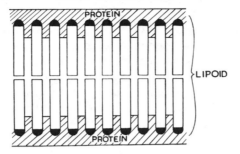

WATER OUTSIDE CELL

LIPOID

WATER INSIDE CELL

FIG. 5.4 Classical representation of plasma membrane (Davson and Danielli, 1952.)

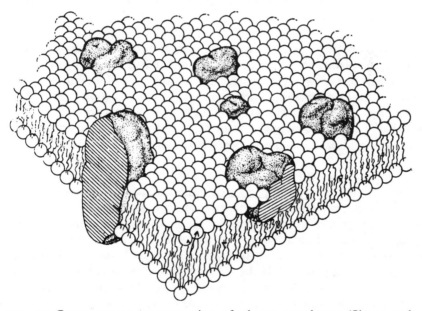

FIG. 5.5 Contemporary representation of plasma membrane (Singer and Nicolson, 1972.)

in conjunction with electron microscopy). Plant cells (onion root, yeast), examined after freeze-etching, gave the impression that each membrane was organized partly as extended bimolecular layers and partly as globular units in free equilibrium with one another (Branton, 1966). Other techniques (fluorescence and ultraviolet spectroscopy, optical rotatory dispersion in polarized light, and low-angle X-ray diffraction), used to investigate moist animal membranes (e.g. ascites tumour), suggested that some protein layers bounded part of the membrane above and below (as in Fig. 5.4), but that other strands of protein penetrated the lipid layer, some of them bunched together to form water-filled microtubules (Wallach and Zahler, 1966).

The current opinion, widely held, is that all biological membranes, including mammalian plasma membranes, have as a structural framework a phospholipid bilayer of which the characteristic feature is a parallel array of hydrocarbon chains, averaging 16 carbon atoms in length. This bilayer has some of the properties of a two-dimensional fluid in which individual lipid molecules can diffuse rapidly in the plane of their own monolayer, but cannot easily pass into the other monolayer. This lipid matrix provides the basic structure of the membrane, and specific proteins are inserted into it asymmetrically. These proteins are responsible for most of the membrane's functions, e.g. receiving and transducing chemical signallers such as hormones, neurotransmitters, growth factors, and antigens, and also forming the three main types of cell junction, namely: tight, small gap, and synaptic. Moreover, these proteins are concerned in the transport of ions and molecules.

This fluid-mosaic membrane model allows proteins their freedom to diffuse in the plane of the lipid membrane and hence to become distributed over the cell surface in a pattern that is sometimes random and sometimes homogeneous (Singer and Nicolson, 1972). There are (a) integral proteins running perpendicularly to the plane of the lipid layer, some passing right through the bilayer, others only half way, and (b) extrinsic proteins that have become adsorbed on one or other of the surfaces of the bilayer and are easily lost.

Some of the proteins that span the bilayer seem to be coiled rods, as detected by freeze fracture, whereas others appear to be globular (see Fig. 5.5). Most, possibly all, of these penetrating proteins have an attached carbohydrate molecule, which remains on the cytoplasmic side, apparently serving as a hydrophilic anchor for the protein. Membrane proteins at the site of junction between two cells appear to have little mobility.

Some important details of the composition of plasma membranes will now be discussed. Calcium is abundantly present, and plays an important part in membrane stabilization, and in controlling the pores (Danielli, 1937). The stability of biological membranes is considerable as the following experiment shows. Membranes from erythrocytes, mitochondria, and endoplasmic reticulum, when treated with phospholipase, lost about 70 per cent of their phosphatidylcholine (4.38). This loss changed the area of the membrane, but the proteins remained bound to it and their conformation (as measured by circular dichroism) was little changed (Trump et al., 1970).

The lipids consist of lecithin (phosphatidylcholine), triglycerides (ordinary fats), fatty acids, and cholesterol (see Section 4.3 for lipid chemistry). The phospholipid seems to predominate. Phospholipid bilayers have a characteristic 'melting point', namely a phase transition where they pass abruptly from a rigid to a fluid condition. This temperature depends on the nature of the head-group as well as on the length, and degree of un-saturation, of the hydrocarbon chain. The highest melting point is found for lipids with long, unsaturated hydrocarbon chains.

In many, possibly all, biological membranes, the lipids are distributed asymmetrically. The outer half of the bilayer consists mainly of neutral lipids, whereas the inner half contains the negatively charged examples, particularly phosphatidylserine. The interior of such a membrane can be 300 mV more positive than the solution that bathes the outside. Such differences in potential can be measured by the potassium nonactin probe (Latorre and Hall, 1976) (see Section 14.1 for nonactin). Such potential differences indicate the source of some typical membrane properties such as the gating potentials of nerves.

When cholesterol is present, its plate-like steroid rings intercalate between the long chains of the phospholipid molecules, restricting their motion, and hence increasing the rigidity of the membrane as well as raising its melting temperature (Coleman, 1973). Both n.m.r. and spin-label e.s.r. studies in artificial phospholipid membranes confirm these conclusions (Gent and Prestegard, 1974).

The proteins of membranes often include enzymes, e.g. adenosine tri-phosphatase which occurs in the plasma membrane of yeast where it assists uptake of aminoacids (Post *et al.*, 1960); and permeases (Section 2.1) are commonly found in membranes. It is logical to suppose that the pro-truding parts of the membrane proteins are made mainly of aminoacids with *polar* side-chains, whereas the embedded parts are rich in aminoacids with *non-polar* side-chains.

The proportion of lipid to proteins in different kinds of membranes varies greatly. Myelin membrane (which shields the nerve fibre) is at one extreme with a molar ratio of lipid to protein of 9:1, whereas the mito-chondrial membrane lies at the other extreme with a 1:1 ratio. Myelin membrane lipid is composed of cholesterol, phosphatidylethanolamine, and cerebrosides (the latter are phosphorus-free condensation products of ethanolamine, fatty acids, and a hexose), whereas mitochondrial membrane lipid consists mainly of phosphatidylethanolamine, lecithin, and cardiolipin (diphosphatidyl glycerol).

Animal membranes. Mammalian plasma membranes are particularly rich in the phospholipids, namely phosphatidyl -choline, -serine, and -ethanolamine. Each membrane enzyme seems to need a specific phospholi-pid in order to function (Coleman, 1973). The principal residue in the 2-position of the glycerol moiety is that of arachidonic acid. Cholesterol is also present. The excitability of the cytoplasmic membranes of muscle and nerve are well known; but it appears that *all* cytoplasmic membranes possess a small degree of irritability, responding to tactile stimuli and making small holes to allow the passage of particles (pinocytosis), whereas to dissolved molecules they remain selective (see Section 3.1). The highly excitable axon membranes, which may be built on slightly different principles from those used solely to govern permeability, are discussed in Section 7.5a.

Plant membranes.   The plasma membrane of plant cells is called the plasmalemma and, in spite of earlier doubts, is well established as the osmotic barrier of the cell (Greenham, 1966). Plant cells are unique in containing large vacuoles which often consist largely of water isotonic with the cytoplasm, and are generally used as a repository for waste. However, at some phases of the cell's growth, the vacuole can become rich in enzymes. The tonoplast which surrounds each vacuole seems to be very like the plasma membrane in composition and properties.

A myoinositol-containing lipid is present in all the membranes of the fungus *Neurospora crassa*, and in an inositol-less mutant of this mould all the membranes are degenerate. Myoinositol is essential for balanced growth in yeast, and analogues of this inositol antagonize growth (Shatkin and Tatum, 1961). L-Myoinositol 1-phosphate, which appears to be the form in which myoinositol exists in the membrane lipid, has structure (*4.39*).

Fungi, including yeast, have an absolute requirement for ergosterol in the plasma membrane. The polyene antibiotics, such as amphotericin (*5.7*), used clinically, make this membrane leaky, or even rupture it, by entering alongside the sterol, and spoiling the continuity (see, further Section 14.2).

Amphotericin B
(*5.7*)

Bacterial membranes.   The cytoplasmic membrane of bacteria has both usual and unusual features. When the cell wall is completely hydrolysed by lysozyme, this membrane becomes the outer layer. It is 60–100 Å thick and sometimes extends into the cytoplasm as a few simple protrusions (Mitchell and Moyle, 1956b; Hughes, 1962). It forms about 10 per cent of the dry weight of the cell and has a lipid content of about 25 per cent. There is usually little lipid elsewhere in the cell. An analysis of the lipid of *M. lysodeikticus* shows that 80 per cent is phospholipid, which is mainly diphosphatidyl glycerol, but some phosphatidyl inositol is also present.

The diphosphatidyl glycerol (a GPGPG-lipid) has C-15 branched, aliphatic groups (Macfarlane, 1961). Sterols are completely absent from bacteria.

The proteins have all the common (and no uncommon), aminoacids. By chromatography on a lipophilic surface (cadmium lauroylsarcosinate), the plasma membranes of various bacteria yield many protein fractions, to one of which the DNA of the solitary bacterial chromosome is firmly attached (Daniels, 1971). Ribonucleic acid, too, is a normal component of the membrane (Hughes, 1962; Yudkin and Davis, 1965).

Plasma membranes of bacteria also contain permeases and the enzymes which synthesize cell wall (Crathorn and Hunter, 1958). Because of their small size, bacteria have no room for mitochondria; hence many mitochondrial enzymes are incorporated in the bacterial plasma membrane. The presence of so many vital enzymes in such an exposed position makes bacteria particularly vulnerable to selectively toxic agents (see further under nucleus and mitochondria in Section 5.3). For further reading on bacterial membranes, see Rogers and Perkins (1968); Gale *et al.* (1972).

Although bacteria have no sterols, another class of prokaryotes, the mycoplasmas (which lack all walls), have plasma membranes that depend for their integrity on the presence of a sterol, usually ergosterol. They cause disease in plants and animals, but are susceptible to polyene antibiotics and the tetracyclines.

Cancer cell membranes.   When a healthy cell undergoes a cancerous change, its surface structure becomes recognizibly different. It has been shown, by intracellular electro-techniques, that cells form an orderly tissue by being able to recognize the presence of one another and to exchange 'messages' between their plasma membranes (Loewenstein and Kanno, 1967). This regulatory mechanism, which prevents unrestrained growth, is lacking in malignant cells. See also under 'transformation' in Section 5.0.

The increased content of sialic acid (5.8) in the surface layer of malignant cells (e.g. human leukaemic and lymphosarcoma cells) not only changes the glycoprotein composition, but makes a visible structural change (van Beek, Smets, and Emmelot, 1975).

$$CH_2OH$$
$$|$$
$$HOCH$$
$$|$$
$$HO_2C \quad HOCH$$

OH
OH

NH·COMe

N-Acetylneuraminic acid
(Sialic acid)
(*5.8*)

Artificial membranes.   Much work on these is being carried out, some of it to obtain excitable membranes (e.g. Mueller and Rudin, 1976), some to study the permeability of ions (e.g. Bangham, Standish and Weissman, 1965). A favoured procedure is to ultrasonicate a mixture of lecithin and water, which produces a suspension of vesicles with a bilayer structure (Huang, 1969). These vesicles lend themselves to studies of transport across natural membranes (Papakadjopoulos, Nir, and Ohki, 1972).

★   ★   ★   ★

For further reading on the structure and function of biological membranes see Gomperts (1977); Chapman and Wallach (1973, 1976); or for a short account, read Finean, Coleman, and Michell (1974). Surface chemistry is discussed in Chapter 14.

5.3 The intracellular organelles

The nucleus.   Except for bacteria, all cells have a large, often spherical, nucleus in which one or several nucleoli can often be seen under the optical microscope. The nucleus is surrounded by an inner and an outer membrane each about 80 Å thick but several hundred Å apart. The nucleolus is a web of threads with no surrounding membrane and is rich in RNA. The nuclear sap contains chromatin threads which, at mitosis, become more densely organized and are seen as chromosomes (DNA + proteins). The total length of DNA in a nucleus is about 1 m, made up of about 3×10^9 nucleotides each with a mol. wt. of about 350. F. Sanger has compared the amount of information stored in this quantity of DNA to that available in a large library.

The 23 pairs of chromosomes in a human nucleus contain, together, about 200 000 genes; at the other end of the scale, a virus may have as few as ten. [A gene is a strip of DNA that completely specifies a particular RNA, which itself completely specifies one protein (mRNA) or one amino-acid (tRNA)].

Instead of a nucleus, bacteria store their genetic material as a single chromosome which is seen as a loop of DNA, lying unprotected in the cytoplasm, but attached to the plasma membrane at one point (Ryter and Jacob, 1964). For example, radioautography of *E. coli* that had been pulsed with ³H-thymidine showed that the DNA formed a two-stranded circle, about 800 μm long (Cairns, 1963). A strand of this length has about three million base pairs, enough to form about 10 thousand genes. The replication points of the bacterial chromosome are bound to the cytoplasmic membrane (Smith and Hanawalt, 1967; Sueoka and Quinn, 1968). Bacterial DNA is more vulnerable to selective agents than that of higher forms of life because it is unprotected by a nuclear membrane, or even by histone molecules (Zubay and Watson, 1959). The highly selective action of the aminoacridines against bacteria in wounds provides an example (see Sections 2.2

and 10.3a). See Fig. 5.2 for the relative sizes of a bacterium and a mammalian nucleus.

A plasmid is an extrachromosomal genetic structure, found in most of the bacterial species, but not constantly present. It varies in size from 1000 to 400 000 nucleotide pairs, the latter size corresponding to about 600 genes. Plasmids can pass from bacterium to bacterium, even between members of different species. They are frequently responsible for introducing resistance to drugs (Section 6.5). For a review of plasmids, see Cohen (1976).

Mitochondria. Mitochondria, the energy generators-and-storers of the living cell, are present in all cells except bacteria. Mitochondria, which are the site of all oxidative phosphorylation, form rods or nearly spherical cylinders, from 0.2 to 3.0 µm in diameter. Often as many as a thousand mitochondria are present in a cell.

Under aerobic conditions, as most cells grow, mitochondria are the site of (i) the tricarboxylic acid cycle which transforms (to carbon dioxide, water, and energy) the acetyl Co-A which is produced by the metabolism of both carbohydrates and fatty acids; (ii) the enzymes that oxidize and convert fatty acids to acetyl Co-A; (iii) the respiratory chain enzymes which transmit, to atmospheric oxygen, the electrons removed from all the various metabolic substrates, and store part of the energy, obtained in this way, as adenosine triphosphate. The enzymes of carbohydrate glycolysis, the Meyerhof sequence, are in the cytoplasm.

Mitochondria are surrounded by two lipoprotein membranes, together about 180 Å thick. The inner membrane is folded into the cell as a series of invaginations known as cristae. About one quarter of the protein part of the cristae consists of oxysomes (respiratory assemblies), i.e. ordered arrangements of riboflavine-protein, coenzyme Q, cytochromes b, c_1, c, a, and a_3 (in that sequence) together with their specific proteins (Yamashita and Racker, 1968). The tricarboxylic acid cycle ensures the reduction of the first two members of the above chain, and each member is oxidized by the member on its right (in the above list), and so on to the end of the chain at cytochrome a_3 which is in equilibrium with atmospheric oxygen.

Some biologists think that the mitochondrion in eukaryotic cells arose from a respiring bacterium that had been engulfed by a fermenting ameoboid cell, and that the metabolism and reproduction of the invader and host were harmonized with the passage of time (Margulis, 1970). Those who refute this hypothesis point out that many vital components of mitochondria are coded by the DNA of the cell's nucleus, even though others are under the control of the mitochondrion's own DNA (Raff and Mahler, 1972).

Mitochondria contain about 20 soluble and 20 insoluble proteins, most of them enzymes. Many of these proteins are made in the cytoplasmic ribosomes, but others are synthesized by the mitochondrial ones (Haldar, Freeman and Work, 1966). Both DNA and RNA are present, the former as single-stranded rings with a mol. wt. of about 10 million (Sinclair and

Stevens, 1966). Mitochondria reproduce by forming buds which break free.

Mitochondria undergo cycles of swelling and contraction. Swelling, corresponding to an energy-discharging phase, is initiated by calcium ions, also by thyroxine and other hormones; contraction is brought about only by adenosine triphosphate. Swelling corresponds to the conversion of chemical energy (from electron transport) to mechanical work (Hackenbrock, 1968), but excessive swelling corresponds to damage. The cristae are studded with patches of the enzyme adenosine triphosphatase, similar to that which constitutes the myosin fibrils of muscle. Although normal mitochondria take up calcium ions to the point where oxidative phosphorylation becomes uncoupled, ascites tumour cells do not react in this way, and hence it seems that the calcium-controlled uncoupling mechanism does not exist in these cancer cells (Thorne and Bygrave, 1974). For more information on calcium in mitochondria, see Section 11.0.

Large differences in structure can be seen between the mitochondria of various organisms (Palade, 1952). But even within a single organism, there are notable differences in the structure. In any mammal, mitochondria from different organs have different numbers of cristae: thus the mitochondria of the heart and kidney, rapidly respiring tissues, have numerous cristae whereas those of the liver are much fewer (Lehninger 1971). Mammalian brain contains at least two populations of mitochondria, each with its own series of functional enzymes (Blokhuis and Veldstra, 1970). All mitochondria in the rapidly growing hepatoma 3924A (in contrast to those from the host cells: rat liver) were found to have deleted an important enzyme β-hydroxybutyrate dehydrogenase, also the matrices had lost affinity for stains although both membranes were intact (Pedersen et al., 1970). Liver mitochondria of both rat and chick have been separated into two populations of differing densities; the denser preponderates in embryos, the lighter in adults (Pollak and Woog, 1971). In some cases, the inner mitochondrial membrane has invaginations differing from normal cristae. These are 'pillow-case' in the beef heart (Penniston et al., 1968), scalloped tubes in the adrenal cortex (Allmann et al., 1970), or tubes that are circular, triangular, or hexagonal in cross section (Korman et al., 1970). The tubular types are more resistant to damage.

Tissue distinctions can also be made on the basis of swelling. Brain tissue, confined as it is in the rigid, heat-retaining skull, has mitochondria which, through internal cross-bracing, can undergo no more than a one per cent increase in volume in response to swelling agents, whereas the mitochondria of liver and kidney can expand to two or three times their normal volume (Lehninger, 1971). Thyroxine makes isolated rat liver mitochondria swell greatly whereas, under the same conditions, heart mitochondria are little affected (Tapley and Cooper, 1956). Chlorpromazine inhibits oxidative phosphorylation in intact mitochondria of brain, but not of liver (Berger, 1957).

The various structural differences mentioned above provide scope for the discovery of selective drugs, particularly when assisted by selective organ permeability (Siekevitz, 1963).

Mitochondria and unicellular organisms. Bacteria have no mitochondria. Being of mitochondrial size, the bacterium has to function as its own mitochondrion; its plasma membrane, although it lacks cristae, has to attempt to carry out as many as it can of the complex activities of eukaryotic mitochondria. Hence many of the typical enzymes of eukaryotic mitochondria are located in the bacterial plasma membrane (De Ley and Docky, 1960; Mitchell and Moyle, 1956a). In particular, the enzymes of the tricarboxylic acid cycle are found there. More than 90% of the cell's succinic, malic, lactic, and formic dehydrogenases, as well as the cytochrome oxidase, are present in the plasma membrane of typical bacteria, e.g. *Staphylococcus aureus* and *Micrococcus lysodeikticus* (Mitchell, 1961, 1963).

The exposure, on the bacterial plasma membrane, of so many enzymes that, in the host, are well protected behind mitochondrial membranes, makes bacteria particularly susceptible to selectively toxic agents. The case of oxine, and other chelating drugs that act similarly, was discussed in Section 2.2 (p. 34). Similarly, the activated halogen antibacterials, such as bronopol (5.9) (2-bromo-2-nitropropan-1,3-diol), selectively attack superficially exposed, but vitally important, mercapto (-SH) groups in bacteria, without harming the corresponding but better protected structures in higher forms of life (Clark, *et al.*, 1974; Stretton and Manson, 1973). Bronopol is particularly effective against *Pseudomonas pyocyanea* which is insensitive to the majority of antibacterials.

$$HO \cdot H_2C - \overset{\overset{\displaystyle NO_2}{|}}{\underset{\underset{\displaystyle Br}{|}}{C}} - CH_2OH$$

Bronopol
(5.9)

Some organisms which lack mitochondria under certain conditions will now be mentioned. When yeasts are grown anaerobically, the mitochondria are replaced by a thin network and all oxidative phosphorylation ceases (Linnane *et al.*, 1962); but an adequate oxygen supply stimulates the production of cytochromes and the enzymes of the citric acid cycle; shortly after this, some mitochondria appear. Thus form and function are related.

In some protozoa the mitochondria are few, in others numerous, and more often filled with tubules than with cristae. The solitary kinetoplast of trypanosomes, which contains DNA, arises by division of an earlier kinetoplast, and contains all the information needed to produce mitochondria (and a cytochrome system) when these parasites infect their second host (an insect) where they reproduce as 'crithidia' (Steinert, 1960; Vickerman, 1962). This alternation of forms continues as a cycle in the two hosts. The natural factor which transforms crithidial to trypanosomal forms is urea, and this inhibits the synthesis of DNA (Steinert and Steinert, 1960). Because the kinetoplast is so unique an organelle, it has lent itself to selective attack. The following antitrypanosomal drugs bind irreversibly to, and disintegrate, the kinetoplast of *Trypanosoma rhodesiense* (in the mouse) without any effect on the cell's nucleus: diminazine, ethidium, pentamidine, hydroxystilbamidine, and trypaflavine (Macadam and Williamson, 1972). The lack of a histone covering over the kinetoplast makes it more vulnerable than the nucleus to these drugs (Steinert, 1965). For more about these trypanocidal drugs, see Section 10.3d.

For further reading on the structure and properties of mitochondria, see Lehninger (1971); Munn (1974); also Lloyd (1974) (micro-organisms only).

Chloroplasts, the green photosynthetic organelles of plants, resemble mitochondria. Chloroplasts are about 0.2 µm in diameter and surrounded by a double-layered lipoprotein membrane about 100 Å thick. The two major components of chloroplasts are the membrane system and the stroma. The membrane system contains grana and interconnecting lamellae which carry the chlorophyll molecules, whereas the stroma contains ribosomes ($70S$) and both RNA and DNA. In spite of the presence of DNA, chloroplasts (like mitochondria) are not autonomous but depend for many of their proteins on nuclear DNA and cytoplasmic ribosomes (Ellis, 1971). Liposoluble spheres containing carotinoids are also present (Mercer, 1960). See Section 4.5 for the many herbicides whose selectivity is exerted on the chloroplasts.

Those few bacteria that are capable of photosynthesis have bacteriochlorophyll contained in chromatophores which resemble chloroplasts.

For further reading on chloroplasts, see Goodwin (1966).

The endoplasmic reticulum. 'Microsomes'.   Most cells have a highly convoluted internal membrane, which forms an extensive network of tubules that seems almost to fill the cytoplasm. This membrane, called the endoplasmic reticulum (or *e.r.* for short), is a lipoprotein mosaic very much like the plasma membrane.

There are two kinds of *e.r.*, a smooth-surfaced form and one that appears rough because of the large number of ribosomes attached to it. The two varieties of *e.r.* can be separated, although only in a somewhat degraded form, by homogenization followed by differential ultracentrifugation. This treatment converts the smooth *e.r.* to spherical artifacts known as 'microsomes', which are much used in experiments because they behave like native *e.r.* The *e.r.* is a storage organelle. In mammalian lymphocytes it stores the antibodies, whereas in the liver its membrane is the site of a host of enzymes which degrade foreign liposoluble substances (Section

3.4). Although in bacteria the *e.r.* is lacking, it is abundantly present in fungi.

See Section 3.4 for selective aspects of the endoplasmic reticulum.

Ribosomes. The ribosomes, which are the site of protein synthesis, consist of particles of 100–200 Å in diameter, built up from many different kinds of proteins and RNA. Whereas the ribosomes of higher organisms form a sediment at 80S, those of bacteria do so at 70S. The latter are rich in magnesium, upon withdrawal of which (e.g. with EDTA), they split at once into two particles, one of 30S and one of 50S. Eukaryotic (80S) ribosomes have much less magnesium, and are much harder to split (Taylor and Storck, 1964). These properties argue for a structural difference between prokaryotic and eukaryotic ribosomes, even though the process of protein synthesis follows a similar course with both (Vazquez, 1964).

About 60 per cent of the 70S (bacterial) ribosomes consist of RNA, and most of the remainder are proteins, of which *E. coli* has 55 kinds but only one molecule of each (Gale *et al.*, 1972, p. 279). Bacterial ribosomes account for about one third of the dry mass of rapidly growing *E. Coli* cells.

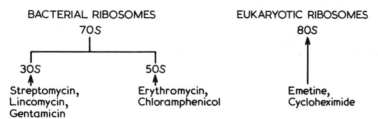

FIG. 5.6 Selective binding to ribosomes of several inhibitors of protein synthesis.

Many drugs that inhibit protein synthesis are able to distinguish between bacterial and eukaryotic ribosomes, even in intact cells. This is illustrated in Fig. 5.6. The aminoglycoside antibiotics, such as streptomycin, bind to the 30S subunit exclusively, whereas chloramphenicol and erythromycin bind only to the 50S subunit. Through having no affinity for the host's 80S ribosomes, these antibiotics exert great selectivity. The tetracyclines, which bind equally to 30S and 80S material in isolated ribosomal fractions, do not reach the 80S ribosomes under therapeutic conditions, on account of a highly selective distribution effect (see Introduction to Chapter 3). Finally, counter-selective properties are shown by emetine and cycloheximide which bind to eukaryotic, but not to prokaryotic, ribosomes. (See Section 4.1 for more on drugs that act by inhibiting protein synthesis).

The synthesis of proteins on ribosomes is shown diagrammatically in Fig. 5.7. The messenger RNA becomes bound to the smaller subunit, most likely in the cleft between the two subunits. The transfer RNA makes contact with the mRNA and, as a result, a polypeptide chain is biosynthesized on the larger subunit.

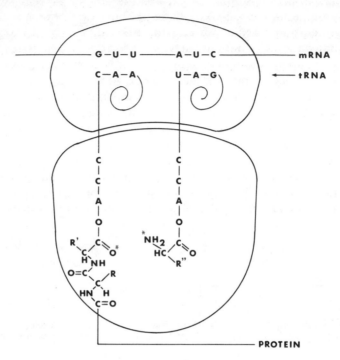

FIG. 5.7 Diagrammatic representation of protein synthesis taking place on the surface of a pair of ribosome sub-units. The peptide bond is being formed between two groups marked with an asterisk.

The mitochondrial ribosomes of mammals are small (about $55S$) and insensitive to erythromycin and lincomycin, although these antibiotics penetrate freely into the mitochondria. These ribosomes are sensitive to chloramphenicol which, fortunately, does not normally penetrate into mammalian mitochondria (Towers, Kellerman, and Linnane, 1973; Huang *et al.*, 1966). Chloroplasts have ribosomes that are sensitive to most of the protein synthesis inhibitors that injure bacteria (Küntzel and Noll, 1967).

Viruses have no ribosomes and are completely dependent for reproduction on those of the host.

For further reading on ribosomes, see Nomura, Tissières, and Lengyel (1974).

Dictyosomes. These organelles, collectively termed the 'Golgi apparatus', are sack-shaped bodies of variable outline and cohesiveness, and are surrounded by a lipoprotein membrane. The known functions of dictyosomes are the partial synthesis and the assembly of glyco- and lipo-proteins, the formation and packaging of secretory granules, the synthesis of lysosomal enzymes, and the assembly of membrane components. For a review, see Dauwalder, Whaley, and Kephart (1972).

Lysosomes, formed by the endoplasmic reticulum, can penetrate the cytoplasmic membrane and hence leave the cell, whereupon their membrane ruptures and liberates proteolytic and other hydrolytic enzymes such as acid phosphatase and acid deoxyribonuclease. In some one-celled organisms, lysosomes help nutrition by providing extracellular digestion. In higher organisms they assist in the reorganization of tissues by the destruction of aged or merely superfluous cells. Lysosomes are labilized by vitamin A, an effect reversed by chlorpromazine (Guth *et al.*, 1965). Because they are more exposed than other organelles, they are thought of as promising sites of action for membrane-stabilizing and -destabilizing drugs. In inflammation and degenerative diseases, the therapeutic aim is to stabilize or repair the containing membrane of the lysosome (see Section 14.3). However, to attack tumours, lysosome rupture is being attempted, as in the combined use of vitamin A and cyclophosphoramide in the treatment of mammary carcinoma (Brandes *et al.*, 1966; see, for further examples of rupturing agents, Section 14.2).

For a review on lysosomes, see Dean and Barrett (1976).

Microfibrils. Actin and myosin, which were once thought to be present only in muscle cells, are now being found in microfibril organelles in many types of cell, including vertebrate and protozoan. For example, micro-fibrils, about 50 Å in diameter, play the leading role in such common cellular phenomena as protoplasmic streaming, cytokinesis, ruffling of membranes, nerve outgrowths, phagocytosis, and pinocytosis. This knowledge has accrued through the use of a fungal product, cytochalasin B, which is a specific inhibitor of microfilament movement (Carter, 1967). (Cytochalasins are isoindol-1-ones).

The non-muscle myosins share with muscle myosin the ability to hydro-lyze ATP and to form cross links between actin filaments, but there is considerable variation in their other physical, chemical and enzymatic properties. This variation in the myosins may be related to the diversity of movements which different cells exhibit.

Microtubules are widely distributed, e.g. in nerve cells, ciliated cells, leucocytes, and sperm cells. They play an important part in moving chromosomes (together and apart) during mitosis. The alkaloid colchicine specifically and reversibly combines with tubulin, the protein (of sedimentation constant $6S$) which normally polymerizes to form these tubules (Borisy and Taylor, 1967). The powerful action of colchicine (*5.10*) in blocking mitosis at metaphase by arresting formation of the mitotic spindle, is due to its selective binding to tubulin. Colchicine causes disappearance of microtubules in granulocytes and other normally mobile cells. Its rapid anti-inflammatory effect in the treatment of gout is thought to be due to a similar action on leucocytes. Colchicine is a drug of low selectivity, hence the treatment of gout is usually continued with allopurinol (see Section 9.4, p. 319). Nocodazole (5.11) is a simple synthetic compound with a strong, specific, and reversible inhibitory action on the polymerization of tubulin, to which it binds at the same site as colchicine. Its biological use is under investigation. Another substance interfering with the poly-merization of tubulin is maytansine, an ansa-molecule (cf. rifamycin, p. 117) occurring in an African plant (Meyers and Shaw, 1974). It is under-going clinical trial in leukaemia (Rebhun, 1975).

Colchicine
(5.10)

Nocodazole
(5.11)

   The vinca alkaloids, notably vincristine and vinblastine, isolated from the garden plant 'periwinkle' (*Vinca rosea*), have a complex non-sym-metrical structure based on the indole nucleus. They inhibit mitosis in metaphase by binding to tubulin, but *not* at the colchicine site (Marantz and Shelanski, 1970). Vinca alkaloids are used in the first days of a course of drug treatment for leukaemia; they give a powerful start to the treat-ment, after which their place is taken by more selective drugs such as methotrexate.

   For further reading on microtubules, see Gaskin and Shelanski (1976).

   Miscellaneous organelles and particles. Many are known, but only those of possible interest in therapy will be mentioned here. Acetylcholine, synthesized in motor nerve terminals, is stored there in minute *vesicles* (Whittaker, 1963), which become ruptured when the arrival of a nervous impulse releases calcium ions. *Synaptosomes*, which are much larger, are the snapped-off pre-synaptic ends of nerves, and can be isolated by centrifugation (Blaschko, 1959). Depending on their source, they may contain noradrenaline, dopamine, serotonin, the corticotrophic-releasing factor, and other transmitters, but never acetylcholine. Catecholinergic synaptosomes actually synthesize catecholamines (Patrick and Barchas, 1974). The rupture of presynaptic vesicles in the insect is thought to play an important part in the insecticidal action of DDT (see Section 7.6e).

Liposomes arise physiologically after a meal, when they are seen in the blood as finely divided fatty particles. The use of artificially produced liposomes as carriers of therapeutic material was discussed in Section 3.6.

5.4 Viruses

Viruses are non-cellular forms of life, structurally simpler than bacteria. They vary in size from rounded particles as small as 200 Å, to others that form long rods ($10\,000 \times 100$ Å).

The *virion* (the complete infective virus, such as exists extracellularly) consists of a core of either DNA or RNA (but not both) surrounded by a protective capsid (= shell) of one, or sometimes two, proteins. These two components are arranged in a highly ordered fashion that is characteristic of the particular kind of virus. Most of the viruses that infect animals are icosahedral (20-sided) and hence roughly spherical. But the viruses of measles and influenza are spirals. In the latter virus two kinds of protein (neuraminidase and haemagglutinin) form the capsid which is embedded in lipid, and this lipoprotein envelope encloses a coiled ribonucleoprotein tube. Poxviruses, the largest known, are brick-shaped and of very complicated structure. Many types of virus have a protein core around which the nucleic acid is arranged.

Phages have a special shape, consisting of a head and a tail. The head of T2 coliphage, for example, contains a single molecule of DNA (mol. wt. = 10^8), which weighs 2×10^{-10} µg and contains 2×10^5 nucleotide pairs. This molecule, neatly folded into an approximately spherical mass and surrounded by neatly packed (non-genetic) protein molecules, constitutes the 'head'. To this is attached a 'tail' built of a series of five structures: (1) the outer sheath consisting of a contractile, myosin-like protein with about 110 molecules of adenosine triphosphate, (2) a solid core, (3) a tip consisting of a spiked plate, (4) a few molecules of endolysine, a lysozyme-like enzyme, (5) a series of fibres which are wound around the distal end. A typical T-even coliphage, such as T2 or T4, is shown diagrammatically in Fig. 5.8.

Chemical components.   Individual members of the various classes of virus contain from 1 to 20 kinds of proteins, some of which are enzymes (see below).

The molecular weights of nucleic acids, in various types of virus, varies from 2 to 160 million. RNA and DNA types are about equally common in viruses infecting man. Typical DNA viruses are the adenoviruses (causing infections of the respiratory tract), the poxviruses, and the herpesviruses. Typical RNA viruses are the myxoviruses (including influenza), paramyxoviruses (mumps and measles), and those causing yellow fever and encephalitis. The nucleic acids are double-stranded in some types, but single stranded in others.

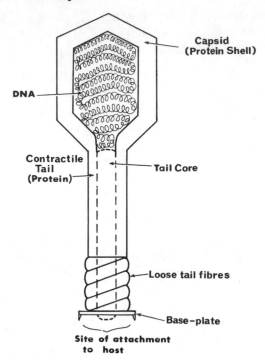

FIG. 5.8 Diagram of T-even coliphage. (After Kozloff *et al.*, 1957.)

Phages (viruses that infect bacteria) contain aliphatic diamines such as putrescine [$H_2N(CH_2)_4NH_2$] and spermidine [$H_2N(CH_2)_3NH(CH_2)_4NH_2$], in quantities sufficient to neutralize from 30 to 50 per cent of the DNA present. These amines seem to be stabilizers of the folded state of DNA (Mahler *et al.*, 1961); but they are non-specific cations as they can be replaced by an excess of magnesium ions without disturbing the functioning (Ames and Dublin, 1960). Many other viruses, e.g. poliovirus and tobacco mosaic virus, lack these organic bases. All T-even phages infecting *E. coli* contain a folic acid derivative, dihydropteroyl-pentaglutamic acid, localized near the tail-plate. These phages also induce formation of this acid in the bacterium after infection (Kozloff, *et al.*, 1970).

Although lipid barriers are common outside the capsids of viruses (and inside as well for poxviruses), no lipids are associated with adenoviruses or reoviruses. Enzymes are frequently present. Neuraminidase, in myxo-viruses, releases sialic acid (*5.8*) from a glycopeptide widely present in mucus. Vaccinia virus (a poxvirus) contains the enzyme RNA-polymerase which enters the host cell at the time of infection. A herpesvirus has adenosine triphosphatase. Lysozyme is common in phages. Carbohydrates, other than the pentose that forms part of the nucleic acids, have often been found. Analysis of purified herpes simplex virus showed proteins (70 per cent), phospholipids (22 per cent), DNA (6 per cent), and carbohydrates (1.6 per cent) (Russell, Watson and Wildy, 1963).

In viruses, no device for producing energy is present, nor is there any cell wall. Nevertheless each type of virion has considerable individuality and complexity, and it is hard to recall that 25 years ago each virus was thought to consist only of one molecule of nucleic acid and one of protein.

When a virus particle infects a cell, the nucleic acid (which is the sole infectious part) passes into the host and not only reorganizes the host's supply of intermediates to produce fresh viruses, but can also command the synthesis of new intermediates which it may require. A typical RNA virus such as *Vaccinia* enters the host cell's cytoplasm and, by means of reverse-transcriptase, it brings about the synthesis of complementary DNA and the host cell's DNA is repressed. As soon as the new DNA makes viral RNA and the host's ribosomes begin to translate the latter into viral proteins, the virus particles multiply fast in the host cell.

Coliphage attacks *E. coli* in a series of steps. First the long tail fibres come to rest on the surface of the cell, then the spiked base-plate is brought into contact with this surface. The lysozyme-like enzyme in the plate then depolymerizes a small area in the murein of the bacteria cell wall. The myosin-like sheath of the virus then contracts and the solid core pierces the bacterial membrane; finally the viral DNA is injected into the cytoplasm (Lwoff, 1961).

During the short period of its life-cycle when a virus is extracellular, it is susceptible to chemicals, even to dilute soap solution. However, no useful attack can be made on virus diseases unless the viruses can be killed in the parasitized cell without harm to uninfected host cells. The unique structure of virions encourage the hope that a selective attack on them can be devised.

For more on the sequence of virus invasion of the host cell and reproduction there, and for chemotherapy with the new antiviral drugs, see Section 6.3b. For further reading on viruses, see Fenner *et al.*, 1974.

6 Chemotherapy: history and principles

concl. ?

Discussion in the last three chapters of the three principles that govern selectivity, provides the scientific basis for a review, in the present chapter, of the history and principles of chemotherapy and (in the next chapter) of pharmacodynamics. The study of history grows in interest the more we realize that our best drugs are losing their value, due to drug resistance and metabolic destruction, grim phenomena that continue to plague the drug designer's best efforts. History helps us go back in time to the period just before a discovery was made so that we can see how it was achieved, sometimes in a most unfavourable climate of opinion. Thus we may hope, by reviewing the circumstances in which remarkable new discoveries were made, to learn better how to make others.

6.0 The early history of chemotherapy

Micro-organisms were discovered by Antonie van Leeuwenhoek in Delft (Holland) in 1676, but their role in causing infections, plagues, and epidemics was established only two centuries later, by Robert Koch through his work on anthrax. Koch, and his four postulates for ensuring that a suspected microbe actually caused a given disease, made it possible for biologists to study infectious diseases experimentally for the first time. This set the scene for the discovery of chemotherapy, but it was slow to arrive as we shall see.

In 1891, Romanovsky made a most significant observation in St Petersburg (Russia). By the use of his special microscopic stain (eosin-methylene blue) he showed that the malarial parasite was damaged in the blood of patients undergoing treatment with quinine. The greatest effect was on the asexual intracorpuscular forms, whose nuclei quickly disintegrated. After two days, no parasites could be seen in the blood. This led Romanovsky to state that quinine cured malaria *by damaging the parasite more than the host*. This conclusion had great historical importance, because no one had previously thought that a drug could act in this way, (The protozoon which caused malaria had been discovered by Laveran in 1880). Romanovsky predicted that specifics for other diseases would eventually be found, substances that would cause minimal damage to the tissues of the host, and maximal damage to the parasites (Romanovsky, 1891). This line of thought was so little in tune with the intellectual climate of the times that it was not further pursued, until Ehrlich resumed it with energy and insight, and discovered chemotherapy.

The term *chemotherapy* was coined by Paul Ehrlich (1854–1915), who defined it as *the use of drugs to injure an invading organism without injury to the host*. As his pupil Carl Browning wrote in 1929: (pg 181)

'Chemotherapy is a term coined by Ehrlich to indicate the treatment of infections by compounds, of known chemical constitution, which effect cure by leading to destruction of the pathogenic organisms or their products. Thus a contrast is implied between chemotherapeutic substances and the class of antibodies, which represent highly complex, specific products of the biological reaction to the infecting organisms.'

The essence of chemotherapy is the achievement of a differential effect whereby the host, in his struggle with a parasite, gains some advantage through the introduction of a drug. This leaves the majority of the struggle to be done by the host's leucocytes and other natural defensive forces, but a useful drug can tip the balance in the host's favour.

The progress of chemotherapy was greatly speeded by the non-identity of the economic and the uneconomic species (see Section 1.0), for this gave the possibility of examining (and even culturing) the parasite independently of the host. As a result, the governing principles of chemotherapy have been brought to light much sooner than those of pharmacodynamics

(Chapter 7). The present chapter is concerned with the nature of these principles and the historical background which led to their discovery.

A few chemotherapeutic agents were known before Ehrlich's time. These were cinchona bark and ipecacuanha rhizome, for the cure of malaria and amoebic dysentery respectively, and mercury for alleviation of the symptoms of syphilis. Mercury began to be used in this way in the sixteenth century, cinchona and ipecacuanha in the seventeenth. Santonin and male fern have been used as anthelmintics since classical times. In view of the many centuries during which medication had been practised, this list is remarkable only for its brevity.

6.1 Ehrlich's fundamental contributions

It is customary to take 1899 as the start of Ehrlich's interest in chemo-therapy. At that time he was 45 years old, and had just been appointed Director of the Königliches Institut für experimentelle Therapie, in Frankfurt (Germany). Up to that date, his work had consisted of applications of chemistry to the furthering of biological knowledge, and selectivity was his guiding light. His earliest work, on the distribution of lead in the body, revealed preferential accumulation in the central nervous system. Next came his discoveries of the differential staining of tissues by dyes. His technique and his division of the stained leucocytes into acidophil, basophil, neutrophil, and non-granular, is used by clinical pathologists to this day. Belonging to this period is his discovery of vital staining (using methylene blue and neutral red), and his ranking of the different tissues of the body by their comparative oxygen requirements.

All of this work he capped by outstanding discoveries in immuno-chemistry. He showed, by the first test-tube experiments to be done in

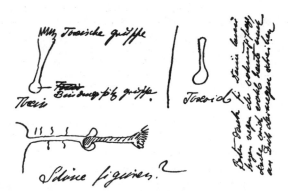

FIG. 6.1 Ehrlich's explanation of immunochemistry in his own symbols (from a letter to Carl Weigert, 1898, in which he gives the first pictorial representation of his side-chain theory). (Heymann, 1928.)

the field of immunity, that the neutralization of toxin by antitoxin, and antigen by antibody, are direct reactions which do not require the presence of a living mammal, as had been thought. He then went on to state his side-chain theory, a chemical interpretation of the immune process, as follows. An antigen has two active areas, namely the *haptophore* (anchorer) and the *toxophile* (poisoner). Mammalian cells, he believed, have 'side-chains' which contain *receptors*, i.e. groups or regions that are complementary to the haptophores, and hence anchor them (see Fig. 6.1). This combination, he taught, was in itself harmless but brought the toxophile close enough to the cell to poison it. He believed that the normal function of the receptors was to anchor nutrient molecules. [For more on antibodies, which have a mol. wt. of 150 000, see Nisonoff, Hopper and Spring, (1975)].

His experimental investigations on immunity, begun in 1893, led to discovery of an accurate method for standardizing diphtheria antitoxin. This prompted the State to create the Royal Institute for Experimental Therapy*, for the statutory control of sera and vaccines. When Ehrlich assumed the Directorship in 1899, his reputation as a chemical pathologist had already been established internationally. He could well have rested on his laurels, but the chemist in him made him eager to launch out in an entirely new direction: the cure of infectious diseases with *small* molecules, specific enough to be 'magic bullets' that could harm only the invader.

In visits to the Hoechst works near Frankfurt, Ehrlich was brought face to face with the German synthetic chemical industry and saw the manufacture of a profusion of synthetic analgesics, antipyretics, and anaesthetics (see Section 7.1). It seemed logical to him that, because the factories were turning out simple substances that differentiated between various tissues in man, it should be possible to synthesize other small molecules which would differentiate between man and his parasites. The emphasis on low molecular weight illustrates the contrast which Ehrlich made between immunotherapy and chemotherapy. He realized that immunotherapy was a matter of strengthening the defence forces of the body, but he conceived of chemotherapy as a direct attack upon the parasite. The problem, as he saw it, was to find chemicals with very much stronger affinities for the parasites than for the tissues of the host.

Many of Ehrlich's contemporaries did not think his new line of research was reasonable or likely to succeed. The State, in particular, had expected him to confine his research to immunology in the new institute, and noted that chemotherapeutic research would be very expensive because of the large number of experimental animals required. A compromise was reached that Ehrlich might investigate the therapy of cancer with small molecules. He took up this cancer work late in 1901, pursued it for a few years and made some interesting observations, but realized that in many ways the

* Originally in Berlin, later moved to Frankfurt at that city's request.

time was not ripe for this kind of work, and dropped it without publishing.

From 1904 onwards Ehrlich concerned himself chiefly with chemotherapy, selecting trypanosomiasis in the mouse as his principal model.
Conditions for this work were poor in his Institute, and became steadily
worse. However, in 1906 his gloom was dispersed by the splendid action
of a benefactor, Frau Franziska Speyer who had come to regard Ehrlich's
work with the greatest affection. In memory of her late husband, she
purchased a large house near the University, and named it the Georg
Speyer Haus which she equipped and handsomely endowed for Ehrlich
to pursue his research into chemotherapy. These chemical and biological
laboratories became the Mecca for the cream of Europe's young drug
scientists. Ehrlich thus became, virtually, Director of two Institutes.

Ehrlich's first chemotherapeutic experiments were performed with
dyes. Three series gave good results in the chemotherapy of trypanosomiasis
in the mouse, namely the acridines, the triphenylmethanes, and the azo
dyes, but none was outstanding. True, in 1904 Ehrlich cured trypanosome-
infected mice with trypan red (a polyazo dye), which thereby became the
first man-made chemotherapeutic agent. This aroused interest, but unfortunately the drug was inactive in man, and his thoughts turned to organic
arsenical compounds.

The status of arsenicals in infectious diseases at the beginning of the
present century can be judged from the following. In 1902, Laveran and
Mesnil injected arsenious acid (HO·As:O) into mice infected with trypanosomiasis. All the mice died, but they 'died cured' which was considered
a great advance at the time. In 1905, Thomas and Breinl (in Liverpool) had
shown that an arsenical drug, 'Atoxyl' (6.1), had a slight, favourable action
on human trypanosomiasis.* This discovery influenced Ehrlich to commence prolonged experimentation with aromatic arsenicals.

Atoxyl   Arsphenamine (monomer)   Oxophenarsine
(6.1)   (6.2)   (6.3)

In 1908, a Nobel Prize in Medicine was awarded Ehrlich, 'in recognition
of his work on Immunity'. Chemotherapy was not mentioned. Even in
Germany, many of his colleagues thought that his interpretations were
wild, and had completely outrun the evidence. It could not be denied that

* The rather optimistically-named 'Atoxyl' (p-aminophenylarsonic acid) was discovered in
1860 by Béchamp, whose wrongly assigned constitution was corrected later by Ehrlich and
Bertheim (1907).

Ehrlich had been working intensely on his self-chosen, seemingly improbable subject for ten years without producing even one result of use in human medicine.

Yet this run of bad luck was suddenly to change, for in 1910 a discovery of utmost significance was made, namely the antisyphilitic drug arsphenamine (6.2), whose laboratory code number had been '606' (Ehrlich and Hata, 1910). It happened as follows. In 1905 Schaudinn had discovered that the causative organism of syphilis was a highly motile bacterium (a spirochaete)

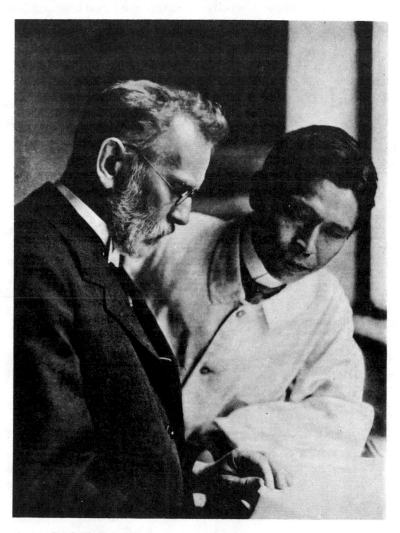

PLATE 3   Paul Ehrlich (1854–1915) and Sahachiro Hata (1873–1938), who together discovered the curative action of arsphenamine ('Salvarsan') in syphilis.

which he named *Treponema pallidum*. Hata, working in the Kitasato Institute for Infectious Diseases in Tokyo, followed by discovering how to produce this disease in rabbits. Hence, for the first time, an experimental model was available for laboratory work in this disease. (Parenthetically it must be noted that, over and over again, progress in chemotherapy was to await discovery of a suitable laboratory model, in one disease after another). Hearing of Hata's discovery, Ehrlich lost no time in bringing him to the Georg Speyer Haus (see Plate 3).

It may seen a vast leap for Ehrlich to transfer his interest from a protozoon (*Trypanosoma*) to a bacterium (*Treponema*), but there was this in common: both were incessantly motile organisms, precariously dependant on a widly racing metabolism. Ehrlich had an intuition* that *Treponema* would yield to his new arsenicals. Of these, he now had examples with increased selectivity, thanks to the collaboration of Professor A. Bertheim and Drs Kahn and Schmitz, chemists who had learnt to synthesize a wide variety of organic arsenical compounds, difficult though this task turned out to be (Ehrlich, 1909).

The synthesis of arsphenamine was reported by Ehrlich and Bertheim (1912) and it was patented and then manufactured by the firm Hoechst (DRP 224 953), and sold by them under the name 'Salvarsan'. The initial announcement of a cure for syphilis was taken up by the newspapers, and Ehrlich became a world celebrity overnight. This affected him little, for he had worries that arose from the discovery. For example, arsphenamine was oxidized in the air to a more toxic product, now known to be oxophenarsine (*6.3*) a much more selective and desirable drug, and one that would in time replace arsphenamine (see Section 6.2). However, at that time, the uncontrolled oxidations were causing deaths, so that Ehrlich decided that arsphenamine must be issued only as single doses, and in sealed tubes from which all oxygen had been removed. He also issued directions for the preparation of solutions in sterile distilled water, neutralization, and intravenous injection without delay. These directions were often departed from, and the resulting disasters attracted unfortunate publicity. Ehrlich later introduced neoarsphenamine ('914'), a more soluble derivative.

Ehrlich always had entertained hopes of his 'magic bullets' curing with a single dose, but arsphenamine was not selective enough for a sufficiently large dose to be given. Hence treatment with it had to be spread over several months (Ehrlich, 1911).

From the observation point of today, there can be no doubt that arsphenamine, with all its faults, was the opening event in the chemotherapeutic revolution which transformed all treatment of infectious diseases. This happy result owes much to Ehrlich's quantitative approach.

---

* H. Uhlenhuth had noticed a slight, favourable effect of atoxyl in human syphilis, but increasing the dose caused blindness (Ehrlich, 1909).

In seeking drugs which would have a great affinity for the invader and little for the host, Ehrlich introduced the 'Chemotherapeutic Index' which he defined as the ratio:

$$\frac{\text{minimal curative dose}}{\text{maximal tolerated dose}}$$

Thus a substance which was curative of trypanosomiasis in mice at 2 mg/kg, and did not kill below 50 mg/kg, would have an Index of 1/25 (Ehrlich, 1911). Thus the idea of selective toxicity* was provided with a yardstick for measuring the degree of selectivity. How this measure was later developed and refined will be seen in Section 6.2.

When Ehrlich had transferred his interests from large molecules to small ones, he drew on part of his 'side-chain' (immunological) hypothesis to explain the mode of action of chemotherapeutic agents. They too, he supposed, had distinct haptophoric and toxophilic groups (he demonstrated this for arsenicals; see the end of this Section), and they combined with cellular receptors whose normal function was to take part in cellular nutrition or respiration.

Ehrlich insisted that drugs acted upon cells by ordinary chemical reactions. This is substantially the present-day view, although the phrase 'ordinary chemical reactions' conjures up a much wider variety of bonds than was known in Ehrlich's time (see Section 8.0). Ehrlich's highly original concepts, of chemically reactive groups on drugs and of chemically reactive receptors for them on cells, made an important advance in biological thought. His thesis that the most effective drugs would have a fairly low molecular weight has been well substantiated. Table 6.1 shows a representative selection of chemotherapeutic drugs. The molecular weights range from about 140 to 1400, the latter being unusually high. On the other hand, γ-globulin, of which antibodies are fashioned, has a molecular weight of 150 000.

The work done by Ehrlich and his band of collaborators in the Georg Speyer Haus did not stand high in the esteem of all contemporary scientists. Many people of this period thought that his interpretations had outrun the experimental evidence. Chief among Ehrlich's critics was Uhlenhuth, an influential and respected pathologist. Uhlenhuth contended that drugs had no direct action on the parasite, but worked by stimulating the natural defences of the host. He made the most of the fact that 'Atoxyl' and trypan red can cure trypanosomiasis in the animals and yet do not attack trypanosomes in the test-tube (Uhlenhuth, 1907). This objection was taken seriously because these substances were two of Ehrlich's most important experimental agents. But in 1909 Ehrlich discovered that *tri*valent arsenicals

* The phrase 'selective toxicity' was born long after Ehrlich's time. I first heard it in an entomology symposium in Australia, about 1940.

Table 6.1

THE LOW ORDER OF COMPLEXITY OF TYPICAL CHEMOTHERAPEUTIC AGENTS

Substance	Number of atoms per molecule	Molecular weight
Isoniazid	17	137
Oxine	18	145
Sulphanilamide	19	172
Aminacrine	25	194
Oxophenarsine ('Mapharside')	16	199
Pyrimethamine	30	249
Sulphadiazine	27	250
Chloroquine	48	320
Chloramphenicol	32	323
Quinine	48	325
Pentamidine	49	332
Penicillin	41	356
Tetracycline	56	408
Emetine	75	480
Streptomycin	79	582
Suramin	126	1429
For comparison		
Glucose	24	180
γ-Globulin	32 000	150 000

were trypanocidal in the test-tube and he suggested that pentavalent arsenicals would also be found active if it were possible to keep trypanosomes alive in culture until they had time to reduce the drug. That this was actually so was not proved until (15 years after his death) a better culture method became available. However, Ehrlich did show that pentavalent arsenicals became active *in vitro* if they were first incubated with a reducing tissue (e.g. liver), and this result served to explain their activity *in vivo*.

The discovery of drug-resistance (discussed in Section 6.5) in Ehrlich's laboratories gave welcome support to his chemical hypothesis of absorption and combination. Ehrlich observed that those trypanosomes which were resistant to trypan red did not absorb it, whereas susceptible trypanosomes were stained red by the dye. Thus the resistant parasites, by selective breeding, had lost one of the chemical groups that combined with the dye. Later, Ehrlich found two strains of trypansomes, each resistant to a different kind of organic (aromatic) arsenical. There was no cross-resistance between these strains. Because no trypanosomes are resistant to inorganic arsenic (e.g. $HO \cdot As : O$), Ehrlich concluded (i) that the resistance was directed against certain substituents in the benzene ring, (ii) that these substituents (e.g. $-NH_2$) were responsible for the uptake of the aromatic arsenicals by the parasite, and (iii) that the arsenoxide group ($-As : O$) was responsible for the death of the parasites. These results indicated the chemical composition of both haptophoric- and toxophilic-groups in those arsenicals which have selectivity (only *aromatic* arsenicals are selective, see Section 12.0).

For an account of Ehrlich's aims, and a sample of his rather rhetorical style, see his address to the German Chemical Society in 1908 (Ehrlich, 1909). For more biographical material, see Muir, (1921); Browning (1955); Himmelweit (1956); also the 'Paul Ehrlich Centennial' issue (1954) of the *Annals of the New York Academy of Sciences* which includes assessments by various authors of Ehrlich's work and its present-day developments.

6.2 Chemotherapeutic drugs available before 1935. The chemotherapeutic index

Although the discovery of sulphonamides in 1935 immensely quickened the pace of chemotherapeutic research, the principles that govern chemotherapeutic action had been brought to light before that date. Before Ehrlich died in 1915, the following advances bore witness to the faith in chemotherapy that he had treated. Antimony, in the form of tartar emetic, was shown to cure trypanosomiasis in mice (Plimmer and Thompson, 1907) and to influence the disease favourably, but without cure, in man (Manson, 1908). In Ehrlich's Institute 'Optochin', a simple derivative of quinine, cured pneumonia in the mouse, but was ineffective in man (Morgenroth and Levy, 1911). Next, tartar emetic (*12.5*) was introduced as a clinical treatment for the protozoal disease leishmaniasis by Vianna (1912) in Brazil. About this time, Rogers found that emetine (*4.34*) was the most active principle in ipecacuanha, and used it to cure advanced amoebiasis in man (Rogers, 1912). Ehrlich had just shown that euflavine ('Trypaflavin') (*6.4*), which Benda had synthesized for him at the Hoechst works, could cure trypanosomiasis in mice, but it was useless in man (Ehrlich, 1912). Thus the only clinically useful drugs discovered by Ehrlich were arsphenamine ('Salvarsan') and its solubilized derivatives. His influence on the development of chemotherapy came not so much from these discoveries as from his clear delineation of the principles involved in treating infectious diseases with chemicals of low molecular weight.

Euflavine ('Trypaflavine')
(*6.4*)

Proflavine
(3,6-diaminoacridine)
(*6.5*)

In 1913, Browing, a former pupil of Ehrlich, discovered the remarkably selective antibacterials, acriflavine and proflavine (6.5), which were chemically allied to euflavine (Browning and Gilmour, 1913). Apart from an extensive use of these acridines in wounds, the First World War passed without any notable advance in chemotherapy. The control of bacterial infection in the blood-stream was still an unrealized dream, and the feeling was widespread that chemotherapy had promised more than it was likely to give. This pessimism was premature, particularly as research on protozoal diseases was prospering. To begin with, Christopherson worked out dose schedules that made antimonials, for many long years, the drugs of choice in schistosomiasis (Christopherson, 1918), and other important remedies quickly followed.

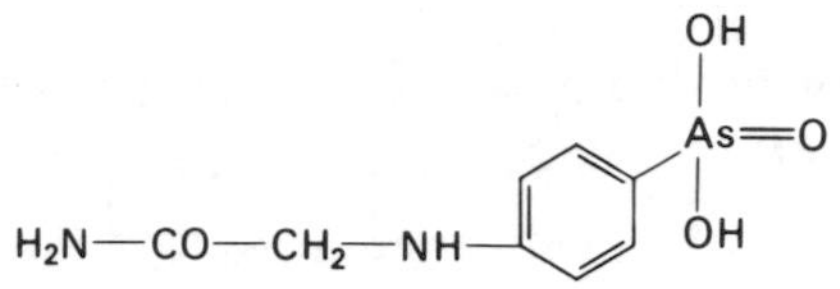

Tryparsamide
(6.6)

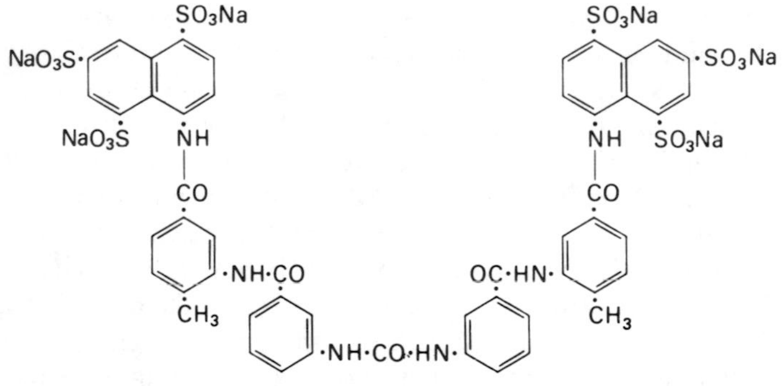

Suramin
(6.7)

In 1920, two drugs were discovered which became the basis of a successful treatment of sleeping sickness. These were (a) tryparsamide (6.6), a pentavalent arsenical derived from, but less toxic than, 'Atoxyl' (Jacobs and Heidelberger, 1919; Brown and Pearce, 1919), and (b) suramin ('Bayer 205', 'Germanin'), a colourless and highly effective analogue of trypan red (Heymann et al., 1917). Suramin (6.7) was later used for prophylaxis after it was found that a single dose gave immunity for three months (Roehl, 1920; Heymann, 1924). The next notable advance was the introduction of the first synthetic antimalarials, pamaquine ('Plasmoquine') (6.8) (Roehl, 1926a;

Schulemann *et al.*, 1932), and mepacrine (*6.9*) ('Atebrin') (Kikuth, 1932; Mauss and Mietzsch, 1933). They were inspired by the weak antimalarial action that Guttmann and Ehrlich (1891) had found in methylene blue (*6.10*), but systematic work had to await discovery of a test object, and Roehl found this in malaria-infected finches.

In 1930, Leake introduced carbarsone (*6.11*) for the treatment of amoebiasis, a less nauseating drug than emetine which was henceforth reserved for the severer cases. Interestingly, this organic arsenical (4-ureidobenzenearsonic acid) had been synthesized by Bertheim in 1907, and found unsuccessful by Ehrlich against trypanosomiasis and syphilis (Leake, Koch and Anderson, 1930). Until the discovery by Laidlaw, *et al.* (1928) of a method of cultivating entamoebae *in vitro*, the experimental study of amoebicides had been severely handicapped.

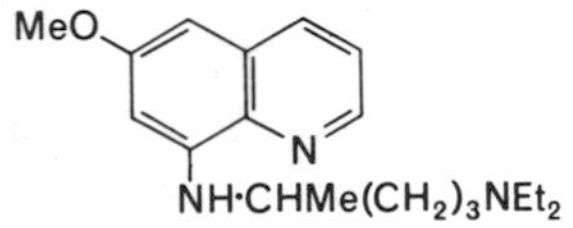

Pamaquine
(*6.8*)

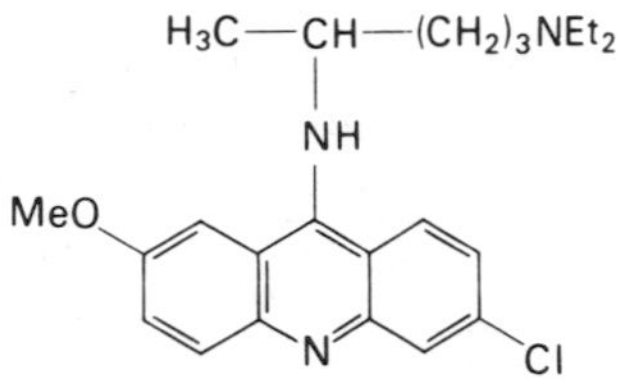

Mepacrine
(Quinacrine, 'Atebrin')
(*6.9*)

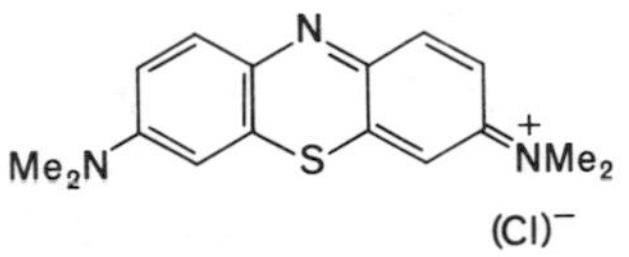

Methylene blue
(*6.10*)

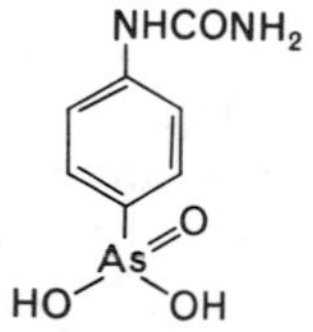

Carbarsone
(*6.11*)

All these discoveries were made by pursuing clues which Ehrlich and his school had revealed. Indicative of the impact that chemotherapy was now making was the German State's ban of any disclosure of the constitution of suramin and mepacrine, because of the potential they lent to tropical warfare. This was a complete swing of the pendulum from the State's apathy in 1899. (Parenthetically, the secrecy was short-lived: the constitution of suramin was solved by Fourneau *et al.* in 1924 at the Pasteur Institute in Paris, and Maghidson and Grigorovski, in Moscow, published that of mepacrine in 1933).

The year (1932) was notable not only for the introduction of mepacrine, but for the discovery by Tatum and Cooper of a much safer arsenical drug for use in syphilis, namely oxophenarsine (6.3) ('Mapharside') (Tatum and Cooper, 1934). This drug had been discovered by Ehrlich and his colleagues and undervalued by them in experimental work, so that the clinical application was not foreseen (see Section 12.0).

Yorke, Adams and Murgatroyd (1929) had found how to keep trypanosomes alive and unmetamorphosed in the test-tube for two days, whereas Ehrlich had only moribund parasites *in vitro*. With the help of this new technique, Yorke, Murgatroyd and Hawking (1931) showed that when normal trypansomes were treated with a solution of a trivalent arsenical, they were rapidly killed and the solution would not kill fresh trypanosomes. On the other hand, when arsenic-resistant trypanosomes were treated with a trivalent arsenical, they were not killed, and the residual solution would still kill susceptible trypanosomes. It was then shown that the bodies of the killed parasites contained measurable amounts of arsenic and that the resistant parasites contained none (Reiner, Leonard and Chao, 1932). Advances in technique made it possible for others to show that fixation of drugs by the parasite could take place while the latter was actually circulating in the host's blood-steam. Thus v. Jancsó (1932) used the fluorescent microscope to show that 'Trypaflavin' was taken up in this way. These discoveries confirmed the idea that accumulation of the drug by the parasite was a necessary step in the drug's lethal action, thus fulfilling one of Ehrlich's main predictions, one that had been controversial in his lifetime.

Another prediction confirmed in this period was the co-operation between drug and the host's defence forces. Ehrlich had held the view that the function of a drug was to disorganize the parasite's metabolism, after which the natural defence forces of the body would complete the actual destruction of the invader. This was confirmed when Kritschewsky (1927, 1928) showed that the host's reticulo-endothelial system provided such co-operation, because when this was artificially damaged, the efficiency of chemotherapeutic drugs was lowered greatly.

That a parasite need not be harmed merely by taking up a foreign substance, followed from Ehrlich's teaching that the haptophoric (anchoring) and toxophilic (poisoning) portions of a substance were distinct entities. Techniques of vital staining have now made this concept familiar.

As momentous as any discovery in the period we are considering, was the first demonstration of the chemical nature of the union between a drug and a parasite. This was accomplished by Voegtlin and his colleagues in the United States Public Health Services, who showed that the toxic action of arsenicals was due to the formation of As–S bonds with essential thiol-groups in the parasites (see Section 12.0). This, too, had been predicted by Ehrlich (1909).

Thus, at the end of this period, the scientific principles of chemotherapy, as foreshadowed by Ehrlich, had become established. It was now generally agreed that substances of relatively low molecular weight make the most satisfactory chemotherapeutic drugs, that their action is directly on the parasite, and that their reaction with the parasite is chemical in nature. Ehrlich's division of a drug into haptophoric and toxophilic portions still reminds us to look closely at the structure of every agent and to ask what each group is contributing to the total effect. But today we know that the properties of a molecule also depend on the electronic interaction of its component parts which, according to well-known laws of chemistry, augment or diminish one another's influence in fairly predictable ways (see Appendix III).

The Chemotherapeutic Index.   Ehrlich's Index (Section 6.1) has under-gone some changes. In the course of time, it came to be used as a reciprocal *refer back* (i.e. 25 instead of 1/25). It was found later that more repeatable results can be obtained if the LD_{50} (dose killing 50 per cent of the test animals) was used instead of the maximal tolerated dose, and if CD_{50} (dose curing 50 per cent of the animals) replaced the minimal curative dose. The Chemotherapeutic Index makes it clear that it is no advantage to find a new substance with half the toxicity to the host unless the new substance is *more* than half as active. With this idea to guide them, chemists and biologists have discovered drugs of tremendously improved Chemotherapeutic Index in the last 40 years. The toxicity of the best sulphonamide antibacterials to mammals is so low that it is difficult to measure accurately; that of penicillin is almost negligible.

The adoption of the LD_{50} was due to the English mathematician J. W. Trevan, who showed that there is a Gaussian distribution of variations in the intensity of cellular responses to a given dose of a drug. Fig. 6.2 makes this clear. When these intensities were summated for increasing dosage in accordance with the percentage of cells responding, a sigmoid relationship was obtained (Fig. 6.3; Trevan, 1927; Trevan and Boock, 1926).

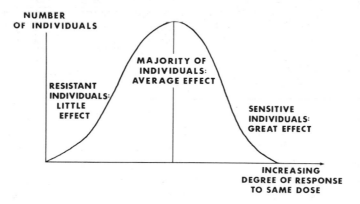

FIG. 6.2 A normal distribution curve.

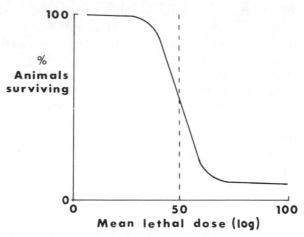

FIG. 6.3 A sigmoid dose response curve.

Many aspects of the relationships between dose and effect, particularly as regards time and concentration, were analysed by Clark (1933, 1937). Further statistical analysis showed that the safety of a drug is better established by comparing CD_{99} with LD_1, namely the dose which cures 99 per cent of the hosts is compared with the dose which kills 1 per cent of them. Judged by these high standards, several drugs now in use, particularly the cardiac glycosides, are seen to require a substitute with a better Chemotherapeutic Index.

6.3 1935 and afterwards

The year 1935 forms a natural division in the history of chemotherapy because of Domagk's discovery of the chemotherapeutic properties of 'Prontosil', the first of the antibacterial sulphonamides. This discovery refuted a prejudice that chemotherapy applied mainly to protozoal diseases, and it opened a new era in medical and surgical treatment. Wood's later discovery (1940), that sulphonamides blocked the use by bacteria of one of their essential constituents (p-aminobenzoic acid), gave detailed support to Ehrlich's postulate that drugs combined with receptors in such a way as to prevent normal nutrients from reaching them (see Section 9.3a).

(a) *Antibacterials*

Antibacterial sulphonamides.   The discovery of sulphachrysoidine, (*3.16*, p. 87) ('Prontosil'), followed a strange course. Gerhard Domagk (1895–1964), who later received a Nobel prize for this work, was a pathologist, studying the phagocytosis of streptococci by the Kupffer cells of the liver. This he was doing in the research laboratories of the Bayer company in Elberfeld, Germany. Needing to weaken the pathogenicity of the bacteria, he recalled a technique of Ehrlich's and asked for a selection of azo-dyes. Among those given him was 'Prontosil' which Mietzsch and Klarer had recently synthesized for textile adornment. Noting how well his animals survived injection of the dye-treated streptococci, Domagk tried the effect of 'Prontosil' on established streptococcal infection in mice. The result was dramatically successful (Domagk, 1935). However his employers, reflecting the current climate of opinion, moved very slowly: they had seen many candidate drugs, including azo-dyes, fail as systemic antibacterials.

Domagk was immensely disappointed, but fate played a remarkable trick. On the fourth of December 1935, his little daughter who was making a Christmas present, punctured her hand with a needle while running down stairs for her mother to rethread it. Although she was rushed to hospital, and received the best treatment available in those times, severe inflammation and fever soon set in. Four days later, she seemed likely to die from streptococcal septicaemia, as was not at all uncommon in those days. Domagk begged for permission to administer 'Prontosil': the speed of her recovery confounded the physicians (Domagk, 1936). Almost ignored in Germany, the first large and controlled clinical application of 'Prontosil' took place in London, where Colebrook and Kenny (1936) demonstrated its power in saving moribund mothers from puerperal sepsis. The drug was now truly launched.

A discovery of great importance for perfecting Domagk's discovery was made late in 1935 by Tréfouël and his co-workers in the Institut Pasteur, who showed that the inactivity of 'Prontosil' towards bacteria in test-tube experiments could be overcome by adding a reducing substance. In devising this experiment, they were guided by Ehrlich's parallel activation of pentavalent arsenicals (Section 6.1). Later, they were able to show that not only did the mammalian body reduce 'Prontosil' to give sulphanilamide* (*3.17*, p. 87), but that this substance was equally active (and helpfully much more soluble) in the treatment of bacteraemia. Had the French workers not made this discovery, the evolution of sulphonamides would very likely have continued on 'hit-and-miss' lines, with immense resources squandered in the search for new types of *coloured* sulphonamides.

An important scientific advance was made when Marshall (1937) showed that the effect of sulphanilamide was proportional to the concentration reached in the blood of the patient being treated, and that, for a given dose, this varied from patient to patient. This was the beginning of the analytical control of blood levels during chemotherapy, although it was soon found

---

* Sulphanilamide, synthesized by Gelmo in 1908, was not known to have any biological activity. Yet, because 'Prontosil' was made from it, its antibacterial nature could easily have been observed in Elberfeld.

that the activity of some substances (e.g. mepacrine) is not proportional to their concentration in blood if greater concentrations exist, loosely bound, in the tissues.

The mode of action of sulphonamides was greatly clarified by Woods in 1940. It had been shown that tissue extracts, pus, bacteria, and particularly yeast extract contained a heat-stable substance of low molecular weight which would inhibit the action of sulphonamides on bacteria (Stamp, 1939). Woods, recalling that enzymes are inhibited by substances which chemically and sterically resemble their substrates (see Section 9.3a), adopted this hypothesis: that the inhibitory substance in yeast is the substrate of an enzyme widely distributed in nature, and that it resembles sulphanilamide chemically. He found activity was concentrated in an alkali-soluble fraction of yeast, and that it ran parallel to a colour test for an aromatic amino-group. Activity was lost on esterification or acetylation, recovered on hydrolysis, and lost again on treatment with nitrous acid (Woods, 1940). Thus he made it clear that the active substance was an aromatic aminoacid. Because p-aminobenzoic acid (pAB) (*2.13*, p. 28) is the aromatic aminoacid that most resembles sulphanilamide (*2.12*) he tried it as an inhibitor of bacteriostasis, and found that one molecule could prevent 5000 to 25 000 molecules of sulphanilamide from functioning.

Next, pAB was isolated (as the benzoyl-derivative) from yeast by Rubbo and Gillespie (1940), who showed that it was a growth-factor for a bacterium (*Clostridium acetobutylicum*), i.e. it was essential for this bacterium in the way that vitamins are for human beings. Since 1940, it has been found to be essential for many families and genera of micro-organisms, including the malarial parasite; most micro-organisms do not require an *external* source of pAB because they synthesize it. That the antagonistic action of pAB was exerted also *in vivo* was shown by Selbie (1940), who found that simultaneous administration of this acid prevented sulphanilamide from curing mice infected with streptococci.

Knowledge of this antagonism between sulphonamides and pAB, of Voegtlin's work on the mode of action of arsenic (see Section 12.0), and of his own similar work with mercurials, led Fildes (1940a) to appeal for a more rational approach to chemotherapy. He pointed out that the action of a drug on a parasite had much in common with the inhibition of an enzyme by a foreign substance, and that many of the most successful enzyme inhibitors were analogues of substrates. [This relationship was already well established in pharmacodynamics (see Sections 2.0 and 9.2).] Fildes discussed two main types of enzyme inactivation as models for new drugs: (a) the inhibitor combines with the enzyme, and displaces a similarly constituted substrate or coenzyme, and (b) the inhibitor combines with the substrate or coenzyme.

This visualization of some of Ehrlich's receptors as enzymes provided an incentive for biochemists to study the enzymes of parasites, to discover the nature of the substrates, and to synthesize molecules that would be like enough to these substrates to be accepted by the bacterium, and yet different enough to interrupt its vital processes. By developing Fischer's analogy that enzymes and their substrates have a lock-and-key relationship, a chemo-therapeutic agent could be seen as a key that fits the lock only well enough to jam it (see Section 9.1). This thought was received with too much enthusiasm! Countless analogues of natural metabolites were synthesized, but the majority of these proved to be as toxic to the host as to the parasite. Why these misfortunes occurred, and how they were overcome, is discussed in Chapter 9.

Antibiotics. Seven years after the sulphonamides appeared on the scene, penicillin, the first chemotherapeutic antibiotic, began to be used in the clinic. Antibiotics are toxic substances, of low molecular weight, secreted by few bacteria but by many other prokaryotes, and by a few fungi, most of them the lower fungi known as moulds. Most antibiotics are insufficiently selective to be used in medicine, but some twenty highly selective kinds are right in the forefront of current prescribing.

The name 'antibiotic' is a misnomer because it implies that organisms secrete these substances to fight their natural enemies. However, if penicil-lin were of survival value to *Penicillium notatum*, the few strains which manufacture this substance would be the commonest examples of this species whereas, in nature, they are actually the most uncommon. The fact is that bacteria and fungi produce what we call antibiotics at the time when they have completed the fast, logarithmic phase of growth, and stasis has set in. To get the highest yields, manufacturers of antibiotics make full use of this static phase, hastening its commencement and prolonging it arti-ficially. Woodruff (1966) thought that stasis allowed existing enzymes to act on substrates which would normally have been used for growth and whose production, in higher forms of life, would be suppressed at this stage by feedback mechanisms. This, he suggested, was the origin of most of the antibiotics. Among true bacteria, only sporulating organisms produce antibiotics (all of which are polypeptides), and this production occurs only at the end of logarithmic growth (Schaeffer, 1969). It has been suggested that antibiotics are made by the bacteria to switch off normal metabolism, thus preparing the cell for sporulation (Schazschneider *et al.*, 1974). These authors note, for example, that tryocidin combines with DNA, in a way that inactivates many of the genes responsible for vegetative growth.

Before mentioning the principal types of antibiotics now available, the discovery and application of these substances will be briefly described. In 1929, Fleming discovered that a particular strain of the mould *Penicillium notatum*, which landed in, and lysed, a culture of staphylococci in his Lon-don laboratory, secreted a substance of low molecular weight that was highly toxic to Gram-positive bacteria, and had a low toxicity to mammals. However, he found it too unstable to isolate and did not persevere further.

In 1938, it occurred to Florey that much more potent antibiotics should be obtainable from bacteria and fungi than the known but feebly active examples: hydrogen peroxide, alcohol, pyocyanase, and acetic acid. Systematic investigations by Florey, Chain and their colleagues at Oxford led them back to penicillin and they discovered how to isolate it in a pure state (Florey, *et al.*, 1940, 1941, 1949; Chain, 1948). They also demonstrated its remarkable clinical usefulness. At first penicillin was used as the mixture of naturally occurring homologues; later it was found that the best of these, benzyl-penicillin (see Section 12.1), could be produced exclusively if a related mould (*Penicillium chrysogenum*) was grown in the presence of phenylacetic acid (Moyer and Coghill, 1947). Industrial improvements in the fermentation and extraction procedures eventually made penicillin one of the least expensive of chemotherapeutic remedies.

The outstanding success of penicillin, in both local and systemic bacterial infections, followed from its high selectivity, the reason for which is discussed in Section 12.1. The mammalian toxicity is so low that it has come to be regarded as the most innocuous of all antibacterial drugs (however, a small proportion of patients become sensitized to it). In 1948, Brotzu found (in a sewage outfall on the Sardinian coast) another mould, *Cephalosporium*, which gave rise to the related cephalosporin series of antibiotics (see Section 12.2).

The world-wide search for antibiotics led to the discovery of many other antibacterials in cultures of lower organisms. The majority of these proved to be too toxic to mammals. Most of those which have achieved widespread clinical use have been derived not from moulds but from the actinomycetales, a distinct class of prokaryote organisms which, from the nature of their cell walls, are related to the true bacteria. From various species of *Streptomyces*, a genus of the actinomycetales, the following clinically useful antibiotics were obtained: (a) *chloramphenicol*, isolated by Bartz (1948) from a culture obtained from a mulched field in Venezuela, (b) chlorotetracycline ('Aureomycin'), the first of the tetracyclines (Duggar, 1948), in a culture from a Missouri farmyard, (c) *streptomycin* by Waksman, in a culture from the gizzard of a chicken, and later from soils (Schatz, Bugie, and Waksman, 1944). Later, many other examples were derived from yet other actinomycetes, such as adriamycin, amphoteracin, the bleomycins, cycloserine, erythromycin, gentamicin, kanamycin, lincomycin, neomycin, nystatin, oleandomycin, paromomycin, the rifamycins, spectinomycin, vancomycin, and viomycin. From the true bacteria (the eubacteriales) came bacitracin, colistin, the gramicidins and tyrocidins (Dubos, 1939), and the polymixins. A fungus (*Penicillium griseofulvum*) yielded griseofulvin (Oxford, Raistrick and Simonart, 1939) which, like amphotericin and nysatin, has purely antifungal properties (all three are used medicinally). Many antibiotics are undergoing trial as anti-cancer agents (see Section 4.0). Antibiotics act in many ways, but principally:

(a) by interfering with the synthesis of nucleic acid or protein (e.g. actino-
    mycin, the rifamycins, chloramphenicol, streptomycin, the tetra-
    cylines; see Sections 4.0 and 4.1);
(b) by interfering with mucopeptide synthesis and hence the formation of
    new bacterial cell wall (e.g. cycloserine, penicillin, cephalothin; see
    Sections 5.1, 12.1 and 12.2); or
(c) by injury to the cytoplasmic membrane (e.g. amphotericin, polymixin;
    see Section 14.2).

The few that act by interfering with oxidative phosphorylation, or energy-
releasing metabolic steps, e.g. antimycin, oligomycin (see Section 4.4) are
unselective and lack clinical value.

For further reading on the mode of action of antibiotics, see Gottlieb and
Shaw (1967), Franklin and Snow (1975), Gale *et al.* (1972), and the journal:
Antibiotics and Chemotherapy.

New synthetic antibacterials.   The success of antibiotics and sulphonamides as antibacterials encouraged new exploration of simple synthetic
compounds. Isoniazid (*6.12*), a very simple substance (*iso*nicotinic hydrazide), has played the leading part in reducing human tuberculosis from a
dreaded scourge to an easily treated disease. It was discovered simultaneously by three independent laboratories (Offe *et al.*, 1952; Grunberg
and Schnitzer, 1953; Fox, 1953). An even simpler substance, *p*-aminosali-
cylic acid, is a valued adjuvant in this treatment.

$$\underset{\text{N}}{\bigcirc}\overset{\overset{\text{O}}{\parallel}}{\text{C}}-\text{NH·NH}_2$$

Isoniazid
(*6.12*)

Antiseptics active against Gram-negative bacterial rods are uncommon,
but two excellent examples have been introduced in recent years. Of these,
nalidixic acid (*4.14*), is highly active against Gram-negative bacteria in the
urinary tract, but is inactive against Gram-positive species. How it acts by
suppressing the synthesis of DNA was outlined in Section 4.0. The other
example is a nitro-heterocycle. Until about 1945 it was thought that a nitro-
group was too dangerous a substituent to introduce into a drug. This prejudice arose from the many cases of methaemoglobinaemia seen in munitions
works where substances, such as trinitrotoluene, were absorbed through the
skin and became reduced to derivatives of aniline in the body. However,
non-benzenoid nitro-derivatives do not give this reaction. The introduction
of nitrofuran drugs, all of them derivatives of nitrofurfural (*6.13*), by Dodd
in 1946 opened up a rich vein in chemotherapy. Nitrofurantoin(*6.14*)('Fura-

dantin'), given orally as a urinary antispetic, is active against both Gram-positive and -negative organisms. More about nitro-heterocycles will be found under antiprotozoal agents on p. 205.

O₂N—○—CHO

Nitrofurfural
(6.13)

Nitrofurantoin
(6.14)

(b) *Antiviral agents*

Antiviral chemotherapy seems now to have reached the stage which antibacterial chemotherapy had attained in 1940 when, following the discovery of the sulphonamides, only a few effective drugs were available, and yet clues were on hand that were to lead to the discovery of a whole wealth of effective remedies.

When a virus infects a cell, several events occur that are specific for the invader and hence offer opportunities for selective attack. First of all, there is the contact with the cell, then the penetration of the cell's plasma membrane and the (often simultaneous) rejection of the viral coating-protein. If the virus is of the RNA type, reverse transcriptase is soon in manufacture, but in any case the synthesis of nucleic acid polymerases dominates this early stage of invasion. Next follows the synthesis of viral nucleic acids, structural proteins, and yet more enzymes, followed by the assembly of these components to form the complete virus. Finally, some thousands of these virions are liberated from each cell. Apart from the possibilities for finding selective inhibitors for each of these stages, the patient could also be helped by other drugs to control the secondary (non-viral) symptoms, which are often of an inflammatory or anaphylactic character.

Already many substances have been found that show selective antiviral action in cell culture, and several of these have demonstrated prophylactic or therapeutic action *in vivo*.

Kethoxal, 3-ethoxy-2-oxobutanal hydrate [CH₃.CH(OEt).CO.CH-(OH)₂] was the first substance, selectively, to inactivate complete virions, namely those causing Newcastle bird disease and influenza tested in embryonated eggs (Tiffany *et al.*, 1957). 2-Thiouracil (*12.44*), a potent inhibitor of the reproduction of plant viruses, also decreases the infectivity of poliovirus by reaction with a mercapto-group in the capsid (Steele and Black, 1967). However agents such as these which act on the complete virion have not yet proved clinically successful.

Hence it is worth listing, in this paragraph, those antiviral agents which have had some success in human medicine. First, there are the two chemoprophylactic agents: amantadine for the prevention of influenza and methisazone for preventing smallpox. These were intended for use during epidemics when it is too late to vaccinate a population that is at risk. Next come the successful therapeutic agents, idoxuridine for herpes infections of the eye, and the arabinosides of cytosine ('Ara C') and adenine ('Ara A'). for systemic use in generalized herpes.

Chemically, amantadine (*6.15*) ('Symmetrel') is 1-aminoadamantane. Adamantane is tricyclodecane ($C_{10}H_{16}$), a cage-like hydrocarbon. The 1-amino-derivative is a strong base of pK_a 10.1 (Perrin and Hawkins, 1972). Prophylactic treatment with amantadine gives immediate protection as effective against influenza during epidemics as that which would have been provided by immunization, which must be begun two months earlier (Oker-Blom, *et al.*, 1970). The prophylactic dose (0.2 g) is taken orally each day for up to 3 months, and it is excreted unchanged in the urine. Unluckily, it acts on only the A-2 strains of influenza virus, although epidemics with these strains are common, and can be dangerous. In one experiment, 238 volunteers in matched groups were given this drug, in a double-blind test. When challenged with a live vaccine of Asian influenza virus, the protected individuals showed a 60 per cent lower incidence (Jackson, *et al.*, 1963). In a similar experiment on 850 volunteers, this substance was found to be a highly effective preventive and also to decrease symptoms in infected subjects (Wendel, 1964).

Amantadine, at least in fowl-plague virus infections, exerts its effect by inhibiting the uncoating of the virus that has to accompany penetration into host cells (Kato and Eggers, 1919). Non-basic analogues of amantadine (especially alcohols, ketones, esters, and nitriles) are also antiviral and many of these, when tested against Newcastle disease virus on a monolayer culture of chick embryo fibroblasts, showed better selectivity (Aigami *et al.*, 1975). Derivatives of a related cage-nucleus, 4-homo*iso*twistane, also showed good *in vitro* antiviral properties (Aigami *et al.*, 1976). For more on the chemoprophylaxis of influenza, see Oxford (1977).

1-Aminoadamantane
('Amantadine')
(*6.15*)

Methisazone
(*6.16*)

Methisazone (*6.16*) (1-methylisatin-3-thiosemicarbazone, 'Marboran') inhibits the multiplication of vaccinia virus in tissue culture and also in experimental animals. The antiviral action is extraordinarily high. Mice infected intracerebrally with 1000 mean lethal doses (LD_{50}) of vaccinia (cowpox) virus required only 0.5 mg/kg for protection, and only 10 mg/kg was needed for protection against variola major (smallpox) virus. The protective effect is immediate, whereas that of vaccination take 7–10 days to develop. The antiviral spectrum of this drug is wide, *in vitro*. It inhibits multiplication of all pox-viruses, and other DNA viruses too (e.g. the adenoviruses, and varicella), as well as several groups of RNA viruses (e.g. poliomyelitis, common cold, influenza A and B, and some arboviruses).

The oral administration of methisazone was acclaimed as the greatest advance in prophylaxis against smallpox since Jenner's time. During an outbreak in Madras, the drug was given to 1100 people who had been in intimate contact with cases of smallpox. Only three cases, all mild, occurred amongst them, but, in a similar number of untreated people, 78 contracted smallpox and 12 died of it. The drug gave protection even when administered too late in the incubation period for vaccination to be of any use (Bauer *et al.*, 1963). However, it could not cure established infections. Now, following the recent elimination of smallpox from the world, methisazone is little used. It causes such intense nausea that it is never given in virus diseases that are not life-threatening (Turner, Bauer and Nimmo-Smith, 1962).

When both of the hydrogen atoms at the end of the side-chain of this drug are replaced by methyl-groups, the action against vaccinia is completely lost, but higher activity against another poxvirus, ectromelia, is found. Similarly, 'type 2' poliovirus, in tissue-culture, was selectively inactivated by 1-methyl-4′,4′-dibutylisatin thiosemicarbazone (Bauer and Sadler, 1961).

Methisazone does not interfere with the replication of viral DNA, the synthesis of viral mRNA, or the functioning of early viral mRNA. However, by disorganizing the formation of 'late' proteins, it prevents assembly of complete, infectious virions (Woodson and Joklik, 1965; Prusoff, 1967).

The antiviral action of 5-iododeoxyuridine (IUdR) (*4.9*) has already been described in Section 4.0. It is widely prescribed for herpetic infections of the conjunctiva. Cytarabine ('Ara C') (*4.10*), more selective, is used for severe generalized herpes in man (see Section 4.0). Vidarabine ('Ara A') (*4.11*), a newer drug, has given useful clinical results in viral pneumonia and herpetic encephalitis (Section 4.0). The action of all these substances is to block stages in the synthesis of viral nucleic acids.

Striking examples were given in Section 4.0, where extra selectivity can be derived from the fact that the enzymes responsible for the replication of viral nucleic acids are different from the normal host-cell's polymerases, and absent from the uninfected cell (see also Tamm and Eggers, 1965). Sodium phosphonoacetate [$(OH)_2P(:O)CH_2.CO_2Na$], which inhibits DNA polymerase but only the one that is virus-induced (Overby, Duff, and Mao, 1977), is undergoing clinical trials. 'HBB' (2-α-hydroxy-benzylbenzimidazole) (6.17) blocks the synthesis of viral RNA in the host's cells (laboratory animals) without disturbing the host's own RNA synthesis. The picornaviruses (including poliovirus) are specially sensitive to this agent. Selectivity and activity were little changed by alkylating the NH-group, or by acylating, or even alkylating, the hydroxy-group (Tamm et al., 1969).

Considerable outpatient use is being made of a photodynamic treatment of recurrent herpes simplex (lips and genitals) in Man. The lesion is painted with 0.1% proflavine (6.5), and then irradiated with visible light. The attack is specifically on the viral DNA and leads to deletion of the guanine moiety (Felber et al., 1973).

Rifampin (4.20b), discussed in Section 4.0, inhibits replication of vaccinia virus in mouse cells (Heller et al., 1969). Also rifamycin SV (4.20a) inhibits reverse transcriptase, the RNA-dependent synthesizer of DNA in viruses. Unfortunately, no clinical applications of these discoveries have been made. Apart from these and the phleomycins (Section 4.0, p. 115), antiviral action has rarely been found among antibiotics.

Tamm's 'HBB'
(6.17)

Tilerone
(6.18)

An exciting new approach to virucides is to make use of the porosity that infection confers on the cytoplasmic membrane of the host's cell, employing, for example, those protein synthesis inhibitors to which the cells are normally impermeable (Carrasco, 1978).

Synthetic antiviral agents discovered so far, tend to be specific for a limited range of viruses; even so, they are usually wider in spectrum than available vaccines, and less expensive. Moreover their ability to treat an *established* viral infection injects new hope into the very area where viral immunotherapy fails.

A quite different approach to antiviral drugs is to seek small molecules which can stimulate the formation of interferon in the host. Interferon is a small protein whose production in the human body is normally stimulated by the presence of a virus, and which causes the host cell to produce an antiviral protein. Human interferon is non-toxic to man and has a broad spectrum of antiviral activity. Small, and inadequate supplies can be obtained from the pooled leucocytes of blood banks. Interferon from other mammals is ineffective in man. Although polynucleotides and some other polymers are effective artificial inducers of interferon, they are inactive orally. Tilerone (6.18) 2,7-bis(2-diethylaminoethoxy)fluoren-9-one, given by mouth, induces formation of interferon, but in a low concentration that is only marginally effective, even as a prophylactic (Krueger and Mayer, 1970). The search for stronger and more selective analogues of tilerone is being vigorously pursued.

Levamisole (6.35) reputedly helps the body fight chronic viral infection (e.g. warts, facial herpes) by stimulating multiplication of the hosts' leucocytes (Helin and Bergh, 1975).

For further reading on medical virology, see Fenner and White (1976); for a review of the chemotherapy of virus diseases, see Tilles (1974); and for an essay on the rational designing of antiviral agents, see Grollman and Horwitz (1971).

(c) Antiprotozoal drugs

Diseases caused by sporozoa. For the prevention and treatment of malaria, quinine came to be replaced, during the Second World War, by mepacrine (6.9). After the war, the latter was replaced for prophylaxis by the more effective pyrimethamine (4.7). For *treatment* it was replaced by chloroquine (10.28), at least among Caucasian people, many of whom disliked the temporary yellow colouration of their skin during mepacrine treatment. Chloroquine was discovered in the Elberfeld (Germany) laboratories of the Bayer Company, who had been responsible for the first synthetic antimalarials: mepacrine ('Atebrin') and pamaquine ('Plasmochin') (Schönhöfer, 1938); but it came to light independently in the U.S.A. during the large-scale 'Antimalarial Survey' of 1941–1945 (Wiselogle, 1946).

The less host-toxic primaquine (3.27) replaced pamaquine (6.8) as a gametocide, used as an auxiliary drug to prevent the patient from infecting new mosquitos (Elderfield, 1946). The first potent antimalarial prophylactic proguanil (3.25) ('Paludrine') was discovered in England towards the end of the 1939–1945 war (Curd, Davey and Rose, 1945), and was tested on volunteers in North Queensland, Australia (Fairley, 1946). It has now largely been replaced by the still more potent and selective prophylactic pyrimethamine (4.7) ('Daraprim'), discovered by a combined American and British team (Falco et al., 1951). Quinine is now reserved for cases of malaria resistant to chloroquine. The emergence of resistant strains of *Plasmodium falciparum* has brought about a renewal of the long-shelved synthetic work designed to find new antimalarials.

Coccidiosis in poultry and cattle, a group of diseases caused by various species of *Eimeria* (a sporozoon), has been a cause of tremendous economic loss in the poultry industry. The chances of infection have been greatly increased by contemporary battery methods of raising the birds, namely in a house of up to 30 000 birds with an earth floor covered by wood shavings.

Excellent prophylaxis, and even cure, of the disease can be obtained with the following drugs mixed with the food: (a) sulphonamides, especially sulfaquinoxaline, (b) amprolium (*9.27*), a metabolite analogue of thiamine, or (c) nitrofurazone (*4.25*).

Diseases caused by flagellates. Notable advances have occurred since 1935 in managing diseases caused by flagellates. Pentamidine (*10.25*) has proved the best of a series of aromatic diamidines for both prophylaxis and treatment of African sleeping sickness, although suramin (*6.7*) still finds a use for both purposes. The diamidines were synthesized by Ewins *et al.*, (first described in 1942), and biologically investigated by King, Lourie and Yorke (1938), and Adler and Tchernomoretz (1942). Diminazene (*10.27*) has since been established as another valuable diamidine for treatment. In advanced cases, where the brain has been invaded, the best treatment is with one of these two specific arsenicals: tryparsamide (*6.6*) and melarsoprol (*12.4*).

For the trypanosomiasis of quadrapeds, that causes such large economic loss in Central Africa, a single injection of an aminophenanthridinium salt can effect a cure, in horses, cattle, and camels (Browning *et al.*, 1938; Carmichael and Bell, 1944). [See the review by Walls (1951) who did the first syntheses, and maintained interest in phenanthridines during a long period of neglect.] Homidium (*10.22*), better known under its trade-name 'Ethidium', seems the best of these phenanthridine trypanocides. Quina-pyramine (*10.26*) is used as a prophylactic (Curd and Davey, 1949; Wilson, 1949). For more on trypanosomiasis, see Sections 1.1 (p. 9) and 10.3d.

Pentamidine (*10.25*) is the drug of choice in leishmaniasis, but organic antimonials still find a useful place in its treatment.

In human medicine, the most troublesome flagellate diseases of *temperate* climates is vaginal trichomoniasis, cured by the oral administration of metronidazole (*6.19*) ('Flagyl'), which is free from side-effects (Keighley, 1962). By its inhibition of hydrogen production by *Trichomonas vaginalis*, metronidazole was shown to interfere with a ferredoxin system of E_0 about -400 mV (Edwards, Dye and Carne, 1973; O'Brien and Morris, 1972). See also nitrofurazone in Section 4.0 (p. 120).

Diseases caused by amoebae. Many useful new amoebicidal drugs have been found which exert their action by contact with colonies of amoebae, and on trophozoites present in the colonic lumen. Metronidazole (*6.19*)

$$N \underset{CH_3}{\overset{NO_2}{\underset{}{\bigcirc}}} N \cdot CH_2CH_2 \cdot OH$$

Metronidazole
(*6.19*)

is the most clinically used example. Trophozoites not accessible to contact (e.g. those in liver abscesses) require systemically acting amoebicides. Here the physician's choice is no longer restricted to nauseating emetine, because chloroquine (*10.28*) has proved clinically effective.

(d) *Fungicides*

Of the fungal diseases of Man, tinea capitis (ringworm of the scalp) is now successfully treated with salicylanilide (*6.20*), a substance first recommended as an anti-mildew agent for cloth by the Shirley Textile Institute in England. Tinea pedis (athlete's foot) usually yields to tolnaftate (*6.21*) ('Tinactin', 'Tinaderm') which is the 2-naphthol ester of *N*-methyl-*N*-*m*-tolythiocarbamic acid. Tinea corporis and capitis can be cured in about 3 weeks with oral doses of the antibiotic griseofulvin (*6.22*), relief being experienced after the second day. However it takes about 6 months for griseofulvin to cure tinea of the fingernails, and no better remedy is known. For more on griseofulvin, see the introduction to Chapter 3.

Some rare, but often fatal, systemic fungal diseases, such as histoplasmosis and North American blastomycosis yield to injections of amphotericin B (5.7, p. 166), but its selectivity is only moderate (for mode of action, see Section 14.2). A related substance, nystatin, is used for superficial candiasis and for those infections of the gut with *Candida albicans* that sometimes follow tetracycline therapy.

A new substance with promise of high systemic antifungal activity coupled with good selectivity is the German drug clotrimazole (*6.23*), which is 2′-chlorophenyl-1-imidazolylbisphenylmethane (Plempel *et al.*, 1969). Its tendency to induce *e.r.* destructive enzymes as readily as phenobarbital does (see Section 3.4, p. 86) may interfere with other medication (Schwacke, 1970). The excellent systemic fungicidal activity of 5-fluorocytosine was mentioned in Section 4.0 (p. 114).

Plant-protecting fungicides are in Section 6.4.

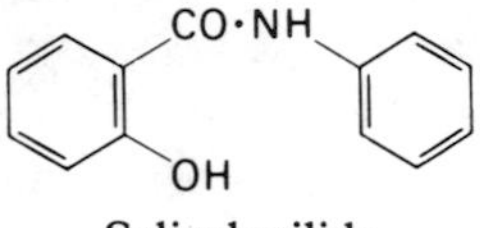

Salicylanilide
(*6.20*)

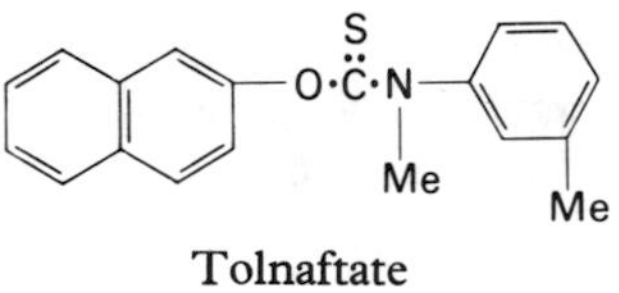

Tolnaftate
(*6.21*)

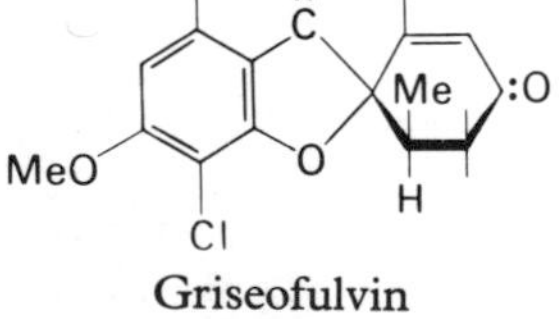

Griseofulvin
(*6.22*)

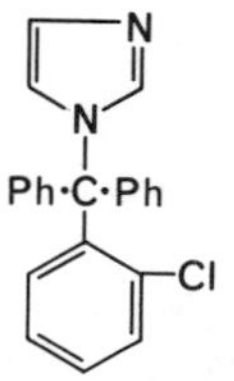

Clotrimazole
(*6.23*)

(e) *Anthelmintics*

Worms that parasitize man belong to widely separated zoological families (see Table 1.1, p. 17) and hence have very different anatomy, physiology, and susceptibility to drugs. The screening of various materials on worms was practised by Francesco Redi in 17th century Tuscany (Redi, 1684). In spite of this early start, very few substances now used against worms were employed before 1935, and those with the highest chemotherapeutic index have been discovered much more recently. The high degree of selectivity shown by contemporary anthelmintics contrasts with the number of infested inhabitants in our World: about 1000 million, or every fourth person. Most of the parasitic worms, in an infected host, are found to be in the adult, non-growing stage of the parasite's life-cycle. Hence they present a problem quite different from bacteria and protozoa which, because they are rapidly growing and multiplying, fall easy victims to drugs which interfere with nucleic acid or protein synthesis. Because in adult worms, these biosynthetic reactions are going at a slow pace, the most vulnerable biochemical pathways are those concerned with motor activity and the generation of metabolic energy. In some cases the selective toxicity shown by anthelmintics depends on a biochemical peculiarity of the parasite; in other cases a high concentration of a drug unabsorbable by the host is built up in the neighbourhood of the worms.

Beginning with the flat worms, and proceeding at once to the flukes, we come to the most devastating worm diseases of all, those caused by flukes in the blood, particularly schistosomiasis, whose natural history is sketched in Section 1.1 (p. 11). Depending on the species, the remedy of first choice is either niridazole (*6.24*) or an organic antimonial (see Table 4.4, p. 132; also Section 12.0). Also an organic phosphate, metriphonate (*12.24*) (dimethyl 2,2,2-trichloro-1-hydroxyethylphosphonate), which selectively inhibits the worm's acetylcholinesterase, provides a useful supplement to the treatment. The greatest need is to find an efficient and safe prophylactic.

Niridazole ('Ambilhar') [1-(5-nitro-2-thiazolyl)-2-imidazolidinone] is preferred over antimony for the bilharzial form of the disease. Treatment need last only one week (Lambert and Ferreira, 1965; Blair *et al.*, 1969). The drug is concentrated in, and destroys, the gonads of the worms and also embryonated eggs. Niridazole is metabolized too quickly in low dosage to be used as a prophylactic. There are indications that niridazole exerts its selectivity by inhibiting the natural inactivation of the enzyme glycogen phosphorylase in the male worms so that an excess of this enzyme accumulates, the rate of glycogenolysis increases, and the glycogen reserves of the worms are severely depleted (Bueding and Fisher, 1970). This occurs to a much smaller extent in the host. The muscular weakness arising from lack of glycogen as an energy reserve has been demonstrated in the isolated worms and also in those recovered from the treated host.

Lung flukes, common in the Americas and the Far East, yield well to the Japanese drug bithionol [2,2'-thio*bis*(4,6-dichlorophenol)], and chloroquine (*10.28*) is also effective. The Chinese liver fluke, *Clonorchis sinensis*, widely distributed in East Asia, yields to a protracted course of chloroquine. The common liver fluke, *Fasciola hepatica*, rarely infests man, but is common in all herbivores, throughout the world. Favoured remedies are nitroxynil (*6.25*) (4-hydroxy-3-iodo-5-nitrobenzonitrile), hexachlorophane (*11.37*), rafoxanide (3'-chloro-4',*p*-chlorophenoxy-3,5-diiodosalicylanilide), and other phenols thought to work by uncoupling oxidative phosphorylation (Corbett and Goose, 1971; see also Section 4.4, p. 135). A new remedy, the first one active against young flukes, is diamphenethide (*6.26*), which the host's liver activates by removing the acetyl group (Rowlands, 1973).

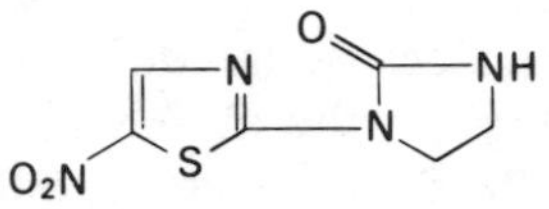

Niridazole
(*6.24*)

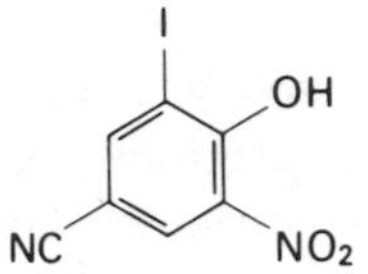

Nitroxynil
(*6.25*)

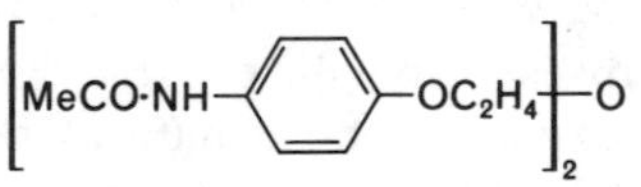

Diamphenethide
(*6.26*)

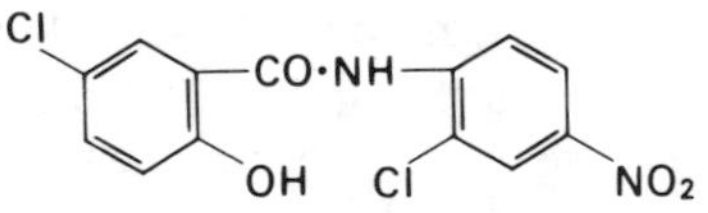

Niclosamide
(*6.27*)

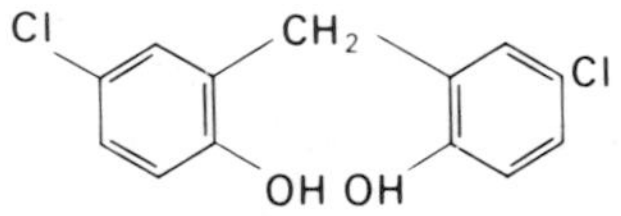

Dichlorophen
(*6.28*)

Turning now to the other division of flat worms, the cestodes or 'tapeworms', it is heartening to note that niclosamide (*6.27*) effects a prompt and painless cure for all four main types (Gönnert and Schraufstätter, 1960); dichlorophen (*6.28*) is also very good. The hydatid-forming worm, *Echinococcus granulosus* can be eliminated from sheep dogs with bunamidine ('Scolaban') (*NN*-dibutyl-4-hexyloxy-1-naphthamidine), and is also an effective one-dose cure for tapeworm in dogs and cats (Gemmell and Shearer, 1968).

The nematodes (round worms) are a large group, of which the various members need individual approaches. Filariasis, a mosquito-borne nematode infestation of the human bloodstream, occurs in Central Africa, South America, India, South China, and the Pacific Islands; when neglected, it leads to gross, swollen limbs, a condition known as elephantiasis. It is satisfactorily treated with diethylcarbamazine (6.29b) ('Hetrazan') (I-diethylcarbamoyl-4-methylpiperazine), which is remarkably selective (Hewitt et al., 1947). For the related West and Central African disease caused by *Onchocerca*, which has a special predilection for skin and eyes, diethylcarbamazine and suramin (6.7) in alternation are very effective, but a long treatment is needed. Another, but larger, tropical skin-infester, the Guinea worm, yields to niridazole (6.24).

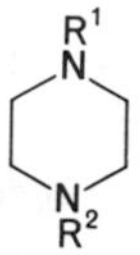

(a) R¹ = R² = H (piperazine)
(b) R¹ = Me; R² = CO·NEt₂ (diethylcarbamazine)
(6.29)

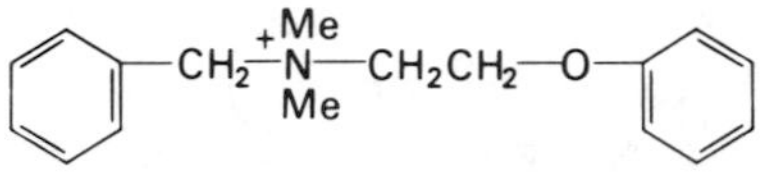

Bephenium (cation)
(6.30)

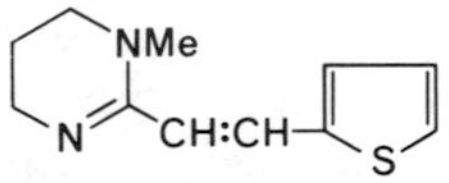

Pyrantel
(6.31)

Hookworm disease, described in Section 1.1 (p. 12), is caused by *Necator americanus* in tropical America and *Ancylostoma duodenale* in Asia and Africa. It is very effectively treated with a single dose of bephenium (6.30) or pyrantel (6.31), and these have replaced the longer, hazardous treatments with chlorinated hydrocarbons. Bephenium is an acetylcholine analogue, particularly selective against the worms (Goodwin, Jayewardene, and Standen, 1978; Standen, 1963). It is given as the 2-hydroxy-3-naphthoate or as the pamoate (= embonate), i.e. 1,1′-methylenebis-2-hydroxynaphth-3-oate: the insolubility of these salts ensuring sustained absorption. Pyrantel ('Banminth') is a depolarizing neuromuscular-blocking agent and inhibits the cholinesterases as well. It also is given as the pamoate and is therapeutically incompatible with piperazine (6.29a) Austin et al., 1966; Desowitz et al., 1970).

Roundworm (*Ascaris lumbricoides*) infestations, described in Section 1.1 (p. 12), respond readily to piperazine (6.29a), a simple and remarkably selective compound (Fayard, 1949; White and Standen, 1953). The high selectivity of piperazine depends on its ability to inhibit the normal contractile action of acetylcholine at the neuromuscular junction in nematodes without having any effect on the corresponding junction in mammals. Conversely, tubocurarine (2.6), which blocks this junction in mammals, has only a very weak action on this site in worms (del Castillo, Mello, and Morales, 1964). Frog muscle, intermediate between that of worms and mammals, is blocked by both drugs (Bueding, 1962). Because the action of piperazine on the junction is hyperpolarizing, it is therapeutically incompatible with pyrantel (6.31), which, on its own, is almost as effective a treatment for roundworm.

The threadworm, common in tropical regions including the southern part of the U.S.A., yields readily to the American drug thiabendazole (6.32), a highly selective benzimidazole (2,4'-thiazolylbenzimidazole) (H.D. Brown, et al., 1961). It is thought that fumarate reductase is essential for the regeneration of NAD from NADH in all those adult parasitic worms (whether flat or round) that live in environments low in oxygen. Although thiabendazole inhibits this enzyme at 10^{-4}M in *Haemonchus contortus* (Prichard, 1970), a more sensitive target probably exists because this drug is completely larvicidal, *in vitro*, at the extraordinary dilution of 1 in 10^{11}, surpassing by far the dilution at which penicillin is still active against bacteria (H.D. Brown et al., 1961). Equally useful for threadworm, but disliked by patients because of its blood-red colour which it imparts also to the faeces, is viprynium (also known as pyrvinium) (6.33), usually dispensed as the poorly soluble pamoate (Sawitz and Karpinski, 1956).

The pinworm (*Oxyuris vermicularis*), common in young children in every community of the world, yields readily to pyrantel (6.31), but piperazine is almost as good. The whip worm (*Trichuris trichuria*), common in warm, humid climates, but distressing mainly to children, is readily overcome by the Belgian drug mebendazole (6.34) (Brugmans et al., 1971). It is thought to work by selectively inhibiting glucose uptake in the worms (Fierlafijn, 1971). For *Trichinella spiralis* infestations (Section 1.1), so common in Europe, the United States, and Canada from eating undercooked pork foods, the most commonly used drugs are the corticoids as palliatives during the agonizing migration of the worm from gut to the host's muscle; thereafter thiabendazole is moderately effective.

Successful *veterinary anthelmintics* include many organic phosphates

Thiabendazole
(6.32)

Pyrvinium, or Viprynium (cation)
(6.33)

Mebendazole
(6.34)

Tetramisole
(Levamisole)
(6.35)

such as dichlorvos (*12.22*) and haloxon (*12.25*) (See Section 12.3). Except for the use of metriphonate in schistosomiasis, this field has not yet supplied selective drugs for human use. For nematode worms, thiabendazole enjoys widespread use. It has a wide range of activity against both adult and immature worms in cattle, horses, pigs and sheep. It is so selective, and so rapidly eliminated, that animals can safely be slaughtered, and milk from cows used, soon after administration.

Tetramisole (and levamisole, the more selective laevorotatory isomer obtained by optical resolution) (*6.35*) ('Nilverm'), is 2,3,5,6-tetrahydro-6-phenylimidazo[2,1-*b*]thiazole. Much used for many kinds of nematode infections in cattle, pigs, and sheep (Raeymaekers *et al.*, 1966), in human medicine it has proved satisfactory only for ascariasis. However it has found two other human uses: for treating low-grade virus infections (see Section 6.3b) and in arthritis: but here its true value remains to be proved. Levamisole inhibits fumarate reductase, but it also causes muscular paralysis in *Ascaris* (van den Bossche and Janssen, 1969).

Mebendazole (*6.34*), and its variants in which the 5-benzoyl-group is replaced by a butyl (parbendazole), phenylthio (fenbendazole) or propylthio (albendazole) group are highly selective variants of thiabendazole. Albendazole has a particularly broad spectrum of activity (Theodorides *et al.*, 1976). Phenothiazine, the first of the selective anthelmintics for sheep, is now little used because of the large dose needed.

For a study of the comparative biochemistry of parasites, see van den Bossche (1972).

(f) *Drugs against cancer*

'Cancer' is a collective word which embraces more than 100 different diseases, each responding to therapy differently, but all characterized by unrestrained growth. The treatment of cancer by drugs is essentially pharmacodynamic because both economic and uneconomic cells are part of the same organism. However, the treatment has this in common with chemotherapy: it aims to exterminate the uneconomic cell completely. Hence the phrase, 'The chemotherapy of cancer' was introduced by Ehrlich, and its use is now well established.

After Ehrlich's rejection of cancer chemotherapy as a suitable research topic for his times, the subject languished. About 1935, the Bayer Company in Germany very cautiously put out a candidate drug for clinical trial, but it proved unselective. The goal remained elusive until Alfred Gilman and his colleagues, about 1942 and in conditions of wartime secrecy, adapted the nitrogen mustards (candidate chemical-warfare vesicants) to this purpose (Gilman and Philips, 1946; Goodman, et al., 1946). This launched the era of modern cancer chemotherapy.

The first substance to win clinical approval for the treatment of cancers was chlormethinum* (4.19), which is still called mechlorethamine in the U.S.A. and mustine in Britain. It was the progenitor of the following alkylating agents currently used in cancer therapy: busulphan, chlorambucil, cyclophosphamide, melphalan, nitromin, and thiotepa (see Section 12.4 for details). Analogues of purines and pyrimidines soon arrived on the scene, and the following are being used clinically to-day: 8-azaguanine, cytarabine, fluorouracil, 6-mercaptopurine, and thioguanine (see Section 12.5); also the important pteridine (folic acid) analogue, methotrexate (Section 9.3c). Miscellaneous synthetic compounds used in treatment include hydroxyurea (Section 4.0, p.116), dacarbazine (4-dimethyl-triazenoimidazole-5-carboxamide) for melanoma, and mitotane (an analogue of DDT) used exclusively in adrenal carcinoma. Of natural products, the most clinically used are the antibiotics adriamycin (Section 10.3b), bleomycin (Section 4.0, p.115), and dactinomycin (Section 4.0, p.118), the male and female sex hormones and the various corticosteroids, some of them partly synthetic (Section 5.0, p.154), an enzyme (asparaginase), the retinoids related to vitamin A, and the tubule-inhibiting Vinca alkaloids (Section 5.3, p.176). Some of these remedies have inbuilt selectivity, but most of them need to be used in conjunction with knowledge of the cell cycle (Section 5.0), or through enforcing a selective distribution.

At no time has interest in the chemotherapy of cancer stood higher than to-day, and this enthusiasm reflects current achievements (see Section 1.1, p.13). This use of drugs enables the physician to reach out beyond what surgery and radiation can accomplish. Patients with widespread metastatic cancers can have these lesions reached and cured by chemotherapy even in situations where their presence is unsuspected and undetectable. In 1975, the Division of Cancer Treatment of the National Cancer Institute in Bethesda (U.S.A.) estimated that drugs are now curing about 8% of otherwise fatal cancers each year in the U.S.A., and are allowing lengthened survival in a great many other cases.

6.4 Parallel developments in insecticides and crop-protecting agents: Agrochemicals.

Progress, parallel to that discussed for the chemotherapy of mammals, has also taken place in agriculture where the farmer must prevent, and

* Internationally accepted name (WHO).

even cure, the invasion of his crops by weeds, insects, and fungi. Interest in insecticides has a still broader base, because insects are also ectoparasites of man and his domestic animals, and the vectors of infectious diseases. Insects have been wasting about 14 per cent of the world's annual crop production, moreover plant diseases (caused by fungi or worms) waste another 12 per cent, weeds another 9 per cent, and rodents perhaps another 10 per cent, an estimated total of 1800 million tons (see Cramer, 1967).

Insecticides. The destruction of insect pests on crops was long attempted, but with rather dispiriting results, using lead arsenate, tobacco dust, soap, and light petroleum. But in 1939, the dramatic possibilities of a potent and selective chemical for insect control were made evident by Paul Müller's discovery (in the Swiss firm, Geigy) of the insecticidal action of DDT. With this event, the modern era of insecticides was born.

DDT (*3.37*) has the internationally accepted name (WHO) of clofenotanum, but is still known in Britain as dicophane and in the U.S.A. as chlorophenothane. For his discovery, Müller was awarded a Nobel prize in medicine, and the early uses of this agent (mainly by the Allied armies in the Second World War) were to control malaria and typhus during campaigns. Because of the war, very little was published about DDT until Läuger, Martin, and Müller (1944) gave their historical account. It turned out that DDT had been known since 1874 when Zeidler first synthesized it, yet its biological properties remained unsuspected for more than six decades, until Müller's preliminary results in 1936.

At the end of the Second World War, DDT was introduced as an agricultural and domestic insecticide, and it was distributed prolifically over farms and premises in the belief that it was completely selective. By increasing crop yields, it played an important part in alleviating the needs for food and clothing of an ever-expanding world population. In 1962, however, there was a sudden realization that, because of its poor biodegradability, DDT constituted an ecological risk, namely a potentially harmful effect of the residues on wildlife (mainly fish, large birds and bees) and possible toxiocological effects on man through chronic overdosage. As a result, many countries banned the use of DDT in agriculture, or limited it to particular crops where no adequate substitute existed.

The medical, as distinct from the agricultural, uses of DDT did not come under this ban. In the constant battle against mosquitos that spread malaria in the tropics, the persistence of DDT after an annual spraying (a year is the smallest economic interval) is a distinct advantage, and the World Health Organization successfully fought complete suspension of its use, while replacing it, wherever practicable. The principal replacements are: the biodegradable analogue methoxychlor (*6.36*), the more persistent of the carbamates [such as propoxur (*6.37*)] and the phosphates [such as diazinon (*12.19*)], and abate (the tetramethyl ester of thiodi-4, 1-phenylenephosphorothioic acid)]. Other candidate phosphates are undergoing trial [particularly fenitrothion (dimethyl 3-methyl-4-nitro-phenyl phosphorothionate) and chlorphoxim (diethyl 2-chloro-α-cyano-benzylideneamino phosphorothionate)]. In places where resistance to chlorinated insecticides had set in, the change to carbamates or phosphates was imperative.

Methoxychlor
(6.36)

Propoxur
(6.37)

The World Health Organization has reported on the long-term effects of DDT on spraymen, exposed to it through their work in India and Brazil. Surveying a total of 1200 sprayman-years, no ill effects due to DDT could be found, although blood-levels remained above normal for several years after the men took on other work (World Health Organization, 1974). [For more on the chronic exposure of men to DDT, see Section 7.6e.]

Discovery of the insecticidal action of DDT was followed by the market-ing of other chlorinated hydrocarbons; but all of these perform in a different way from DDT (see Section 7.6e) and are active on some DDT-resistant strains. The first of these new products was γ-hexachlorocyclohexane (6.38), variously known as BHC, gamma benzene hexachloride, and lin-dane. Introduced in England by Slade (1945), this substance acts with greater speed and power than DDT, but being more volatile, it soon vanishes without residue. In the same year, Hyman (California) introduced the highly potent and persistent cyclodiene series, which included aldrin (6.39), dieldrin, chlordane, heptachlor, and endrin (Hyman, 1949). After a long period of widespread use, these unbiodegradable (and sometimes even carcinogenic) substances were considered in many countries to be insufficiently selective and their use has been limited or even suspend-ed. For the action of chlorinated insecticides on nerves, see Section 7.6e.

At the present time there is much concern over the pollution of waters by polychlorobiphenyls (PCB) which are used as plasticizers, fire-retardants, high-temperature lubricants, and transformer oils; but these are not insecticides.

The introduction of the organo-phosphorus insecticides, about 1945, greatly widened the spectrum of available types. Like the chlorinated hydrocarbons, these are also nerve poisons, but they act in a quite different way, namely by inhibiting esterases. Unfortunately the early examples, discovered in Germany by Schrader, were as toxic for those who sprayed

Gamma benzene
hexachloride
(6.38)

Aldrin
(6.39)

the crops as for the insects themselves. How this defect was overcome is told in Section 12.3. The molecules of the organo-phosphates can be altered at will to produce short-, medium-, and long-acting forms, so that the quality of persistence has come completely under control. As a class, the organo-phosphates are less lipophilic than the chlorinated hydrocarbons. In fact there is quite a range of hydrophilicity and the most hydrophilic examples are taken up by plants, through which they diffuse. This discovery launched the first of the systemic insecticides which have made a noteworthy contribution to selectivity: while completely harmless to the plant because of its lack of a nervous system, their attack on insects is confined to those that bite the plant. The organo-phosphates were soon joined by the organic carbamates, which have similar properties (see Section 12.3).

Rotenone (4.40), an oxygen-heterocycle of plant origin, is another suitable agent for leaf-biting pests. Unfortunately it is destroyed by light. For the source of its action on the respiratory chain, and its selectivity, see Section 4.4. Preliminary attempts have been made to find selective inhibitors of α-glycerophosphate metabolism, of extreme physiological importance to the insect for flight, and controlled by enzymes which are merely analogous to their mammalian equivalents (Marquardt and Brosemer, 1966).

The pyrethrins, esters of plant origin, long used as domestic insecticides, suffer from two defects: ease of destruction by light, and provision of 'knockdown' (a reversible general anaesthesia for the insect) rather than 'kill'. How these defects have been overcome in recent years, through modification of the pyrethrins into pyrethroids, is told in Section 7.6e.

The modern farmer has found that the more selective of the phosphate and carbamate insecticides come in such a large range of persistence-times, that there is one to suit every need. Unfortunately, resistance to these insecticides is mounting, including some cross-resistance with chlorinated hydrocarbons. For this reason, much hope is placed in the successful performance of the pyrethroids on a larger scale than their present use (limited, so far, by their comparative expensiveness) has demonstrated.

In practice, the selectivity and success of insecticides is greatly enhanced by proper timing and restricted distribution. There is a pressing need for a still more intense study at the molecular level of the activity and selectivity of insecticides. In spite of frequent and optimistic statements to the contrary, it is evident that chemicals will have to be our major means of controlling insects in the foreseeable future.

Much hope has been entertained for analogues of the juvenile hormone, such as hydroprene (ethyl 3,7,11-triethyldodeca-2,4-dienoate), which have an absolute selectivity against insects. They have proved useful where the *adult* insect is the nuisance-form, as with biting flies and mosquitos; but as for 'crop protection', they keep the insect at the larval stage where it is at its most voracious (see further Section 4.7). *Inhibitors* of the juvenile hormone (mentioned in Section 4.7) may turn out to be more valuable. Some growth-regulator analogues have been found which selectively inhibit synthesis of the insect cuticle, notably: 1-(4-chlorophenyl)-3-(2,6-difluorobenzoyl) urea (Post *et al.*, 1974), and 2,6-di-*t*-butyl-4(α,α-dimethylbenzyl)phenol (Hollingworth, 1975). The former (diflubenzuron, 'Dimilin') inhibits egg hatching. It also affects larviporous insects, such as tsetse flies, so that they have no viable offspring. It seems to be as powerful as DDT, and harmless to man (Jordan and Trevern, 1978).

For background information on insect biochemistry and physiology, see Casida (1973); Corbett (1974); Wilkinson (1976). For an account of the scientific principles of crop protection, see Martin (1973); for the various methods available for insect pest management, see Metcalf and Luckman (1975); and for discussions of pesticide selectivity, see Street (1975). The following handbooks give the chemical composition of all insecticides: Frear (1975); Martin and Worthing (1977).

Ectoparasites.   Scabies in man is now rapidly curable by local application of either benzyl benzoate or lindane. Pediculosis (infestation with one or other kind of lice) is similarly cured with carbaryl (*12.28*), isobornyl thiocyanate, lindane, or DDT.

Insect repellants.   The medical welfare of human beings is safeguarded by insect repellants, such as dimethyl phthalate and *m*-diethyltoluamide against mosquitos, and dibutyl phthalate against the mites that carry scrub typhus (see Christophers, 1947, for the physical principles involved).

Plant fungicides.   Fungi, far more than bacteria, viruses, or worms, are the main agents of plant disease. Pathogenic fungi cause the well-known blights, wilts, mildews, scabs, and rusts to which Man's economic crops are prone and they have, throughout history, played havoc with his food supplies. The economic and social devastation wrought by such fungal diseases as blight in potatoes, mildew on vines, and rust and smut in wheat, have been graphically recorded (Large, 1940). These depredations of fungi were traditionally fought by crop rotation, open planting, and the use of disease-free seeds and resistant varieties. Yet so adaptable are fungi that these methods do not suffice, and fungicides remain the most important method of controlling fungal diseases.

Until recently most available fungicides were biochemically non-specific, and depended for their selectivity on favourable distribution coefficients (see Chapter 3). They were usually routed to the fungus (rather than to the plant) by providing them with extra lipophilic character, often by means of adding a hydrocarbon side-chain to the molecule. The basis of this selectivity was the protection given to the plant by its cuticle which does not readily permit the passage of either lipophilic substances or the cations of heavy metals, whereas fungi (particularly their conidia or sporulating structures) easily accumulate substances of these types. For example, apple leaves absorbed only 1 µg/g (dry weight) of captan (*6.40*) from a 25 µM aqueous solution in 30 minutes, whereas the conidia of *Neurospora crassa* took up 7000 times as much under the same conditions (Richmond and Somers, 1962). Glyodin (2-heptadecyl-imidazoline) and dodine (*n*-dodecylguanidine) behaved similarly. In the fungus, such substances tend to be non-specific, attacking *many* enzymes or other vulnerable cell constituents. As a class they have little toxicity for vertebrates, and they do not incite fungi to produce resistant strains.

In most cases these substances kill the fungus before it has penetrated the plant. Recently more selective substances have been found which penetrate into the plant and either prevent penetration of fungi, or kill those have already penetrated. This systemic use of agents, 'plant chemotherapy', is more difficult than animal chemotherapy because plants have no true circulation, no phagocytes to assist the agent, and no mechanism for the detoxication or excretion of the agent when its work is done. Horsfall (1972) has suggested several ways in which the biochemical interactions between plants and fungi might be disturbed so as to favour the plant. (1) The basic metabolism of the plant may be so altered that it becomes a less attractive host; for example, when plant growth substances lower the sugar level in foliage, resistance to fungi usually increases. (2) Systemic agents may inactivate fungal toxins and tissue-destroying enzymes, as diaminoazobenzene inactivates the toxin produced by *Phytophthora cactorum* (Howard, 1941), or as rufianic acid protects tomato plants from the pectase secreted by *Fusarium oxysporum* (Grossmann, 1962). (3) The agent can protect the plant by lignifying the point of attack; phenylthiourea (*6.41*), which has no fungitoxic properties, seems to act in this way (Sijpesteijn and Sisler, 1968).

Spray-protection of crops is still practised, often with inexpensive, traditional inorganic agents. Basic cupric calcium sulphate (Bordeaux mixture), introduced by Millardet in 1885, is highly selective and still much employed, as is elemental sulphur which has been used for this purpose during some 2500 years. Sulphur, by contact with living tissues, forms two mildly antifungal substances: hydrogen sulphide and

Captan
(6.40)

Phenylthiourea
(6.41)

Chlorothalonil
(6.42)

pentathionic acid. A great advance was made in 1934 when Tisdale and Williams reported the high antifungal action of dimethyldithiocarbamic acid (3.41) as its iron and zinc salts, ferbam and ziram. These have no toxicity for man, cattle, or the higher plants, but show a wide spectrum of toxicity for fungi, and are made and sold in enormous quantities.

Another agent with specialized uses is captan (6.40) (N-trichloromethyl-thio-4-cyclohexene-1,2-dicarboximide), introduced by Kittleson (1952); this and the related agent, folpet, in which a benzene ring replaced the cyclohexene ring, are used mainly on fruit trees. These are alkylating agents which block metabolically important -SH groups, particularly in coenzyme A and glyceraldehyde-3-phosphate dehydrogenase, but their total action is coarser than this. Other antifungals which act on sites bearing a solitary mercapto-group are: the mericurials, and the salts of ethylene-1,2 -bisdithiocarbamic acid (nabam, zineb). A precise attack on the SH-group of cysteine-149 in glyceraldehyde-3-phosphate dehydrogenase is made by chlorothalonil (6.42) (2,4,5,6-tetrachloroisophthalonitrile) (Long and Siegel, 1975).

The modes of action of these and other sprayed-on antifungal agents have been classified by Sijpesteijn (1970). The paired mercapto-groups in lipoic acid and lipoic dehydrogenase, which are important for the oxidation of pyruvate in fungi (Wren and Massey, 1965), as in other forms of life, are inactivated by dialkyldithiocarbamates, and 8-hydroxyquinoline. Of these agents, which require copper as a co-toxicant, the former is sprayed on crops and the latter used for the mould-proofing of canvas, wood, and outdoor equipment (see, further, Section 11.7). Oxidative phosphorylation (Section 4.4) is the target for trialkyl-tin salts, and dini-trophenols. Antibiotics which expand, or disrupt, plasma membranes have mainly medical uses (see Section 14.2). Azauracil (4.24), a pyrimidine antimetabolite which interferes with uracil metabolism (Section 4.0, p.ooo), is much used to control powdery mildew in cucumber.

A startling improvement in fungicides was heralded by the introduction in 1966 of benomyl (3.42a, p.93) (methyl 1-butylcarbamoyl-2-benzim-idazolecarbamate) 'Benlate'). After the careful report of Delp and Klopping (1968), it was realized that, not only was benomyl a fungicide of unprecedented selectivity and potency, but that it could be used in a new and very advantageous way, namely systemically. This ushered in the age of chemotherapy for fungus-infected plants. The agent is usually placed in the soil, gains access to the transpiration stream through the root hairs and ends in the leaves. In this way, deeper penetration and a more even application are possible than with spraying techniques. Benomyl exerts its antifungal effect at concentrations as low as 0.02 parts per million, and it is active against a very wide range of fungal diseases (Selling et al., 1970). As recounted in Section 3.4, benomyl is hydrolysed by water to methyl 2-benzimidazolecarbamate (3.42b), which is the actual agent; methyl thiophanate (3.43) is also used in the fields as a precursor of this carbamate (see Section 3.5, p.93).

Unfortunately, resistance to benomyl soon set in, although resistance to fungicides was previously unknown. As a result, larger doses had to be used, and fewer species of fungus could be subjugated. This led to a vigorous search for other systemic fungicides. Thiabendazole (6.32), which had been introduced in 1961 as a veterinary vermifuge (see Section 6.3e), was found to be a good systemic fungicide for plants. The primary site of action seems to be inhibition of electron transport in fungal mito-chondria (Allen and Gottlieb, 1970).

Another successful systemic agent, ethirimol (5-n-butyl-2-ethylamino-6-methylpyrimid-4-one) (6.43) ('Milstem') is much used against powdery mildew which formerly caused great loss in cereal crops (particularly barley) throughout Europe (Bebbington, et al., 1969). It acts by inhibiting folic acid metabolism, somewhat similarly to pyrimethamine in Section 9.3c (Bent, 1970).

Ethirimol
(6.43)

Carboxin
(6.44)

The disinfection of stored seeds prior to planting has traditionally been accomplished with mercurials and, in recent times, with hexachlorobenzene. Unfortunately if, as does happen, the seeds are mistakenly eaten, these chemicals can cause severe illness. Hence there has been a search for substances that injure fungal spores but are selective enough not to hinder germination or harm humans. Benomyl meets these criteria. Another substance that has been outstandingly successful, although specialized to act only against basidiomycetes (such as smuts and rusts in barley and wheat), is carboxin (6.44) ('Vitavax') (5,6-dihydro-2-methyl-1,4-oxathiin-3-carboxanilide) (Edgington, Walton and Miller, 1966). The essential structure in carboxin is a methyl-group placed ortho to an anilide group;

the nature of the nucleus is not of prime importance and a benzene ring will suffice (Carter, Huppatz, and Wain, 1975). These anilides attack succinic dehydrogenase in the basidiomycete mitochondria (White and Thorn, 1975), and act systemically in the emergent plant.

For killing fungi in the soil, salts of methyldithiocarbamic acid and various chloronitrobenzenes have been found suitable; for soil fumigation more volatile substances such as chloropicrin and methyl *iso*thiocyanate are preferred.

In practice, it is found that every species of plant can protect itself from all but a very few species of fungi, most of which are highly specific for particular varieties of plant. Many higher plants protect themselves against fungal invasion by producing phytoalexins, substances absent from healthy plants. Thus *Leguminosae* synthesize isoflavonoid protectants; the *Solanaceae*, diterpenes; and the *Compositae*, polyacetylenes (Cruickshank, 1963).

Much of the damage caused by fungi arises from fungal toxins such as tentoxin, the cyclic tetrapeptide secreted into fruits and grains by *Altenaria tenuis* which inhibits photophosphorylation (Steele *et al.*, 1976). Herein lies a possibility for another kind of selective attack on fungal infection.

In spraying crops, many of the affected tissues cannot be reached directly, but depend on receiving fungicide by slow *translocation*. As Rich (1954) has shown, the particles of copper-containing fungicides are positively charged and cling more readily to the negatively charged leaf than to one another. As the wind and the rain dislodge particles from each residual clump, they move to aspects of the leaves not covered by the original spraying.

For further reading on fungicides, see Lukens (1971), and Corbett (1974); and for a treatise on systemic fungicides, Marsh (1972). For chemical formulae and uses of all fungicides, see Martin and Worthing (1977).

Herbicides (weed killers).   Only in recent times have farmers become receptive to the idea of selectivity in eliminating uneconomic plants (i.e. weeds). In 1895–7 it was demonstrated independently by Bonnet in France, by Bolley in America, and by Schultz in Germany that a solution of cupric sulphate killed the ubiquitous charlock (*Sinapis arvensis*) without injury to the crop in which it was a weed. While continuing to use their traditional fungicides and insecticides, farmers turned a deaf ear to this news of the world's first selective herbicide. In 1911 a Frenchman showed that a solution of sulphuric acid could be safely used on crops to destroy the weeds (Rabaté, 1927). So slowly did thinking about herbicides move, that not until 1932 were systemic trials of Rabaté's method made in England and the U.S.A. (see Plate 1, page 52). These trials established the high selectivity of this simple acid, but problems arose from corrosion of equipment, and the increased acidity of the soil. Soon two more Frenchmen discovered the selective weed-killing properties of dinitro-*o*-cresol (*6.45*), a substance which had been known since 1866 (Truffaut and Pastac, 1932, 1944).

By the middle 1930s, a good deal of the prejudice against selectively toxic weed killers had been overcome, and the agricultural industry became receptive to the phenoxyacetic acids. These substances were designed to resemble the natural auxin, indoleacetic acid (*4.52*) but, unlike the latter, to resist destruction by the plant. At first they were used only for their hormone-like action, to promote the setting of unfertilized fruits, and to promote the growth of roots (Zimmerman, 1942). When using them in excess as leaf sprays, Templeman found that they acted as herbicides (Sexton, *et al.*, 1941; Templeman and Sexton, 1946). This discovery led eventually to the use of these substances in colossal amounts throughout the world, killing weeds as the result of inducing excessive growth. The two most used herbicides in this class are 2-methyl-4-chlorophenoxyacetic acid (*6.46*), and 2,4-dichlorophenoxyacetic acid. See, further, Sections 4.7 (p. 148) and 13.2.

DNOC
(6.45)

MCPA
(6.46)

By 1950, herbicides were being employed in farming on a tremendous scale, and with a great gain in yield. Research was now directed to finding examples that had other types of selectivity. Few of them have shown biochemical specificity. Selectivity, when it occurs, is often based on distribution such as differential wettability of leaf surfaces, ease of uptake and translocation, or relative access to root systems. In other cases, selectivity depends on different capacities of plants to degrade the herbicide to a less toxic derivative.

Of these later discoveries, picloram (*6.47*) ('Tordon'), 3,5,6-trichloro-4-aminopyridine-2-carboxylic acid, resembles the phenoxyacetic acids in mode of action, but is much more potent, and highly persistent. It is being widely used (Kefford, 1966).

The cyanophenol herbicides, conceived as a variant of the nitrophenol types, have some special properties. A typical example is 2,6-diiodo-4-cyanophenol (*6.48*) (ioxynil, 'Actril'), introduced simultaneously by Wain (1963) and Carpenter and Heywood (1963). It is a contact herbicide which, like DNOC (*6.45*), powerfully uncouples oxidative phosphorylation (Section 4.4), in fact much more strongly than 2,4-dinitrophenol does (Kerr and Wain, 1964). It is selective against young dicotyledonous weeds in cereal crops and is often used synergistically with MCPA (6.46). Useful specificity is shown by 2,4-dinitro*sec*butylphenol, a homologue of (6.45), which is widely used to eliminate dicotyledonous weeds from peas which are themselves dicotyledons (Roberts, 1954). Both in the nitro- and the cyano-phenols, 2,6-disubstitution greatly increases the potency. The ionization and penetration of nitrophenols is discussed in Section 10.5.

Picloram   Ioxynil
(6.47)   (6.48)

Some other substances, whose action is quite the contrary of MCPA, can eliminate monocotyledonous weeds from a dicotyledon crop. For this purpose 2,2-dichloropropionic acid (dalapon, 'Dowpon') is much used. Its mode of action is discussed in Section 9.4. The carbamates, which are mitotic poisons, introduced by Templeman and Sexton (1945), are also available for this purpose. The most selective example is barbane (6.49) (4-chlorobut-2-ynyl N,3'-chlorophenylcarbamate), which suppresses the growth of wild oats in cereal crops (Crafts, 1964).

The bipyridylium herbicides diquat and paraquat, used as an alternative to ploughing, and acting through the formation of free radicals, are described in Section 4.5.

An ingenious method for increasing the selectivity of herbicides in the phenoxyacetic acid series, by β-degradation of intrinsically harmless homologues, was recounted in Section 3.5 (p. 93) and illustrated in Plate 2.

A distinction will now be made between herbicides that are sprayed on the foliage, as the above types are, and those that are applied to the soil. In recent years, the latter have become more used at the expense of the former. *Soil-applied herbicides* have to be strongly adsorbable on soil particles, and readily taken up by the root hairs of plants. They are selective against quick-growing weeds which usually have the most copious surface roots, and they are more sparing of economic crops because the latter usually have roots that are slow-growing, tougher, and deeper. Many are available for use in the soil at seed-sowing time, to exert 'pre-emergence control'. The triazines, such as simazine (4.41), are the most used of all soil-applied herbicides; small changes in the substituents give excellent control over selectivity and persistence. These substances [and the phenyl-ureas, such as diuron (4.42), which are also soil-types] act by interfering with the Hill reaction in photosynthesis (see Section 4.5).

The most prized herbicides are those which, after eliminating the undesired weeds, become degraded (to harmless material) by sunlight, air, rain, bacteria, or the soils (Kearney and Kaufman, 1968).

Some substances retard the growth of plants by suppressing transport of the natural growth hormone, indoleacetic acid. The simplest of these is 2,3,5-triiodobenzoic acid, which is used to dwarf a soya-bean crop and so increase the yield of beans. The morphactans, a series of fluorene derivatives of which the best seems to be 2-chloro-9-hydroxyfluorene-9-carboxylic acid (6.50) (Schneider, 1964), are used to retard the growth of dicotylendonous weeds in a grain crop until, overgrown by the crop, these weeds are finally destroyed by lack of light, meanwhile serving a good purpose by protecting the soil from drying (Ziegler, 1970).

$$Cl \quad \text{—} \quad NH \cdot CO \cdot O \cdot CH_2C \vdots C \cdot CH_2Cl$$

Barbane
(6.49)

$$HO \quad CO_2H \quad Cl$$

A morphactan
(6.50)

Glyphosate (N-phosphonomethylglycine) is proving effective for killing woody or fleshy plants that are little affected by other herbicides (Barrett, 1974).

For further reading on herbicides, see Ashton and Crafts (1973); Audus (1976); Büchel (1977); and Corbett (1974).

Defoliants.   The aerial spraying of defoliants was introduced in East Africa to eliminate tsetse flies, which carry the trypanosomes of sleeping sickness (Blackman, 1954). The most used substances are aliphatic arsenicals (e.g. sodium cacodylate), 3-amino-1,2,4-triazole, and the phenoxyacetic acids and their *n*-butyl esters. When a defoliation campaign moves near to agricultural land, ominous ecological problems, such as soil erosion, arise. An unsuspected hazard of defoliation by 2,4,5-trichlorophenoxyacetic acid (2,4,5-T) in the Viet Nam war, was the presence of a small percentage of 2,3,7,8-tetrachlorodibenzo-*p*-dioxin (6.51), a by-product of synthesis. It is outstandingly toxic to mammals and is teratogenic (foetus-deforming) as well. The use of 2,4,5-T is at present out of favour. Picloram (6.47) is used to defoliate conifers.

A defoliant is essentially a substance that causes rapid senescence, and there is no more effective way to do this than to increase the level of ethylene in the leaf. 2-chloroethanephosphonic acid (6.52), which liberates ethylene in the cell, effects this and is also being used (at lower concentrations) to accelerate ripening of fruits. For a review, see Osborne (1968).

Plant antiviral agents.   Low concentrations of the antibiotic blasticidin S selectively inhibit virus multiplication in bean and tobacco plants (Hirai

Tetrachlorodibenzodioxin
(6.51)

$$ClCH_2CH_2\overset{O}{\underset{O}{P}}\cdot OH$$

Chloroethane-phosphonic acid
(6.52)

et al., 1966). This was the first success in the difficult subject of viral chemotherapy in plants.

Agricultural anthelmintics.   Nematodes can impoverish soil and attack
roots. 1,2-Dibromo-3-chloropropane (DBCP) ('Nemagon') is a volatile
nematocide used to rid soil of these undesirable worms. Plants are remarkably tolerant of it, but it has been suspected of suppressing spermatogenesis
in the adult human male.

Molluscicides.   By killing the worm-carrying snails in the watercourses
of Egypt and other countries where bilharzia in man is widespread (see
Section 1.1), an essential stage in the life-cycle of this parasite can be broken.
The traditional use of copper sulphate for this purpose has been replaced
by the more efficient amides such as 2,5-dichloro-(4-nitrosalicyl) anilide
('Bayluscid'). *N*-Tritylmorpholine ('Frescon'), another potent mollusci-
cide, is very selective; other forms of aquatic life are little affected by it
and mammals unharmed (Boyce, Jones and van Tongeren, 1967). In a
field test in Brazil, *bis*tributyltin oxide (Bu$_3$Sn-O-SnBu$_3$) (hexabutyl-
distannoxane), in an asphalt base, retained strong molluscicidal activity
when immersed in a stream for a year, and was not inactivated either
by immersion in mud or drying in the sun (Gilbert *et al.*, 1973). The
Ethiopian water plant *Phytolacca dodecandra* is useful to grow in infested
streams because it secretes a molluscicidal glycoside.

Rodenticides.   Annually huge amounts of crops and food stacks are
spoilt by rats, and many people die from such rodent-borne diseases as
bubonic plague, rickettsiosis, leishmaniasis, spirochaetosis, leptospirosis,
and (through rat-borne lice) typhus. Because of the rat's habit of fighting
his brethren to the point of drawing blood, anticoagulants were introduced
as (chronic) rodenticides, namely the indanediones and hydroxycoumarins.
Of the latter, warfarin (6.53) has given outstanding service, although resistance to its action has developed among many scattered populations of the
the common rat (*Rattus norvegicus*). This resistance has been partly overcome by incorporating calciferol (vitamin D) with it in the bait. Of the
acute rodenticides, norbormide (4.59) is absolutely specific but rats soon
become 'bait-shy' because of its characteristic odour. See Section 4.8 for
more about this agent, and a related development. *N*-3-pyridylmethyl-*N'*-
p-nitrophenylurea ('Vacor') kills both rats and mice, after a single dose, by
inhibiting their nicotinamide metabolism. The rats die from paralysis and
pulmonary arrest. Mice are not so easy to poison as rats, for the mice eat

a little here and there, and not much from any single bait. The weak point of a mouse's defence is the habit of compulsory self-grooming, which can be utilized by strewing a selectively-medicated powder to cling to its paws and fur. Such traditionally-used rodenticides as arsenic, thallium, zinc phosphide, and naphthylthiourea (antu) are now little esteemed.

Since the early 1900s, biological control of the rat and field mouse has been attempted, on a large scale, from one end of Europe to another. Usually a species of *Salmonella* bacteria (sometimes misbranded 'rat virus') was used, and false claims were made that the organism was specific for the rat. Actually these bacteria are pathogenic to Man and several epidemics have been started in this way (Wodzicki, 1973). A joint WHO/FAO expert committee strongly condemned this form of 'biological control' in 1967.

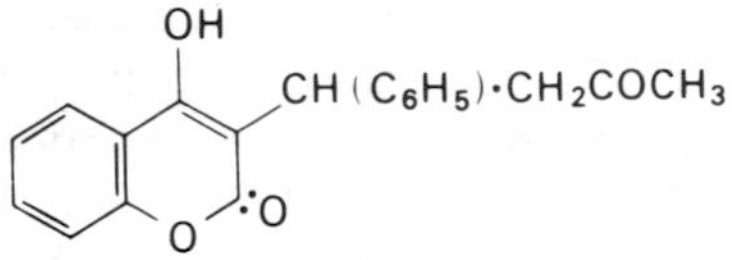

OH

CH(C₆H₅)·CH₂COCH₃

Warfarin
(6.53)

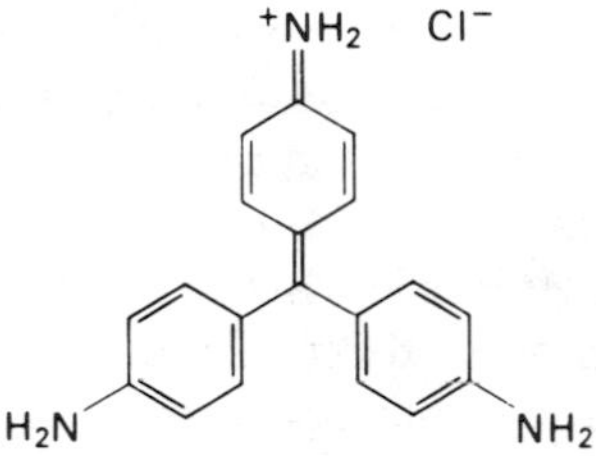

Parafuchsin
(6.54)

Biological control of rabbits, using *Myxoma* virus, has been successful in Australia, where it was first undertaken. Although a moderate degree of resistance has now set in, the survivors are easily exterminated with sodium fluoroacetate (non-selective).

6.5 Resistance to drugs and other agents

In 1905 Franke and Roehl, while working with Ehrlich, doscovered the phenomenon of *drug-resistance* in the following way. Mice, suffering from trypanosomiasis, were treated with drugs in doses that were too small to cure; inevitably a relapse took place but, surprisingly, the renewal of treatment with normally curative doses of the drug also failed. The trypanosomes had developed a resistance which was hereditary, and usually irreversible. As Yorke later observed, resistant trypanosome strains may require up to 250 times the normal concentration of drug before they are injured. Such massive dosage is usually more than the host can tolerate.

Ehrlich (1909) thought that resistance was caused by stepwise withdrawal, or masking, of the receptor by the organism. However, this is not the case, and it remained for Yorke *et al.* (1931) to show that, at least in trypanosomes, resistance is caused by diminution of uptake by the parasite.

Ehrlich encountered several distinct types of resistance in trypanosomes.

Parasites which had become resistant to trypan red resisted all other azo-dyes. Some other strains, which were resistant to 'Atoxyl' (*p*-amino-phenylarsonic acid) (*6.1*), resisted all other phenylarsonic acids, and a third type, resistant to parafuchsin (*6.54*), resisted all other triphenylmethanes. Yet a strain resistant to one of these three classes of drugs did not resist the other two classes unless specially trained to do so.

Later, Ehrlich recognized two classes of arsenical agents between which there was no cross-resistance, and today three classes are known. The first of these, typified by (*6.3*), is distinguished by the presence of water-attracting substituents, which may be $-OH$, $-CONH_2$, or $-SO_2NH_2$ (in place of NH_2, or in addition to it), but only such as are not ionized (as anions) at pH 7. Nearly all the arsenical drugs that have achieved clinical use belong to this sub-class, members of which usually have a favourable therapeutic index. It was also found that the acridine, trypaflavine (*6.4*) belonged to this sub-class because trypansomes made resistant to it were automatically resistant to arsenicals of type (*6.3*). The second class of resistance-prone arsenicals lacked hydrophilic substituents, the third class had substituents (e.g. $-CO_2H$) which ionized as anions at pH 7.

In these three classes of arsenicals, the initial state of oxidation of the arsenic is of no consequence. The eventual toxic action of the drug follows on biological conversion to the arsenoxide group ($-As:O$), whether in an organic arsenical or in arsenious acid ($HO.As:O$) (see Section 12.0). These facts, taken in conjunction with the knowledge that no resistance to arsenious acid could be achieved (although carefully sought), show that the non-arsenical part of the molecule is responsible for the uptake of the drug and that the resistant parasite is able to block this uptake. There are at least three distinct mechanisms for the uptake of aromatic arsenicals, corresponding to the three types of arsenical resistance (King and Strange-ways, 1942). These examples show how a study of resistance can contribute to knowledge of the uptake of drugs.

As far as is known, resistance in trypanosomes always takes the same form: the parasite so modifies the chemistry of its surface that the drug is no longer taken up but remains behind in the medium (Yorke *et al.*, 1931). On the other hand, a susceptible trypanosome can accumulate in its interior a 500 times greater concentration of arsenic than exists in the external medium (Eagle, 1945).

To-day a rough distinction is made between natural and acquired resistance, as illustrated by the following three cases. The *Mycobacterium* that causes human tuberculosis has natural resistance to penicillin; *Staphylo-coccus aureus* (the common yellow pus organism) has many strains that are susceptible to penicillin but can easily acquire resistance to it; *Streptococci* lack natural resistance to penicillin and do not acquire it either.

Resistance arises mainly by natural selection, namely by the outgrowth of a naturally resistant strain after the drug has killed all the susceptible strains. Resistance seldom arises by induction. In the laboratory some organisms have been induced to resist steadily increasing concentrations of some agent, but resistance acquired by induction can rarely be detected in the progeny. Again, resistance seldom arises by drug-provoked mutation, because the use of mutagens as drugs and agrochemicals is avoided. In addition to natural selection, drug resistance can be conferred by gene-transfer as in the mating of insects, the conjugation of Gram-negative bacteria, and the transformation of pneumococci.

In the commonest form of drug resistance, namely that arising by selection of a naturally-arisen mutant, the situation is as follows. A culture of about ten million bacteria may contain only one organism resistant to a particular drug. The chance of finding an organism resistant against two different drugs is often put at 1 in 10^{14}, and against three drugs 1 in 10^{21}. Hence the great success of using several drugs simultaneously when the uneconomic cell is known to be able to acquire resistance. On the other hand, attempted elimination of a susceptible organism by one solitary drug gives the resistant cells an opportunity to proliferate.

The ingenious technique of replica-plating was devised to show that organisms resistant to a drug need have had no previous contact with it (Lederberg and Lederberg, 1952). Bacteria (*E. coli*) were grown on an agar plate, and replicas of the colonies were transferred to several other agar plates by printing with velveteen. One such plate contained streptomycin. When (after incubation) the position of a colony resistant to streptomycin was found in the antibiotic-containing plate, colonies were harvested from identical positions in the streptomycin-free plates. This process was repeated, and finally an entire plate was obtained of streptomycin-resistant organisms that had never been in contact with streptomycin. Another proof of the pre-existance of resistant organisms was provided by the bacteriologist's habit of freeze-drying and storing cultures, from which viable specimens can be drawn after the passage of whole decades. Many bacterial strains that were stored, long before currently used antibacterials were developed, have been found to be immediately resistant to them. The explanation of these results is that an agent usually attacks just one metabolic step, and that a resistant organism does not use this step but has an alternative pathway (which is not always advantageous to it).

Resistance is a widespread, but not universal, phenomenon. Its possibilities, although frightening in special cases [insects to most known insecticides; the gonococcus to most of the formerly useful antibiotics (Saunders, 1977)], are not unlimited. Replica-plating discloses that *E. coli* can be made to achieve only a threefold increase in resistance to chloramphenicol (Cavalli-Sforza and Lederberg, 1956), and this seems to be representative of what natural selection usually accomplishes.

The five main types of resistance (the first four of them arising by natural selection, the fifth by gene-transfer) will now be described.

(a)   *Type 1 resistance : Exclusion from site*
As exclusion of the drug was the first recognized method by which an organism (actually, the trypanosome, see Yorke's work, above) acquired resistance, this type is mentioned first. Among many known examples, *Staphylococcus aureus* becomes resistant to tetracycline when the drug-accumulating mechanism of this organism (see introduction to Chapter 3) ceases to function, even though the drug's target (protein synthesis on ribosomes) remains as sensitive as ever (Sompolinsky, *et al.*, 1970). This effect has also been demonstrated in a Gram-negative bacterium (*E. coli*).

In mouse leukaemia, the survival time of the leukaemic cell suspensions is inversely proportional to the rate of uptake of methotrexate (4.6), but this rate begins to decline soon after treatment is instigated (Kessel *et al.*, 1965). This phenomenon has not been demonstrated in human leukaemia.

The physical basis for Type 1 resistance is suggested by the work of Haest *et al.*, (1972) who showed that the cell membrane can adjust its net charge by varying the proportion of phosphatidyl-glycerol (anionic) to lysylphosphatidyl-glycerol (cationic). It is easy to see how, in this way, either anionic or cationic drugs can be excluded by the operation of Coulomb's law.

(b)   *Type 2 resistance : Increased enzyme production*
Quite the commonest way for an organism to achieve resistance is to let the susceptible clones be replaced by others that have an increased production of an enzyme, either the target (if that is an enzyme) or else a drug-destroying enzyme.

In this way *Staphylococcus aureus* becomes resistant to penicillin in the clinic. Penicillin-resistant strains isolated from patients secrete the enzyme β-lactamase ('penicillinase')*. This enzyme hydrolyses the drug to penicilloic acid, which is biologically inert (see Section 12.1). Penicillinase-producing staphylococci are inherently quite sensitive to penicillin. Hence *small* inocula can be inhibited by low concentrations of the antibiotic. It is, in effect, a race between the speed with which penicillin can kill the bacteria and the speed with which they can produce enough of the enzyme to destroy the penicillin (Knox, 1962). Actually penicillin can be made to induce some strains of *Staph. aureus* to produce penicillinase. No permanently resistant population of this bacterium has arisen in this way, and the organisms return fairly rapidly to the 'uninduced' susceptible state when the penicillin is withdrawn. Much of the detail of penicillinase-induction was first worked out in *Bacillus cereus* (Pollock and Perret, 1951).

In many hospitals, over 90 per cent of the nursing staff harbour penicillinase-containing, penicillin-resistant *Staph. aureus* in the nose, a

*In some cases this happens when the bacterium acquires a plasmid that produces this enzyme (see Type 5, below) (Richmond and Curtis, 1974).

state of affairs that is quite rare outside of hospitals. This has been attributed to the continual inhalation of traces of penicillin, which destroys the sensitive strains and thus liberates the nostrils as ideal culture-areas for growth of resistant strains (Gould, 1957).

The treatment of acute leukaemia with cytosine arabinoside (4.10) fails in proportion as malignant cells with a higher concentration of cytosine deaminase appear (Steuart and Burke, 1971). Acquisition of insensitivity to 6-mercaptopurine by acute lymphocytic leukaemia cells in man, and by murine sarcoma 180/TG, was shown to be due to an increase in alkaline phosphatase which causes degradation of the tumour-inhibiting nucleotide to which the cell converts this pro-drug (Rosman et al., 1974).

Insects usually become resistant by a Type 2 mechanism, most often through the acquisition of a mixed function oxidase (Casida, 1973), very similar in nature to the combined oxidases of the human endoplasmic reticulum (see Section 3.4). This genetic change brings with it resistance to all the main types of chlorinated hydrocarbons, to the phosphates and carbamates, and (though in reduced degree) to some of the newer pyrethroids and the pyrethrin synergists (Tsukamoto and Casida, 1967). Resistance to organophosphates can, alternatively, be effected by organophosphate esterase and, sometimes, by glutathione S-transferase (Casida, 1973).

In addition, two different types of resistance to chlorinated hydrocarbons occur in insects, particularly flies: one is to DDT and the other is to dieldrin, chlordane, and benzene hexachloride (BHC). DDT-resistance in flies is commonly due to the increased rate of conversion of DDT (dichlorodiphenyltrichloroethane) (3.37) to DDE (dichlorodiphenyldichloroethylene), which is inactive (Sternburg, Kearns and Moorefield, 1954; Busvine, 1957). This is achieved by an increased production of the enzyme 'DDT-dehydrochlorinase' (Winteringham and Barnes, 1955). The normal function of this dehydrochlorinase is unknown in the mutant which the agent has caused to be selected. Resistance to BHC in houseflies has been traced to its conversion to water-soluble sulphur-containing derivatives, probably mercapturic acids (Bradbury and Standen, 1959).

In human leukaemia, the malignant blood cells readily develop resistance to methotrexate (4.6). The reason is not known but may be connected with the observed excess of dihydrofolate reductase (the enzyme that methotrexate is employed to block) that forms in the patient's leucocytes (Bertino, et al., 1965). The 200-fold increase in reductase found in murine sarcoma and lymphoma cells which became resistant through methotrexate treatment, has been traced to induction, by the drug, of extra copies of the gene (Alt et al., 1978).

Type 2 resistance to any agent can be overcome by blocking the destroying enzyme, when suitable inhibitors are found. Thus DMC, 1,1-bis-(p-chlorophenyl)ethanol, 'Kelthane' (6.55), which is structurally related to

DDT, overcomes resistance in flies by blocking the enzyme which degrades DDT to 1,1-*bis*-(*p*-chlorophenyl)-2,2-dichloroethylene (DDE). Typical results are given in Table 6.2.

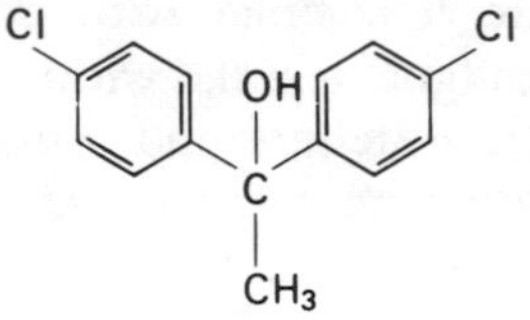

DMC
(6.55)

Table 6.2

EFFECT OF DMC (6.55) IN OVERCOMING
THE RESISTANCE OF HOUSEFLIES TO DDT

Amount applied to fly in μg		Inhibition of enzymic conversion of DDT to DDE (per cent)	Mortality of flies (per cent)
DDT	DMC		
0.65	0.0	0	0
0.65	0.06	20	2
0.65	0.65	49	50
0.65	1.30	65	72
0.65	6.50	84	100

(Perry *et al.*, 1953.)

(c) *Type 3 resistance : Decreased enzyme production*

Human neoplasm cells in culture show a different type of resistance to 6-mercaptopurine from that cited above, in that they delete the enzyme responsible for converting this pro-drug to the therapeutic nucleotide (6-thioinosine-5′-phosphate) (Brockman, 1963). The deleted enzyme is inosine-5′-phosphate pyrophosphorylase. Similarly, resistance to 8-azaguanine is accompanied by loss of the enzyme guanosine-5′-phosphate pyrophosphorylase in human epidermoid carcinoma cells (Brockman *et al.*, 1961). Resistance to 5-fluorouracil also depends on the uneconomic cell's ceasing to convert this pro-drug to the nucleotide.

A related kind of resistance, 'target withdrawal', falls somewhere in between Type 2 and Type 3. In an example, the clinical resistance of *Staphylococcus aureus* to erythromycin, the 50*S* ribosome subunits were found to have been methylated by an enzyme peculiar to the resistant strain

(Lai and Weisblum, 1971). Also, in some examples of clinical resistance of pneumococci to sulphonamides, the target enzyme, dihydrofolate synthetase, has been found chemically altered (Ortiz, 1970).

The widespread resistance, recently encountered in rats, to the anticoagulant rodenticide warfarin (6.53), seems to be of this type. Ribosomes from resistant animals contain less warfarin than normal, due to replacement of the usual binding protein by one with less affinity (Martin, 1973).

It will be realized that in Type 3 resistance, and much of Type 2, the uneconomic cells have to make increased use of an alternative biochemical pathway.

(d) *Type 4 resistance: Increased metabolite production*

Type 4 resistance takes the form of secretion by the organism of an excessive amount of the substance to which the drug is a metabolite-antagonist. Several workers, for instance, have shown that staphylococci, pneumococci, and gonococci become resistant to the usual concentrations of sulphonamide drugs by secreting extra quantities of *p*-aminobenzoic acid (cf. Landy and Gerstung, 1944). The *p*-aminobenzoic acid produced in this way has been isolated chromatographically (Moss and Lemberg, 1950; Lemberg *et al.*, 1948).

(e) *Type 5 resistance: Gene-transfer*

The following is the classical example. When sensitive pneumococci were cultivated in a medium to which an extract of penicillin-resistant pneumococci had been added, a proportion of the resulting organisms were penicillin-resistant and continued so on sub-culture. The transforming factor was found to be a DNA, and is the active part of a bacterial gene. In this way sensitive cells can be made resistant to penicillin without ever having been in contact with that drug (Hotchkiss, 1951), and streptomycin-resistance can be induced in the same way (Hotchkiss, 1955).

Another aspect of gene-transfer, known as *infectious multiple drug resistance*, has, in some localities, undermined the usefulness of a wide range of drugs normally able to cope with serious intestinal infections. As was first suspected about 1960, many Gram-negative bacteria in the intestines carry a plasmid (i.e. a transferable particle of DNA), also called the 'R Factor' or episome. This can invade other bacteria if two species conjugate, and thus transfer drug-resistance from the first to the second species. The bacteria in question are those that cause dysentery, cholera, typhoid fever, tularemia, and plague. This R Factor often confers simultaneous resistance to sulphadiazine, streptomycin, the tetracyclines, and analogues of all these, by chemical elaboration of the drug to give an inert substance. Thus *E. coli* plasmids use adenylic acid to esterify streptomycin (Takasawa *et al.*, 1968), and those from *E. coli* and *Staph. aureus* inactivate chloramphenicol by acetylation, and kanamycin by phosphorylation (Doi, *et al.*, 1968). Usually plasmid-caused resistance is chemically different from that caused by mutation.

The R Factor is a unit of non-chromosomal inheritance that exists independently of any exposure to drugs. It is mainly a centre for detoxification of foreign substances similar in function to the endoplasmic reticulum of mammalian liver (see Section 3.4). It can be inactivated *in vitro* by short exposure to simple aminoacridines and phenanthridines (Mitsuhashi *et al.*, 1961; Bouanchaud *et al.*, 1968); but clinically the problem, of ever increasing magnitude, is unsolved. Plasmid-conveyed drug resistance has raised serious problems in the treatment of infections caused by the enterobacteria. Chief among such infections are shigellosis, often called bacillary dysentery, and salmonellosis, which is often referred to as food poisoning and may be caused by any of 1200 serotypes of *Salmonella*. Typhoid fever is also caused by *Salmonella* (*S. typhi*). The resistance problem was first recognized in Japan in 1959–60, when *Shigellae* were shown to have become resistant to tetracyclines, streptomycin, sulfonamides, and chloramphenicol. The Central American outbreak due to *Shigella dysenteriae I*, which was resistant to these drugs, caused over 12 000 deaths in Guatemala in 1968–69 and also spread to Mexico. In 1972, similarly resistant strains of *S. typhi* appeared in India, Mexico, and Viet-Nam (Anon., WHO, 1974).

General remarks on resistance in the clinic. A useful distinction can be made between resistance acquired (a) in the patient and (b) apart from him. Thus, in patients undergoing treatment for tuberculosis with streptomycin, isoniazid, or *p*-aminosalicylic acid, the causative organism (*Mycobacterium tuberculosis*) often becomes resistant to one or more of these drugs. This has been found to take place, stepwise, by a selection of resistant strains within the patient's body. Resistant staphylococci, on the other hand, are very often acquired from other infected people (Knox, 1962).

The discovery of multiple resistances in his experimental organism (the trypanosome), and the existence of multiple receptors which this finding indicated, led Ehrlich (1909) to suggest *multiple therapy*, the treatment of the sick patient with two or more drugs, simultaneously, each aimed at a different receptor. When applied at the start of the treatment, this strategy can greatly delay the onset of any kind of resistance. In current therapy, this approach is much used in tuberculosis, leukaemia, and antibacterial therapy in general. In practice, it usually effects a vast decrease in the parasite/host ratio before resistance has had time to set in.

Resistance is often a purely regional phenomenon, at least at first. When the malarial parasite *Plasmodium falciparum* had become insusceptible to chloroquin in South-East Asia and South America too, it remained highly susceptible elsewhere. A population of inadequately dosed sufferers forms a dangerous reservoir of resistant organisms.

When one pauses to think how widely drugs and other selective agents are used, and how widespread the resistance phenomenon has become, it is gratifying to find some organisms that remain universally susceptible (see above, p. 226).

In pharmacodynamics, the parallel phenomenon to resistance is the loss of effect of a drug, either through the body having learnt to degrade it (as happens with barbiturates, Section 3.4) or by the sensitivity of the receptor apparently declining (as happens with nicotine and morphine).

For further reading on the biochemical basis of drug resistance, see Mihich (1973), and for infectious multiple drug resistance, see Falkow (1975).

6.6 Therapeutic interference

The term *therapeutic interference* was coined by Browning and Gulbransen (1922) to describe the following phenomenon which they discovered. Mice suffering from trypanosomiasis could not be cured by injection of the usual dose of euflavine (6.4) if they had previously been fed para-fuchsin (6.54). Although parafuchsin is itself slightly trypanocidal, it was used here in an ineffective dose. The phenomenon has often been confirmed and a typical experiment is shown in Table 6.3. Organisms cannot pass the interference effect on to the next generation, a point of difference from drug-resistance.

Table 6.3

THERAPEUTIC INTERFERENCE
INJECTIONS INTO
TRYPANOSOME-INFECTED MICE

Parafuchsin	Euflavine	Result
Nil	Nil	Died 5th to 7th day (parasites + + +)
0.05	Nil	Died 5th to 7th day (parasites + + +)
0.25	Nil	Died 5th to 7th day (parasites + + +)
Nil	0.5	Cured on 3rd day
0.05	0.5	Died 6th to 7th day (parasites + + +)
0.25	0.5	Died 7th day (parasites + + +)

(Schnitzer, 1926.)

It can be seen from this Table that one part of parafuchsin can prevent 10 parts of euflavine from acting. Interference between these substances has been demonstrated *in vitro*, where the parafuchsin again prevents the euflavine from killing the organism (v. Jancsó, 1931). The same antagonism has also been demonstrated respirometrically (Scheff and Hasskó, 1936); both substances separately depress consumption of glucose, but a mixture does not.

The term therapeutic interference has been confined to cases where there is chemical similarity between the two substances and hence no likelihood of their reacting chemically with one another. The phenomenon brings to mind the often-met situation in pharmacodynamics where an agonist can be converted, by an increase in molecular weight, to an antagonist of low or zero efficacy, but with a greater affinity for the receptor (see Section 7.5b, p. 257).

In the clinic, the current situation is that many pairs of interfering drugs are known. The wise physician prescribes as few drugs as possible at any one time, while warning the patient against self-medication while treatment is in progress. For a handbook of drug interactions, see Swidler, (1971).

7 Pharmacodynamics

The word pharmacodynamics, as used in this book, means the study of those examples of selective toxicity where the economic and uneconomic species are constituent cells *in the one organism*. Thus it stands in contrast to chemotherapy, where the uneconomic species is a different organism from the economic one.

The beginnings of pharmacodynamics as a science is traceable to the efforts of Rudolf Buchheim (1820–1879), born in Saxony, the son of a physician. Four years after graduating in medicine, he was promoted to full professor at the (Baltic) University of Dorpat, where he established the world's first pharmacological laboratory and attracted many brilliant young men to work in it. In 1867, he transferred to a comparable position in Giessen (Germany), where he remained until his death from a stroke.

Buchheim taught that the mode of action of drugs should be investigated by scientific means in order to introduce a more rational basis for therapy. This way of thinking was, at that time, revolutionary, yet he went on to write (Buchheim, 1872):

'If we translate our often obscure ideas about drug actions into an exact physiological language, this should without doubt be a considerable achievement. However, scientific recognition of the action of a given drug would imply our ability to deduce each of its actions from its chemical formula'.

Buchheim also pressed for the study of metabolism and of statistical methods to raise pharmacology to the level of an exact discipline, equal in status to chemistry and physiology. He placed special emphasis on experimentation with simple models.

Although no great discovery can be connected with Buchheim's name, he was a great teacher and introduced into pharmacodynamics the methods that were essential for its later achievements. A forerunner whose writings may have influenced his early thinking was the French physiologist François Magendie (1783–1855).

For further reading on Buchheim, see biographies by his disciple Schmiedeberg (1912), and by Habermann (1974).

7.0 Pharmacodynamics and chemotherapy compared

In pharmacodynamics at least three problems arise which have little or no counterpart in chemotherapy.

In the first place, pharmacodynamic results are usually required to be reversible. The patient who submits to an anaesthetic does not expect to be deprived of feeling permanently. In chemotherapy, on the other hand, the toxic action is most esteemed when it is most irreversible.

In the second place, pharmacodynamic drugs are expected to act with a *graded* response. In proportion to the severity of a spasm or excessive secretion, so should various doses of the remedy exactly neutralize what is morbid without inflicting upon the patient any further loss of function. The reverse of the graded response, namely the all-or-nothing effect so desirable in chemotherapy, must be avoided in pharmacodynamics.

In the third place, the worker in pharmacodynamics finds his biological testing material harder to isolate in quantity and in a uniform condition. Ideally he should begin with the simplest system possible, namely the selectively toxic agent and a uniform population of the cells on which it is to act. Once these fundamental relationships have been explored, the natural complicating factors may be added gradually so as to enable the work eventually to serve a utilitarian end. Thus he should progress from effector cells to the tissue in which they occur, from these to the organ and, eventually, to the entire plant or animal.

However, the student of pharmacodynamics finds difficulty in studying cells in isolation. It is often not practicable to obtain a uniform population of these, undamaged and functional. Moreover, he may be interested in the communication mechanism (e.g. a synapse) between two different kinds of cells. But it is a sad fact that most pharmacological test-objects contain a high percentage of entirely extraneous cells which are rich 'sites of loss' (as defined in Section 3.3). This makes it difficult to obtain results that are significantly quantitative. Moreover, the tradition has been to begin most exploratory work in perfused organs or even with an intact animal.

Fortunately, from time to time some progress has been made in the direction of A. J. Clark's ideal: single-cell pharmacology. Thus the intra- and extra-cellular response of single nerve or muscle cells can be recorded while electrophoretic administration of a drug is being made into the extraneuronal environment (del Castillo and Katz, 1957; Katz, 1966).

In general, pharmacodynamic drugs would be expected to have less specificity than chemotherapeutic ones, because of the greater difficulty of discriminating between receptors *in the one organism* (especially as many of them happen to be receptors for a single neurotransmitter, acetylcholine). As a consequence of this, pharmacodynamic drugs often fail to reverse the disease process, but merely arrest or retard its progress; when this is the case, the prolongation of therapy is likely to be accompanied by long-term side-effects.

From these considerations, it might be concluded that the study of chemotherapy is immeasurably simpler than that of pharmacodynamics. However, those who study chemotherapy have to perform pharmacodynamic work also in order to follow the side-effects of their drugs on the host. Even drugs, such as piperazine and penicillin, which have no side-effects at all in the average patient, nevertheless need to be studied pharmacodynamically to discover their pattern of distribution in the body, and the origins of their favourable selectivity.

7.1 Early history of the use of synthesis to find new drugs

The use of pharmacodynamic remedies had its remote origins in tribal practices, but even the great civilizations of antiquity knew of only a few drugs acceptable today (notably opium, ergot, and belladonna). Early in the seventeenth century, the pragmatic flavour of Baconian philosophy led to the publication of pharmacopoeias, books which listed the most valued drugs and set standards for them. Among the very first of these works the *London Pharmacopoeia* of 1618 contained several remedies that are still in use, but also many quaint and futile items such as the fat of dogs, eels, storks, and hedgehogs, the excrement of various animals, and stones from a patient's bladder. The first isolation of an alkaloid (morphine, by Sertürner in 1803) turned attention to the value of obtaining pure active substances from the vegetable or animal mass in which they were commonly dispersed.

Chemical synthesis did not seem, at first, a likely source of useful remedies. However, after Wöhler's synthesis of urea, in 1828, a whole range of synthetic organic chemicals was introduced into medical practice. After several false starts, some relatively simple substances were adopted as inhalation anaesthetics, namely nitrous oxide, ether, and chloroform (1844–7) which, by giving the surgeon adequate time for his task, initiated a tremendous refinement and extension of the possibilities of surgery.

What is so odd, from our present-day point of view, is that these anaesthetics were first tried on man, not on laboratory animals. Later it was found that the changes induced in man could be reproduced in experimental animals and this altered the method of testing new substances as potential anaesthetics. For human trials, those compounds were selected which had shown maximal activity without injurious side-effects in laboratory animals. This change of approach initiated a procedure which is now traversed in the search for all new remedies.

Between 1860 and 1905, organic syntheses were energetically pressed into the service of finding hypnotics, i.e. drugs to induce sleep in the sleepless patient. The first hypnotics were relatively simple substances, such as chloral hydrate (Liebreich, 1869) and paraldehyde (Cervello, 1882), and progressed in complexity to barbitone ('Veronal') (Fischer and von Mering, 1903). The immaturity of organic chemistry not only conditioned the choice of substances used as sedatives but, through them, it selected the type of sedation which came to be regarded as desirable (cf. McIlwain, 1957). How limited this type was, has been made clear by relatively recent discoveries of the kinds (and proportions) of sleep regarded as normal, and of drugs which sedate different regions of the brain quite selectively.

In the last quarter of the nineteenth century, a vigorous search for temperature-reducing drugs, with quinine as a vague model, brought to light a whole class of mild synthetic analgesics, such as acetanilide (Cahn and Hepp, 1887) and antipyrine or phenazone (Knorr, 1887). Sodium salicylate was introduced as a combined analgesic and antirheumatic in 1875 by Buss, and aspirin by Dreser in 1899.

The alkaloid cocaine, the first local anaesthetic, was introduced by Koller (with some help from Sigmund Freud) in 1884. Caught up in a contemporary urge to simplify natural products as described in Section 7.3, Einhorn (1905) produced the synthetic (and in many ways more useful) local anaesthetic, procaine.

Mention has been made (in Section 6.1) of how these pharmacodynamic discoveries led Ehrlich to seek simple synthetic remedies for infectious disease: this initiated his opening up the subject of chemotherapy in 1899. For the next 50 years or so, its rate of progress far outpaced that of pharmacodynamics, largely for the reasons given at the beginning of this section. Pharmacodynamics, in short, is much the more complex of the two divisions of pharmacology. Fortunately, in the last few decades, a more quantitative and molecular approach to pharmacodynamics has enabled it to forge ahead once again. This new progress is important because most serious illnesses in the more industrialized countries are non-infectious in nature (Section 1.1).

7.2 Some common molecular patterns in pharmacodynamic drugs

It is one of the curiosities of nature that many plants find it convenient to excrete waste nitrogen in molecules that have patterns which affect

vertebrate nerve and muscle, although these two kinds of tissue
are completely lacking in the plant kingdom. Alkaloids are typical waste
products of plant metabolism, allowed to accumulate only in those parts
of the plant which can easily be shed, such as the bark, leaves, and fruit.
The majority of alkaloids are biologically inert in mammals. Of the 25
alkaloids of opium, only 4 show an effect on man.

Inspection of the formulae of medicinal alkaloids shows that a certain
pattern of atoms is repeated. This pattern consists of the tertiary amino-
group connected by two or three (rarely four) saturated carbon atoms to
another tertiary amino- (or to a secondary alcoholic, or an ether) group,
or to an unsaturated ring, for example (7.1), (7.2), and (7.3). This pattern
occurs in lobeline, atropine, cocaine, quinine, strychnine, and morphine,
to give a few of the many examples. These complex alkaloids have other
groups and rings, to be sure, but the heart of their pharmacological action
seems to reside in the above patterns which can, in whole or part (although
this is almost immaterial) occur in a heteroaliphatic ring such as piperidine.
The hydroxyl-group, when present, is often acylated. This pattern is
somewhat reminiscent of those found in such potent mammalian nitrogenous hormones as acetylcholine (7.4), noradrenaline (7.5), adrenaline, and
histamine (7.6).

$$R_2N \cdot CH_2 \cdot CH_2 \cdot NR_2 \qquad\qquad R_2N \cdot CH_2 \cdot CHR \cdot OH$$

(7.1)   (7.2)

$$CH_2 \cdot CH_2 \cdot NR_2$$

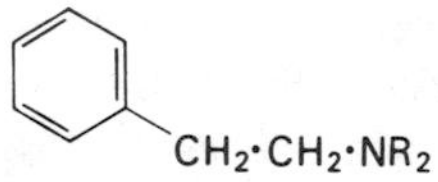

(7.3)

$$CH_3 \overset{O}{\underset{}{\overset{\|}{C}}} \cdot OCH_2 \cdot CH_2 \cdot N^+(CH_3)_3 \} Cl^-$$

Acetylcholine chloride
(7.4)

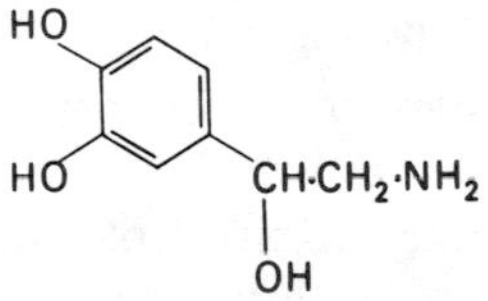

Noradrenaline
(7.5)

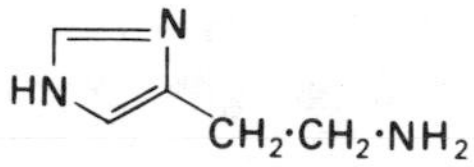

Histamine
(7.6)

Further, this pattern turns up often in contemporary pharmacodynamic
agents, especially in local anaesthetics, antihistamines, anti-emetics,
tranquillizers, and in drugs intended to replace one or more uses of atropine. This is not a chance occurrence, because Fourneau and Bovet,

working in Paris in the Institut Pasteur, began about 1935 to explore the pharmacodynamic effect of attaching this pattern of atoms to aromatic and heteroaromatic rings. The discovery of antihistamines and tranquillizers, two novel and highly valuable classes of drug, was an early reward for this inspired approach.

It may at first seem bold to suggest that all these substances, whether alkaloids, neurotransmitters, or the newer synthetic drugs, are acting on a few, chemically similar, receptors. The pattern itself allows of considerable variation without loss of a particular biological effect, e.g. local anaesthetics may be either type (7.1) or (7.2), the number of connecting carbon atoms may be two or three, and these may carry small substituents such as methyl-groups. This points to a conclusion that the receptors of vertebrates have not so great a specificity for their substrates as many enzymes have (Ariëns, 1960; Fastier, 1964).

In line with this conclusion is the fact that few pharmacodynamic drugs have *complete* biological specificity. They usually give results suggestive of combination principally with a single, fairly specific, receptor, but in addition show a number of side-effects indicative of combination with other receptors. For example, it is reasonable to think that each of the following six properties of a drug would involve a different kind of receptor: local anaesthetic, antihistaminic, spasmolytic, analgesic, antiacetylcholine, and prolongation of the refractory period of the heart. Yet each of the seven following substances displays *all* of these properties (although each possesses one of them in an enhanced degree): procaine, mepyramine, papaverine, pethidine (meperidine), atropine, quinidine, and sparteine. It has been suggested that the basis of these common properties is that such substances can antagonize acetylcholine, histamine, and possibly adrenaline too, in a number of tissues (Burn, 1950).

Although the specificity of receptors is not so strict as that of the most important anabolic and catabolic enzymes, it is at least as strict as the degradative enzymes of microsomes (see Section 3.4). Thus at ganglia, nicotine (7.18) [but not muscarine (7.39)] can take the place of acetylcholine, whereas at postganglionic parasympathetic synapses, muscarine (but not nicotine) can take its place (see Table 7.1). Further specificity is shown in acetylcholine *antagonism*, for which tubocurarine is specific at the neuromuscular junction, hexamethonium at ganglia, and atropine at parasympathetic postganglionic synapses.

Although it seems that receptors have only a moderate specificity, it should still be possible to find specific drugs by (a) arranging their ionic (Chapter 10) and lipophilic (Section 3.2 and Appendix II) properties to give them the best possible access to the site, and (b) providing them with such blocking groups as sterically prevent their access to other sites (Fastier, 1964). At the same time, the structure should be kept as simple as possible to avoid side-effects.

7.3 Simplification of the structure of natural products

Late in the last century, a beginning was made in the task of simplifying the molecular structure of natural products while retaining the therapeutic action. It was hoped in this way to obtain substances which could be more easily synthesized and which might be free from toxic side-effects introduced by unwanted parts of the molecule. The introduction of salicylic acid into medicine in 1875 was one of the earliest results of this endeavour, and this acid and its salts and derivatives such as aspirin replaced the use of willow bark, and the glucoside of salicyl alcohol which this bark contained.

In the last century, many plant alkaloids were found to have powerful pharmacological actions. The simplification of the structure of cocaine (7.7) to give the local anaesthetic, procaine ('Novocain') (7.8), was the first notable success in modifying the structure of alkaloids to suit the combined needs of manufacturer and clinic (Einhorn, 1905). Procaine, unlike cocaine, does not penetrate mucous membranes but is non-addictive and lacks other side-effects of cocaine. It at once achieved widespread use as a dental anaesthetic, and is still much used. The guiding principle in these alkaloidal simplifications is that *saturated* heterocyclic rings are to be broken open (mentally, that is), a process which affects physical and chemical properties very little. Thus cocaine (7.7), which has a tertiary amine group in two saturated rings which bear an alcoholic group esterified with benzoic acid, was simplified to an isomer (7.9) of benzamine without loss of local anaesthetic properties. Next, the other saturated ring was opened to give 3-diethylaminopropyl benzoate (7.10). The basic strength, which had gone up, from loss of the methyl ester group of cocaine, was advantageously (see Section 10.5) lowered by deleting a methylene group, thus restoring better penetration of the nerve plasma membrane. One final change led to procaine (7.8): an amino-group was inserted in the benzene ring to achieve an effective hydrophilic/lipophilic balance. It must not be supposed that the physical principles behind each of these changes could be so clearly expressed in 1905 as to-day. Yet they must have been understood intuitively, because they were soon being applied to the molecules of other alkaloids.

Cocaine
(flattened formula)
(7.7)

Isobenzamine
(7.9)

$Et_2N \cdot CH_2 \cdot CH_2 \cdot O \cdot \overset{..}{\underset{O}{C}} - C_6H_4(p-NH_2)$

Procaine
(7.8)

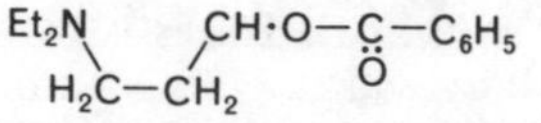
Et₂N
CH·O—C—C₆H₅
O
H₂C—CH₂

3-Diethylaminopropyl benzoate
(*7.10*)

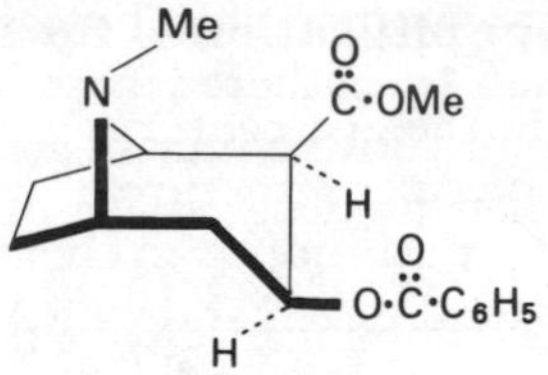
Me
N
O
C·OMe
H
O
O·C·C₆H₅
H

Cocaine
(conformational formula)
(*7.11*)

It is now known (Fodor, 1960; Sinnema *et al.*, 1968) that the molecule of cocaine has a very rigid three-dimensional conformation*, whereas that of procaine (*7.8*) is loosely jointed, which is no disadvantage, for it allows better adaptation to the receptor.

Later the structure of procaine was modified to obtain, for particular medical uses, a substance which could easily penetrate mucous membranes. A redistribution of lipophilic groups gave the much-used local anaesthetic amethocaine (tetracaine, 'Decicain') (*7.12*). This simple solution to the problem was reached after many false clues had been followed (reviewed by Barlow, 1964). It is now known that a tremendous number of chemicals have local anaesthetic activity. The ester-group can be replaced by an amide-group [or even a reversed amide-group as in lignocaine (*7.13*)]. A good feature of esters is that they are soon hydrolysed by serum esterases, so that the duration of the anaesthesia is self-limited.

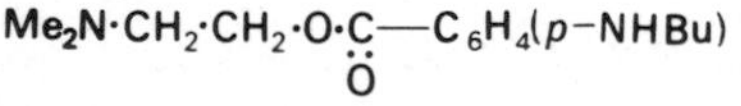
Me₂N·CH₂·CH₂·O·C—C₆H₄(p–NHBu)
O

Amethocaine
(*7.12*)

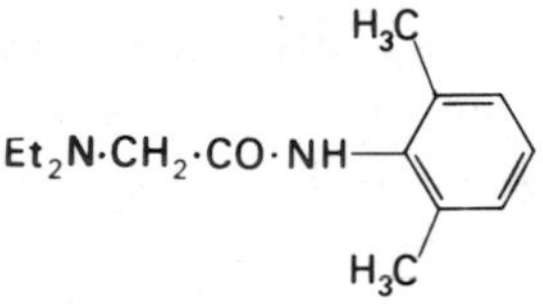
H₃C
Et₂N·CH₂·CO·NH
H₃C

Lignocaine ('Xylocain')
(*7.13*)

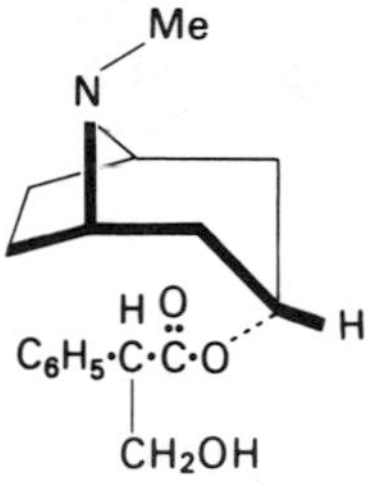
Me
N
H O
C₆H₅·C·C·O
H
CH₂OH

Atropine
(conformational formula)
(*7.14*)

* A refresher on molecular structure: when every second bond is a double-bond (e.g. benzene) the molecule is flat and rigid. A saturated ring (no double-bonds), as in cocaine, is three-dimensional and fairly rigid. A saturated aliphatic molecule without a double-bond (e.g. ethanol) is three-dimensional and flexible. For conformation, see Section 13.3.

It was remarkable how successful some of these simplifications were. As may be gathered from Section 7.5b, there was a risk of turning an antagonist into an agonist if the process were taken too far; another risk was that the drug, shorn of sterically hindering groups, might act on too many receptors.

The simplification of atropine (DL-hyoscyamine) (7.14) was begun at the start of this century. Although both atropine and cocaine have a tropine ring-system, the conformations are different, as can be seen by comparing (7.11) and (7.14) (Fodor, 1960). Many attempts were made to prepare a stripped-down analogue that would conserve the typical anti-muscarinic action on the gut (and hence be a good antispasmodic) without the CNS-stimulating, pupil-dilating, and throat-drying side-effects of atropine. As was realized at the start, the greater bulk of the esterifying acid in atropine (versus cocaine) was significant, but the first substances produced, even with this knowledge, had more local anaesthetic than parasympathetic-blocking action, e.g. adiphenine ('Trasentin'). Improvements, which came slowly, were to increase the bulk of the esterifying acid still further, and either to quaternize the basic group, as in oxyphenonium ('Antrenyl') (7.15), or to conserve a ring structure for it, as in oxyphencyclimine ('Daricon') (7.16). The former has acquired some ganglion-blocking activity through the quaternization, but this is not very evident at the low dose used (Barrett et al., 1953). The latter (7.16) is purely anti-muscarinic. Benzhexol (trihexyphenidyl, 'Artane') 1-cyclohexyl-1-phenyl-3-piperidinylpropan-1-ol, is used in parkinsonism for its anticholinergic effect. The quaternized types are poorly absorbed from the gut and hence affect the CNS very little. Many similar 'simplified atropines' such as tropicamide and cyclopentolate (7.17) have the full mydriatic effect of atropine on the pupil of the eye, and are used in ophthalmology as alternatives to atropine, homotropine, and ephedrine. It can be seen that cyclopentolate ('Cyclogyl') is simply the ester of dimethylaminoethanol with a large hydroxyacid, similar to that used in (7.15).

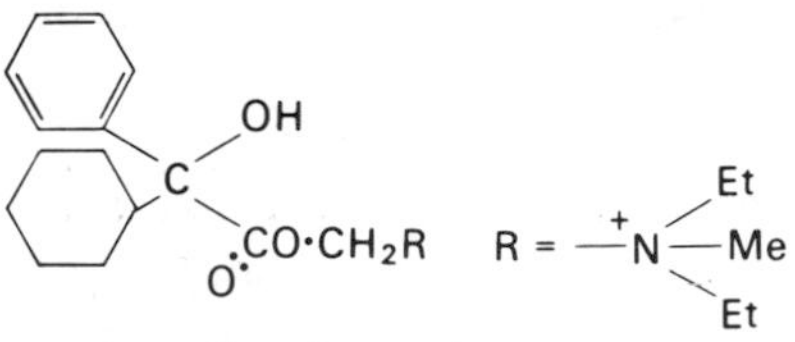

Oxyphenonium
(7.15)

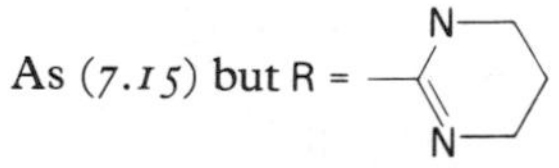

As (7.15) but R =

Oxyphencyclimine
(7.16)

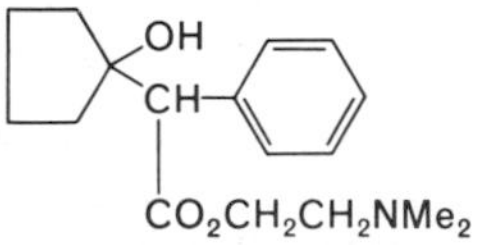

Cyclopentolate
(7.17)

The neurotransmitter actions of acetylcholine are imitated by nicotine (*7.18*) at both the ganglionic and the voluntary neuromuscular synapses (Table 7.1). It is a potent insecticide, and attempts to simplify the molecule have mainly had that property in mind. The nature and potency of its action are hardly changed by quaternization (further methylation) of the nitrogen in the saturated (pyrrolidine) ring. When the quaternary salt was modified by opening the saturated ring, as was done for cocaine, the product, and its homologues, had typical nicotine-like activity, e.g. at the neuromuscular junction (rat and chick). Substance (*7.19*, $n = 1$) was as potent as nicotine, and substance (*7.19*, $n = 2$) was 2.6 times as potent (Barlow and Hamilton, 1962). [The conformation of the nicotine molecule was worked out by Hudson and Neuberger (1950)].

Me

$-(CH_2)_n-N^+(CH_3)_3$

Nicotine
(conformational formula)
(*7.18*)

(*7.19*)

Attempts to simplify the molecule of tubocurarine were made while it was still thought to have two quaternized amino-groups, whereas it has in fact only one (Everett, Lowe, and Wilkinson, 1970). In spite of this misconception, some very useful drugs were developed. It was related in Section 2.0 how Crum Brown and Fraser (1869) had shown that various alkaloids acquire curare-like properties by methylation to quaternary ammonium bases. Even simple aliphatic quaternary amines, so long as they possess at least one methyl-group, have this curare-like action, but they are far too weak to be useful adjuncts to surgical anaesthesia. Reviewing the evidence, Ing (1936) came to the conclusion that tubocurarine (*2.6*), and similarly acting quaternary amines, worked by blocking the action of acetylcholine on the muscle end-plate of the neuromuscular junction.

In 1948, many substances with two or more quaternary nitrogen atoms were synthesized and some were found to produce neuromuscular block, e.g. decamethonium (*7.20*) (decane*bis*trimethylammonium iodide) (Paton and Zaimis, 1948; Barlow and Ing, 1948). Close examination showed that this substance not only acts durably as an acetylcholine blocking agent (as tubocurarine does), but first acts momentarily as an acetylcholine analogue, causing depolarization which is easily demonstrated with non-polarizable silver electrodes (Burns and Paton, 1951). Suxamethonium (*7.21*) also has this type of action (Bovet and Bovet-Nitti, 1949). After brief muscular contraction, prolonged relaxation follows the use of these drugs because they are strongly adsorbed and hence prevent newly liberated acetylcholine from reaching its receptors. Decamethonium was used for some years to secure muscular relaxation during light anaesthesia, but suxamethonium is preferred because its effect is self-terminating thanks to hydrolysis by esterases (in the serum of normal patients). There is no antidote for these depolarizing-curarizing agents whereas the action of tubocurarine or gallamine can be promptly terminated by neostigmine. The disulphide (7.22) is another ingeniously self-terminating agent, the disulphide bond being easily broken by cysteine (Khromov-Borisov *et al.*, 1969).

Gallamine (7.23) gallamine triethiodide) is one of the simplest substances with a true tubocurare-like action, although it has no *N*-methyl-group (Bovet, 1947). It is much used as a muscle-relaxant in surgery.

In the course of investigating the homologous series of *bis*onium compounds which led to the discovery of decamethonium, hexamethonium (7.24) was found to block the receptors for acetylcholine within autonomic ganglia, a type of activity which tubocurarine shows only weakly. At first these *bis*onium ganglion-blocking drugs were used clinically to treat hypertension, but drugs which block the sympathetic nerve endings, e.g. propranolol, give fewer side-effects and are now preferred.

$$I^-\{Me_3N^+-(CH_2)_{10}-N^+Me_3\}I^-$$

Decamethonium iodide
(7.20)

$$(Me_3N^+-(CH_2)_2-O-\overset{\overset{O}{||}}{C}-CH_2$$
$$(Me_3N^+-(CH_2)_2-O-\underset{\underset{O}{..}}{C}-CH_2$$

Suxamethonium (cation)
(7.21)

$$Me_3N^+ \!-\!\!\left\langle \right\rangle\!-\!S-S-\!\left\langle \right\rangle\!-\!NMe_3$$

(7.22)

$$Me_3N^+-(CH_2)_6-{}^+NMe_3$$

Hexamethonium (cation)
(7.24)

$$O-CH_2\cdot CH_2\cdot N^+Et_3$$
$$O-CH_2\cdot CH_2\cdot N^+Et_3$$
$$O-CH_2\cdot CH_2-N^+Et_3$$

Gallamine (cation)
(7.23)

The action of naturally secreted acetylcholine can be reinforced by drugs which acylate, and hence block, the enzyme acetylcholinesterase (see Section 12.3). The organic phosphates and carbamates do this. Of the carbamates, the alkaloid physostigmine (7.25), also known as eserine, has long been used for therapeutic results which can now be defined as 'giving the patient a much enhanced effect from his own acetylcholine'. Even at a dilution of 10^{-7}M, it strongly inhibits this enzyme, and is pharmacologically active at both nerve-nerve and nerve-muscle synapses (see Table 7.1) Stedman (1926) came to the conclusion that the methylcarbamate-group of physostigmine was responsible for its action, and he esterified simple derivatives of phenol with (mono- and di-)methylaminoformic acid. The presence of a basic group, ionized at pH 7, was found to be necessary also, and so he took the only possible way of increasing the low basic strength of an aromatic amino-group, namely by quaternization. The pharmacological results led to the introduction of neostigmine ('Prostigmine') (7.26) as a substitute for physostigmine (Aeschlimann and Reinert, 1931). It is free from some of the side-effects of the latter and has, in addition, a small ACh agonist action. It is much used in the treatment of myasthenia gravis, a disease characterized by muscular weakness, and in overcoming postoperative bladder atony.

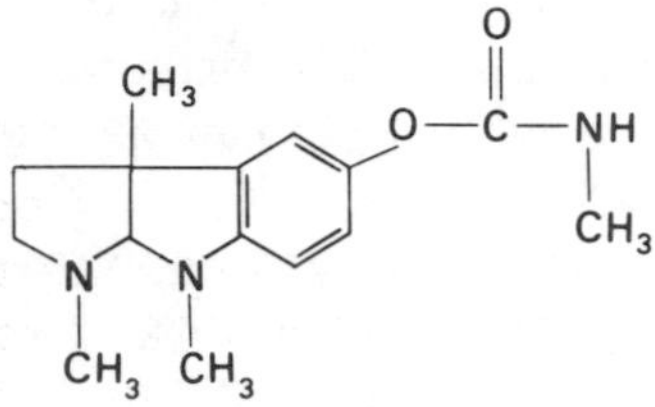

Physostigmine (eserine)
(7.25)

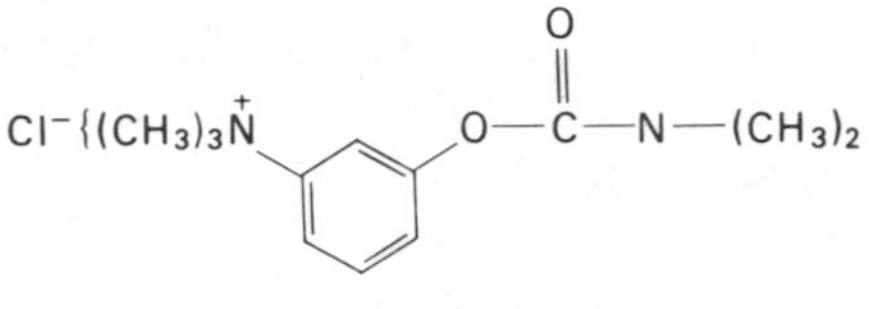

Neostigmine
(7.26)

A simple analogue for the alkaloid morphine (7.27, 7.28a) was sought in vain until Eisleb and Schaumann (1938), in Germany, produced pethidine (meperidine) (7.29) while engaged in a search for antispasmodics. Although only one-tenth as powerful as morphine, pethidine is widely used in childbirth where it causes less respiratory depression. This discovery made it clear that the molecule of morphine could be drastically simplified without qualitative loss of the morphine-type analgesic action. During the Second World War, the Hoechst company discovered the non-heterocyclic analgesic methadone (amidone) (7.30), which is quantitatively and qualitatively as effective as morphine, and still much used. For the history of the discovery of these, the first synthetic opioids, see Bergel and Morrison, 1948.

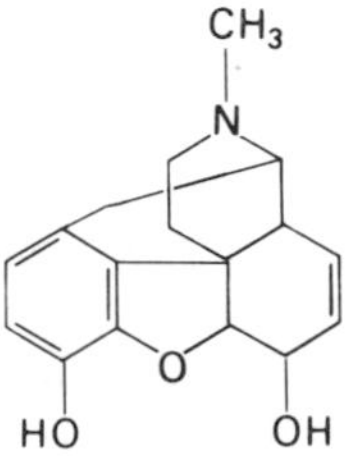

Morphine
(flattened formula)
(7.27)

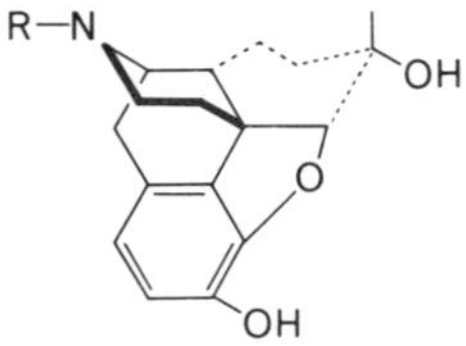

(a) Morphine (R = CH_3)
(b) Nalorphine (R = —$CH_2CH : CH_2$)
(conformational formula)
(7.28)

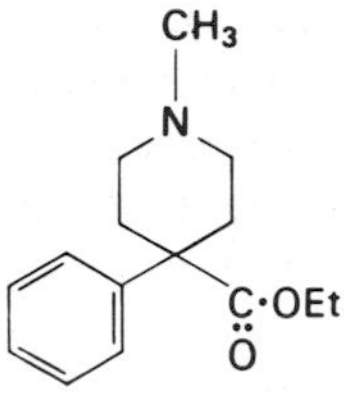

Pethidine (Meperidine)
(7.29)

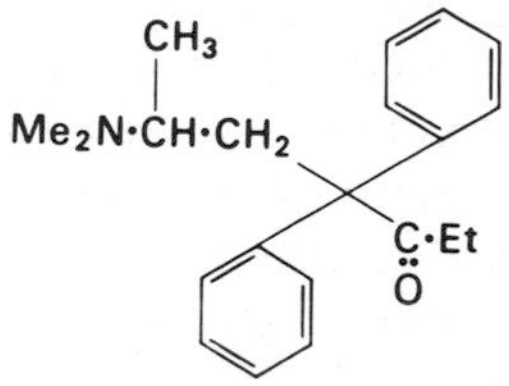

Methadone
(7.30)

Most of the synthetic analogues of morphine resemble it in producing euphoria, and hence are liable to cause addiction. An important non-addictive analogue of morphine is the partial agonist nalorphine (7.28b) (allyl*nor*morphine). It is highly analgesic and non-addictive, but tends to cause delirium. Nevertheless it gave the clue to the discovery of pentazocine (7.31) ('Fortral', 'Talwin') which is nearly as analgesic as morphine, but causes less euphoria and has less tendency to addiction (Bellville and Forrest, 1968). The molecule of pentazocine is closely related to that of morphine, but two rings have been eliminated, and a weighty group added to the ring nitrogen atom. A recent and more powerful analgesic of this type is butorphanol (17-cyclobutylmethyl-3,14-dihydroxymorphinan) (Dobkin, 1975). In hospital wards, the preferred analgesics for managing the postoperative patient are those with euphoric properties, although a switch is made later, if analgesia has to be maintained.

A quaternary carbon, such as that in the 4-position of the piperidine ring of pethidine (7.29), used to be thought indispensable for analgesic activity. However, a tertiary nitrogen atom in, or attached to, an aromatic ring is a good substitute. For example, the Swiss compound etonitazine (7.32) has exactly the same type of analgesic action as morphine but is 1500 times more potent (Gross and Turrian, 1957); it is tremendously addictive too (Winkler *et al.*, 1960).

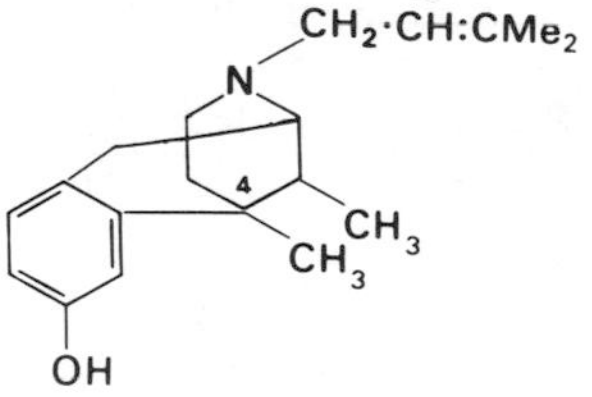

Pentazocine
(7.31)

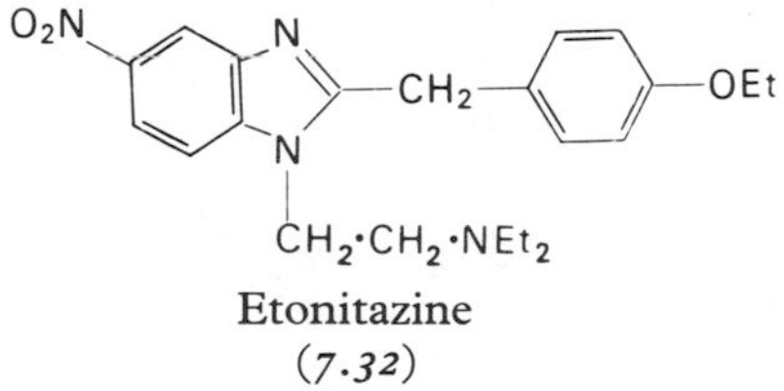

Etonitazine
(7.32)

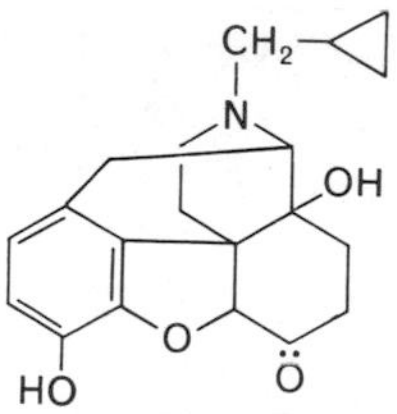

Naltrexone
(7.33)

Heroin addiction is usually treated in special Government centres where out-patients are given oral methadone; this is itself addictive but is thought to avoid the emotional swings characteristic of heroin and hence to favour gradual withdrawal. A longer acting derivative known as LAMM (1-α-acetylmethadol) is beginning to take the place of methadone in these centres. Only addicts with a strong motivation to recovery derive benefit from the faster but more painful treatment with opiate antagonists, of which naltrexone (7.33) seems to be the best.

The convulsant strychnine has been simplified to N-acetylindoline with a tertiary amine on a side-chain in the 3-position (Hershenson et al., 1977).

7.4 Recognition of the importance of measurement

The standardization and quantification of technique, and the rigorous application of statistics to the results has, in the last three decades, provided pharmacodynamics with a solid base such as it had not previously known. The use of experimental and control groups in tests on laboratory animals followed by similar tests on the human subject, have made it possible to evaluate the efficacy and side-effects of drugs reliably, for the first time, and also to make meaningful comparisons with established remedies.

No less revolutionary in the quantification of pharmacodynamics was the insistance on size relationships which Alfred Joseph Clark (London) introduced in his book, 'The Mode of Action of Drugs on Cells' (Clark, A.J., 1933). The mnemonic diagram that forms the frontispiece of the present book will serve to introduce this aspect. In it we see a typical mammal (dog) followed by a typical insect (flea) which is a thousand times smaller, and this is followed by a typical microbe (streptococcus) which is yet a thousand times smaller, and finally a typical bioactive molecule (p-aminobenzoic acid) which is one thousand times smaller still. Thus we have familiar reference objects staked out over a size-range of 10^{12} (a million-millionfold).

To proceed further, a molecule of muscle protein, if unfolded, would be about 8 nm long. This could be compared with the length of a muscle cell (about 60 μm). If a model of some common pharmacodynamic drug, one with a molecular weight in the usual range of 150–300, is built from a molecular model kit (of the scale in which 0.1 nm is reproduced as 1 cm), the molecule of the drug will seem to be about 2 in (5 cm)long, the molecule of protein 10 yd (9 m) long, and the muscle cell $3\frac{1}{2}$ miles (5.5 km) long by 200 yd (180 m) wide. These size-relationships show that many useless collisions are likely to take place before a drug hits the desired receptor, and that the drug has many opportunities to land on a 'site of loss' (defined in Section 3.3). Nevertheless, given sufficient specificity between drug and receptor, the receptor is eventually reached and combined with. In favourable cases combination occurs even at a dilution of 10^{-9}M, a dilution at which hardly any substances can be recognized in the test-tube by ordinary chemical tests.

Calculations of this kind help us realize what a prodigious number of molecules are present in one microgram of a drug (namely three thousand million million, assuming a molecular weight of about 200). It would need only four million molecules to cover a staphylococcus which has a surface area of about 2 μm^2. However, to cover a cell is unnecessary for pharmacodynamic purposes. The amount of acetylcholine, adrenaline, and histamine taken up by frog heart, frog stomach, and rat uterus (respectively), when the organs are markedly inhibited by these hormones, corresponds to about 10^{14} molecules per gram moist weight. This quantity of hormone can cover only 1 cm^2. The surface area of the cells in 1 g of frog's heart is about 6000 cm^2, and hence these hormones are active when only about 1/6000 of the surface is covered. This shows that they act by uniting with certain specific receptors, which form only a minute fraction of the total cell surface (Clark, 1933).

It is rewarding to apply these simple calculations to experimental data, in order to build a mental picture of the proportion of drug to target. For example, the lowest effective concentration for acetylcholine on the frog's heart was found to be a 5×10^{-19}M solution (Boyd and Pathak, 1965). This is equivalent to only 330 molecules per ml and must be approaching the very limit of physiological detectability. Actually Hahnemann, the founder of homeopathy, claimed therapeutic effects from various drugs at a dilution of 1 in 10^{60}. This claim strains credulity because it corresponds to one molecule in a sphere of circumference equal to the orbit of the planet Neptune (A.J. Clark, 1940, quoted by Wilson and Schild, 1968).

An example of how a test-preparation can be refined, so as to present fewer sites of loss for the drug, is afforded by the neuromuscular junction. Until recently, this had to be studied in an isolated 'nerve-muscle' preparation (such as the rat phrenic nerve diaphragm) which contained much extraneous material. But in 1957, it was found that drugs could be applied electrophoretically, from a point-source, right on to the motor end-plate of a frog's sartorius muscle. This close-range application of acetylcholine set up transient potential changes of several millivolts (del Castillo and Katz, 1957). This proved to be the best model system for obtaining correlations between structure and activity of drugs at the neuromuscular junction.

New aspects of structure-activity relationships came into view when new techniques enabled a further advance in measurement to be made. For example, Merrit and Putnam (1938) discovered the clinically useful antiepileptic drug phenytoin *15.4*), by first seeking a substance capable of suppressing electrically-induced convulsions in laboratory mammals. This discovery was a great advance in antiepileptic therapy because phenytoin has no hypnotic action; and so it was suddenly realized that anti-epileptics need not cloud the consciousness, as had been thought inevitable. Hence this work came to be widely discussed in a broader context, and gave encouragement to those using physical methods of measurement in seeking remedies for other diseases, whether with intact animals, isolated organs, cells, or cell constituents.

How dose-effect relationships came to be more accurately measured and judged is outlined in Section 6.2.

7.5 How agonists and antagonists act on receptors

The concept of a 'receptor' was explained in Section 2.1. For most chemo-therapeutic agents it has been satisfactory to assume that the observed physiological response occurs as soon as the agent becomes adsorbed on the receptor, and that (short of death of the cell) the response continues so long as the agent remains adsorbed. This is usually satisfactory also in pharmacodynamics. Several pharmacodynamic drugs, e.g. organic phosphorus derivatives, are known to act by inhibiting identifiable enzymes, and often the very atom with which a drug combined covalently in such an enzyme has been identified (see Section 12.3). When, as is more usual, the combination is not covalent, combination follows the law of mass action and can generally be described by the same relationships as are used in the Langmuir adsorption isotherm (see Section 8.1, also Gaddum, 1926). In all these cases, the response of a tissue seems to depend on the proportion of its specific receptor-groups occupied by the drug. This assumption can be referred to as *simple occupation theory*. The action of most *inhibitors* can be fairly well described by this theory.

However, drugs which *activate* receptors are more complex in their actions. The structural requirements for these activators are much more specific than those for antagonists. Many *agonists* (= activators*) are naturally occurring physiological substances, or else synthetic substances which mimic their action because of structural similarity. Other agonists prevent destruction of the natural substances or liberate them from storage sites, as tyramine liberates noradrenaline (see Section 7.6c). Because the behaviour of such drugs is complex, several hypotheses have been evolved which will be discussed a little later in this Section. As there can be no action without expenditure of the chemical energy that is stored in nature as complex phosphates, agonists work by liberating energy from energy-stores, even if only indirectly.

(a) *Chemical and electrical conduction compared*
At least 80 per cent of known pharmacodynamic agents act exclusively on

---

* The term 'agonist' was introduced by Reuse (1948).

nerve or at nerve-muscle junctions. Hence it is desirable to preface further discussion with a brief account of the propagation of an impulse along nerves, and across synapses. Nerve cells (*neurones*) consist essentially of a central, roughly spherical portion, which is drawn out into fibres, one of which (the *axon*) is much longer than the others. At the junction with a muscle fibre or a second nerve, the axon is swollen into a synaptic *terminal* which lies about 20–400 nm from specialized receptors on the muscle or nerve with which it has to communicate. Thus, at the synapse, there is a gap (*synaptic cleft*) between pre- and post-synaptic structures. Neurones of similar function are often collected together and such groupings are called *ganglia*. Fig. 7.1 shows, diagrammatically, a nerve-nerve synapse and a nerve-muscle junction which are essentially similar. For a general article on synapses, see Eccles (1965), for a book, Katz (1966).

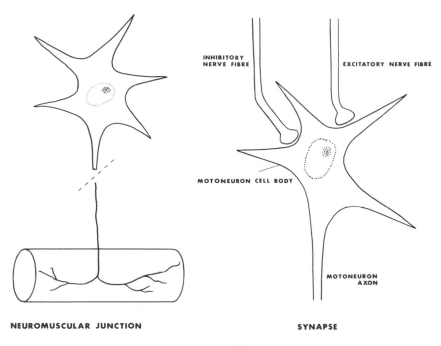

INHIBITORY NERVE FIBRE

EXCITATORY NERVE FIBRE

MOTONEURON CELL BODY

MOTONEURON AXON

NEUROMUSCULAR JUNCTION

SYNAPSE

FIG. 7.1

The main cation inside cells is potassium (K^+), and that outside is sodium (Na^+). Because of the difference in ion concentrations across the cytoplasmic membrane of nerve and muscle cells, there is usually a resting negative potential of 50 to 100 mV (compared to the outside, defined as 0V). It is as though the membrane were a miniature battery with the negative terminal on its inside. When it loses this potential, it is said to be depolarized.

This membrane is lipoprotein and permits active transport (see Section 3.1). in both directions.

The passage of a nerve impulse along a nerve fibre is a complicated physicochemical event which follows upon the depolarization of the fibre at one end, either within the nervous system (for a motor fibre) or at the peripheral sense organ (for a sensory fibre). This change in potential brings about a transient increase in the membrane's permeability to sodium ions, which pass rapidly into the nerve fibre, thus reversing the resting level of membrane potential. This process is immediately followed by a transient increase in the permeability to potassium ions which pass out of the fibre, thus restoring the membrane potential. This sequence of changes is confined to a very small area, but the associated ionic currents depolarize the next portion of the membrane which goes through the same sequence of events. In this way the impulse, which is essentially this transient reversal of membrane potential, is propagated along the fibre at a rate that depends upon the fibre diameter. The conduction velocity varies from 0.1 to 100 m s^{-1} (Hodgkin, 1964).

This rapid entry of sodium can be selectively prevented by tetrodotoxin (7.34), a spherical perhydroquinazoline molecule from which a highly basic guanidinium group protrudes like a tongue. It occurs naturally in various species of fish, amphibia, and molluscs. By excluding sodium ions, tetrodotoxin blocks the generation of a potential (and hence of transmission) in both nerve and muscle. Because transmission at synapses is unaffected, mammals die by a purely peripheral toxicity, usually by respiratory paralysis (Narahashi *et al.*, 1964). Potassium transport is unaffected.

Tetrodotoxin
(7.34)

As guanidinium is one of the few cations that can replace sodium ions in the production of action potentials (Watanabe *et al.*, 1967), it is reasonable to suppose that the guanidinium group of tetrodotoxin enters a sodium channel which the rest of the molecule then blocks. Saxitoxin, a perhydropurine with two guanidinium groups, (obtained from unicellular ocean dinoflagellates) acts almost identically. For a general review on tetrodotoxin (and the related saxitoxin), see Gage (1971), and for the chemistry, see Goto, *et al.* (1965).

Returning now to the normal firing of a nerve, it is inevitable that the passage of a single impulse leaves behind a small elevation of the intracellular $Na^+:K^+$ ratio, which is eventually restored to normal (without change in the resting potential) by a slow, energy-consuming process of ion transport called the 'sodium-potassium pump' (Hodgkin and Huxley, 1952). There are separate channels for sodium and potassium ions distinct from the shared channel mentioned above, and usually only one (or neither) of these is open. Either can be blocked independently of the other with foreign ions, and both can be kept open together with veratridine or DDT (Baker, 1968). In vertebrate cardiac muscle and vertebrate smooth muscle, Ca^{2+} replaces Na^+ for carrying the inward current (Reuter, 1973). The transport of cations consumes much energy, of which adenosine triphosphate is the source (Hokin and Hokin 1963). (Information on the transport of inorganic cations through membranes by small ionophores will be found in Section 14.1).

When a nerve impulse arrives at a synapse, it causes the release of a minute amount of a chemical substance called a neurotransmitter (or synaptic transmitter) which is a localized hormone. This substance diffuses across the gap and, on reaching the far side, it interacts with receptors on the post-synaptic membrane of a muscle or nerve cell. As soon as it has acted, the neurotransmitter is removed from the synaptic cleft, either by reabsorption into the pre-synaptic store (noradrenaline) or by enzymatic destruction (acetylcholine). The synapse is thus rapidly restored to its resting state, ready for another impulse. The most familiar transmitters of the peripheral nervous system are acetylcholine (7.4) and noradrenaline (7.5). It has been suggested that ATP is the neurotransmitter released by the non-adrenergic inhibitory innervation of the gut (Burnstock et al., 1970). In many invertebrates, such as crustaceans, molluscs, and flat worms, dopamine and 5-hydroxytryptophan have been observed playing the roles that belong to acetylcholine and noradrenaline in mammals.

Historically, it was T. R. Elliot who, while still a student at Cambridge, concluded that sympathetic nerve impulses must release minute amounts of an agent that was taken up by a receptor on the other side of the synapse. Hence he was the first to postulate that transmission across synapses was chemical (Elliott, 1905). Henry Dale (1914) proposed acetylcholine as the parasympathetic neurotransmitter and, because of its short life, he added that an enzyme must be on the spot to hydrolyse it. Otto Loewi (1921) achieved the first convincing proof of chemical transmission of a nervous impulse across a synapse, and in 1926 (with Navratil) identified the commonest neurotransmitter as acetylcholine. Dale (1914) noted that some of the actions of acetylcholine can be imitated by nicotine (7.18) and others by muscarine (7.39), and the terms nicotinic and muscarinic have turned out very useful in classifying the sites at which this neurotransmitter acts.

In mammals, histamine (7.6) and adrenaline (epinephrin) [the N-methyl derivative of (7.5)] are tissue hormones, but not neurotransmitters. The mammalian central nevous system has many neurotransmitters: acetylcholine, noradrenaline, dopamine (7.35), 5-hydroxytryptamine (7.36) and the following aminoacids: glycine, glutamate (7.37), and gamma-aminobutyric acid (GABA) (7.38). The undecapeptide known as Substance P is widely distributed in brain neuroterminals where it acts as an excitatory neurotransmitter (Iversen, 1974). The enkephalins (Section 13.7), other polypeptides and taurine are at present being canvassed as possible central neurotransmitters. The functions of some of these central neurotransmitters are defined below (p. 257).

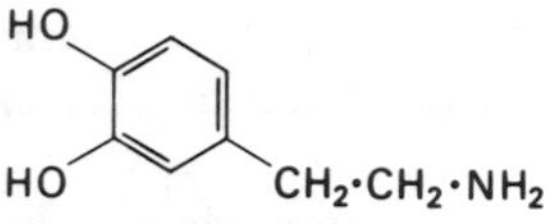

Dopamine
(7.35)

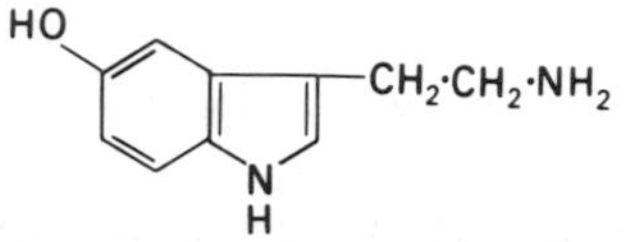

5-Hydroxytryptamine
(7.36)

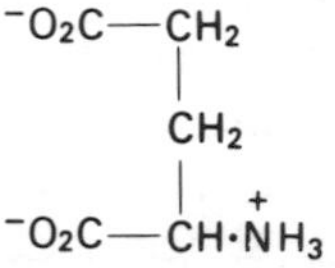

Glutamate anion
(7.37)

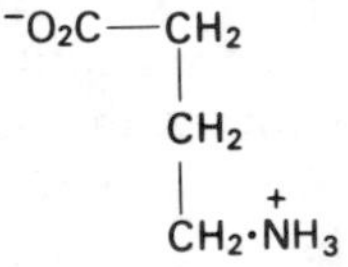

GABA
(7.38)

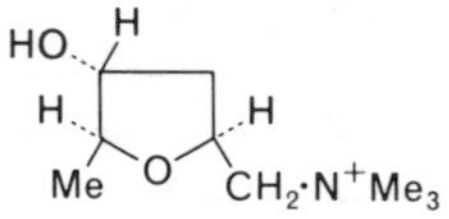

L(+)-Muscarine
(cation)
(7.39)

Events happening at the neuromuscular junction (see Fig. 7.1) on the arrival of a nerve impulse will now be described. The topography of this junction, already explored with the light microscope, has become even better known through the electron microscope (Katz, 1962). In a typical example (the junction of voluntary nerve with the sartorius muscle of the frog), the nerve-tip gives off slender branches (total length about 1 mm) which lie in gutters formed in the tip of the muscle fibre. Nerve and muscle are separated by a *synaptic cleft* of about 100 Å, and it is only this part of the muscle (the *end-plate*) which is ordinarily sensitive to acetylcholine. This transmitter is stored in the presynaptic terminal within synaptic vesicles which are about 200–500 Å in diameter. In the frog there are about three million vesicles per junction.

At the neuromuscular junction, acetylcholine interacts with receptors on the muscle end-plate. The resultant depolarization triggers an action potential which is similar to a nervous impulse (described above). For about one millisecond, acetylcholine opens channels that allow sodium ions to flow inwards, there is a temporary loss of membrane potential, and the muscle begins to contract. The acetylcholine is then destroyed by acetylcholinesterase, which is located elsewhere in the end-plate. This process occupies only a few milliseconds and can be reproduced by administering acetylcholine close to the end-plate region. However, injection directly into the interior of the muscle cell produces neither depolarization nor contraction.

The amount of acetylcholine released by a nerve terminal in one impulse is 1.5×10^{-10} µg (as found in both cat and frog). This is 5×10^6 molecules, or 200 times as much as is needed to depolarize the end-plate. However, enough acetylcholinesterase exists at the neuromuscular junction to split 10^9 molecules of the transmitter every millisecond. The dissociation constant of the complex formed by acetylcholine with its destructive enzyme is 2.6×10^{-4} (Nachmansohn, 1959).

The muscle end-plate is thus a *chemically excitable* membrane, and stands in contrast to the *electrically excitable* membrane which covers the bulk of every nerve fibre as described above. The conductance (permeability to ions) of a chemically excitable membrane is changed only by the specific chemical messenger (synaptic transmitter). These changes in ionic conductance produce membrane potential changes that are proportional to the concentration of the transmitter.

Acetylcholine is also the transmitter at sites other than the neuromuscular junction (see Table 7.1), namely at all autonomic ganglia (whether sympathetic or parasympathetic), at parasympathetic end-organs, and some synapses in the central nervous system. A hypothesis that acetylcholine is concerned in transmission within all nerve cells (Nachmansohn, 1959) is not widely entertained.

Noradrenaline is the transmitter at sympathetically innervated end-organs (see Table 7.1). After initiating synaptic transmission, it is inactivated mainly by re-absorption into the synaptosomes of the presynaptic terminal which secreted it (Axelrod *et al.*, 1959; Iversen, 1967). A little of the noradrenaline is metabolized, in the neurones by monoamine oxidase, and extraneuronally by catechol-*O*-methyltransferase which effects 3-*O* methylation.

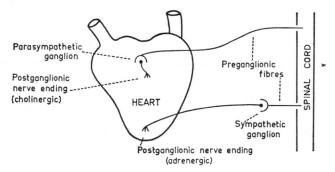

FIG. 7.2 Diagram showing examples of control by autonomic nervous system.

Fig. 7.2 summarizes the anatomical features of the autonomic nervous system. This differs from the voluntary system (exemplified by the neuromuscular junction in Fig. 7.1) in that one extra control point exists for each fibre, namely an extra synapse (situated in a ganglion). In sympathetic fibres, these ganglia are not far from the spinal cord: in parasympathetic fibres, the ganglia are near the end-organ, i.e. the one which the nerve is to influence. As was pointed out, all such ganglionic synapses are activated by acetylcholine. The postganglionic nerve endings (those which make contact with the end-organ) transmit each impulse to the organ by means of acetylcholine in parasympathetic fibres, but by noradrenaline in sympathetic fibres.

Table 7.1

DRUGS ACTING AT PERIPHERAL SYNAPSES

Synapses	Stimulants			Antagonists of natural transmitter
	Natural transmitter	Mimic of natural transmitter	Protector of transmitter from destruction	
1. Voluntary muscle (neuro-muscular junction)	acetylcholine (7.4)	nicotine (7.18)	physostigmine (2.7)	tubocurarine (2.6)
2. Ganglionic (sympathetic and para-sympathetic)	acetylcholine	nicotine	physostigmine	hexamethonium (7.24); tubocurarine (weak); nicotine (if in excess)
3. Postganglionic nerve-endings (para-sympathetic)	acetylcholine	muscarine (7.39)	physostigmine	atropine (7.14)
4. Postganglionic nerve-endings (sympathetic)	noradrenaline (7.5)	phenyl-ephrine (7.46)	β-phenyl-ethyl-hydrazine (9.36); pyrogallol	propranolol (13.41)

The distinction between *excitatory* and *inhibitory* transmitters will now be outlined. At the neuromuscular junction, and within autonomic ganglia, acetylcholine is an excitatory transmitter which depolarizes and hence fires neurones or causes muscle to contract. However, within the heart, acetylcholine is an inhibitory transmitter. In mammals, inhibitory transmission plays a very important role in the central nervous system where the continual interplay of inhibitory and excitatory inputs, into each single neurone, results in very fine control (Eccles, 1964). Glycine and gamma-aminobutyrate are central inhibitory transmitters; it seems likely that asparate and glutamate are excitatory transmitters in the mammalian brain and spinal cord (Curtis and Johnston, 1970). Acetylcholine is an important central excitatory transmitter (Curtis, Ryall and Watkins, 1964; Krnjević, 1966), and so, apparently, are dopamine and 5-hydroxytryptamine (Gaddum, 1963); noradrenaline has either action, depending on the region studied. [Some evidence suggests that inhibitory transmitters act by driving chloride ions into the cell while potassium ions escape (Boakes *et al.*, 1971).]

The brain is a highly complex organ with many distinct regions; it may be a long time before all the functions and interplay of its neurotransmitters can be discovered. For further reading on neurotransmitter-receptor interactions, see Section 13.4 and 13.6, also Triggle and Triggle (1977), For brain cell biology, see Watson (1976).

(b) *The principal hypotheses of drug action*
The classical work of Clark (1937), based on the application of Langmuir's adsorption isotherm (see Section 8.1), assumed that the effect of a drug is proportional to the fraction of receptors occupied by drug molecules, and that a maximal effect is obtainable only when all receptors are occupied by the drug. As a statement of the action of inhibitors (so important for work in chemotherapy and agriculture) this *simple occupation theory* can hardly be bettered. However, it is inadequate to explain the kinetics of agents which elicit a positive response: substances like the synaptic transmitter acetylcholine and innumerable artifical agonists.

Clark realized this, and said: 'The action of acetylcholine depends on at least two separable factors, firstly the fixation of the drug by certain receptors, and secondly the power to produce its action after fixation' (Clark, 1937). Further experimental work in Holland established these concepts firmly under the names *affinity* and *intrinsic activity* respectively (Ariëns, 1954). An inhibitor (e.g. a chemotherapeutic drug, insecticide, or fungicide) requires only affinity; but many pharmacodynamic drugs must have intrinsic activity as well, namely the ability to produce a natural physiological response as soon as combination between drug and receptor has occurred. The affinity is a measure of the attraction between the stimulant and the receptor: numerically it is the reciprocal of the dissociation constant of the complex so formed. The intrinsic activity is a measure of the ability of the complex to evoke a positive biological response, and it is expressed as the amount of response recorded for the fraction of receptors occupied (Ariëns, 1954).

The equation defining the dose-response curve is first-order with respect to both drug and receptor, and there is often a close agreement between the theoretically and experimentally obtained curves (Ariëns, van Rossum and Simonis, 1957). These authors compared the intrinsic activities of various neuromuscular depolarizing drugs by plotting their elicited degree of muscular contraction against increasing concentrations of the drug. It was found that when some drugs reached their maximal effect (i.e. one which no higher dosage could increase) they produced much less contraction than did other drugs. The dose required to obtain the maximal effect was used as a measure of the affinity of the drug. (The curves obtained were usually hyperbolas, similar to that in Fig. 8.2).

Traditionally, help in understanding drug-receptor interaction has been sought from (apparently) parallel phenomena in enzymology. It was recalled that enzymes have two types of specificity which are exerted independently of one another, (a) different substrates are *bound* with different affinities, and (b) different substrates *react* at different rates. To Ariens in 1957, it seemed that intrinsic activity corresponded to the constant that governs the transformation of an enzyme-substrate complex into products [see Section 9.1, Equation (iii)]. Because the drug was not changed by the receptor, it was assumed that the drug catalyses the breakdown of a receptor-substrate complex, and that it is this breakdown which triggers the response. The drug was thus seen as an equivalent of the co-factor in enzyme chemistry (cf. Welsh, 1948). A somewhat related thought was entertained at this time: that the membrane surrounding the receptor is opened by the agonist and sealed by the antagonist, as in Levine's hypothesis of the action of insulin which he supposed to open membranes that normally bar the passage of glucose (Levine and Goldstein, 1955, p. 360). This was the beginning of all our contemporary thinking that agonists produce conformational changes.

The Ariëns *composite occupation theory* was soon supplemented by that of Stephenson (1956). Using new, and more precise data for the effect of acetylcholine and histamine on guinea-pig ileum, Stephenson found, from the slope of the concentration-versus-effect curve, that the activity was not proportional to the number of receptors occupied. He was led to conclude, (a) that a maximal effect can be produced by the occupation of only a small proportion (even an exceedingly small proportion) of available receptors, (b) that response was not *linearly* proportional to the number of receptors occupied, and (c) that different drugs have different capacities to initiate a response, and hence that they occupy different proportions of the receptors when producing equal responses. This property, Stephenson called *efficacy*. This was defined as the reciprocal of the fractional occupancy required to produce a response equal to 50% of which the tissue is capable. A drug had high efficacy if it occupied a very small proportion of available receptors when it gave the maximal response of which the test-organ was capable.

There is a general resemblance between the Ariëns concept of intrinsic activity and the Stephenson concept of efficacy, but the latter needs more data for its calculation and seems to be a more fundamental attribute. Dose, for example, is one of the parameters of efficacy because all reasonably efficacious members of a homologous series can elicit the maximal activity of the test-organ, but at different doses. Stephenson extended the old idea, that all drugs were either agonists or antagonists, to include a third class: *partial agonists*. These have only moderate efficacy coupled with high affinity. Hence they can elicit a feeble response from the test-organ, but they can also prevent an agonist from eliciting its full activity. Table 7.2 shows the distribution of efficacy and affinity in a homologous series. Unfortunately, the efficacy of many common pharmacodynamic drugs has yet to be determined. The much-used concept of *spare receptors* (receptors unoccupied when the concentration of a drug is just enough for it to exert its maximal effect) sprang naturally from Stephenson's work.

Table 7.2

EFFICACY CONTRASTED WITH AFFINITY
COMPARISON OF ACTIVITY OF ALKYL TRIMETHYLAMMONIUM
IONS ON GUINEA-PIG ILEUM

Alkyl group	Me	Et	Pr	Bu	Pent	Hex	Hept	Oct	Non	Dec
Efficacy	94	31	4.3	200	200	21	2.2	1.4	1.0	0.6
Affinity $\times 10^{-3}$	0.2	0.6	1.6	3.8	8.5	19	41	63	110	190

(Stephenson, 1956.)

Knowledge of the free energy of association of ions permits calculation of the equilibrium distance separating the two centres of charge. This is so because the work done in removing a unit charge from another charge to an infinitely distant position is equal to this free energy. The work done can be found from the Coulomb equation (Pressman *et al.*, 1946). Using this relationship, Burgen (1965) calculated the equilibrium distance of the quaternary nitrogen atom of acetylcholine, from the negatively charged group in the receptor, as 3.29 Å. This calculation was based on the difference of free energy of interaction of acetylcholine (*7.4*) and dimethylbutyl acetate (*13.45*) as calculated from the response of guinea-pig ileum. He showed similarly that the basic centre, of acetylcholine and similarly acting analogues, makes a closer fit on the receptor than does that of chemically related antagonists (presumably because the intense van der Waals bonding of the 'tail' dislocates the positioning of the 'head'). Hence the distinction between agonists and antagonists was suggested to lie in the agonists' greater intimacy of receptor-association and consequent ability to induce conformational changes. Similar calculations and conclusions were made by Belleau, Tani and Lie (1965).

Ephedrine
(7.40)

Phentolamine
(7.41)

The association of increasing molecular weight with increasing antagonistic power is well known. An antagonist is always bulkier than the corresponding stimulant, and it is obvious that the likelihood of forming extra van der Waals bonds with the receptor increases the chances of the bulkier molecule having a longer retention time (see Sections 8.0, 8.1, and 10.3b). Among the sympathomimetic amines, a gradation can be traced from members with a strong stimulant action plus a tendency to tachyphylaxis* (e.g. ephedrine) (7.40), through members that are in turn both strongly stimulant and antagonistic (e.g. ergotamine), to drugs which show only a trace of excitatory action followed by sustained depression (e.g. phentolamine) (7.41). Again, with parasympathomimetic drugs examined at the neuromuscular junction, a similar sequence can be traced as molecular complexity increases from members with a strong stimulant but occasionally small antagonist action, through the type that is first stimulant and then antagonistic (e.g. tridecamethonium), to tubocurarine (2.6) which is primarily antagonistic but retains the ability to excite the end-plate under special conditions. Another example is afforded by the dialkyl-glutaramides, e.g. bemegride (15.3), which can be analeptic and convulsant when the alkyl-group is ethyl, hypnotic and anticonvulsant when it is larger then propyl; but when it is propyl, the drug is convulsant in small doses and hypnotic in large ones (Shulman, et al., 1965; Laycock and Shulman, 1967). These graded series correspond to diminishing rates of dissociation from the receptor.

It has been proposed that hypnotics and analeptics act on the same

---

*Tachyphylaxis (desensitization) is the steadily dwindling response of some tissues to the repeated application of the same dose of a drug.

lipophilic neuronal membrane; the hypnotics, being more lipophilic, are supposed to bind to lipids, increasing their cohesion and thus preventing permeability to sodium ions; the analeptics, being more hydrophilic, are supposed to bind to protein, rendering it more permeable to these ions. Drugs with both depressant and stimulant action are considered to act on both lipid and protein components of the membrane. Substances like phenytoin (15.4) and 5-ethyl-5-(1,3-dimethylbutyl) barbituric acid exhibit either stimultant or depressant action on the central nervous system (intact mouse), depending on the dose (Shulman and Laycock, 1967).

Two hypotheses, which differ from those described, have been put forward: the rate hypothesis and the allosteric hypothesis, which will now be outlined. The *rate hypothesis* suggests that the biological effect, produced by agonists, is proportional to the rate of combination of the drug with its receptor, but not to occupancy (Paton, 1961). This conclusion followed from some meticulous kinetic studies with histamine, acetylcholine, and related stimulants on the isolated guinea-pig ileum, which showed that each contraction declined immediately after it had reached its peak. Rate theory attempts to answer the often-asked question, why do repeated doses of a stimulant usually produce steadily diminishing responses? It suggests that when time has not been allowed for the release of all the drug first applied, insufficient receptors are available for subsequent doses, and stimulation is proportional to the rate of drug-receptor combination. The fading of response of guinea-pig gut to repeated doses of acetylcholine, histamine, and a homologous series of quaternary amines is cited in support of this argument (Paton, 1961). Similar results had been obtained with a homologous series of *S*-alkyl*iso*thioureas (Fastier and Reid, 1952), but the phenomenon seems to be rare, and is opposed to the common finding of 'spare receptors' (see above). An ideal system for investigating rates must not offer any barrier to diffusion of the drug, and it must not impose any delay between the application of the stimulus and the registration of the response. Few pharmacodynamic systems have these requirements. The historic importance of the rate hypothesis is that it has made pharmacologists more conscious of kinetic aspects.

The *allosteric hypothesis* postulates that only two conformational states of the receptor exist, in equilibrium with one another. It is supposed that one state (called T) can initiate no physiological action whereas the other (R) can do so. Drugs are presumed to act as antagonists or agonists, depending on whether they are so constituted as to bind to (T) or to (R) respectively (Karlin, 1967). This hypothesis grew out of the Monod-Wyman-Changeux (1965) discovery of allosteric transitions in enzymes (see Section 9.0). The strongest evidence in support of the idea of allosteric receptors is possibly the co-operative effect (i.e. a sigmoid, instead of the usual hyperbolic, response) at the motor end-plate (frog) after stable cholinergic drugs (e.g. carbachol) have been applied to it. The classical composite occupation theory assumes that agonists, at least, produce conformational changes, and that these often open an ion channel, thus initiating the physiological response. However, it assumes that different drugs produce different kinds of conformational change, some not so effective as others: this was done to explain why chemically similar drugs could differ in efficacy. That there can be more than two conformational states of the receptor was later shown by current measurements on four agonists at the frog's muscle end-plate (Colquhoun *et al.*, 1975).

Some other conformation-related phenomena will be mentioned. Many test-objects, exposed to a large dose of an agonist, temporarily lose their sensitivity after the drug has been washed out. The rate of recovery of sensitivity is constant for the tissue, regardless of the drug used. In one explanation, it is suggested that desensitization depends on a change of the agonist-receptor complex (AR) to a different conformational state (AR′) which then dissociates, leaving the altered receptor (R′) free to revert slowly to the original receptor (Katz and Thesleff, 1957). Study of the kinetics of development and recovery from desensitization by cholinergic drugs in chick and frog muscle indicated that the physiological effect of the drug was proportional to the fraction of receptors in the active conformation (Rang and Ritter, 1970). The 'metaphilic effect' is a related phenomenon: the affinity of receptors for cholinergic antagonists (tubocurarine, gallamine) was increased when a relevant agonist (carbachol) was applied shortly beforehand (Rang and Ritter, 1969). This was interpreted to mean that the agonist generates more (R′), the form with which it is supposed the antagonist preferentially binds.

For reading on conformational changes induced by drugs (e.g. chlorpromazine, streptomycin, cardiac glycosides), see Levitzki (1973).

7.6 The natural divisions of pharmacodynamics

Various classifications of pharmacodynamic action are practised. Sometimes drugs are classified according to their main therapeutic use, and thence subdivided according to the pharmacological pathway by which this goal is reached. Thus drugs for use in hypertension are divided into (a) those with mainly central action (e.g. reserpine), (b) those which block sympathetic ganglia (e.g. pentolinium), (c) those which block sympathetic nerve-endings (e.g. propranolol), (d) those which relax the muscle of the blood-vessels (e.g. nitrites), and (e) those which attack the molecular cause by blocking the angiotensin-forming enzyme (e.g. SQ 14,225). In what follows, drugs are classified according to their site of action, without previous classification by therapeutic uses.

(a) *Drugs acting on the central nervous system*
These are further divided into depressants and stimulants. Typical of central nervous *depressants* are the general anaesthetics such as ether and

chloroform (see Chapter 15). These depress the higher centres before the lower ones; but at high concentrations, centres in the medulla become blocked and respiration ceases. (The introduction of muscle-relaxant drugs, about 1940, abolished the need for deep anaesthesia during operations.) The hypnotics (e.g. chloral hydrate, and barbiturates) are central depressants usually administered by mouth to achieve much less depression than is required in surgical anaesthesia. Some quicker-acting barbiturates (e.g. thiopentone) are commonly injected intravenously for the rapid induction of surgical anaesthesia, which is then continued by volatile anaesthetics. Alcohol is also a depressant, but its central action is more complex: in some people, it depresses the sensory system more than the motor system and produces restlessness.

Other drugs, which are not general nervous system depressants, effect *specific* centres in the central nervous system. Some important examples are (i) morphine and morphine-like analgesics, which can relieve pain without inducing sleep, (ii) the antalgics such as phenacetin and aspirin, which relieve *mild* pain only, (iii) anticonvulsants used in treating epilepsy without inducing sleepiness, e.g. phenytoin (diphenylhydantoin), (iv) substances acting specifically on brain centres that lack dopamine due to Parkinson's disease, e.g. L-dopa, (v) central relaxants, which quell anxiety, acting mainly on the spinal cord, e.g. meprobamate and diazepam ('Valium'), (vi) major tranquillizers, such as chlorpromazine (Section 13.8) which block dopamine receptors in the corpus striatum, (vii) the tricyclic antidepressants, e.g. imipramine, which seem to act mainly by preventing uptake of noradrenaline and 5-hydroxytryptamine into the presynaptic terminal after the passage of a nervous impulse, and (viii) the hallucinogenics, e.g. LSD, which disturbs 5-HT metabolism in the brain stem. There are many hypotheses as to how these various, and often highly selective, effects are brought about, but so complex is the central nervous system that little of a definitive nature is yet known. For one brave attempt at integrating the flimsy clues, see Dewhurst (1968).

Stimulants of the central nervous system are divided into (i) those that antagonize general central (drug-induced) nervous depression, such as leptazol, which are convulsants in larger doses, (ii) those which stimulate the respiratory centre in the brain, e.g. lobeline, (iii) psychomotor drugs, which increase capacity for work at the expense of the body's energy reserves, such as (a) caffeine which also stimulates the heart directly and causes diuresis, (b) amphetamine ('Benzedrine') which drives noradrenaline and dopamine out of their stores*, it also stimulates the sympathetic nervous system (see below) and curbs appetite for food, and (c) inhibitors, e.g. phenelzine, of monoamine oxidase which allow high concentrations

* When the synthesis of these two transmitters is blocked by a low dose of α-methyltyrosine, the central effects of amphetamine disappear (Sulser and Sanders-Bush, 1971).

of 5-HT and other amines to build up, (iv) antagonists of central inhibition, e.g. strychnine which blocks the inhibitory action of glycine on the spinal cord (Curtis and Johnston, 1970; Eccles, 1957), and bicuculline which, like picrotoxin, blocks the inhibitory action of γ-aminobutyric acid (Curtis *et al.*, 1971), and (v) diuretics, like α-methyl-dopa through its metabolic product α-methylnoradrenaline. Electroconvulsive therapy seems to act by liberating dopamine and 5-HT in the brain (Green *et al.*, 1977).

CH$_2$·CH(CH$_3$)·NH$_2$

Amphetamine
(*7.42*)

(b) *Drugs acting on peripheral nerve fibres*
Only depressant drugs are known in this class. These drugs are the well-known local anaesthetics, used also in dental and spinal anaesthesia. In general, they preferentially affect the smaller fibres; hence sensory nerves are affected more than motor nerves. They elevate the threshold for excitation and thus block propagation of the nervous impulse without depolarizing the fibre.

Local anaesthesia is not (except in a homologous series) correlated with lipid/water distribution coefficients, nor do local anaesthetics have any hypnotic or general anaesthetic action, even in excess. The view that local anaesthetics act by competition with acetylcholine for a receptor (Nachmansohn, 1959) has been replaced by the concept, first put forward by Straub (1956), that local anaesthetics act by decreasing sodium conductance in the rising phase of the nerve potential. Taylor (1959), using voltage-clamp technique on the squid giant nerve fibre, showed that this was true for the action of procaine. Similarly, in frog sartorius muscle, implanting microelectrodes in a single fibre showed that procaine competed with external sodium ions, and that the sodium-derived increase in conductance, which normally follows a stimulus, was suppressed (Inoue and Frank, 1962). Again voltage-clamp current analysis on the Ranvier node of single myelinated frog nerve fibres showed that the actions of lignocaine (*7.13* and tetrodotoxin (respective pK_a values: 7.9, 12.5) resided in the cations. Both drug blocked the sodium ion channels, presumably by combining with anionic groups lining these channels. The potassium ion channels were unaffected (Hille, 1966).

For the effect of the ionization of the drug on these events, see Section 10.5. For a review of local anaesthetics, see Ritchie and Greengard (1966).

(c) *Drugs acting on peripheral nerve-endings*
Stimulation of *sensory* nerve-endings occurs in tasting and smelling, and by electrical, thermal, and mechanical means. Veratrine and the amidines stimulate nerve-endings in heart and lungs, resulting in a reflex lowering of blood-pressure. Apart from this, little is known of the chemical stimulation of sensory nerves by drugs.

Chemical stimulation at *motor* nerve-endings, on the contrary, has an immense literature to which Section 7.5 may serve as an introduction. See also Table 7.1.

Cholinergic synapses. Drugs with an acetylcholine-like action, but of higher selectivity and longer acting, and those which prolong the action of this neurotransmitter by blocking acetylcholinesterase, are used in treating disordered heart rhythms, glaucoma, myasthenia gravis, or to stimulate the bladder and gastro-intestinal tract after operations. See Section 7.3 for notes on the discovery of some of these drugs, Section 13.6 for further discussion of the agonists, and Sections 12.3 and 13.5 and more information on the cholinesterase inhibitors.

As explained in Section 7.3, there are two different ways in which the action of acetylcholine can be blocked at the neuromuscular junction: with or without depolarization. Drugs with either kind of action are much used to secure muscular relaxation during anaesthesia. Similarly, there are two different types of ganglion-blocking drug: those (e.g. tetraethylammonium salts, hexamethonium, or tubocurarine) which block the receptors for acetylcholine but cause no depolarization, and other (e.g. tetramethylammonium salts, or excess of nicotine) which block these receptors *and* cause prolonged depolarization (Paton and Perry, 1953). Clinical interest in ganglion-blocking drugs has waned because insufficient selectivity between ganglia led to unpleasant side-effects. For drugs blocking postganglionic release of acetylcholine, see under atropine in Section 7.3.

Other inhibitors depress the *synthesis* of acetylcholine in the motor nerve terminals, e.g. triethylcholine (*7.43*) (Bull and Hemsworth, 1965) and the more complex hemicholinium (Schueler, 1956). These agents interfere with choline transport and hence deprive acetyltransferase of its substrate; also their action is reversed by choline (cf. Macintosh, Birks and Sastry, 1956). Glycollic acids bearing liposoluble substituents (e.g. *p*-phenylmandelic acid) inhibit this enzyme in the brain (Holan, 1965).

$(Et_3N^+ \cdot CH_2 \cdot CH_2 \cdot OH)$

Triethylcholine cation
(*7.43*)

Metaraminol
(*7.44*)

Adrenergic* synapses.   Since the pioneering work of Barger and Dale (1910), the many pharmacological effects of β-phenylethylamines have become much better understood. As explained in Section 7.5a, the arrival of an impulse at a presynaptic terminal releases noradrenaline, which transmits the impulse to the receptor. This action is terminated mainly by reabsorption of the noradrenaline into the presynaptic terminal and the two destructive enzymes (MAO and COMT) play little part. Drugs have been discovered which prevent this uptake by becoming adsorbed on the terminal. The structural features optimal for this adsorption have been worked out by Burgen and Iversen (1965). It appears that a hydroxyl-group in position 3 or 4 increases uptake as does α-methylation, whereas O-methylation, N-substitution, and β-hydroxylation decrease it. That these specifications differ from those needed for combining with either an α- or a β-sympathetic receptor (defined in Section 13.4) points up the complexity of structure-activity studies in this area. Of the substances which prevent the uptake of noradrenaline by the presynaptic terminal, metaraminol (*7.44*) has four times the affinity of the natural substrate. Cocaine (*7.11*) and amphetamine also show this effect, although it is only a part of their total spectrum of activities.

Another common activity for a substituted β-phenylethylamine** is to accumulate in the presynaptic terminal and push the local stores of noradrenaline out into the synaptic gap. If this is done rapidly, the action must necessarily be of limited duration, as the stores eventually become depleted. Ephedrine (*7.40*) acts principally in this way (Schümann, 1961), and provides an excellent morning treatment for hay-fever, but its stimulant effect on the CNS causes disturbance of sleep if it is taken later in the day. The next morning, when noradrenaline stores have built up again in the adrenergic terminals, the patient can derive benefit from another dose. (Ephedrine, unlike noradrenaline is not destroyed in the stomach and may be given orally.) Amphetamine (*7.42*) has this combination of peripheral and central actions but with the latter preponderating. Tyramine, on the other hand has a purely peripheral action.

Comparing the two actions described in the last two paragraphs (prevention of re-uptake of noradrenaline by presynaptic terminal, and enforced release of noradrenaline from this terminal), it is notable that, although many substances like metaraminol, tyramine, and ephedrine show both effects, they exercise these properties quite independently. In other words, when put into ranking order for one effect, they are not in order for the other

---

* Dale's original name is still in use, although 'Noradrenergic' would more accurately reflect current knowledge.

**This use of β for 'on the side-chain, in the position next to the benzene ring' and α for 'on the side-chain in the position next to the amino-group' have nothing to do with Ahlquist's division of all sympathetic receptors into α or β types (see Section 12.4).

(Burgen and Iversen, 1965). However, both classes of drug give the patient a temporary overdose of his own noradrenaline (Burn and Rand, 1958).

Another class of substance that accumulates in the presynaptic terminal pushes the stored noradrenaline out no faster than it can be destroyed by monoamine oxidase. Examples are guanethidine (7.45), which is much used medicinally, in blood pressure of moderate severity, to block, then slowly deplete these noradrenaline stores (Boura and Green, 1965), and the more dangerous reserpine, which is now little used.

Many β-phenylethylamines can not only compete with noradrenaline, in binding at the presynaptic terminal, but can themselves be liberated by each nervous impulse and activate the postsynaptic receptor, thus functioning as *false transmitters*. Usually the efficacy of a false transmitter is less than that of noradrenaline (this is the case for metaraminol and α-methyldopamine), but a few, notably α-methyladrenaline have a higher efficacy than noradrenaline (Kopin 1968).

Some false transmitters are known which are not taken up by the presynaptic terminal, but display a direct noradrenaline-like effect on the receptor. The most used of these is phenylephrine (7.46) ('Neo-synephrine') which is applied to inflamed mucous membranes. Whereas phenylephrine acts exclusively on α-receptors, isoproterenol (isoprenaline) (13.35) affects only β-receptors, and salbutamol (13.42) only one type of β-receptor (more about this in Section 13.4).

Guanethidine
(7.45)

Phenylephrine
(7.46)

Some depressants of the sympathetic system act by interference with synthesis of noradrenaline, as α-methyltyrosine does (not used medicinally), whereas others, such as propranolol (13.41), compete with noradrenaline at the postsynaptic receptor, and are clinically highly successful for reducing high blood pressure (see further Section 13.4).

From the above outline, it becomes clear that modes of action of adrenergic amines are highly varied, which allows for specialized applications in therapy. Some are used to raise blood-pressure, others to lower it, or else as central stimulants in narcolepsy, as nasal decongestants, for treating asthma or allergies, to curb appetite, and to control bleeding. For further reading on release, uptake and destruction of noradrenaline and its analogues, see Iversen (1967); Schümann and Kroneberg (1970); for a book on false transmitters, see Thoenen (1969), for the stereochemistry of catecholamines see Section 13.1, then the review by Patel, Miller, and Trendelenburg (1974).

In discussing the pharmacodynamics of postganglionic nerves, should the vague words 'sympathomimetic' and 'parasympathomimetic' be avoided? Because most parts of the body are innervated by both sympathetic and parasympathetic nerves, opposing one another, a 'parasympathomimetic' drug may be acting by stimulating the parasympathetic, or by blocking the sympathetic, receptors.

For further reading on chemical aspects of the nervous system, see Triggle and Triggle, (1977); Cooper, Bloom, and Roth, (1974).

(d) *Drugs acting on muscles, glands, and elsewhere*

Most of the pharmacodynamic drugs act on nerves, and most of the remainder act on muscles. When a nervous impulse reaches the nerve-muscle junction (see Section 7.5a), the acetylcholine, secreted by the nerve-ending, liberates calcium ions from the sarcoplasmic reticulum (a membranous structure in muscle somewhat like the endoplasmic reticulum discussed in Section 5.3). Magnesium ions then activate the ends of the myosin molecules to function as an ATPase which, by hydrolysing ATP released from the numerous mitochondria of muscle cells, supplies the energy needed for contraction. Of course, not all muscular action is acetylcholine-activated. Quite apart from the noradrenaline-activation of much involuntary muscle in response to postganglionic sympathetic stimulation, there is the action of adrenaline to be considered. This tissue hormone, constantly secreted by the suprarenal gland, maintains the normal tone of involuntary muscle, relaxing lung muscle by activating the B_2 receptors and stimulating heart muscle by its action on B_1 receptors.

For further reading on the structure of the actomyosin complex, see Smith (1972), Bourne (1973). Microfibrils, which are primitive equivalents of muscles, were discussed in Section 5.3.

Several drugs act on smooth muscle, seemingly quite independently of the nervous impulse. Histamine (7.6), a tissue hormone, causes contraction of the intestine and uterus, and dilatation of the muscular fibres of blood-vessels. A number of excellent antihistaminic drugs have been synthesized and are dealt with in Section 9.4. 5-Hydroxytryptamine (*7.36*), another widespread hormone, whose peripheral functions are obscure, causes strong contractions in smooth muscle.

Ergometrine powerfully stimulates the smooth muscle of the uterus, and constricts the muscular fibres of blood-vessels. Papaverine, a poppy alkaloid, has a direct antispasmodic action on gut muscle. A number of simple aliphatic amidines, guanidines, *iso*ureas, and *iso*thioureas, all of which are strong bases, raise blood-pressure and contract the intestine by direct action (Fastier, 1949). These substances are not blocked by antihistaminics.

The principal cardiac glycosides (from digitalis, strophanthus, and squill) have a direct and selective action on heart muscle, increasing the force of the contraction (for details, see Section 14.1). Quinidine, and innumerable substances in which an aromatic ring is linked (by an ester, ketone, ether, or carbinol bridge) to a basic group, have a therapeutically useful depressant effect on certain portions of the heart (Dawes, 1946), and are used to correct arythmias.

Several drugs used in reducing moderately high blood pressure directly relax the vascular muscles in the capillary bed throughout the body (examples: hydrallazine (*11.43*), the organic nitrates, the inorganic nitrites, and prazosin (*7.47*) (Stokes and Weber, 1974).

Prazosin
(*7.47*)

Many antagonists of hormones are known. For example, some substances decreased the biosynthesis of the thyroid hormones by inhibiting the process of concentrating iodine in the thyroid gland, others by preventing the iodination of tyrosine. The clinically useful thio-drugs, such as propylthiouracil and carbimazole (*3.36*), have the latter type of action.

Many drugs cause diuresis by influencing the secretory and resorptive properties of the kidneys which were discussed in Section 3.1. Several drugs are known which act directly on the haematopoietic system (e.g. phenindione, warfarin, sodium calcium edetate, amethopterin), on fibrous tissues (e.g. salicylates, prednisolone, cortisone), and on tumours.

＊   ＊   ＊   ＊

For wider reading on systematic pharmacodynamics, see Goodman and Gilman (1975); Barlow (1964); and for the principles of pharmacodynamics, see Goldstein *et al.*, (1968).

(e) *Insect nerves and insecticides*
Of the most-used insecticides, the chlorinated hydrocarbons bring about death by initially stimulating and then exhausting the nervous system. The insect central nervous system consists essentially of a double nerve cord situated ventrally and punctuated by segmental ganglia from which the peripheral nerves arise. The axon of such a nerve measures up to 10 μm in diameter and is enclosed in a thin non-myelinated lipoprotein sheath. These axons are bundled into nerves which are surrounded by dove-

tailed layers of neuroglial cells, and the whole is enclosed by a protein lamella. The polarization of a resting nerve is very similar to that of vertebrate nerve (see Section 7.5a). On electrical stimulation, successive spikes can be obtained at intervals of a millisecond; but the action potentials are propagated only at about $2\,m\,s^{-1}$, i.e. some 50 times slower than in the larger myelinated axons of vertebrates.

The chemical mediator at insect ganglia is acetylcholine which is abundantly present in the brain. The mediator at the neuromuscular junction is not acetylcholine, as in mammals, but L-glutamic acid (7.37) (Clements and May, 1974; Irving, Osborne, and Wilson, 1976), and for this neurotransmitter, no selective antagonist has yet been found. The receptors for both neurotransmitters are well protected by selectively permeable membranes.

The principal action of DDT (3.37) is to stimulate the sensory, central, and motor axons (Roeder and Weiant, 1948). It does not inhibit acetylcholinesterase as the phosphorus insecticides do (Section 12.3). However, the net effect is a large increase in free acetylcholine which seems to come from a bound form (e.g. presynaptic vesicles) (Lewis, Waller and Fowler, 1960); it is not due to any increased rate of acetylcholine synthesis (Rothschild and Howden, 1961), but to a disorganization of the axonal membranes (Mullins, 1956) through DDT forming electron-transfer complexes (Section 8.0) (Holan, 1971). This causes disruption of the ion-transport mechanism in nerve cells, DDT simultaneously increasing Na^+ influx and blocking K^+ influx (Narahashi and Haas, 1968). The electron-transfer complexes dissociate about $30°$, thus exempting warm-blooded animals (Holan, 1971). The Holan hypothesis led to the discovery of several DDT analogues with high insecticidal activity (see below). It did not seem to apply to unsymmetrically-substituted analogues, until the assumption was made that the DDT molecule fits into a flexible pouch (and not a rigid cavity) in the membrane (Fahmy et al., 1973).

The action of the other chlorinated insecticides is not so well understood, and is clearly different in detail: nevertheless they resemble DDT in liberating vast stores of acetylcholine without blocking acetylcholinesterase. Aldrin trans-diol is thought to be the active form of dieldrin, for it brings about the multiple axonal discharges and inhibits the sodium and potassium activation mechanisms of nerve membranes just as dieldrin does, but much faster (van den Bercken and Narahashi, 1974).

The onset of DDT poisoning is slow, and the legs (but not wings) make useless movements. Death is not owing to exhaustion from these movements, because anaesthetized insects die just as fast. Lindane (BHC) and the dieldrin-aldrin group of chlorinated insecticides produce a still slower onset, and useless wing (but not leg) movements are seen.

The intoxication produced in insects by DDT or by the phosphorus insecticides is fatal of itself if the dose is high enough. However, if death does not occur, because of under-dosage or resistance, a secondary effect occurs, namely a release of abnormal amounts of a neurophysiologically active substance which can also be released by vibration or electric shock. The ventral nerve-cord seems to be the principal source of this endotoxin which often eventually causes death (Sternburg, *et al.*, 1959). Lindane does not seem to cause this effect. The nature of the substance is still unknown: it is not acetylcholine, and it is toxic to other insects if injected into them.

After examination of 106 chlorinated cyclodiene insecticides on six selected types of insect, Soloway (1965) concluded that a strict geometry governs ability to react with insect receptors. Two electron-rich sites are required (Cl, O, N, S, or double-bond) for electrostatic adsorption (di-hydro-aldrin has only one such site, and has only a low toxicity to insects). Aldrin (*6.39*, *7.48*) is a typical example. Chemically it is *endo-endo*-1,2,3,4, 10,10-hexachloro-1,4:5,8-dimethano-hexahydronaphthalene. The critical outline which these nearly spherical molecules require for activity is shown in (*7.49*); it was produced by viewing molecular models along a line joining the bridgehead (methano) atoms. Lindane, which has a similar mode of action, has a similar outline.

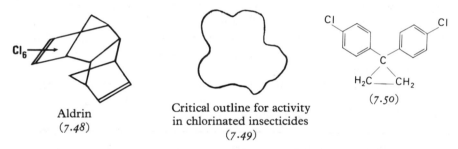

Aldrin
(*7.48*)

Critical outline for activity
in chlorinated insecticides
(*7.49*)

(*7.50*)

Similar examination of models of DDT and its analogues (including the related, more stable diphenyl*cyclo*propanes, e.g. (*7.50*), which produce identical symptoms in the housefly), indicated that activity was lost if the distance between the insertion points of the electron-releasing groups (halo-, alkyl-, alkoxy-) in the benzene rings exceeded 11 Å; other limiting dimensions were specified (Holan, 1969, 1971).

In Section 6.4, the discovery of the principal insecticides was outlined, and an indication given of the stern control under which the chlorinated insecticides have come in some of the most highly developed countries where they have been applied too liberally. The World Health Organiza-tion, on the other hand, found DDT safe in its malaria-eradication program-me, when used in the recommended concentrations (WHO, 1971, 1973a). In a sober and well-documented review of the toxicity of pesticides, Hayes (1967) concluded that 20 years of experience with DDT has provided no evidence that it injured people who were much more heavily exposed to it than are the general population. In 1956, Hayes, Durham, and Cueto, of the U.S.A. Public Health Service, fed 35 mg of DDT per man per day (i.e. 200 times the highest average dietary intake of that time in the U.S.A.) to human volunteers for 18 months. None of the subjects developed any symptom related to this chemical.

Workers employed in the formulation of DDT since 1945 have absorbed doses many hundred times greater than the average public intake without incurring ill-health. In a study of 35 men who had 11 to 19 years of exposure to DDT in the Montrose plant in California (which has produced it continuously since 1947), careful medical examination disclosed no ill-effects attributable to this agent. The storage of DDT and its metabolites in the men's fat was found to be 38 to 647 p.p.m., as compared to an average of 8 p.p.m. in the surrounding population. It was estimated that the average daily intake was 18 mg per day as compared to 0.04 mg in the public at large (i.e. at that time, for it is now much less). No sign of cancer was found in any of the workers (Laws, Curley, and Biros, 1967; Warnick and Carter, 1972). Experiments on the CFI strain of mice, which have a 22% incidence of spontaneous liver cell tumours, showed an increase when fed 2 mg/kg of DDT (Tomatis *et al.*, 1972). The BALB/C strain, which is not prone to spontaneous tumours, showed no incidence at this dose, but some at a tenfold higher dose (Terracini, *et al.*, 1973). For the logic of extrapolating from rodents to man, see Section 12.5. Government bans on DDT are less concerned with its effect on man than on its accumulation in the food chain of fish and birds.

For an account of the carbamate and organophosphorus insecticides, see Section 12.3; for nicotine, Section 13.6. These are the synapse-blocking insecticides. Nicotine is relatively little used.

The pyrethrins (*7.51*), extracted with petroleum from Dalmatian Insect Flowers (a species of Chrysanthemum) resemble the chlorinated hydrocarbon insecticides in being axonal blockers. They act on both central and sensory components of the nervous system. However, and this is quite unlike what happens with the chlorinated hydrocarbons, the insects merely fall down in a stupor. There are no useless movements and a high rate of recovery occurs. Mammals detoxify pyrethrins very quickly by both hydrolysis and oxidation, hence the selectivity of these agents, but

Pyrethrins (flattened formula)
Pyrethrin I   (R = —CH$_3$)
Pyrethrin II (R = —CO$_2$CH$_3$)
(*7.51*)

Pyrethrins (conformational formula)
(R as in 7.51)
(7.52)

they are toxic to fish. Chemically, each pyrethrin is an ester of chrysanthemic acid (a *cyclo*propane derivative) with a lipophilic, flat, rigid alcohol derived from *cyclo*pentane. The conformation is as (7.52).

Changing the molecular structure of the pyrethrins to overcome their tendencies to destruction by light and ephemeral action, has produced the more lipophilic pyrethroids which have greatly increased potency (without rapid 'knockdown', however) and useful outdoor persistance. Decamethrin (7.53), probably the best of the pyrethroids, has an ED_{50} against the housefly of 2 µg/kg (when synergized, as described in Section 3.4), truly a remarkable potency, particularly as it is non-toxic to mammals (Elliott, *et al.*, 1974).

Decamethrin
(7.53)

The toxic effect, to insects, of both the pyrethrins and the pyrethroids depends on the presence of gem-dimethyl groups on the *cyclo*propane ring, and on unsaturation in the alcoholic component of the ester. Halogen substitution of the acidic component of the ester greatly increases stability to sunlight. The pyrethroids stimulate nerves to produce repetitive discharges and subsequently cause paralysis. Like DDT, they open up the sodium channel and close the potassium channel, and there is a huge negative temperature dependence. However, the complete action of pyrethroids is more complex than this, and much is unknown.

For reading on the neurochemistry of arthropods, see Treherne (1966). For more reading on the chemistry and mode of action of pyrethrins and pyrethroids, see Yamamoto (1970), and Elliott (1977).

PART TWO

Studies, in depth, of topics from part one

8 The nature of chemical bonds. Adsorption

As soon as the forces of distribution (Chapter 3) have brought a drug molecule close to a receptor, the two are sure to be hurled into a fleeting contact by thermal agitation. How durable and how selective that contact may be depends on the chemical nature of both drug and receptor, and on the type of bonds they can form.

In what follows, the various types of chemical bond will be discussed with reference to the part that each can play in drug-receptor unions. This outline will lead to a discussion of adsorption, which is much the same phenomenon described in different terms. The Chapter will conclude with examples of highly selective binding found in non-biological settings, serving to remind us that selectivity flourishes independently of life.

8.0 Types of chemical bonds

In the past, it used to be claimed that some drugs acted by 'physical' and some by 'chemical' means. It was also suggested that the physical properties of a drug were responsible for getting it to the site of action, but there it reacted chemically. In these connotations, the word 'chemical' was strangely limited to the formation of covalent bonds.

Such a contrast between 'physical' and 'chemical' now seems unreal. Langmuir (1916, 1917) made it clear that physics and chemistry are interwoven: every substance has physical properties, and the physical properties which it has are the inevitable result of its particular chemical structure. Thus 'physical' and 'chemical' are not alternate sets of properties, but different aspects of the same set. For example, in raising a kettle of water to the boiling-point we may seem to be carrying out a purely physical process, but, as Langmuir pointed out, it is actually a depolymerization, involving the rupture of countless millions of hydrogen bonds: in short it is a chemical reaction.

The appearance of Pauling's book *The Nature of the Chemical Bond* in 1939 did much to codify knowledge of the various types of bonds between atoms. The four most important chemical bond-types for the student of drugs to understand are: covalent bonds, hydrogen bonds, electrostatic bond, and van der Waals forces. Within these main types, special varieties can be recognized. To make or break any of these bonds, whether covalent or otherwise, is a true chemical reaction often involving much energy. Modern knowledge of bonds rests on the fundamental basis of quantum mechanics and the understanding of valence that has come from the application of quantum mechanics to atomic orbitals. Bond strengths are usually experimentally determined, but can often be calculated too. The principal bond types will now be discussed in turn.

(a) *The covalent bond*

This is formed from two electrons, one contributed from each of the atoms forming the bond between them. They are the typical bonds of the organic chemist who spends so much of his time making and breaking them. They are usually much stronger than other types of bond, having bond-strengths lying between 50 and 150 kilocalories* per mole. Thus a single-bond between two carbon atoms (C–C) is 59 and a double-bond (C = C) is 100; a single-bond between carbon and oxygen (C–O) is 70 and a double-bond (C = O) is 150; a single-bond between carbon and nitrogen (C–N) is 49 and a double-bond (C = N) is 94 (kcal/mol). The greatest strength of bond that can be broken readily (i.e. non-enzymatically) in the 20–40° range is 10 kcal. Very few agents act by forming covalent bonds with the receptor; those that do (e.g. penicillin and the organic phosphates) are dealt with in Chapter 12. Most drug effects are reversible if the agent is simply washed away, as in Fig. 2.1, and this easy reversal indicates that the activity does not depend on the formation of a covalent bond.

However, it must not be supposed that difficulty encountered in washing a drug out of a tissue necessarily implies covalent bond formation. The drug molecule may simple be *clathrate*, i.e. physically imprisoned in the folds of a macromolecule (biopolymer). The textile industry has long made use of this principle in dyeing cotton fabrics with long, narrow molecules (mol.wt. 200–400), which require no mordant (Lapworth, 1940).

A variant of the covalent bond, usually much weaker, is the *co-ordinate bond* formed when both electrons of the bond have to be provided by the

---

* Division by 4.18 gives kilojoules.

one atom, for reasons of valency. A familiar example is the union of a hydrogen ion with an anion to give a non-ionized acid, or of a hydrogen ion with an amine to give an ammonium ion (e.g. $CH_3.NH_2 + H^+ \rightleftharpoons$ $CH_3.^+NH_3$). This is the phenomenon known as ionization, which covers quite a range of bond-strengths and is discussed quantitatively in Chapter 10. In a related example of co-ordinate bond formation, a metal cation can replace the hydrogen cation in the previous examples. The metal complexes which arise in this way are discussed quantitatively in Chapter 11. Other examples of the co-ordinate bond are to be seen in nitrogen oxides, e.g. (2.23), and the nitro-group.

Covalent bonds are non-localized in *conjugate systems*. A conjugated system is a molecule (or portion of a molecule) in which every second bond is conventionally written as a double-bond. Conjugated systems are quite planar; butadiene, benzene, and pyridine are examples. In benzene, six of the valency electrons (one from each carbon atom) unite in forming the π-layer which completely covers both faces of the molecule. This condition is maintained by *resonance*. However, resonance can exist without conjugation, as in amides, which have a structure intermediate between (8.1) and (8.2), but not otherwise representable. The double-headed arrow is the accepted sign for resonance. Note that in the canonical forms [such as (8.1) and (8.2)] which make up the resonance hybrid, no atom ever moves position, only the electrons move. The flatness of the amide group, like that of the benzene ring, was demonstrated by X-ray diffraction.

$$
\underset{(8.1)}{R-C\overset{O}{\underset{NH_2}{\diagdown}}} \longleftrightarrow \underset{(8.2)}{R-C\overset{O^-}{\underset{\overset{+}{N}H_2}{\diagup}}}
$$

(b) *The electrostatic bond*

These are bonds between two ions, or an ion and a molecule, in each case maintained by purely electrostatic forces, which are long-range, falling off by only the second power of the distance. Of these two types, the *ionic bond*, formed between two ions of opposite charge, has a strength of about 5 kcal/mol. Sodium chloride ($Na^+ Cl^-$) is a typical example, and explains why this type of bond was formerly called a 'salt bond'. The characteristic feature of ionic bonds is the readiness with which they interchange. Thus in a biological environment they may last only 10^{-5}s because of the large amount of inorganic salts present and the opportunities thus afforded for ion-exchange. Nevertheless, when an ionic bond is reinforced by the simultaneous presence of shorter-range bonds, the union becomes stronger and more permanent. For example, the cations of all amines, except quaternary amines, simultaneously form hydrogen bonds and ionic bonds with the anions of carboxylic acids, as in (8.3) where the charge of the carboxylate anion is shown in mesomeric form, rather than as one of the canonical forms of the resonance hybrid. These hydrogen-bonded salts are credited with 10 kcal/mol of bond-strength. Amidines form even more tightly bound salts (8.4). Again, two molecules can be held together at one point by an ionic bond and elsewhere by van der Waals bonds, as in the intercalation of 9-aminoacridine by DNA (Section 10.3b). These reinforcements greatly increase the permanence of the bond.

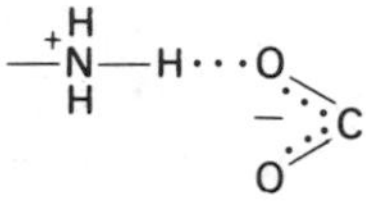

Salt of amine
(8.3)

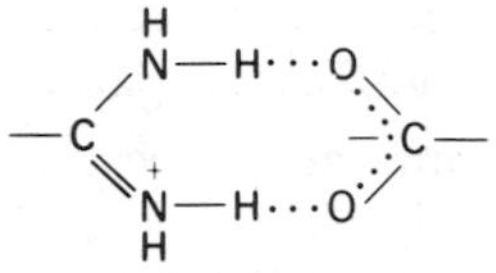

Salt of amidine
(8.4)

The stabilization of ion-pairs (i.e. pairs of oppositely charged ions) by short-range bonds is admirably illustrated by a modern analytical method known as ion-extraction analysis. For example, picric acid (8.5), in aqueous solution, can be readily determined by titration with an aqueous solution of methylene blue (8.6) if a layer of chloroform is present. Neither methylene blue (a chloride of a very strong base) nor picric acid dissolves appreciably in chloroform, whereas methylene blue picrate is quite soluble in this solvent. The end-point is taken as the first appearance of a faint, permanent blue colour in the aqueous phase (Bolliger, 1939). Normally a salt has no properties other than those of the ions of which it is composed. But when large areas of the two ions can be brought into intimate contact, and both (8.5) and (8.6) have flat structures, the total bonding (ionic + secondary) is so strong that the water of hydration which all ions possess is squeezed out, and the salt becomes liposoluble. Similarly cationic organic drugs, like mepacrine (6.9), can be determined, in the presence of an im-miscible solvent, with coloured sulphonic acids such as methyl orange (8.7) (Brodie et al., 1945) or bromothymol blue. Such ion-extraction is a model for the uptake of drug cations by receptors, and for the carrier-aided passage of agents through semi-permeable membranes (see Section 3.1).

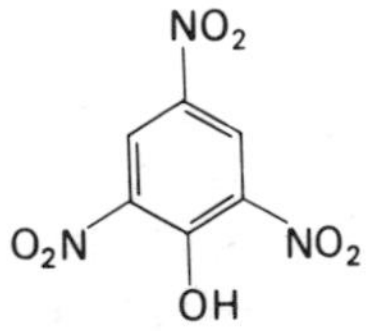

Picric acid
(8.5)

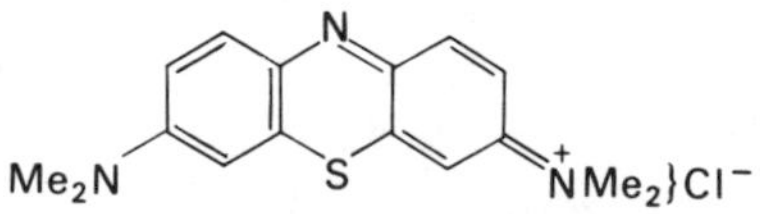

Methylene blue
(8.6)

Methyl orange
(8.7)

To picture an *ion-dipole bond*, one must first recall that many molecules which are not ionized have dipole moments and hence carry a (fractional) positive and a negative charge on some of their constituent atoms. For example, electron-attracting groups have a fractional negative charge (see Appendix III for a classified list of groups). These charges can attract ions of the opposite sign, thus forming bonds only slightly weaker than ionic bonds.

Finally there are *dipole-dipole bonds* whose strength declines with the third power of the distance. Perhaps the most familiar example of an ion-dipole bond is that which unites all anions (and cations) to water, in aqueous solution, and makes the properties of these hydrated ions so different from those of the anhydrous ions in a crystal. In the Wilson-Bergmann model of acetylcholinesterase (Fig. 13.3), a dipole-dipole bond was postulated between the doubly-bound nitrogen atom of the imidazole ring (of the enzyme) and the fractional positive charge of the carbon atom in the ester group (of acetylcholine). Better examples exist among the antibacterial sulphonamides. Although these inhibit the enzyme (dihydrofolate synthetase) best if they are anions, a useful if mild potency is available in members that are incapable of ionization [examples: dapsone (9.9) which is the best sulphonamide for leprosy, and sulphaguanidine (*10.34*) which, although since bettered, was considered an immense step forward when introduced into the Armed Forces in 1941 for treating severe bacterial dysentery].

These various kinds of electrostatic forces are thought to be very important for attracting substrates and coenzymes to enzymes, and agents to their receptors. This is because they are long-range forces that begin to act from far away. But they make highly exchangeable bonds, and hence the unions which they facilitate are only short-lived unless the uniting surfaces are so constituted that short-range forces can come into play, namely hydrogen bonds and van der Waals bonds.

(c) The hydrogen bond

The high concentration of positive charge in an uniquely small volume enables the hydrogen atom to act as a bond between two electronegative atoms (mainly O, N, and F): e.g. $-O-H \ldots N-$. Hydrogen-bondable atoms must have complete octets of which at least one electron-pair is unshared. The atoms bound by hydrogen may be in the same or in different molecules. The bond-strength is usually 3–5 kcal/mol. To form a hydrogen bond the atoms must be free to take up a position along the line of the OH or NH axis, and at a particular distance (e.g. 2.7 Å for an O–H ... O bond). They dissociate readily on warming.

The greater the difference in electron affinity of the two atoms linked by hydrogen (even if both atoms are of the same element, say, nitrogen) the stronger the hydrogen bond, whose nature lies roughly between the co-ordinate and the electrostatic bond. Hydrogen bonds involving sulphur are weak, those involving halogens (except fluorine) are weaker still, and those in which carbon participates are barely observable. Hydrogen-bonding is recognized by changes in the infrared spectra, ionization constants, melting-points, volatility, and solubility.

Hydrogen bonds are both short-range and angle-restricted. Because of the stringency of the conditions under which they can be formed, they have a highly selective character. For this reason, hydrogen bonds are considered to be important in drug-receptor interactions, and they are known to play a key role in maintaining the structure of proteins.

Ice, paper, and nylon (and, to some degree, cotton and wool) are typical examples of solids whose mechanical properties are controlled mainly by their hydrogen bonds. For a review of the nature of hydrogen bonding, a state first recognized by Latimer and Rodebush in 1920, see Kollman and Allen (1972).

(d) *Van der Waals forces**
These are the most universal of all attractions between atoms. They operate whenever any two atoms belonging to different molecules are brought sufficiently close together. Van der Waals forces arise from the fact that all molecules possess energy which leads to internal vibration. The temporary dipoles which this vibration creates in the constituent atoms, induce dipoles in neighbouring atoms of other molecules, a process which results in a net attraction. Such forces vary inversely as the seventh power of the distance, so that they are significant only over a short range. (Hence if two atoms are separated twice as far as they were previously, the attraction falls to 1/128 of its former value; cf. the attraction of an ionic bond which would fall to only 1/4 of its former value, and a dipole-dipole bond to 1/8).

Van der Waals attraction increases with rise in atomic weight; it is negligible for hydrogen atoms, and about 0.5 kcal/mol between pairs of atoms of atomic weight 12–16 which are of greatest significance in drug-receptor unions. These forces add up to a significant attraction between any two molecules that can fit one another so well that many atoms in one molecule can touch those in the other molecule. In this way, strong bonding (e.g. 5 kcal/mol) may result from close juxtaposition of an agent and its receptor. Van der Waals bonds are more temperature-sensitive than ionic bonds (Lonsdale *et al.*, 1965).

*Purists withhold the name 'bond' because of incomplete stoichiometry.

No *direct* way of measuring van der Waals forces in isolation is known, but their values can be obtained by orbital calculation or by subtracting other forces from the measured sum-total of all forces between two molecules or between a molecule and the whole of its environment. Of these total forces the following can be calculated reliably: ion-ion, ion-dipole, and dipole-dipole. (Here 'dipole' is used to signify a *permanent dipole* whose magnitude and orientation are known or can easily be determined, whereas van der Waals forces are between *oscillating dipoles*.)

Actually van der Waals forces are the resultant of four kinds of ultimate forces, namely the London attraction, the Debye attraction, the temperature-sensitive Keesom force, and the Born repulsion. The last-named arises as follows. Two atoms in any organic molecule are usually about 1.4 Å apart, but the atoms in *different* molecules cannot get as close as this. Two molecules begin to repel one another strongly as soon as their respective atoms come within about 3.0 Å (for C, H, or N atoms, but only 2.4 Å for two hydrogen atoms). These minimal distances are attributed to the addition of two van der Waals radii (1.2 Å for H, 1.55 Å for N).* These powerful repulsive forces come into play whenever two non-bonded atoms, even in the same molecule, approach to a distance equal to the sum of their van der Waals radii. This repulsion sets the upper limit to van der Waals attraction.

The attraction between an antigen and its antibody consists entirely of short-range forces of the van der Waals and hydrogen-bond type (Pardee and Pauling, 1949).

For reviews on van der Waals forces, see London (1937) and Pitzer (1959).

Electron-transfer complexes are a special manifestation of some non-localized covalent bonds. As was outlined above, molecules with two or more conjugated double-bonds have some highly delocalized electrons which form a π-electron layer covering the conjugated area. Through further delocalization, caused by substituents with powerful dipoles, this π-layer can have either a deficiency or an excess of π-electrons compared to the normal (two π-electrons contributed by each double-bond). Hence, particularly in ring-systems, it is desirable to distinguish between π-deficient substances (e.g. nitrobenzene and pyridine) and 'π-excessive' substances (e.g. aniline and pyrrole) (Albert, 1968). A strongly π-deficient substance can form a very weak complex with a strongly π-excessive substance, seemingly sharing electrons almost as freely as though the two molecules were two adjacent rings in the one molecule. The thermodynamic basis for this effect is poorly understood, and the principal observable fact is the appearance of a new absorption peak in the ultraviolet or visible spectrum.

Interest in electron-transfer complexes began with spectroscopic studies, three decades ago (Benesi and Hilderbrand, 1948). It was then found that

---

* For other van der Waals radii, see Bondi (1964).

riboflavine forms such a complex with tryptophan, and with 5-hydroxy-tryptamine. Some workers think that this type of bonding is likely to prove highly significant in biology (Szent-Györgi, 1960). The term 'charge-transfer complexes', in Mulliken's original sense, referred to electron-transfer complexes *temporarily* formed by the action of light. For further reading on electron-transfer complexes, see Slifkin (1971).

The term *hydrophobic bonding* was invented by Kauzmann (1954) to describe the van der Waals attractions between atoms in the non-polar parts of two molecules immersed in water. Because van der Waals bonds operate over such short distances, there is no room for water molecules in the vicinity of the mutually-bound paraffinic surfaces. Conversely the attraction of water molecules for one another, by hydrogen bonds (see end of Section 3.0), ensured that molecular regions lacking oxygen or nitrogen atoms (which are themselves hydrogen-bondable) tend to be squeezed out of water. Thus no new kind of bond is involved in the term 'hydrophobic bond', and its use served only to remind a reader that the region (of a molecule) under discussion is one free from oxygen and nitrogen atoms. The term lacks the thermodynamic validity of the four principal types of bond discussed above.

That the concept of 'hydrophobic bonding' does not square with the facts, was pointed out by Hildebrand (1960). He showed that no phobia for water forces together the atoms constituting two hydrocarbon chains. He instanced that the energy required to evaporate a mole of butane from its aqueous solution (at 1 atm and 25°) is 0.65 kcal greater than from its own pure liquid. 'This represents attraction not phobia', he wrote. Admittedly, the attraction of hydrocarbons for water is far smaller than that possessed by more polar substances, but it is slightly greater than the attraction of hydrocarbons for one another. This was a flat contradiction of the claim, 'Hydrocarbons actually prefer a nonpolar environment to being surrounded by water' (Nemethy, Scheraga, and Kauzmann, 1960). Hildebrand replied that if you pour some octane on ice, you can see that the ice is instantly wet by it (Hildebrand, 1960).

For more on the lipophilic and the hydrophilic regions of molecules, see Appendix II.

For further reading on bonds formed between molecules, see Pauling (1967), and for information on valency, see Speakman (1968). For the effect of water on modifying molecular attraction, see Salem (1962).

8.1 Adsorption

Many direct and indirect references to adsorption have been made in this narrative. Now that the main types of chemical bond have been reviewed, it is possible to discuss this property at a fundamental level, namely in terms of bonds.

A substance is said to be adsorbed when it is concentrated reversibly at a surface. It was not a well-understood phenomenon until Langmuir (1916, 1917, 1918) clarified the subject in three papers. Adsorption involves exactly the same types of bond (especially van der Waals, hydrogen, and ionic bonds) as are involved in chemical reactions in the bulk phase. Formerly, workers tried to differentiate between 'chemical' and 'physical' adsorption, but it became evident that, because all bonds are chemical bonds, all adsorption is chemical.

A surface has two special features which can make reactions taking place there quantitatively different from analogous reactions taking place in solution. Firstly, a surface presents a 100 per cent concentration of the substance involved. As the substance is sparingly soluble (if it were soluble, it would not be present as a surface), this concentration enormously increases the opportunities for the reaction to take place. For example, a crystal of silver chloride has a surface concentration of 7 M, as one can quickly verify from the molecular weight. On the other hand, a saturated solution of this substance (1×10^{-5} M) contains practically no silver chloride.

The other special feature about a surface is that it is apt to contain unsatisfied valencies, which, elsewhere in the solid, are used to bind similar atoms or molecules together. This is evident from the representation of a piece of carbon in Fig. 8.1. It is obvious that the finer the carbon is ground, the more residual valencies there will be, and the more active an adsorbent it will become.

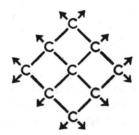

FIG. 8.1 Residual affinity of fragment of carbon.

Except in the rare cases where covalent bonds are made, adsorption is a reversible process, and equilibrium is established according to the mass-action law. In 1918 Langmuir derived the following equation from this law to permit of a more accurate quantitative treatment of adsorption than had been possible.

$$\frac{x}{m} = \frac{abc}{1 + ac}$$

This equation states that, if the temperature is kept constant, the weight (x) of a substance adsorbed per weight (m) of adsorbant is proportional to the term on the right where c is the concentration of *un*adsorbed substance, and a and b are constants. The equation expresses the fact that the adsorbant becomes saturated at high values of c, (because, when c is much larger than 1, the term on the right becomes simply b). This 'isotherm', as it is called, is represented graphically as a hyperbola (Fig. 8.2). It is evident that this equation is a general treatment of a subject which has some familar special cases, e.g. the union of a hydrogen ion with an ammonia molecule (to give an ammonium cation) which follows the same hyperbolic curve and is one of the simplest examples of adsorption by ionic bonds.

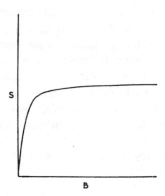

FIG. 8.2 Typical Langmuir isotherm. S, concentration of substance adsorbed (x/m). B, total concentration of substance.

In the adsorption of drugs on their specific receptors, it is very often found that doubling the dose produces smaller and smaller additional responses, and that this falling off corresponds to the shape of a hyperbola (Clark, 1933). This relationship is sometimes complicated by destruction or other loss of the drug (see 'Sites of loss' in Section 3.3).

In general chemistry, Langmuir's isotherm fits the experimental data in a very large number of cases where the adsorbed layer is unimolecular. However, some other patterns of adsorption are known and a convenient general classification has been made, as follows, by Giles *et al.* (1960).

(i) L-curves, normal Langmuir isotherms (e.g. Fig. 8.2) indicative of molecules adsorbed *flat* on the surface. The more solute is adsorbed, the harder it is for additional amounts to become fixed.

(ii) S-curves, indicative of *vertical* orientation of adsorbed molecules. In the initial part of the sigmoid curve, the more solute is already adsorbed, the easier it is for additional amounts to become fixed. This is the co-operative effect.

(iii) H-curves, high-affinity curves which commence at a high value of the 'concentration on solid' axis; often given by solids adsorbed as micelles, and by high-affinity ions that exchange with low-affinity ions.

(iv) C-curves, constant-partition linear curves given by substances which penetrate into the adsorbant more readily than the solvent can.

It is important to bear in mind that 'dissolved' proteins and other large molecules are in the colloidal state. Such suspensions although transparent to the eye, present an enormous surface for adsorption. For example, a cubic centimetre of human serum contains 100 m^2 of protein surface.

8.2 Non-biological examples of selectivity

Chemical selectivity, of a degree comparable with the specificity shown by drugs, can be found in simple non-living material. Thus it is not necessary to assume *new* types of bonds to explain the action of biologically active agents.

Examples will be chosen from two topics, *dyeing* and *flotation*, which require chemicals that can differentiate between rather similar substances. Seemingly irrelevant to the study of selective toxicity, these parallel investigations can throw light on some of biological selectivity's knottiest problems.

In industry, two chemically related fibres, such as cellulose and cellulose acetate, are often woven into an invisible design and dyed in contrasting colours, simultaneously. Thus a dyebath containing both 'Chlorazol Sky Blue FFS' (*8.8*) (in U.S.A.: 'Pontamine Sky Blue 6BX') and 'Dispersol Yellow 3G' (*8.9*) (in U.S.A.: 'Acetamine Yellow CG') will dye the cellulose fibres pure blue and the cellulose acetate fibres pure yellow, giving a fabric with, for example, a yellow design on a blue ground. In short, each fibre has combined very strongly with its selective dye and has rejected the opposite type. The structure of the cellulose fibre consists of long, rather flat molecules, packed together in sheets. Each molecule is liberally studded with hydrogen-bonding groups. Hence it is not surprising that the majority of water-soluble dyes which have an affinity for unmordanted cellulose are also long and flat and are liberally studded with hydrogen-bonding groups (Lapworth, 1940; Ruggli, 1934). 'Chlorazol Sky Blue' is such a substance. In cellulose acetate, however, five out of every six hydroxyl-groups have been blocked by acetylation and the molecule has taken on the general characteristics of a lipophilic ester. Hence it is not surprising to find that the majority of dyes which have an affinity for cellulose acetate are very soluble in esters. The union is not by hydrogen-bonding groups, and the possession of these is disadvantageous (the introduction of a single sulphonic-group has been found to destroy all affinity for cellulose acetate). For further information on the connection between constitution and selectivity in these dyes, see Lapworth (1940) and Green (1937).

'Sky Blue'
(8.8)

(8.9)   (8.10)

In mining technology, flotation agents are commonly used to separate the constituents of a mixed ore. The crushed ore is placed in a tank of water through which a stream of air bubbles is rising. When the specific 'collector' is added, the mineral which it selects will rise to the surface, off which it is mechanically scraped. Thus to float mercuric sulphide, enough potassium *iso*amyl xanthate (8.10) is added to give a 1 in 100 000 solution. Similarly sodium stearate will cause copper silicate to float, and in both examples all quartz (sand) will remain at the bottom of the tank. This and similar processes are familiar to every mining engineer and are used commercially on a immense scale. For further reading on flotation, see Holman (1941); Sutherland and Wark (1955).

Details for carrying out lecture demonstrations of (a) dyeing a mixed fabric blue and yellow simultaneously from the same bath, and (b) separating, by flotation, red mercuric sulphide, followed by green cupric silicate from their mixture with sand, will be found in the first four editions of this book. The degree of selectivity shown, in chromatography, by such substances as alumina and silica also lends itself to demonstrations.

9 Metabolites, enzymes, and metabolite analogues

The smallest change in the chemical constitution of a selectively toxic agent often makes an enormous change in its biological activity, and many examples of this have been given in Chapter 2. The present chapter deals in greater detail with one cause of high specificity, namely a close resemblance between (a) the normal substrate (or coenzyme) of an *enzyme* and (b) an agent which inhibits it. In biochemical nomenclature, the substrate, the precursors of coenzymes, and the products of enzymes are referred to collectively as *metabolites**.

9.0 Enzymes, their substrates and other metabolites

The process of growth and division involves cells in ceaseless chemical activity. For the most part this activity takes the form of chemical reactions between enzymes and substrates, whereby the enzymes remain unchanged, and the substrates are transformed into other metabolites by the breaking or making of covalent bonds. Even the organic coenzymes may undergo

* In pharmacological usage, the word metabolite is often used more narrowly to mean: a product of the degradative action of an organism on a drug. These are *secondary* metabolites.

a covalent change in the course of their functioning, e.g. nicotinamide adenine dinucleotide receives, and then loses, a hydrogen atom on the carbon atom in position 4. Similarly, diphosphothiamine receives, and then loses, an acetyl-group on C-2.

Some coenzymes ('co-factors') are inorganic cations, many others are simple organic molecules, but many enzymes need no co-enzyme. The organic coenzymes are either synthesized by the organism, or by another organism and taken in with food. The protein portion of an enzyme that has a coenzyme is called the apoenzyme. The substrates are either (a) food or (b) simple molecules formed from the food by the action of other enzymes (both degradative and synthetic). In the 1972 survey, 1740 different enzymes were recorded, of which more than 100 had been crystallized (Commission on Enzymes, 1972). Today the numbers are much greater because many enzymes have been found to have isoenzymes (defined below). Some enzymes may be present in cells only to the extent of a few molecules, or even only as 'information' in the DNA which can permit the enzyme to be synthesized when it is needed; but other enzymes may constitute at least 50 per cent of the dry weight of the cell, as myosin (an adenosine triphosphatase) does in muscle cells.

Until recently, the conventional purification of enzymes, e.g. by electrophoresis, was slow and the yields poor. The recent introduction of affinity chromatography enables an enzyme to be obtained pure and in high yield. In this technique, a specific inhibitor of the enzyme is attached, covalently and by a flexible link such as $-CH_2.CH_2-$, to a polymeric adsorbant. The enzyme collects on the inhibitor, from which it can usually be freed by a change in pH (Cuatrecasas, Wilcheck and Anfinsen, 1968).

The first enzyme to be completely synthesized was ribonuclease. This was done both in solution, by the classical chemical methods (Hirschmann et al., 1969), and by Merrifield's solid-support technique (Gutte and Merrifield, 1969).

The most successful method for disclosing enzyme structure is the X-ray diffraction study of a suitable crystal. For definitive results, a resolution of 2 Å is eventually attempted, but this is extremely time-consuming, even with computational aid. The special value of X-ray diffraction is that it reveals the tertiary folding of the enzyme molecule, so that it can be seen which aminoacids are physically close to one another *in the folded state*. It is known that the active site of an enzyme is usually composed of two or three aminoacid residues that would lie far apart if the chain were extended. For example, the action of the enzyme lysozyme (from white of egg) on its substrate in the bacterial cell wall (murein; Fig. 5.3) requires the proximity of residues 35 and 52 (glutamic and aspartic acid, respectively) from two strands of the enzyme (Phillips, 1966). Lysozyme has predominantly a hydrophobic interior and hydrophilic exterior in its tertiary structure, an arrangement quite common in enzymes.

Ribonuclease, another enzyme whose tertiary structure has been found by X-ray diffraction, is compact, hydrophilic outside, hydrophobic inside, with a slot to receive the substrate. The active site makes use of histidine residues (numbers 12 and 119) that would otherwise be remote from one another (Kartha, Bello and Harker, 1967). The dimensions of the folded ribonuclease molecule are about $30 \times 30 \times 38$ Å (mol. wt. 15 000). When charged with a substrate, e.g. cytidine phosphate, one histidine residue binds the phosphate group, the other the sugar. The tertiary structure of α-chymotrypsin has been similarly worked out: the active site depends on the closeness of two aminoacids that are on different strands, namely serine 195 and histidine 57 (Matthews *et al.*, 1967). Human carbonic anhydrase, too, has had its tertiary structure revealed by X-ray crystallography: with the help of an inhibitor (labelled with mercury) the active site was shown to lie in a deep slot and to include the zinc atom essential for activity (Fridborg *et al.*, 1967).

Carboxypeptidase A, an important enzyme of the pancreas which hydrolyses only peptides with hydrophobic side-chains, was examined similarly at 2 Å resolution. The zinc atom, a necessary co-factor, was found to lie in a shallow depression in the surface of the molecule, adjacent to a deep lipophilic cavity. The zinc was bound by the following three residues: two histidines (69) and (196), and glutamic acid (72). The enzyme had 307 aminoacid residues, and the mol.wt. was 34 500. Comparison of the contour maps for the enzyme with and without a typical substrate (glycyl-tyrosine) shows that the phenyl-group fits into the deep cavity and thus forces the peptide carbonyl oxygen atom (of the substrate) against the zinc, which consequently loses a co-ordinated molecule of water. The free carboxyl-group of the substrate forms an ionic bond with arginine (145). This causes the arginine to move through 2 Å, thus disrupting nearby hydrogen bonds. This disturbance causes the free hydroxyl-group of tyrosine (248) to rotate through 120°, so that it enters the shallow depression close to the peptide bond of the substrate, and probably protonates the nitrogen atom in the susceptible peptide bond. Glutamic acid (270) is thought to complete the hydrolysis. This was the first direct evidence that substrates can distort the active sites of enzymes, a conformational change (Lipscomb *et al.*, 1969; Lipscomb, 1970).

The more precise information which X-ray crystallography has provided about active sites has expunged those speculative sketches which, until recently, decorated the literature of enzymology. It seems a safe prediction that the similar sketches of drug receptors, e.g. (*13.3*), will go the same way.

The determination of aminoacid sequences in enzyme-hydrolysates has provided great help in the interpretation of X-ray contour maps, but does not give reliable clues to active sites. However, such clues have often been obtained by allowing the enzyme, before hydrolysis, to react with a substance with which it forms a covalent bond. The organic phosphates

(Section 12.3) have often proved useful for proteolytic enzymes. Thus di*iso*propyl phosphofluoridate (*12.15*), taken up by chymotrypsin as a pseudo-substrate, alkylphosphorylates the enzyme at the active centre, thus making this enzyme unavailable for true substrates. It was found that one molecule of the inhibitor reacts with one active centre in each enzyme molecule. Hydrolytic degradation of the inhibited enzyme produced di*iso*-propylphosphorylated serine, and from this it was concluded that a serine residue played an important part in the active centre of the enzyme (Schaffer, May and Summerson, 1954). Degradative studies of this kind have shown that the sequence asp-ser-gly occurs at the active centre of chymotrypsin (which has 230 aminoacids in each molecule, of which 28 are serine) and trypsin, but glu-ser-ala is found at the active centre of acetylcholinesterase, pseudocholinesterase, and liver aliesterase (Sanger, 1963).

Other information about enzyme active sites has been obtained from the use of molecular probes (Chance *et al.*, 1971). The latter are small molecules of which a measurable property is altered when the probe is adsorbed on an enzyme. Suitable properties are optical absorption, fluorescence, electron spin resonance, and nuclear magnetic resonance.

Koshland (1964) was the first to postulate that substrates and co-factors can change the *conformation* of enzymes and vice versa. This has been confirmed by X-ray diffraction studies of enzymes, examined first without, and then with their metabolites. For example, the apoenzyme of lactate dehydrogenase was seen to be considerably deformed in the presence of its coenzyme NAD, and this coenzyme, which is normally closely folded, was stretched out simultaneously by the apoenzyme (Adams *et al.*, 1970). Conformational changes in an enzyme-substrate complex were described above under carboxypeptidase A. Again, the conformation of an acetyl-glucosamine residue was seen to be distorted from a 'chair' to a 'half chair' when bound to the active site of lysozyme (Blake *et al.*, 1967). For a diagram of conformational change taking place in haemoglobin when it becomes linked to oxygen, see Fig. 13.2.

Enzymes play their vitally important part in metabolism by speeding the numerous chemical reactions occurring within the cell. They act by lowering the energy barrier and thus increase the speed at which a reaction will proceed to equilibrium. For example, the energy of activation for the decomposition of hydrogen peroxide is lowered, from 18 to 2 kcal/mol, by the enzyme catalase which accelerates the reaction ($H_2O_2 \rightarrow H_2O + O$) by a factor of 1.6×10^{11}.

This remarkable catalytic activity of enzymes depends only on ordinary principles of physical and organic chemistry: (a) The substrate molecules are fixed on the enzyme in a particular conformation, often one that is only a minor component of the substrate population but is energetically favourable for the reaction; (b) the enzyme then initiates the reaction by supplying an electric field (+ and −) at unusually close range because of the close contact between 'key' atoms on the substrate and 'lock' atoms on the enzyme; (c) the aminoacid side-chains, lining the active site of the enzyme, form a microenvironment that can alter the stability of the transition state (and hence the reaction rate) by maintaining a low dielectric constant or, conversely, by supplying new sites for temporary bonding. In bimolecular reactions, the enzyme can bring the two substrates together more closely and in better orientation than would be possible in solution.

Enzymes have two types of specificity: (a) various degrees of affinity for the substrate, and (b) various rates at which different substrates undergo reaction after binding has taken place. These are called, respectively, binding specificity and kinetic specificity and each is exerted independently of the other (Koshland and Neet, 1968).

The first to be isolated of those complexes which enzymes form with their substrates was the complex of D-alanine, D-aminoacid oxidase, and its co-factor FAD (riboflavine adenine dinucleotide). It consisted of hexagonal purple crystals and was stable in the absence of air. Electron spin resonance measurements showed that the co-factor, present in these crystals, was in its free-radical monohydro-form (FADH) (Yagi, 1965).

Although all known enzymes are proteins, some simple non-protein models perform just like enzymes. For example, of the *cyclo*amyloses (*cyclo*dextrins) made by the degradation of starch (Cramer and Martin, 1958), *cyclo*hexaamylose is an efficient esterase for various substituted phenyl acetates (Bender *et al.*, 1966). The X-ray diffraction analysis of this pseudo-amylase shows a torus consisting of six α-D-glucose units in the usual conformation; hydroxyl-groups form crowns around top and bottom of the torus, which has an internal diameter of about 5 Å. The carbonyl-group of the acetate 'guest' presses against the secondary hydroxyl-groups of the 'host': the closer the approach, the faster the hydrolysis. The 'guest' ester acylates a hydroxy-group in the 'host', thus releasing phenol. The non-acylated 'host' is then regenerated by intramolecular catalysis, and the cycle can continue indefinitely. The cycle further resembles an enzyme reaction by obeying Michaelis-Menten kinetics (Section 9.1), and by the ease with which it is inhibited by analogues of the normal 'guests'.

This model shows that enzyme-like action can be obtained with a molecule of mol. wt. just under 1000, and a structure of great simplicity and symmetry. For further reading on low molecular-weight synthetic compounds with enzyme-like properties, see Jencks (1969); Bender (1971); and Bruice and Benkovic (1966).

Further light on enzyme action is shed by micelles of amphiphilic molecules, which catalyse many chemical reactions and are often regarded as very simple models for enzymes ('amphiphilic' and 'micelle' are defined in Section 14.0). The disposition of hydrophobic (inside) and hydrophilic (outside) groups in a micelle resembles that of enzymes. Like enzymes, too, micelles are denatured by heat or urea, and they show specificity towards substrates (Jencks, 1969). Reactions that liberate anions, e.g. the hydrolysis of esters, are catalysed by cationic micelles, e.g. those of cetyl-trimethylammonium bromide (*14.10*) (Menger and Portnoy, 1967). The substrate is concentrated around the micelle electrostatically. That van der Waals bonding then occurs is shown by the increasing efficacy of catalysis as the size of the substrate molecule is increased. The charged head groups of the micelle provide a charged environment (that may stabilize a transition state of the substrate) and are thought of as the actual catalysts. The low dielectric constant of the rest of the micelle is bound to destabilize any charge on the substrate, its transition state, and its products.

What a micellar catalyst can achieve is exemplified by sodium dodecyl sulphate which accelerates 500 000-fold the binding of Cu^{2+} by prophyrins (Lowe and Phillips, 1961). For general reading on catalysis by micelles, see Cordes (1973); Fendler and Fendler (1975).

Biological regulation of enzymes.   Enzymes functionally related to one another in a metabolic sequence are organized either in particles, or embedded in membranes (Dixon, 1966). In these systems the enzymes are coupled to one another chemically, thermodynamically, and by physical location. Hence, as soon as a reaction product appears from the first enzyme it can become the substrate for the next one, and so on. Such sequences of enzymes are often controlled by an *allosteric effect*, as follows. Enzymes near the beginning of a chain of reactions may have a second receptor (at some distance) which can combine with a natural inhibitor. (This inhibitor is often the normal product of an enzyme further down in the chain of reactions.) The combination causes a conformational change in the enzyme and as a result its normal substrate cannot get to the active site. This feed-back mechanism plays an important part in the self-regulation of the cell's metabolism (Monod, Changeux and Jacob, 1963). It has been shown that the presence of natural purines in a living cell can prevent further purine synthesis until the concentration falls below a certain level. Similar feedback control has been demonstrated with both natural and unnatural pyrimidines (Bresnick and Hitchings, 1961). The control of catecholamine synthesis by feedback mechanisms is shown in Fig. 9.1.

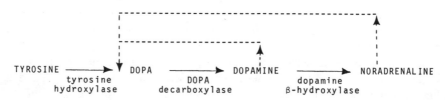

FIG. 9.1 Control of catecholamine synthesis.

Isoenzymes and analogous enzymes.   Many apparently pure enzymes have been separated by electrophoresis into a small number of pure proteins; each of these isoenzymes has a specificity similar to that of the crude enzyme, yet differing subtly in physical properties. One of the best-known examples, lactic dehydrogenase (LDH), exists in animal tissues as five isoenzymes. These are tetramers, formed by the association of two polypeptides A and B, and have the following composition: B_4, AB_3, A_2B_2, A_3B, and A_4. Creatine kinase and arginine kinase similarly have several isoenzymes. Isoenzymic patterns tend to remain constant for a given tissue in various mammalian species, but to differ from tissue to tissue in any one species. For selective inhibition of a particular isoenzyme, see Sections 9.4 (monoamine oxidase) and 9.6 (lactic dehydrogenase). Whereas isoenzymes seem to differ from one another only by a small increment of electric charge, analogous enzymes (which perform the same function in *different* organisms) usually differ from one another in a more fundamental way (see Section 4.6). For further reading on isoenzymes, see Shugar (1970).

Enzymes and drugs.   Many selective agents owe their useful properties to inhibiting particular enzymes. Before any such relationship can be established, the following requirements must be met (Hunter and Lowry, 1956): (a) the enzyme should be inhibited in the intact cell, as well as in the isolated state; and (b) enzyme inhibition must not require concentrations of the agent greater than are commonly used to elicit the pharmacological effect on the cell.

By these standards, organic phosphates, and also urethanes, have been shown to exert their biological effects by inhibiting acetylcholinesterase; and oximes exert their antidotal effect by reversing this inhibition (see Section 12.3). Many of the most interesting and useful examples of agents acting by inhibiting enzymes are those which show a close resemblance, both in structure and in electron-distribution, to a substrate or coenzyme. Such agents are called 'metabolite analogues' and most of the rest of this chapter will be devoted to them.

For a simple introduction to the chemistry of enzyme action, see Williams (1969); for the chemical reactivity and biological role of functional groups in enzymes, see Smellie (1970); for a catalogue of enzymes, see Webb (1972), for a discussion of individual enzymes, see Dixon and Webb (1964); for a multivolume work on enzymes, see Boyer (1970).

9.1 Metabolite analogues: definition, derivation, and mode of action

Those metabolites (substrates or coenzymes) that are present in only small amounts in a cell or tissue can be antagonized by substances known as *metabolite analogues*. The molecules of each such analogue have a region which is similar to that region of the metabolite which makes contact with the enzyme protein. To be effective, this similarity must be not only in dimensions, but also in electron-distribution, because most of the active sites on enzymes are highly polar. Each analogue exerts its antagonism by occupying and blocking the enzyme site used by the metabolite (see Section 9.2).

Although a metabolite can be turned into an analogue by effecting a chemical alteration in the molecule, the change must not be too large or the normal action is lost without any antagonistic action being created. Various additions and subtractions of a methyl-group from thiamine seriously diminish its vitamin properties (see introduction to Chapter 2) but do not create antagonists. In general, the loss or gain of a methyl-group is too great a change to make an antagonist.

Some antagonists are of such a chemically simple nature that their relevance as metabolite analogues is often overlooked. For example, inorganic cations are in competition with other inorganic cations (Sections 9.2 and 11.0). Even the hydrogen ion, itself an important metabolite, is in competition with organic and inorganic cations (Section 10.3a). Alcohol, in beverages, acts by successfully competing with water (for distribution at least). Alcohol can also antagonize the toxic effects of methanol, by displacing it from the enzyme that oxidizes methanol (Röe, 1955).

Several examples of competition between simple anions have been observed. Thus the perchlorate and the thiocyanate anion inhibit concentration of the iodide anion by the thyroid gland, without affecting the oxidative incorporation of the iodide anion into thyroxine (Stanbury and Wyngaarden, 1952). Likewise, the organism *Nitrobacter*, which oxidizes nitrite to nitrate, is inhibited by cyanate or chlorate (anions), an effect easily reversed by washing (Lees and Simpson, 1957).

Some physiological processes are regulated by pairs of analogous metabolites, for example the polyene sex hormones of algae (Kuhn, 1940), and the mammalian sex hormones. Of two prostaglandins present in human lungs, PGE_2 relaxes and PGF_{2a} contracts bronchial muscle (Sweatman and Collier, 1968). Similarly prostaglandin D_1 inhibits the increase of vascular permeability produced in the rat skin by prostaglandins E_1, E_2, and D_2 (Flower and Kingston, 1975).

Very few examples are known of antagonists made by rearranging the order of groups at an asymmetric carbon atom. One such antagonist is D-histidine which inhibits the enzyme histidase which normally opens the imidazole ring of L-histidine (Edlbacher *et al.*, 1940). This method is seldom effective in such small molecules, because the space-relationships required for adsorption on the enzyme are the very ones altered by the rearrangement. For this reason, a mixture of two optical antipodes (or the recemized substance) usually has the averaged potency of both constituents, as happens with atropine and with DL-adrenaline, i.e. there is no antagonism. A reliable method for antagonizing a large metabolite is to use a small molecule which resembles a repeating unit. As long ago as 1910 it was found that amylase, which normally hydrolyses starch, is strongly inhibited by dextrin and maltose (which are products of its action on starch), and also by glucose (which is not). These three inhibitory carbohydrates have the same configuration as the unit of which starch is a polymer. On the other hand, galactose and mannose, which are stereo-isomers of glucose, are less inhibitory; fructose, which is an isomer of glucose but not a stereo-isomer, is not inhibitory at all (Wohl and Glimm, 1910).

Small molecules are sometimes antagonized by their near homologues, e.g. malonic acid (9.1) antagonizes the oxidation of succinic acid (9.2) by succinic dehydrogenase (Quastel and Wooldridge, 1927).

HO$_2$C   CO$_2$H

C
H$_2$

Malonic acid
(9.1)

HO$_2$C   CO$_2$H

C—C
H$_2$ H$_2$

Succinic acid
(9.2)

R

HOCH$_2$—   —OH
    —CH$_3$
N

Pyridoxin (R = —CH$_2$OH)
(9.3)

Another method for obtaining antagonistic analogues is to make a small change in the atoms that form a ring. For example, an antagonist of the vitamin biotin (9.3) has been obtained by replacing the sulphur atom by oxygen, and an antagonist of thiamine (2.1) was formed by replacing the sulphur by an ethylene group (see below); also the reverse change in phenylalanine (replacing an ethylene group by sulphur, giving thienylalanine) produced a very strong antagonist for this aminoacid in micro-organisms (Dittmer, 1949). Moreover, the change of thiophen for benzene is very often effective. For example, α-thienylalkylamines resemble the corresponding phenylalkylamines in hypertensive activity, and 2-thenoic esters of alkylamines resemble the corresponding benzoic esters as local anaesthetics.

One of the best general methods for obtaining antagonists is to substitute one electron-attracting group for another. Thus – COOH may be replaced by – COCH$_3$, by – SO$_2$OH, or – SO$_2$NH$_2$. When designing replacements of this sort, it is important not to alter the ionization of any basic group present in the molecule. Thus the amino-group in p-aminobenzoic acid (anion) (9.4) is not ionized, and hence it is not admissible to replace – COOH by SO$_3$H because the basic group would then become ionized and the new substance too dissimilar to be a good analogue (this has been experimentally verified). As will be described in Section 9.3, a highly satisfactory antagonist for p-aminobenzoic acid (anion) (9.4) is sulphanilamide (anion) (9.5).

Sometimes antagonists have been made by substituting fluorine for hydrogen, e.g. p-fluorophenylalanine as an antagonist for phenylalanine,

and fluorocitric acid for citric acid (Section 12.5). Similarly, replacement of
a methyl-group by chlorine is often effective, as in the riboflavine antagonists (Kuhn, Weygand and Möller, 1943). Table 9.1 shows why these
changes are sterically appropriate, and why the substitution of chlorine or
methyl for hydrogen does not usually give effective antagonists. The unifying
feature is that these analogues must be so similar to the substrate that the
enzyme is deceived into taking up the foreign molecule in place of the
substrate. Yet the analogue must be dissimilar enough to be incapable of
functioning as the substrate does. That is to say, it must either fail to undergo
the very next chemical reaction normal for the substrate, or if it does
undergo this reaction, the product must be unacceptable to an enzyme
later in the sequence of reactions.

Table 9.1

SOME VAN DER WAALS RADII
RELEVANT TO
METABOLITE ANTAGONISM

Substituent	Radius (Å)
H	1.2
F	1.35
Cl	1.8
CH_3	2.0

Antagonistic metabolite analogues have been found for almost every
known vitamin. For example, when the thiazole portion of thiamine (2.1) is
replaced by a similarly substituted pyridine ring, the product ('pyrithiamine') produces characteristic symptoms of thiamine-deficiency in mice
(Woolley, 1950) [see Section 9.4 for a commercially successful thiamine
antagonist (9.24)].

Desoxypyridoxine [(9.3), R = –CH₃] produces signs of vitamin B₆
deficiency in man, chicks, and rats, rapidly reversed by the vitamin [(9.3),
R = –CH₂OH] (Mueller and Vilter, 1950). For most of the vitamins,
several antagonists are known. Metabolite analogues have also been found
for aminoacids, purines, pyrimidines, some hormones, and the participating
acids of the Krebs cycle.

Apparently no molecule is too large to have an antagonist: acetylation
of the thyroid-stimulating hormone (TSH), a protein of the pituitary gland,
gives an analogue which accumulates in the thyroid gland and reduces
hyperthyroidism by blocking the action of TSH (Sonenberg and Money,
1957). Again, very small chemical alterations of other polypeptide pituitary
hormones, such as oxytocin and vasopressin, produce antagonists to the
relevant hormones (Dyckes et al., 1974). Even at this level of molecular

complexity, Nature has evolved many examples of mutual antagonism. A natural polypeptide (mol. wt. 6512) called aprotinin ('Trasylol'), abundantly present in mammalian tissues, inhibits the proteolytic enzymes trypsin, chymotrypsin, and plasmin; it is sometimes used in acute pancreatitis.

In many cases, the site of action of a metabolite antagonist is known. Thus pyrithiamine displaces thiamine from the enzyme which phosphorylates it to give the coenzyme. Again, desoxypyridoxine [(9.3), $R = -CH_3$] seems inactive until it is phosphorylated in animals to a derivative which competes with pyridoxal phosphate, which is the coenzyme of the amino-acid decarboxylases (Woolley, 1952).

Wood's discovery of the mode of action of sulphonamides on bacteria (see Section 9.3a) led to an intense search for metabolite antagonists that would be useful in controlling disease. This proved to be difficult because economic and uneconomic cells share many common biochemical pathways. For some time the principal successes were confined to anti-folic acid drugs, commencing with the sulphonamides. However, little by little many other useful metabolite antagonists were discovered, some by chance but others by design, and these are reviewed in Section 9.4. The position to-day is that comparative biochemistry must provide strong evidence of a reaction uniquely carried out by the uneconomic cell for it to be worth while to make analogues of the metabolite involved. Fortunately some of the innumerable *un*selective agents, synthesized during this long period of misunderstanding, have been adopted by biochemists as specific reagents for blocking various metabolic processes *in vitro*.

For reviews of metabolite antagonists in the widest sense, i.e. without special reference to selective toxicity, see Hochster and Quastel (1963).

Quantitative aspects. The relationship between metabolites and metabolite analogues is usually competitive. That is, if x molecules of metabolite are antagonized by y molecules of analogue, then $10x$ molecules of metabolite require $10y$ molecules of analogue to give the same biological end-point, and so on. As such competitive reactions are freely reversible, the antagonism of x molecules of metabolite by y molecules of analogue can be abolished by another x molecules of metabolite, and so on. Malonic acid and succinic acid have a competitive relationship of this kind; sulphanilamide and p-aminobenzoic acid provide another example.

For each pair of substances there will be a unique index of inhibition, defined as the ratio of the number of molecules of analogue (to those of metabolite) required to give 50 per cent inhibition. This ratio will vary with the biological species, but is always the same for any one species. It is obviously an expression of the relative affinity of analogue and metabolite for a receptor-group, but it also includes a term for differences in the penetration of the two substances when the site of action is not exposed. The amount of inhibition which any analogue can produce therefore depends on two things: firstly, its affinity for the receptor relative to that of the metabolite, and, secondly, the relative amounts of analogue and metabolite available at the site of action.

The affinity of a substrate for an enzyme is represented by Equation (i):

$$[E] + [S] \rightleftharpoons [ES] \tag{i}$$

where [E] is the concentration of the enzyme, [S] is that of the substrate, and [ES] that of the complex which they form. The affinity of coenzymes and inhibitors (I) for an apoenzyme is similarly formulated. Hence the dissociation constant for an inhibitor (K_i) is:

$$K_i = \frac{[E][I]}{[EI]} \tag{ii}$$

Unlike an inhibitor, a substrate is changed by the enzyme into a product (P), and the sequence of events becomes:

$$[E] + [S] \underset{k''}{\overset{k'}{\rightleftharpoons}} [ES] \overset{k'''}{\to} [E] + [P] \tag{iii}$$

The ratio k''/k' equals K_m, the Michaelis constant, which is the dissociation constant of the enzyme-substrate complex [ES] into its components [E] and (S) (Michaelis and Menten, 1913). It pertains to the Equilibrium (iv) which is formally analogous to (ii):

$$K_m = \frac{[E][S]}{[ES]} \tag{iv}$$

The *index of inhibition* of an inhibitor is the ratio K_i/K_m; the smaller the index, the more efficient the inhibitor.

The Michaelis constant is obviously inversely proportional to the affinity of the enzyme for the substrate, and is numerically equal to the substrate concentration when the reaction has reached half its maximal velocity. The dimensions of K_i and K_m are recorded as g mol per litre. However, they are not true equilibrium constants but ratios of velocity constant for the forward and reverse reactions. A suitable determination of K_m is by the graphical method of Lineweaver and Burk (1934), where the initial rate of formation of ES is plotted against substrate concentration, both as reciprocals. This should give a straight line and, if it does, the value of K_m is shown at the intersection of slope and abscissa.

Lineweaver-Burk plots are also used to find if an inhibitor is truly competitive (as defined above). For this purpose, the initial rate is plotted against the substrate concentration (both as reciprocals), and this is repeated several times after the addition to the experimental system of ever-increasing concentrations of inhibitor. If the inhibition is competitive, several straight lines should be obtained, one for each concentration of inhibitor, and these should all pass through one point on the ordinate (Hammett, 1970, p. 82).

Briggs and Haldane (1925) showed that it was unnecessary to assume an equilibrium between [E] and [S], and derived equation (v), formally similar to the Michaelis-Menten equation but free from this assumption and suitable for steady state conditions.

$$K_{bh} = \frac{k'' + k'''}{k'} \tag{v}$$

This constant, more general than the earlier one, is a measure of the simultaneous dissociation of ES in two opposite directions. Where K_{bh} replaces K_m, the index of inhibition becomes the ratio K_i/K_{bh}. All of these calculations assume that the inhibitor is not being partly segregated (or even destroyed) by other biological material which may be present.

It may be appropriate to mention here the concept of a 'dystrophic' complex (Zeller, 1963). If a metabolite does not fit an enzyme well, it must be utilized inefficiently; and if it is so constituted that it is attached to the enzyme more durably than a better fitting and more efficiently utilized metabolite, it becomes a partial inhibitor (see Section 7.5b).

The molar inhibitory index of malonic acid is 1/3 (Thorn, 1953). Even more economical inhibition is shown by carbon monoxide when it replaces oxygen on haemoglobin (1/210). Values below unity, such as these, are uncommon, because it is rare to find an analogue that has a greater affinity for a natural receptor than the normal substrate has. Methotrexate (4.6) owes its unprecedentedly high index of 1/10 000 (against folic acid) to the higher basic strength that results from introducing an amino-group C-4. X-ray diffraction of the complex of dihydrofolate reductase with methotrexate shows the pyrimidine ring buried in a mainly lipophilic pocket in which N-1 is linked, ionically, to the carboxylic group of Asp-27, a link that folic acid is too weak a base to make (Matthews *et al.*, 1977). The larger-than-unity figure (300/1) for the antagonism of p-aminobenzoic acid by sulphanilamide (in streptococci) is more typical (Woods, 1940).

It is not surprising that most inhibitory indices are high, because most enzymes have evolved, under the selection pressure of Nature, to handle their natural substrates efficiently. But another reason for the inefficiency of many competitive inhibitors is the *steady-state* condition of the living cell. The target enzyme is continuously supplied with substrate (from the previous enzyme in the chain) and its product is continuously removed by the next enzyme. Hence target enzymes usually turn out to be *under-saturated* with substrate and so have great reserve capacity. It is true that the addition of a competitive inhibitor to a steady-state system initially inhibits the target enzyme; but accumulation of more of the normal substrate of the inhibited enzyme soon overcomes this inhibition. There then exists a new steady-state situation in which the throughput of the pathway is unaltered because the concentration of the substrate in the target enzyme is maintained at a higher level in order to counterbalance the effect of the inhibitor (Cleland, 1970). This exemplifies the difference between the chemistry of the model systems that are studied in the laboratory and more complex systems that have evolved in the living cell.

9.2 History of metabolite antagonism prior to 1940

Studies of metabolite antagonism were foreshadowed by the London work of Ringer (1883) who found, from a helper's error which he was quick to interpret, that the sodium (cations) in a solution of sodium chloride could not maintain the beat of an isolated heart unless balanced by calcium and potassium. As a result of this work, the physiologically balanced solutions, named after Ringer, Locke, and Tyrode, were developed.

The next relevant discovery was made in 1910, when some enzymes were blocked by substances whose molecular structure resembled that of the normal substrates. Thus amylase, which normally hydrolyses starch, is inhibited by glucose (see Section 9.1). Again, malonic acid (9.1) competitively inactivates the enzyme succinic dehydrogenase by displacing the normal substrate, succinic acid (9.2), from the enzyme (Quastel and Wooldridge, 1927). A similar phenomenon in physiology is the toxic action of carbon monoxide (C–O), which is due to its displacing a similarly shaped molecule, oxygen (O–O), from combination with haemoglobin (Douglas, Haldane and Haldane, 1912).

Next, as has been related in Section 2.0, it was shown how the alkaloid physostigmine (2.7) contracted the pupil of the eye by blocking acetylcholinesterase, thus allowing local ACh (2.8) to stimulate the muscle (Stedman, 1926). It was soon found that the portion of the molecule which inhibited the esterase was the methylcarbamoyloxy-group (2.9) (Stedman and Stedman, 1931). In 1932, it was discovered that carbachol (2.11), which has a carbamoyloxy-group, has much of the biological effect of acetylcholine (2.8). This made it clear for the first time that the reason why physostigmine blocked acetylcholinesterase was because the group (2.9) caused that enzyme to adsorb the physostigmine instead of its normal substrate, acetylcholine.

Although this story proved a little too complex to be widely appreciated, and few were inclined to generalize from the evidence, the topic acquired a new facet when Ing (1936) published his much-quoted review. In this he pointed out that the alkaloid tubocurarine (2.6), which blocks neuromuscular transmission (see Section 2.0), must do so by competing with acetylcholine for a receptor in voluntary muscle (both substances are quaternary amines). In addition, Ing postulated that the somewhat weaker curariform action of innumerable quaternary ammonium, phosphonium, arsonium, stibonium, and sulphonium salts arose from their competition with acetylcholine (Ing, 1936). (For further reading on the physiological functions of acetylcholine and how they are antagonized by drugs, see Section 7.3, 7.6c, 13.6 and 13.7.)

Soon after this, the first antivitamin was discovered by a happy accident. Woolley *et al.* (1938) prepared two analogues of nicotinic acid, namely 3-acetylpyridine and pyridine-3-sulphonic acid. Believing that the analogues would have, at least qualitatively, the biological action of the vitamin, they fed them to dogs suffering from nicotinic acid deficiency. To their surprise, the condition was worsened. A clear picture of what was happening emerged as soon as Woods (1940) demonstrated the reversal of the antibacterial action of sulphanilamide by *p*-aminobenzoic acid, and pointed out that this reversal depends on the structural similarity of the two substances.

p-Aminobenzoic acid (anion)
(9.4)

Sulphanilamide (anion) (R = H)
(9.5)

(9.6)

Sulphanilamide (molecule) (R = H)
(9.7)

9.3 The folic acid antagonists

There are antagonists of the biosynthesis of dihydrofolic acid, and antagonists of its utilization. The history of the discovery of the antibacterial sulphonamides, typical antagonists of biosynthesis, was given in Section 6.3a. In 1940, Woods showed that the antibacterial action of sulphanilamide depended on its competition with *p*-aminobenzoic acid (*2.13*), which is a natural metabolite (Woods, 1940). Later this competition was shown to take place at the site on the enzyme dihydrofolate synthetase, which uses p-aminobenzoic acid to build up the molecule of dihydrofolic acid (2.14) (G.M. Brown, 1962).

The enzyme accepts sulphanilamide in place of its normal substrate because of their close resemblance, electronically and sterically. p-Aminobenzoic acid has an acidic pK of 4.9 and is not a zwitterion like glycine is. The anion (9.4) appears to be the biologically active form. Sulphanilamide is a weaker acid (pK 10.3), little ionized at a physiological pH. The primary amino-group in both substances is weakly basic (pK_a 2.5 and 2.6 respectively) and not ionized at a physiological pH. The dimensions of p-aminobenzoic acid (anion) (9.6) and of sulphanilamide (molecule) (9.7) are similar (see formulae). They have similar length, and width; both molecules are planar, and the amino-group must be both primary and situated $para$ to the other group for there to be any biological activity in each case. The given dimensions are little changed by ionization (Bell and Roblin, 1942).

As soon as the clinical value of sulphanilamide was established, many modifications of the molecule were attempted in the hope of finding more active analogues. It was soon found that the most valuable sulphonamides were those in which the 'R' in (9.5) was a heterocyclic ring. As Bell and Roblin showed (1942), this increased the ionization (as an acid) of the sulphonamide; and those sulphonamides that were completely ionized at pH 7 and hence resembled p-aminobenzoic acid still more closely, were found to be the most strongly antibacterial of all (see, further, Section 10.5). Although antibacterial sulphonamides which cannot ionize (as acids) can show useful antibacterial action (examples: dapsone, sulphaguanidine), it is always much weaker than that given by well-ionizing sulphonamides. Thus the minimal inhibitory concentration of sulphadiazine (2-p-aminophenylsulphonamidopyrimidine) against $E.$ $coli$ is 1.02 µmol/litre whereas sulphanilamide is more than 100 times weaker (Krüger-Thiemer and Bünger, 1965). This correlated with the enhanced ionization of sulphadiazine (pK_a 6.5) which yields 75% of anion, at equilibrium (at pH 7). In all these N-substituted sulphonamides (9.7), the 'R' is out of the plane of the rest of the molecule, and hence it cannot interfere with the adsorption on the receptor normally occupied by (9.6).

The selectivity of the antibacterial sulphonamides depends on the non-utilization of p-aminobenzoic acid by mammals, which do not make their own dihydrofolic acid, but obtain it in food. Pathogenic bacteria, on the other hand, cannot absorb preformed dihydrofolic acid (Wood, et $al.$, 1961), and hence are vulnerable to the sulphonamides which prevent them from synthesizing it.

Sulphapyridine (Ewins and Phillips, 1939), the first heterocyclic-substituent type sulphonamide, was soon superseded by sulphathiazole, which was in turn displaced by the three more selective sulphapyrimidines shown in Table 2.5; these, by 1942, were widely accepted as the most useful and innocuous of the sulphonamides for oral use in a wide variety of severe bacterial infections. In spite of the introduction of newer sulphonamides for special purposes, the sulphapyrimidines have maintained a place (alongside the antibiotics) in the forefront of the systemic antibacterials. The two most used are sulphadiazine and sulphadimidine (sulphamethazine).

Newer types of sulphonamide fall mainly into two classes: (a) those that are eliminated very slowly and so give a long, sustained action, and (b) those that are eliminated very rapidly and so produce a high concentration in the urine. Outstanding examples of class (a) are *sulphamethoxydiazine* ('Durenat'; 2-*p*-aminobenzenesulphonamido-5-methoxypyrimidine), *sulfometopyrazine* ('Kelfizine'; 2-*p*-aminobenzenesulphonamido-3-methoxypyrazine), *sulphamethoxypyridazine* ('Lederkyn', 'Kynex', 'Davosin'; 3-*p*-aminobenzenesulphonamido-6-methoxypyridazine), *sulphadimethoxine* ('Madribon'; 4-*p*-aminobenzenesulphonamido-2,6-dimethoxypyrimidine). Outstanding examples of class (b) are *sulphamethizole* ('Urolucosil'; 2-*p*-aminobenzenesulphonamido-5-methyl-1,3,4-thiadiazole) and *sulphafurazole* (*sulfisoxazole*, 'Gantrisin'; 5-*p*-aminobenzenesulphonamido-3, 4-dimethylisoxazole). Drugs for urological use must be very soluble, and so must their acetyl-derivatives.

Sulphamethoxazole ('Gantanol'; 3-*p*-aminobenzenesulphonamido-5-methylisoxazole) has been selected for use with trimethoprim for sequential blocking (Section 9.5), because both drugs have similar distribution and duration.

Sulphonamides based on pyridine, thiazole, oxazole, and isoxazole are not so long-acting (Krüger-Thiemer, 1962) as many related drugs, with two ring-nitrogen atoms, that are well bound by serum albumin and easily resorbed from the kidney. Binding by albumin is favoured by high liposolubility and/or good ionization as an anion (see Chapter 10). Resorption is favoured by high liposolubility and/or poor ionization as anion. Substituents placed *ortho* to the sulphonamido-group, in the heterocyclic ring, hinder binding to protein because of the steric effect (Seydel and Wempe, 1971).

Before a discussion of how sulphonamides interfere with folic acid metabolism, it is desirable to note that many non-sulphonamides can competitively antagonize *p*AB (*p*-aminobenzoic acid). Some of these substances contain the sulphone $(C-SO_2-C)$ instead of the sulphonamide group, but they may contain no sulphur at all, provided that a marked steric and electronic resemblance to *p*AB is present. The insertion of a methyl-group into the 2- or 3-positions of *p*AB gives intermediate types which have neither *p*AB nor anti-*p*AB activity. However, the insertion of a chlorine atom into either the 2- or 3-positions of *p*AB makes an active anti-*p*AB substance (Wyss, Rubin and Strandskov, 1943).

p-Aminobenzenearsonic acid [atoxyl (*6.1*)] is another anti-*p*AB. In general, arsenic acids are not antibacterial (cf. Albert, Falk and Rubbo,

1944), but atoxyl forms an exception because it resembles *p*AB sufficiently well to be able to compete with it (Hirsch, 1942). Another sulphur-free anti-*p*AB is diaminobenzil (*9.8*). This substance is several times more active than sulphanilamide but slightly inferior to sulphathiazole (Kuhn, *et al.*, 1943). Even the sulphur-containing anti-*p*AB substances need not have a sulphonamide-group, as dapsone (*p,p'*-diaminodiphenyl sulphone) (*9.9*) shows. It is much used in treating leprosy, when its mild, steady action is remarkably effective.

(*9.8*)   Dapsone   (*9.10*)
                 (*9.9*)

What features are required for a molecule to have an anti-*p*AB action? Firstly, it is essential that it should have a primary aromatic amino-group. This *N*-4-group must not be substituted in any way unless by a group which will readily break down in the body and liberate the primary amino-group. An azo- or anil-linkage can be depended on to break in this way (as in 'Prontosil'), but acyl- and alkyl-groups do so only to a limited extent (Northey, 1948). Secondly, an electro-negatively charged group is required, placed *para* to the amino-group, and at the same distance as in *p*-aminobenzoic acid. The necessity for keeping the distances between the amino- and the electro-negative-groups similar to that obtaining in *p*-aminobenzoic acid is illustrated by 4-amino-4'-sulphonamidodiphenyl (*9.10*), which has no anti-*p*AB effect (Kumler and Halverstadt, 1941).

Much work has been done, through infrared (Seydel, 1966) and ultra-violet (Rastelli, *et al.*, 1975) spectra, to attempt correlation of charge localization with antibacterial action.

Two derivatives of sulphathiazole, acylated on *N*-4, have proved of great value in treating bacterial dysentery. These are the pro-drugs succinyl-sulphathiazole ('Sulfasuxidine') and phthalysulphathiazole ('Sulfathalidine', 'Thalazole'). The acyl-group is split off in the colon, from which very little sulphathiazole can be absorbed.

Mafenide (*p*-aminomethylbenzenesulphonamide) (*9.11*) ('Marfanil', 'Sulfamylon'), which has only a 'paper-resemblance' to sulphanilamide, is a highly basic substance with special activity against the *Clostridia* which cause gas-gangrene (Evans, *et al.*, 1944). It is not antagonized by *p*-aminobenzoic acid (Jensen and Schmith, 1942) and appears to play no part in folic acid metabolism.

Many useful drugs contain the sulphonamido-group but are not anti-bacterial because they have not been designed as analogues of *p*AB. Some are diuretics (Section 9.4), and others antidiabetics (Section 13.4).

(a) *How sulphonamide drugs act by antagonizing synthesis of dihydrofolic acid*

The discovery of the folic acids led to a complete understanding of how sulphonamides antagonized *p*-aminobenzoic acid. This discovery took place as follows. A bright yellow substance, that had an anti-anaemic effect in vertebrates, had been isolated some time earlier from liver, yeast, green leaves, and bacteria. Degradation, followed by synthesis, established the constitution as in formula (*2.14*) minus the two hydrogen atoms in the 7- and 8-positions (which had been lost in the handling). This substance was named folic acid (pteroyl-glutamic acid) (Waller *et al.*, 1948). The molecule of dihydrofolic acid (*2.14*) consists of three main regions: these are the glutamic acid, the *p*-aminobenzoic acid, and the 2-amino-4-oxo-6-methylpteridine regions.

Bacteria use *p*-aminobenzoic acid only for conversion to 7,8-dihydrofolic acid (Woods, 1962; Griffin and Brown, 1964). Thus, *E. coli* condenses *p*-aminobenzoic acid (and, alternatively, *p*-aminobenzoylglutamic acid) with 2-amino-4-oxo-6-hydroxymethyl-7,8-dihydropteridine (*9.12*) (as the 6-pyrophosphate) to give dihydropteroic acid (and alternatively, dihydro-folic acid) (Jaenicke and Chan, 1960). The sulphonamides competitively inhibit the isolated enzyme *dihydrofolate synthetase* which catalyses these steps (G. Brown, 1962). From *Lactobacillus plantarum* two enzymes res-ponsible for this synthesis have been isolated in a pure state (Shiota, Baugh, Jackson and Dillard, 1969). The first of these catalyses the esterification of 2-amino-4-oxo-6-hydroxymethyl-7,8-dihydropteridine (*9.12*) to its pyrophosphoryl derivative. The second is Brown's dihydrofolate syn-thetase. This second enzyme has also been isolated from several strains of

Mafenide
(*9.11*)

Pteridine intermediate in
folic acid biosynthesis
(*9.12*)

Pneumococcus, found to have a mol. wt. of 90000, and to need ATP and Mg^{2+} as coenzymes (Ortiz, 1970).

The effects of pteroic and folic acids (also their 7,8-dihydro-derivatives) cannot be antagonized by sulphonamides. This is most clearly demonstrated in the very few strains of bacteria which are capable of absorbing folic acid (e.g. *Streptococcus faecalis*, and some *Lactobacilli*). (These bacteria are non-pathogenic to man.) Table 9.2 demonstrates the exact proportionality between the amount of sulphadiazine required to inhibit Ralston's strain of *Streptococcus faecalis* and the amount of pAB required to reverse this inhibition. In contrast, the amount of folic acid required for reversal is constant, regardless of the amount of sulphadiazine used. This indicates that the sulphadiazine interferes with the synthesis of folic acid from p-aminobenzoic acid, but does not interfere with the utilization of folic acid as, for instance, methotrexate does. Similarly, *L. arabinosus* (which requires an external source of pAB) is inhibited by sulphonamides, and this inhibition is reversed competitively by pAB and non-competitively by folic acid. The amount of folic acid (measured by disintegrating the bacteria, and titrating the homogenized culture against *L. casei* which responds to folic acid but not to pAB) produced by this organism is ordinarily proportional to the amount of pAB in the medium. However, if sulphanilamide is also present, it is decreased in proportion to the amount used, over a 10 000-fold range of sulphanilamide concentrations (Nimmo-Smith, Lascelles and Woods, 1948). The production of folic acid is similarly inhibited in *E. coli* by sulphanilamide (Miller, 1944).

Table 9.2

COMPETITIVE AND NON-COMPETITIVE INHIBITION

Substance	Amount needed for 50% antagonism of effect of Sulphadiazine on Ralston's Strept. faecalis			
SULPHADIAZINE →	I	10	100	1000
p-Aminobenzoic acid	0.003	0.03	0.3	3.0
Petroylglutamic acid (folic acid)	0.0003	0.0003	—	0.0003
Thymine (4.1,b)	0.06	0.25	0.25	0.25

All values are μg per ml. (Lampen and Jones, 1946.)

The above explanation of the action of sulphonamides, namely enzyme-inhibition, seems to account for most of the therapeutic action of these drugs. However, in some experiments the sulphonamide was made to unite with the pteridine intermediate (*9.12*). Thus, Brown's enzyme, in a cell-free system containing the sulphonamide, was incubated for 2 hours; the resulting inhibition was irreversible by pAB, an effect which does not occur in growing cells (G. M. Brown, 1962). In pursuit of this effect, folate-synthesizing enzymes from *E. coli* were made to convert sulphamethoxazole (*9.13*) to the pteroic acid analogue: N'-3-(5-methylisoxazolyl)-N^4-(7,8-dihydro-6-pterinylmethyl)sulphanilamide, which was isolated by chromatography and found identical with a synthetic specimen (Bock *et al.*, 1974).

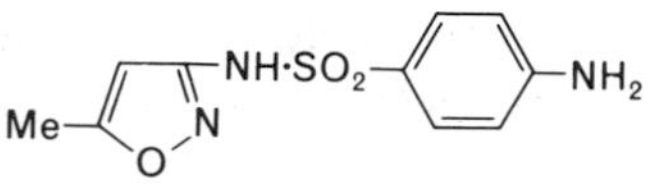

Sulphamethoxazole
(*9.13*)

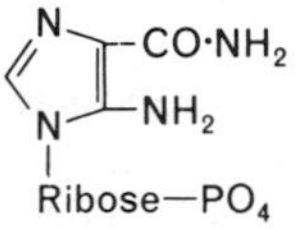

Aminoimidazole
carboxamide ribotide
(*9.14*)

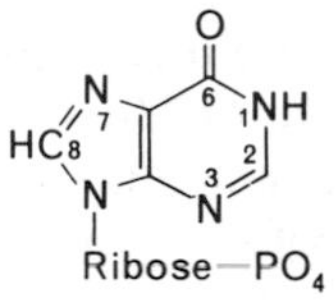

Inosinic acid
(*9.15*)

Of all the reactions catalysed by folic acids, the synthesis of thymine is, in many cases, the most sensitive to a shortage of these acids (see Section 9.3b), although, in some micro-organisms, purine synthesis is inhibited first. It will be observed in Table 9.2 that thymine can antagonize the action of sulphadiazine on the streptococcus and that it does this almost non-competitively. It is not surprising that so large an amount is needed, because thymine is not a catalyst (like pAB and folic acid) but a cell constituent, the demand for which increases as the cell continues to grow.

The action of anti-pAB drugs on most of the *pathogenic* bacteria and protozoa is not reversed by folic acid and its derivatives, because these do not penetrate into the organisms.

(b) *The role of folic acid derivatives in Nature*
As indicated above, derivatives of folic acid play a key role in the biosynthesis of purines and pyrimidines. These pteridines are the coenzymes responsible for inserting the carbon atoms into both positions 2 and 8 of purines, and they also insert the methyl-group into thymine (*4.1*). When bacteria are treated with low concentrations of sulphonamides, 4-aminoimidazole-5-carboxamide ribotide (*9.14*) accumulates in the culture media. This substance is an intermediate in the biosynthesis of inosinic acid (*9.15*) from which all purines are derived (Buchanan, 1957).

The coenzymes are formed from dihydrofolic acid by the enzyme dihydrofolate hydrogenase which gives tetrahydrofolic acid (Osborn, Freeman and Huennekens, 1958), and this is then modified by various one-carbon substituents. The coenzyme for the insertion of C-2 into purines, i.e. for the formylation of the ribotide (9.14) to give (9.15), is $N_{(10)}$-formyl-5,6,7,8-tetrahydrofolic acid. For the earlier stage of the insertion of C-8, i.e. for the formylation of glycinamide ribotide to form (eventually) (9.14), the coenzyme is $N_{(5)}, N_{(10)}$-methenyl-tetrahydrofolic acid (9.16). The coenzyme for inserting the methyl-group into uridylic acid to give thymi-dylic acid is $N_{(5)}, N_{(10)}$-methylene-tetrahydrofolic acid (9.17), the same coenzyme is responsible for the interconversion of two aminoacids, namely serine and glycine. The uridylate $\rightarrow$ thymidylate methylation is effected by thymidylate synthetase (mol. wt. 67 000). The synthesis of methionine and the catabolism of histidine are also effected by pteridine coenzymes, each with its specific apoenzyme. Folic acids with polypeptides formed from the glutamyl portion are found in cells and seem to have coenzymic functions. Humans obtain most of their folic acid from vegetables, as polyglutamyl-folic acid. Liver and yeast are also good sources. Fig. 9.2 shows the biosynthesis and functions of the folic coenzymes.

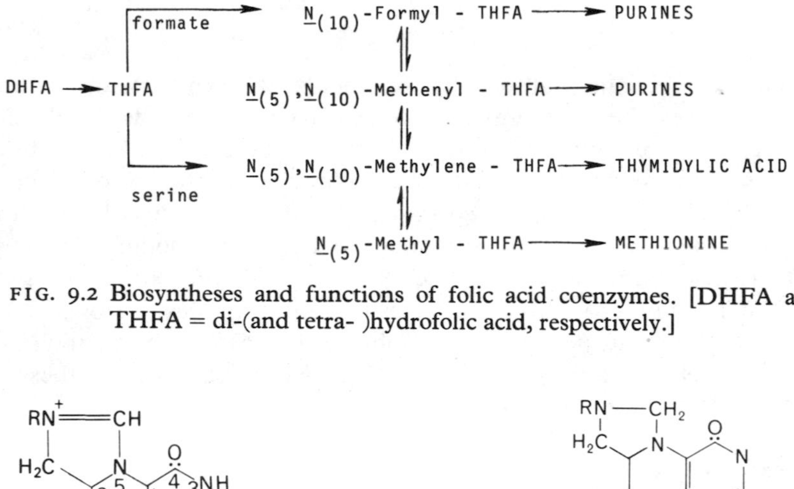

FIG. 9.2 Biosyntheses and functions of folic acid coenzymes. [DHFA and THFA = di-(and tetra-)hydrofolic acid, respectively.]

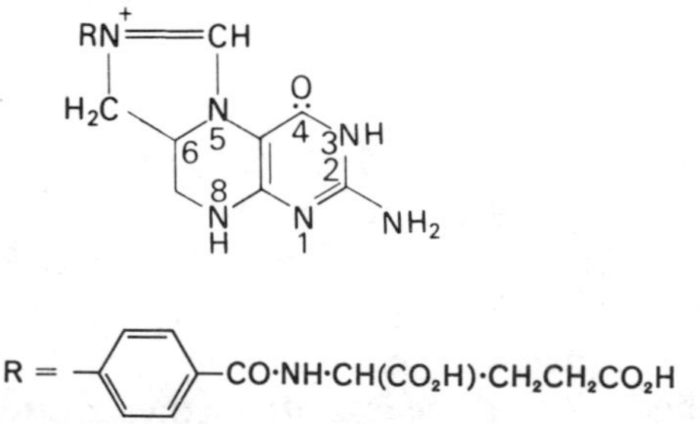

Methenyl-tetrahydrofolic acid
(9.16)

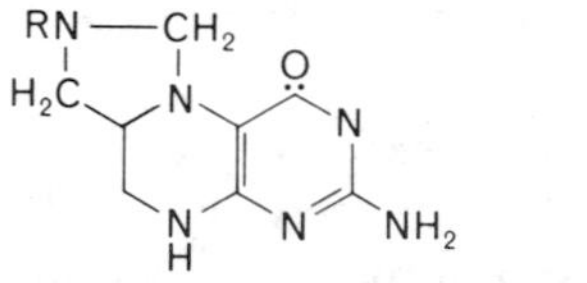

Methylene-tetrahydrofolic acid
R as in (9.16)
(9.17)

The biologically active pteridines are formed in nature by the degradation of the purine, guanine (9.18) (in the form of GTP), to give 2-amino-5-form-amido-4-oxo-6-[(5-O-triphosphato-D-ribosyl-)amino]pyrimidine (Shiota, Baugh and Myrick, 1969). This pyrimidine (9.19) is cyclized by the enzyme dihydro-neopterin triphosphate synthetase (obtainable from *Lactobacillus plantarum*), which forms a new bond between the exocyclic nitrogen atom and C-2′ of the ribose moiety. From the dihydroneopterin,* formed in this way, an enzyme called hydroneopterin aldolase (obtainable from *E. coli*) liberates glycollic aldehyde and leaves 2-amino-4-oxo-6-hydroxymethyl-7,8-dihydropteridine, which is readily built into the molecule of folic acid, as explained in Section 9.3a.

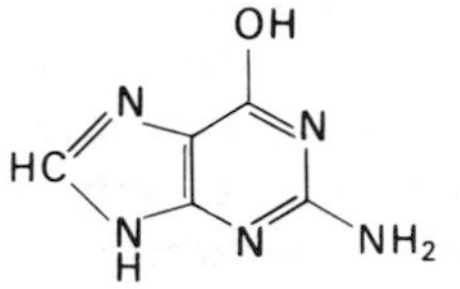

Guanine
(9.18)

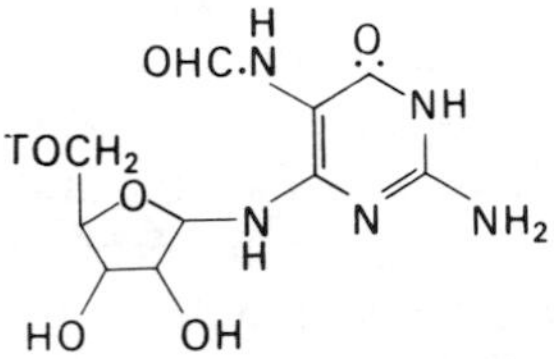

(T = triphosphate-group)
(9.19)

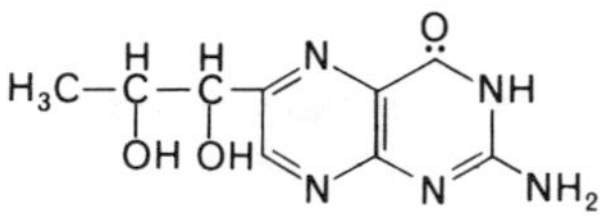

Biopterin
(9.20)

The participation of pteridines in metabolism is by no means restricted to the folic acid derivatives, nor is an amino-group in the 2-position essential for biological activity. The biosynthesis of the vitamin riboflavine takes place via the pteridine 6,7-dimethyl-8-ribityl-2,4-dioxopteridine. In this reaction, one molecule of this pteridine gives and another molecule accepts the four carbon atoms required to form the *o*-xylene ring of riboflavine (Plaut, 1964). The precursor of this pteridine is, once again, GTP of which the ribose-group becomes the ribityl-group of riboflavine.

Biopterin (9.20), an ivory-coloured pteridine, biosynthesized by animals and widely distributed in Nature, is L-erythro-2-amino-4-oxo-6-(1,2-dihydroxypropyl-)pteridine. Once again, GTP is the precursor. A reduced form, 5,6,7,8-tetrahydrobiopterin is the co-factor required for the set of enzymes that use molecular oxygen to oxidize phenylalanine to tyrosine (Kaufman, 1964), tryptophan to 5-hydroxytryptophan, and possibly in in the formation of melanin. This co-factor utilizes oxygen directly from the air.

A pteridine is considered to be the primary receptor of the electrons liberated by light in *photosynthesis* (Fuller *et al.*, 1971); and a pteridine in

*2-amino-4-oxo-6-(D-erythro-1′, 2′, 3′-trihydroxypropyl)-7,8-dihydropteridine.

the *mammalian eye* is presumed to be the agent which protects against the blinding effect of light (Cremer-Bartels, 1975). Cancerous cells break down folic acid to pterin-6-aldehyde which, excreted in the urine, has apparently some diagnostic significance (Halpern *et al.*, 1977).

The biological importance of pteridines has led to a series of international symposia on pteridine chemistry and biology, the sixth of which was held in La Jolla (U.S.A., 1978); for proceedings, see Kisliuk and Brown (1979). The chemistry of pteridines is in many ways unusual, principally because of the strong electron-attracting properties of the four doubly-bound nitrogen atoms, which antagonize the aromaticity implied by the conventional structural formula. The tendency of the pteridine ring to add a molecule of water covalently across a double-bond, even at room temperature (as exemplified by xanthopterin) is further discussed in Section 2.3a, and reviewed by Albert (1967; 1976). Stronger nucleophilic substances, such as acetone, keto-acids, and mercaptans, are added even more readily. Another peculiarity of pteridines and some other nitrogenous heterocycles is the effect of hydrogen-bonding groups (e.g. $-NH_2$) in reducing the solubility in water (Albert, Brown, and Cheeseman, 1952b). Strong chelating properties have been demonstrated and measured in naturally occurring pteridines (Albert, 1953).

For further reading on the biochemistry of folic acid and related pteridines, see Blakley (1969).

(c) *Drugs that act by blocking dihydrofolate hydrogenase*
Folic acid is an indispensable pro-vitamin for man and other mammals, and lack of it quickly causes macrocytic anaemia and gastro-intestinal disorders. Hence it was with some trepidation that chemists began to make metabolite antagonists based on the pteridine nucleus. Nevertheless, several very valuable drugs have been obtained in this way.

Because pteridines play such an important part in catalysing the synthesis of purines and pyrimidines, various analogues of folic acid have been tested as tumour-inhibiting agents. High activity was shown by aminopterin, i.e. folic acid in which the 4-oxo-group was replaced by an amino-group, Clinical trials, from 1958 onwards, showed that methotrexate (*4.6*) was more selective and this has become an important anti-cancer drug. This substance, discovered by Seeger *et al.*, (1949), differs from folic acid in two details, the replacement of the 4-oxo-group by an amino-group, group, and the replacement of the 10-hydrogen atom by a methyl-group.* Methotrexate is in regular use for treating the acute lymphatic leukaemia in the young (Farber, 1952; Zuelzer, 1964). It brings about a remarkable remission of symptoms, but the leukaemic cells can develop resistance to the drug. This is countered by an effective multiple drug

---
* For the molecular basis of folic-methotrexate antagonism, see end of Section 9.1.

approach (Brulé *et al.*, 1973; Skipper, Schabel, and Wilcox, 1964). A very short course of vincrystine (Section 5.3) and a corticosteroid such as prednisolone is given, followed by prolonged treatment with methotrexate and 6-mercaptopurine (*3.12*) (Section 4.0, p. 113). The happy result is a high percentage of apparent cures in what had been, until a few years ago, a rapidly lethal disease.

In two other types of cancer, methotrexate brings about a lasting cure. Choriocarcinoma, a fast-growing tumour of pregnancy with normally a high death-rate, is quickly and completely cured by methotrexate (Ross, *et al.*, 1965). Before this discovery, 5 out of every 6 women struck by this type of cancer had died within one year. A highly malignant lymphoma, discovered by Burkitt in African children living in hot, wet areas, usually begins in the jaw, rapidly spreads throughout the body, and kills the patient within six months. Methotrexate has a dramatic effect in Burkitt's lymphoma and often effects a complete cure (Burkitt, Hutt and Wright, 1965; Bertino and Johns, 1967). Cautious as clinicians are about the use of the word 'cure' in cancer, it is agreed that these are true cures.

Multiple therapy, based on methotrexate, is being tried in other forms of cancer. In breast cancer, although 24% of recurrence is usual after surgery, it seems that a combination of methotrexate, fluorouracil, and cyclophosphamide reduces this to 5%, if treatment is begun 2 weeks after surgery (Bonadonna *et al.*, 1976).

Methotrexate is a drug of only moderate selectivity. Prolonged medication with high doses has an adverse effect on the red blood cells, leading to macrocytic anaemia; later the production of white cells often diminishes. In spite of this, the therapeutic range and the effectiveness of methotrexate have been greatly improved by what is called a 'rescue programme'. In this therapy, the citrovorum factor, 5-formyltetrahydrofolic acid [see (*2.14*) for numbering], is given at weekly intervals while the methotrexate treatment is suspended. For example, the osteogenic sarcoma of young people can be controlled by one thousand times the largest normally safe dose of methotrexate if citrovorum factor rescue periods are introduced. The administration of thymidine along with the methotrexate and citrovorum factor, can protect the host from thymine depletion and allow the therapy to rest on purine depletion, which seems to have a greater selective advantage (Frenkel and Hitchings, 1957; Tattersall, Jaffe, and Frei, 1975).

Methotrexate has also been used successfully in the treatment of psoriasis, a common and rather intractable skin complaint. By repressing biosynthesis of thymine, it decreases the amount of DNA available for the excessive mitotic activity in the epidermal cells. In psoriasis, because of excessive production of dihydrofolate hydrogenase, these cells are shed every 3–4 days, compared to the normal rate of 27 days. This drug must be given systemically and, because of side-effects, is restricted to short-term treatment.

Methotrexate inhibits specimens of dihydrofolate hydrogenase isolated from both mammalian and bacterial cells, although it cannot normally penetrate into the latter (Nichol and Welch, 1950; Werkheiser, 1963). The action of methotrexate is highly specific: 50 per cent inhibition is effected by a 10^{-9} M concentration of the agent which has hardly any effect on any other enzyme. This inhibitor is bound to the enzyme about 10^4 more tightly than the substrate, a most unusual effect (see Section 9.1), and hence is one of the least reversible of reversible inhibitors. The differences between its action on dihydrofolate inhibitors from different species is not large (contrast with the diaminopyrimidines, below) (Werkheiser, 1963).

Aminopterin and methotrexate have little toxicity for most bacteria or protozoa (Wood et al., 1961). To obtain better penetration, the molecule was modified in two ways: either (a) a lipophilic group such as phenyl was introduced, or (b) a good deal of the molecule was cut away, leaving a diaminopyrimidine. Results of both methods (the latter the more successful) will now be given.

2,4-Diamino-6,7-diphenylpteridine is as active as quinine in suppressing malaria due to *Plasmodium gallinaceum* in the chick (Greenberg, 1949), and 2,4,7-triamino-6-phenylpteridine (triamterene) suppresses parasitemia in mice and rats infected with *Pl. berghei* (Aviado, Brugler and Bellet, 1968). 2,4-Diamino-6,7-diethylpteridine is highly effective in laboratory tests against *Vibrio cholerae* (Collier and Waterhouse, 1950), but does not affect many other bacterial species. None of these results led to useful new drugs.

A more successful approach was the simplification of the methotrexate molecule, as initiated by G.H. Hitchings, who found that the omission of the nitrogen atom from position 5 gave better penetrating analogues. These 'simplified amethopterins' were 2,4-diamino-1,3,8-triazanaphthalenes, of which (*9.21*) (2,4-diamino-5-methyl-6-*n*-butyl-1,3,8-triazanaphthalene) is one of the most active (Robins and Hitchings, 1955). The action, on both Gram-positive and -negative bacteria, is assisted by the lipophilic groups in the 5- and 6-positions. When dihydrofolic hydrogenase was isolated from various bacterial species, the inhibitory effect of these triazanaphthalenes was found to be proportional to the effect on intact bacteria (Burchall and Hitchings, 1965; Hitchings and Burchall, 1965). Interesting as these results were, better was to follow.

The diaminobutyltriaza-naphthalene
(*9.21*)

As recounted in Section 4.0 (p. 109) Hitchings, continuing the simplification of the methotrexate molecule, found that quite simple 2,4-diamino-
pyrimidines have a powerful anti-folic acid effect on micro-organisms,
and used this knowledge to develop pyrimethamine (4.7) ('Daraprim')
(Falco et al., 1951). This substance, 2,4-diamino-6-ethyl-5-p-chloro-
phenylpyrimidine, is one of the most powerful antimalarials known, and
has become the most widely used of all prophylactics against malaria.
Its action on specimens of dihydrofolate hydrogenase, isolated from a
variety of living species, and abstracted in Table 4.2, showed great selectivity against the enzyme from the malarial parasite.

As Table 4.2 shows, the plasmodial enzyme is inhibited by pyrimethamine at a concentration about 2000 times lower than that inhibiting the
analogous mammalian enzymes. These data established that the selective
action of pyrimethamine in malaria is due to the extraordinary sensitivity
of the enzyme in the parasite compared to that in the host. The plasmodial
enzyme has demonstrable individuality for, when isolated from Pl. berghei,
it has a mol. wt. of about 200 000, which is 10 times as large as the analogous
mammalian and bacterial enzymes. (The malarial parasite, like bacteria,
cannot absorb preformed folic acid or its derivatives.)

For the highest antimalarial activity in vertebrates, the 2,4-diamino-
pyrimidines require a strongly lipophilic substitution, such as a phenyl-
group in the 5-position and an alkyl-group in the 6-position. But in coccidiosis, a related protozoal disease of poultry, 5-benzyl-derivatives proved
more effective, particularly diaveridine (9.22). Relative crowding of the
5- by the 6-substituent must be avoided in both classes of substance. The
inhibition of isolated dihydrofolate hydrogenase is not greatly altered
when the 5-phenyl-group in pyrimethamine is changed to a n-butyl-, or
even a 4-phenylbutyl-group, but shortening of the butyl-group leads to
progressive loss of affinity for this enzyme (Baker and Shapiro, 1966).

Diaveridine
(9.22)

For the highest *antibacterial* activity in vertebrates, the 2,4-diamino-
pyrimidines require that the massive lipophilic substituent be modified
with a slightly hydrophilic outer area. The best of these compounds proved
to be trimethoprim (4.8) (Roth, Falco, and Hitchings, 1962). It can be seen
from Table 4.2 that pyrimethamine is most selective against the malarial
parasite enzyme, whereas trimethoprim is selective against a bacterial

enzyme as well. Compared with the high selectivity shown by these diamino-pyrimidines, the pteridine (methotrexate) is only poorly selective.

The special uses of trimethoprim as an antibacterial in medical practice are described in Section 9.5 ('Sequential blocking'). Table 4.3 exemplifies the high selectivity that trimethoprim exerts in discriminating against the dihydrofolate hydrogenase of bacteria (both Gram-positive and -negative) while leaving the analogous mammalian enzyme unharmed. It is note-worthy that these useful 2,4-diaminopyrimidine drugs have been discovered mainly by the exercise of scientific reasoning. For biological activity, the basic pK_a value must be at least 6 (maximal activity lies between 7 and 8). This requirement indicates that a cell membrane has to be travers-ed, as discussed in Section 10.5 (Roth and Strelitz, 1969).

The possibility of abortion or damage to the foetus makes it necessary to use antifolic drugs with some caution during pregnancy.

For the much-used pteridine diuretic triamterene, 2,4,7-triamino-6-phenylpteridine, see Section 14.1. For further reading on the biochemistry of anti-folic agents, see Blakley (1969).

9.4 Other metabolite analogues of proven value in prophylaxis and therapy

Introduction. It is not difficult to make metabolite analogues; it has proved very hard to discover ones which are selective, because it is rare to find a metabolite that is important in the uneconomic species and yet unimportant in the economic species. When a metabolite occurs in all living cells, as thiamine does, it must seem unlikely that any selective action of analogues could be achieved. Nevertheless, in favourable cases this selectivity has been demonstrated, and has led to useful and widely employ-ed agents. Success often depends on the analogue being taken up unequally by the two species. Relatively small changes in a molecule can so alter cellular uptake as to make an agent either (a) inaccessible to the economic species, or (b) preferentially absorbed by the uneconomic species, or at least concentrated in the region where the uneconomic species is segregated.

Curiously enough, a metabolite analogue may be treated as a metabolite by one species and as an antagonist by a related species. For example, dethiobiotin is able to replace biotin (*9.23*) as a growth-factor for yeast, yet it antagonizes the growth-promoting effect of biotin on *Lactobacillus casei*. It is known why this should be so: the yeast inserts the missing sulphur atom, but the bacterium is unable to do this (Dittmer and du Vigneaud, 1944). Likewise, the fungus *Endomyces*, when made resistant to pyrithia-mine (*9.24*) by repeated sub-culture in its presence, was found to owe this resistance to its ability to break down the pyrithiamine and synthesize thiamine (*2.1*) from one of the large fragments.

A natural metabolite may function in several enzymes, each of which may be optimally blocked by a different inhibitor. For example, vitamin K (2.2) in the human blood-stream can be antagonized by dicoumarol (9.25), but not by 2,3-dichloronaphthoquinone (9.26), which antagonizes this vitamin in fungi whereas dicoumarol does not.

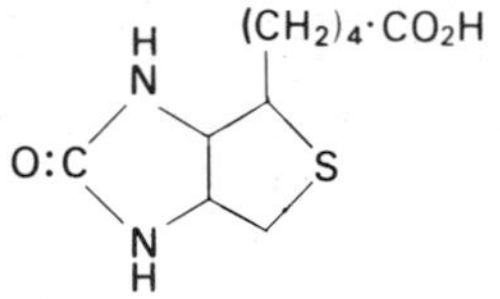

Biotin
(9.23)

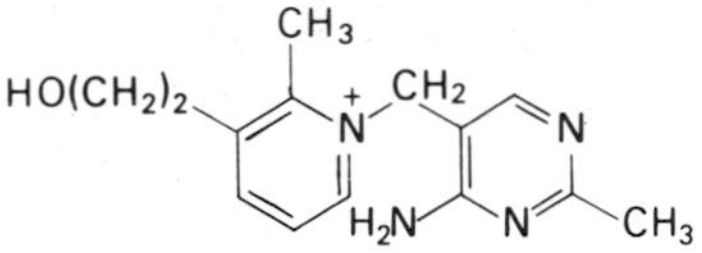

Pyrithiamine (cation)
(9.24)

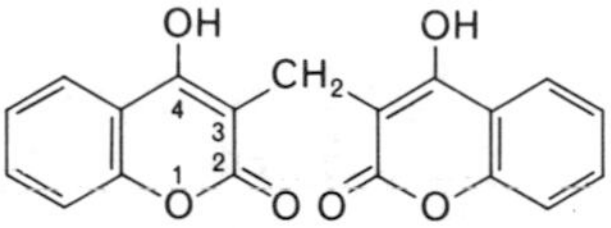

Dicoumarol
(9.25)

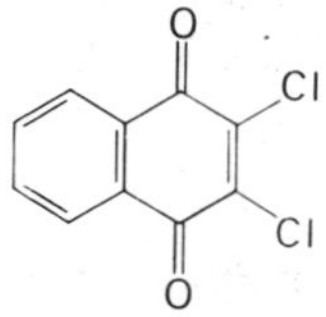

Dichlone
(9.26)

Analogues that antagonize a metabolite in species which require an external source are often less effective in those bacterial species which produce it internally. This is the case with pyrithiamine (9.24). An obvious explanation is that the antimetabolite can be outcompeted by the excess of metabolite in the cell: but in some cases the antimetabolite exerts its antagonism on the uptake of the metabolite through the cell membrane. Alternatively, the cell which makes its own metabolite may lack a mechanism by which an indiffusible analogue could gain entry to the cell. Some other analogues, such as sulphonamides, benzimidazole, 2,3-dichloro-napthoquinone, and phenyl-pantothenone, act against organisms regardless whether or not they require an exogenous source of metabolite.

Examples of success. Metabolite analogues widely used as selectively toxic agents will now be discussed. Analogues of vitamins will first be mentioned. Amprolium (9.27) ('Amprol'), an analogue of thiamine (2.1), has proved highly successful in coccidiosis, a protozoal infection of poultry. Amprolium is thought to antagonize the enzyme thiamine phosphorylase in the protozoal cytoplasmic membrane (Rogers *et al.*, 1960).

Sodium 2,2-dichloropropionate (dalapon, 'Dowpon') is much used for killing grass in dicotyledonous crops such as beet and lucerne. Competitive studies in bacteria (*E. coli*) point to its being an antagonist for the incorporation of pantoic acid [i.e. the left-hand side of (9.28)] into pantothenic acid. This is one of the main sites of its action on grasses and its effect is diminished by external pantothenic acid (Hilton *et al.*, 1959).

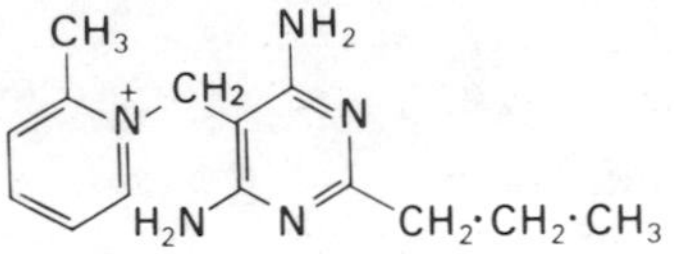

Amprolium (cation)
(9.27)

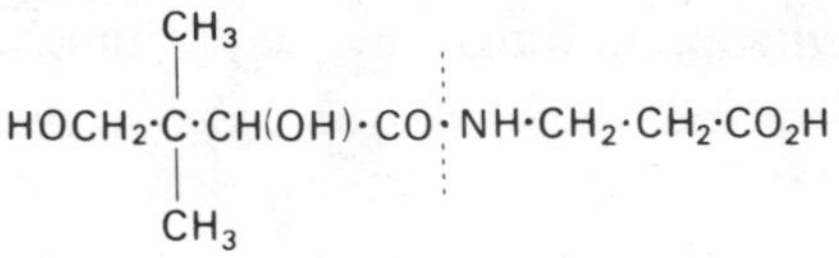

$$HOCH_2{\cdot}C{\cdot}CH(OH){\cdot}CO{\cdot}NH{\cdot}CH_2{\cdot}CH_2{\cdot}CO_2H$$

Pantothenic acid
(9.28)

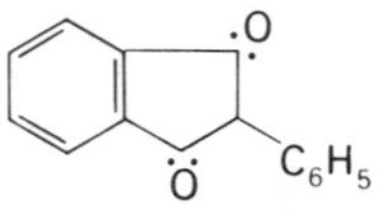

Phenindione
(9.29)

The first of the oral anticoagulant drugs, dicoumarol (*9.25*), had its first clinical trials in 1941. This substance [3,3'-methylene-*bis*(4-hydroxy-coumarin)] had been synthesized 40 years earlier but was not known to have any biological action. However, in 1941, it had just been isolated from a spoilt batch of hay and identified as the factor causing bleeding in cattle eating the hay (Campbell and Link, 1941). Dicoumarol is still very much used as an anticoagulant in the long-term prophylactic treatment of hypertensive patients at risk from coronary thrombosis and stroke. The minimal requirements for anticoagulant activity in coumarins are a 4-hydroxycoumarin nucleus with either hydrogen or carbon in the 3-position. Dicoumarol, and its more powerful analogue warfarin (*6.53*), exert their action by antagonising regeneration of vitamin K (*2.2*) which catalyses synthesis of the clotting proteins, namely the prothrombin-complex factors II, VII, IX, and X. The role of vitamin K is to introduce an extra carboxylic acid group, to assist in the chelation of calcium (Stenflo *et al.*, 1964).

Coumarin anticoagulants are inactive *in vitro* and take 36 hours to develop their action in the body. Although the antagonism that exists between them and vitamin K is very clear (an excess of either neutralizes a dose of the other), it, too, requires the lapse of many hours. These anticoagulants also inhibit release of vitamin K from its storage form, the 2,3-epoxide (Bell and Matschiner, 1972). The indandione anticoagulants, of which the most used member is phenindione (*9.29*), act a little more quickly and were devised in an attempt to find a molecule that resembled the structure of vitamin K more closely (presence of lipophilic group in 3-position; replacement of phenolic by ketonic group).

The antibacterial drug cycloserine (*5.4*) is a structural analogue of D-alanine (*5.5*); the biochemistry of its action has been summarized in

Section 5.1, p. 161. Staphylococci, exposed to cycloserine, accumulate a nucleotide consisting of uridine phosphate linked through acetylmuramic acid to the tripeptide: L-alanyl-D-glutamyl-L-lysine. As soon as D-analyl-D-alanine is supplied to the culture medium, the pentapeptide is completed and becomes available for building new cell wall. Thus cycloserine interferes with the synthesis (but not with the incorporation) of D-alanyl-D-alanine (Strominger, Threnn, and Scott, 1959; Strominger, Ito, and Threnn, 1960). Beyond any doubt, the mode of action of cycloserine is better understood than that of any other antibiotic.

In an extension of this work, it was found that 3-fluoro-D-alanine is highly effective *in vivo* against all the commoner Gram-positive and -negative infections, and is antagonised by D-alanine (see further Section 5.1).

The antibiotic azaserine (*O*-diazoacetyl-L-serine), which is used as a sequential blocking agent in the chemotherapy of cancer, is a structural analogue of glutamine and hence interferes with the biosynthesis of the purine nucleus at one of the earliest stages: amidine formation (Buchanan, 1957).

The well-known herbicide, amitrole (*4.46*) (3-amino-1,2,4-triazole), whose eventual action is to lower the production of chlorophyll, seems to be a metabolite antagonist of natural imidazoles. It causes imidazoleglycerophosphate to accumulate in yeast (Weyter and Broquist, 1960; also histidine (*11.2*) reverses its inhibition of the growth of yeast and of the alga *Prototheca* (Casselton, 1964).

The uses of analogues of natural purines and pyrimidines in cancer and virus diseases is described in Sections 4.0 and 12.5.

Allopurinol (*9.30*) is a metabolite analogue of hypoxanthine (*9.31*). Unlike purines described in Section 4.0, it is not built into a nucleotide, indeed, its action does not involve the formation of any covalent bonds. Allopurinol, 4-oxopyrazolo[3,4-*d*]pyrimidine, is one of the most effective known drugs for reducing the uric acid load of patients with gout or diseases where uric acid is excreted excessively. This drug, which is given orally, is free from side-effects. It acts by blocking the oxidation of hypoxanthine (to xanthine) by the enzyme xanthine oxidase. A small portion of the given dose is oxidized to the corresponding 2,4-dioxopyrazolopyrimidine (alloxanthine), which blocks the oxidation of xanthine to uric acid by the same enzyme Elion *et al.*, 1966).

Allopurinol
(*9.30*)

Hypoxanthine
(*9.31*)

Analogues of the neurotransmitters will now be discussed. Analogues that mimic acetylcholine, either as agonists or antagonists, have been summarized in Section 7.6. Examples of much used *agonistic* metabolite analogues of acetylcholine (*2.8*) are carbachol (*2.11*), methacholine (*13.46*), physostigmine (*2.7*), neostigmine (*2.10*), together with other carbamate inhibitors of acetylcholinesterase (Section 12.3). These agonists are used in myasthenia, glaucoma, and atony of the bladder and bowel. Examples of *antagonistic* metabolite analogues of acetylcholine include the muscle relaxants used in general anaesthesia such as tubocurarine (*2.6*), gallamine (*7.23*), and suxamethonium (*7.21*); and also those partly based on atropine, such as oxyphenonium (*7.15*).

See Section 13.6 for further discussion of the agonists, and Sections 12.3 and 13.5 for the cholinesterase inhibitors. The characteristics which enable an agonist molecule to be modified to give an antagonist molecule have been discussed with special reference to acetylcholine in Section 7.5b.

Adrenergic drugs that were conceived as analogues of adrenaline or noradrenaline are playing a very important part in the treatment of disease. The following examples illustrate the wide range of their usefulness. Metaraminol (*7.44*), by preventing uptake of noradrenaline by the presynaptic terminal, is used to raise lowered blood-pressure and combat the state of shock. Ephedrine (*7.40*), by accumulating in the presynaptic terminal, and steadily pushing stores of noradrenaline out into the synaptic gap, gives valuable relief in hay fever and other allergic states. Some central stimulation can be a troublesome side-effect. Amphetamine (*7.42*) ('Benzedrine') has both actions of ephedrine but the central stimulation is much the stronger. It is used to curb appetite for food and also to promote wakefulness but its addictive properties make for caution in prescribing.

The foregoing three drugs act by giving the patient an overdose of his own noradrenaline, but the following have more individual properties. Guanethidine (*7.45*) accumulates in the presynaptic terminals and steadily pushes out noradrenaline stored there, but at such an abnormally slow rate that it is destroyed as fast as it is liberated. This drug provides an alternative, if insufficiently selective, method for lowering moderate degrees of high blood-pressure. Bretylium (*13.4*) and bethanidine work somewhat similarly and enjoy similar medical use.

Phenylephrine (*7.46*) is not a false transmitter for it is not taken up by the presynaptic terminal; yet it has a powerful noradrenaline-like effect on the receptor. It is sprayed on inflamed and bleeding surfaces as a decongestant and styptic. Salbutamol (*13.42*) has a remarkable selective adrenergic agonist effect in asthma (Section 13.4). Propranolol (*13.41*) is used as an antagonist of noradrenaline, competing with it for a place on the postsynaptic receptor, and effecting reduction in high blood pressure.

Methyldopa (*9.32*) (alpha methyldopa, 'Aldomet') is one of the most used of all drugs for lowering very high blood-pressure. Chemically it is

2-methyl-3′,4′ dihydroxyphenylanine, and is used orally (Gillespie *et al.*, 1962). In the body (presumably in the central nervous system), it is de-carboxylated and hydroxylated (very much as in Fig. 9.1) to α-methyl-noradrenaline (*9.33*) which is the true drug (Iversen, 1967). After many wild guesses as to the mode of action of this methylnoradrenaline, it was found to be an agonist in the brain where it acts on (unspecified) noradrena-line receptors that lower blood-pressure when stimulated (Day, Roach, and Whiting, 1973; Finch and Haeusler, 1973). Another powerful lowerer of heightened blood-pressure, clonidine (*9.34*) ('Catapres') seems to act similarly on central adrenergic receptors (Schmitt, Schmitt, and Fenard, 1973); it is active orally in doses of 0.1 mg. Chemically, it is 2-(2,6-dichloro-anilino)-2-imidazoline; the tautomer shown in (*9.34*) is the one favoured in the crystal as revealed by X-ray diffraction.

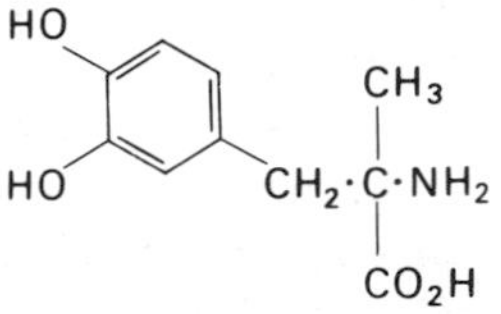

Methyl-dopa
(*9.32*)

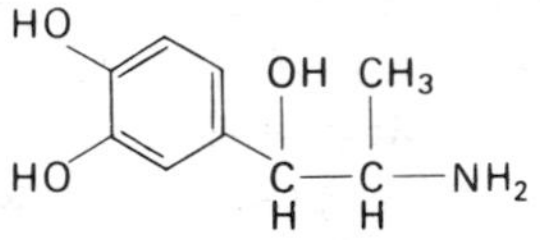

α-Methylnoradrenaline
(*9.33*)

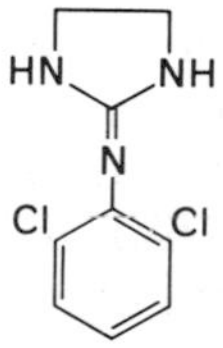

Clonidine
(*9.34*)

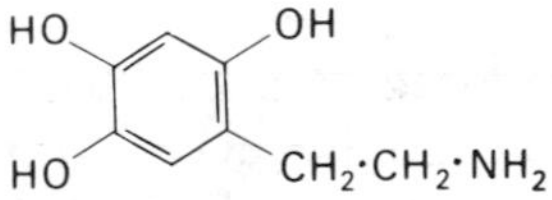

6-Hydroxydopamine
(*9.35*)

For more detail of the various pathways by which adrenergic agonists and antagonists work, see Section 7.6c, and for information on the α- and β-receptors, see Section 13.4. For a book on the biochemical basis of neuropharmacology, see Cooper, Bloom, and Roth (1974).

6-Hydroxydopamine (*9.35*), which is readily oxidized to a *p*-quinone, has been found to destroy all sympathetic nerve-endings in mammals (cat, rat) after a single, small dose. It appears that this compound is distri-buted to the sympathetic endings because of its analogy with noradrenaline, and that it is oxidized there to the quinone which combines covalently with these nerve-endings, thus deactivating them permanently (Thoenen and Tranzer, 1968).

Many hydrazines, e.g. phenelzine (*9.36*) and tranylcypramine, block the enzyme monoamine oxidase and hence allow such blood-pressure raising amines as noradrenaline, dopamine, or tyramine to accumulate. This and similar hydrazines are much used to treat cases of severe mental depression. Unfortunately the inactivated enzyme is re-formed only slowly, so that even quite small doses of these hydrazines can have too long-lasting an effect. The monoamine oxidase (MAO) of human brain consists of four different isoenzymes which show markedly different substrate specificities. Those drugs in common use as inhibitors of monoamine oxidase inhibit various of the isoenzymes selectively (Youdim *et al.*, 1972). About 40 per cent of patients do better on the tricyclic antidepressants (Section, 13.8).

$$CH_2 \cdot CH_2 \cdot NH \cdot NH_2$$

Phenelzine
(9.36)

Pyrogallol (1,2,3-trihydroxybenzene) is a competitive substrate for dopamine (*3.35a*) on the catecholamine-metabolizing enzyme catechol-*O*-methyl transferase. More potent derivatives of pyrogallol are being tried as synergists for laevodopa (*3.35b*) when given in parkinsonism (Section 3.5, p. 91).

Those antihistamine drugs that act on the H_1 receptors must be numbered amongst the most clinically successful of the metabolite analogues. The H_1 receptors may be defined as those that are over-occupied by histamine in coryza (hay fever), urticaria (hives), pruritis (itching), and serum sickness. The first metabolite antagonists of histamine were deliberately sought by Bovet and his colleagues in the Pasteur Institute (Paris) as early as 1937, and the review on structure-action relationships written ten years later is a record of slow but steady progress (Bovet, 1947).

The first example that had any clinical value was antergan (*9.38*) (phenbenzamine, discovered by Halperin in 1942). It is now known that many derivatives of *NN*-dimethylethylenediamine (pK_a values 9.5 and 6.6) have antihistaminic properties. The more basic group in histamine (*9.37*) is the aliphatic amine (pK_a 9.8); the other basic group (pK_a 6.0) is formed by the two ring-nitrogen atoms functioning jointly through imidazole resonance (amidine-type). In antergan, this imidazole ring was represented by the much less basic *N*-benzylaniline group (pK_a about 3.5). Much more active antihistaminics were obtained when a stronger base (2-benzylamino-pyridine, pK_a 6.9) replaced this group. This gave the clinically successful drug mepyramine (pyrilamine, 'Neoantergan', 'Anthisan') (*9.39a*), (Bovet, Horclois, and Walthert, 1944). Parallel work in the Ciba laboratories in New Jersey produced the closely related tripelennamine (*9.39b*) ('Pyribenzamine'), and both of these drugs are still much used.

Meanwhile work in the Parke, Davis laboratories in Michigan had shown the value of drugs based on ethanolamine instead of ethylenediamine, notably diphenhydramine (*9.40*) ('Benadryl'). Members of this class couple an antihistaminic effect with sedative properties, and are used for combined therapy of this kind, and in motion sickness.

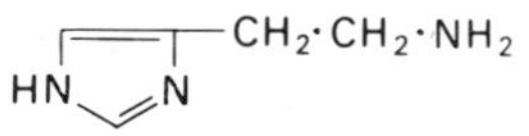

Histamine
(*9.37*)

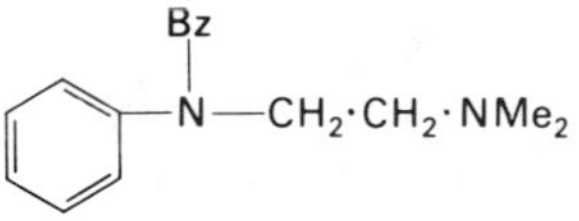

Antergan
(*9.38*)

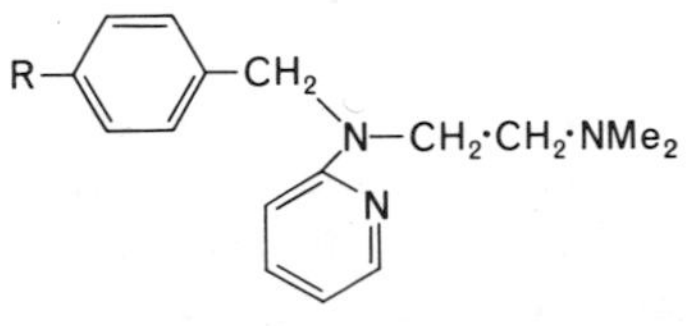

(a) Pyrilamine   (R = OMe)
(b) Tripelennamine (R = H)
(*9.39*)

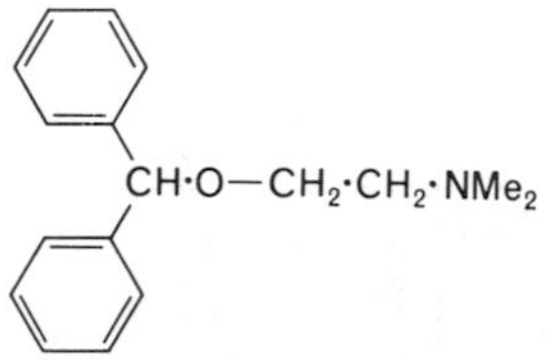

Diphenhydramine
(*9.40*)

Many other minor changes compatible with retention of antihistaminic activity were soon found, but the law of diminishing returns began to operate, and the gains have only been small. In one approach, the two nitrogen atoms of the ethylenediamine model are joined by saturated carbon atoms to form a piperazine ring (the pK_as of piperazine are 9.8 and 5.6). A successful example is chlorcyclizine (*9.41*) ('Histantin'; 'Diparalene'). In another type, exemplified by chlorpheniramine (*9.42*) ('Chlortrimeton'), the carbon-carbon linkage of the side-chain keeps the pK_a down to 5.2 (namely that of pyridine) but this suffices. Chlorpheniramine is a particularly powerful antihistaminic drug with a small, inbuilt centrally-stimulating action that largely overcomes the usual drowsiness produced by anti-H_1 therapy. The dextro-rotatory isomer (dexchlorpheniramine, 'Polaramine') has these qualities in useful balance, and is marketed separately. For a discussion of stereochemical aspects of the structure-action relationships in H_1-antihistaminics, see Casy and Ison, 1970.

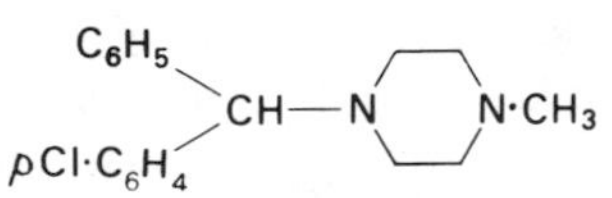

Chlorcylizine
(*9.41*)

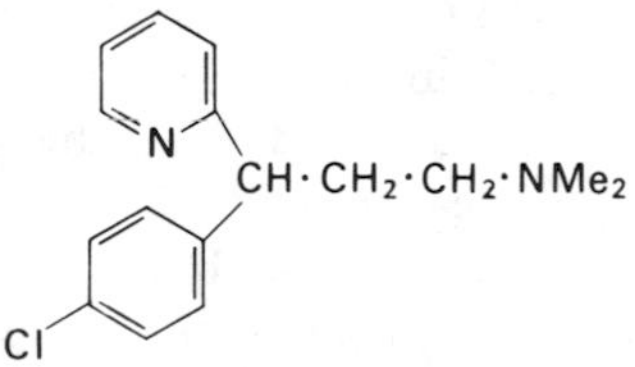

Chlorpheniramine
(*9.42*)

$$Me\underset{HN\diagdown N}{\boxed{\quad}}CH_2\cdot S\cdot CH_2\cdot CH_2\cdot NH\cdot\underset{N\cdot CN}{\overset{H}{\underset{\|}{C}}}\cdot NHMe$$

$$(9.43)$$

In the laboratory, a rapid and perfect antagonism can be demonstrated between histamine and all the above antihistaminics on H_1 receptors such as the bronchii and ileum possess in abundance. However a different type of histamine receptor (H_2) is responsible for stimulation of the uterus, of gastric acid secretion, and of the cardiac atria. A histamine antagonist active at H_2 sites was long sought, but one is now available, namely cimetidine (9.43) ('Tagamet'). This drug is much used to suppress gastric secretion, relieve the pain of peptic ulcers, and to heal them rapidly (Gray et al., 1977). The clue that led to this happy result was the discovery that 4-methylhistamine is an agonist for H_2, but not for H_1 receptors. This situation is reminiscent of the β-methyl-derivative of acetylcholine, which has all the latter's activity at muscarinic receptors, but none at the nicotinic receptors (Section 13.6). It was found that H_2 antagonists act as cations, but if the molecule is too basic, they cannot penetrate to the site of action (Black et al., 1974). The side-chain of cimetidine, which had been much simpler in earlier candidate drugs, took on its present form to avoid side-effects linked to the earlier versions.

The analogue of a quite simple entity, the bicarbonate ion, will now be described. The observation that sulphanilamide caused hens to lay eggs without any shell (Mann and Keilin, 1940), coupled to the observation that this drug also produces an alkaline diuresis (Pitts and Alexander, 1945), led to the discovery that the sulphonamide anion (9.44) can competitively block the access of the bicarbonate anion (9.45) to the enzyme carbonic anhydrase. The $O-O$ separation in a sulphonamide anion is 2.4 Å, and in carbonic acid 2.32 Å. This antagonism prevents dehydration to carbon dioxide. The high concentration of bicarbonate ion which builds up is excreted with an equivalent of sodium ions, causing strong diuresis. This blocking of the receptor cannot occur if the $=NH$-group is substituted, and hence most of the antibacterial sulphonamides do not give this effect. Thus the requirements for 'fit' are much more stringent for competing with bicarbonate anion than for competing with p-aminobenzoic acid (see Section 9.3a). These results led to the decision to insert heterocyclic groups, as R in (9.44), in order to obtain greater anionic ionization than in sulphanilamide, and substances 2000 times as active were found, the activity increasing with the ionization (Miller, Dessert and Roblin, 1950). The best of these substances, acetazolamide (9.46) ('Diamox'), found employment in medicine as a powerful oral diuretic, but it is tachyphylactic (self-limiting) and hence unsuited for prolonged use. It is still prescribed for glaucoma to reduce the intraocular pressure (Maren et al.,

1954). More powerful and tractable diuretics have since been discovered (see Section 14.1).

Sulphonamide ion	Bicarbonate ion	Acetazolamide ion
(9.44)	(9.45)	(9.46)

A simple analogue of glucose, in which the sole change was replacement of the ring oxygen by sulphur (giving 5-thio-D-glucose), inhibited spermato-genesis in low dosage without interfering with libido. It selectively prevented uptake of glucose by the testis and is under consideration as a male contraceptive (Zysk *et al.*, 1975).

9.5 Sequential blocking

The therapeutic usefulness of metabolite analogues can be increased by choosing two of them to achieve sequential blocking (Hitchings, 1952). Growth-factors are gradually built up from components moved along the enzymatic equivalent of a factory's production line, each stage of assembly being carried out by a different enzyme. The arithmetic of sequential blocking is this: if the first enzyme is blocked to the extent of 90 per cent, then only 10 per cent of the partly completed factor reaches the second enzyme. If one is fortunate enough to discover how to block the second enzyme also by 90 per cent, then only 1 per cent of the partly completed factor emerges, and that may be too little to sustain life in the parasite. It may be asked why it is not sufficient to use more of the first drug and block the first enzyme by 100 per cent. The answer is: because of the usual shape of a dose-response curve; increasing the concentration of a drug beyond a certain point seldom leads to much further response. This is because adsorption from solution usually follows a hyperbolic curve (Langmuir's isotherm, see Section 8.1). Thus to increase the blockade of an enzyme from 90 to 100 per cent would usually call for an amount of the drug so excessive that it may endanger the patient's life.

An example of sequential blocking is the use of a sulphadiazine with pyrimethamine ('Daraprim') in the toxoplasmosis of mice and men (Wettingfeld, Rowe and Eyles, 1956). In this sequence, the sulphonamide blocks the incorporation of *p*-aminobenzoic acid into dihydrofolic acid, and the pyrimethamine (4.7) prevents the reduction of this pteridine to tetrahydrofolic acid (Sections 9.3b and c). In humans, too, pyrimethamine and sulphadiazine have been shown to potentiate one another in the three principal types of malaria. Thus less than 0.1 m.e.d. (minimal effective dose) of pyrimethamine and 0.25 m.e.d. of sulphadiazine are together as effective as 1.0 m.e.d. of either drug separately (Hurly, 1959). In tropical medicine, 'Maloprim', a combination of pyrimethamine and dapsone (9.9) (the latter chosen because of its slow rate of excretion which matches that of pyrimethamine), has proved an excellent replacement for chloroquin in cases of malaria resistant to this drug. Another combination ('Fansidar') used for this purpose is pyrimethamine and sulfadoxine, a slowly excreted sulphonamidopyrimidine (Richards, 1970). Similar combinations are used in treating *Eimeria* (protozoal) infections of poultry.

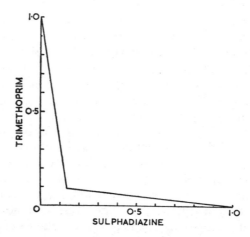

FIG. 9.3 Synergism of trimethoprim and sulphadiazine in treatment of mice infected with *Proteus vulgaris*. The units on the axes represent doses of each drug needed to give half the maximal percentage survival. Each point on the graph represents a combination of fractions of these doses. (The sulphadiazine unit was 0.14 mg, and that of trimethoprim 4 mg, per mouse.) (Hitchings and Burchall, 1965.)

Sequential blocking offers very practical advantages in *antibacterial* chemotherapy also. The synergistic effect of trimethoprim with sulphadiazine, shown in Fig. 9.3, is evident. In medical practice, the most striking and beneficial results have been obtained by selecting a sulphonamide with a similar pattern of distribution and persistence to those of this diaminopyrimidine, namely sulphamethoxazole (9.13), (3-*p*-aminobenzenesulphonamido-5-methylisoxazole), under the name *co-trimoxazole* ('Septrin', 'Bactrim', 'Eusaprim'). This combination, which sequentially blocks first the synthesis and then the reduction of dihydrofolic acid, has been found extraordinarily effective in bacterial dysentery, bronchitis, and long-standing infections of the urinary tract by *E. coli*, *Proteus mirabilis*, *Neisseria gonorrhoeae*, *Klebsiella*, *Streptococcus*, and *Staphylococcus* (Cattell *et al.*, 1971).

The very striking synergistic effect of penicillin and streptomycin on bacteria (Jawetz, 1952), while not sequential, is due to the arithmetical factor described above.

9.6 Analogues that form a covalent bond

Several examples are known where a metabolite analogue is first attracted to the enzyme commonly used by the metabolite and then forms a covalent bond with this enzyme. Thus, penicillin (*12.6b*), as described in Section 12.1, may appear to be a metabolite antagonist for D-alanyl-D-alanine; but instead of these substances being freely competitive at the transpeptidase, the penicillin combines irreversibly with this enzyme by forming a covalent bond. Again, the quaternary ammonium group of pyridine-2-aldoxime methiodide (*12.27*) causes this molecule to come to rest on acetylcholinesterase on the site usually fitted by the quaternary ammonium group of acetylcholine; if this enzyme is already inactivated by phosphorylation, the pyridine antidote brings about activation of the enzyme by transferring the phosphoryl-group to its own hydroxyl-group (see Section 12.3).

It seems reasonable that other useful agents could be made by designing them as metabolite analogues (to bring about concentration on the enzyme), and then giving the molecule one further group which could form a covalent bond with the enzyme which should thus become permanently inactivated. B. R. Baker, working with lactic dehydrogenase as a model, distinguished two kinds of inhibitory alkylating agents, those which alkylate the site which normally combines with the substrate, and those which alkylate adjacent sites. These two classes of inhibitors are called endo- and exo-alkylating agents, respectively. One exo-alkylating agent, 4-iodoacetamido-salicylic acid, is modelled on salicylic acid, which forms a readily reversible complex with L-glutamic dehydrogenase and lactic dehydrogenase. Whereas iodoacetamide does not inhibit these enzymes, the iodoacetamide-group in this acid does so, because the similarity of the rest of the molecule to salicylic acid causes the inhibitor to be concentrated on the enzyme (Baker, *et al.*, 1962a). This inhibition is irreversible because hydrogen iodide is split off and a covalent bond is formed.

This inhibitor can discriminate between isoenzymes. Thus, whereas it irreversibly inhibits the lactic dehydrogenase of skeletal muscle, it does not affect that of the heart. A related compound, 5-(phenoxycarboxamido) salicylic acid, irreversibly inhibits the heart (but not the skeletal) isoenzyme, whereas its 4-isomer irreversibly inhibits the skeletal (but not the heart) isoenzyme (Baker and Patel, 1964; Baker, 1967).

For further reading on active-site-directed irreversible inhibitors, see Baker (1967). This is an idea which, in the long run, may lead to useful new agents.

9.7 Unusual relationships between agonists and antagonists

Some metabolite antagonists are not metabolite analogues. In fact, substances which do not resemble metabolites in any way can be used to combine with or destroy an apoenzyme, a coenzyme, or a substrate (Fildes, 1940a). All that is necessary is a high chemical affinity, hence the combination is often effected by covalent bonds. In contrast to the analogues, these antagonists are not displaceable by the substrate. An example of such an antagonist is the enzyme thiaminase, which splits thiamine into two substances, one containing the pyrimidine ring and the other the thiazole ring. This causes thiamine-deprivation symptoms in animals fed on raw fish, in which this enzyme occurs (Woolley, 1952).

The demonstration of competitive antagonism between two substances does not prove that one of them is a metabolite. Thus the severe contractions of the gut caused by barium chloride are competitively inhibited by sodium sulphate (which is not a normal gut constituent). In this case, there is a chemical reaction between the two substances, and the toxic barium ion is precipitated as the highly insoluble sulphate. Obviously, before a substance can be classed as a metabolite, its presence in nature must be demonstrated, and also its origin and function. Morphine and allyl*nor*morphine are examples of a pair of drugs which compete with one another without either of them being natural metabolites (Unna, 1943) (see Section 7.3). This phenomenon led to discovery of naltrexone (*7.33*) which, although chemically similar to morphine, is used to accelerate withdrawal in addicts (see Section 7.3, p. 247). Similarly 2,4-dichlorophenoxyacetic acid, an artificial plant growth regulator, is strongly antagonized by the equally artifical analogue, 2,4-dichlorophenylthio*iso*butyric acid (Griffiths, *et al.*, 1966). These examples might be classed with the classical 'Therapeutic Interference' effect of Section 6.6.

To assist in the study of pairs of drugs that are antagonistic to one another without either being a metabolite, Schild (1947) introduced the useful concept of pA_x. This is the negative logarithm of that (molar) concentration of an antagonist which reduces the effect of a multiple dose (x) of a drug to that of a single dose. Convenient values of x are 2 and 10. The concept is valid whenever drug and antagonist compete for the same receptor *and* compete according to the law of mass action, as is usually the case. The pA_x can be used to classify drugs, because only those drugs which act on the same receptors are likely to give the same pA_x value with the same competitive antagonist. Moreover, a given drug-antagonist pair can be used to find if receptors in different tissues give the same pA_x values, a coincidence which would heighten the likelihood of these receptors being identical (Arunlakshana and Schild, 1959).

9.8 Pharmacogenetics

In all work on enzyme inhibitors, it must be remembered that individuals do not necessarily possess the same content of enzymes as the population as a whole. Thus many people, particularly in Africa and the Middle East, have a deficiency of glucose 6-phosphate dehydrogenase, a biochemical lesion which does them no harm until they are prescribed the antimalarial drug, primaquine (*3.27*). These patients quickly develop haemolytic anaemia, due to their biochemical lesion which is inherited on an incompletely dominant sex-linked gene (Beutler, 1959). The anaemia is caused by the haemolytic quinone formed in the first stage of metabolism: the enzyme which should destroy the quinone is missing.

Other such enzyme deficiencies have been revealed through an individual's adverse reaction to drugs. More than 90% of Orientals are genetically rapid *N*-acetylators of isoniazid (*6.12*), whereas only 40% of black or white citizens of the United States showed this trait (Kalow, 1962). Rapid acetylators produce acetylhydrazine, which can cause liver damage. The same inheritance controls the acetylation (deactivation) of the sulphonamide antibacterials. The rise of intraocular pressure when glucocorticoids are placed in the eye is another pharmacogenetic effect. Low and high responses are shown by 66% and 5%, respectively, of a sample white population.

For further reading, see Kalow (1962); Goldstein, Aronow, and Kalman (1974, p. 437); and World Health Organization (1973a).

10 Ionization

Quaternary aliphatic amines, such as acetylcholine, must necessarily be completely ionized at all pH values. This follows from their structure: they have no proton to lose, and the nitrogen atom cannot exceed a covalence of 4. However, most biologically active substances are *weak* acids or bases, and hence the extent to which they are ionized is highly dependent on pH. Among such substances, the ionization constants (and hence the degree of ionization at a fixed pH) can be varied widely by making small alterations in the chemical structure. There are two ways of varying the degree of ionization, (a) to employ one substance at various pH values, and (b) to employ several related substances (of varying ionization constants) at a fixed pH. These two ways are valuable to the investigator because ions behave differently from their corresponding uncharged forms. For example, ions undergo different chemical reactions, they penetrate membranes differently, and they become adsorbed to different types of substances.

10.0 The nature of ionization

Many substances are known which do not increase the electrical conductivity of water when dissolved in it. These are called non-electrolytes (chloroform and sucrose are examples) and they depress the freezing-point of water proportionally to their molar concentration. Acids, bases, and salts, on the other hand, increase the electrical conductivity of water. The majority of biologically active agents are acids, bases, or salts, and hence electrolytes. All electrolytes depress the freezing-point of water to a greater extent than would have been expected from their molar concentration. Dilute solutions of hydrochloric acid, sodium hydroxide, and sodium chloride give twice as much depression as would have been expected. This led the Swedish chemist Arrhenius to formulate the theory of ionization of electolytes (1884–7). Thus, in solution, hydrochloric acid consists entirely of hydrogen cations and chloride anions (H^+ and Cl^-), sodium hydroxide of sodium cations and hydroxyl anions (Na^+ and OH^-), and sodium chloride of sodium cations and chloride anions (Na^+ and Cl^-). Sodium sulphate gives three times the expected depression, and it has been shown that, instead of a molecule of Na_2SO_4, three ions are present, namely, two sodium cations and one sulphate anion (SO_4^{2-}).

Salts. In general, salts are completely ionized in dilute solution: of the few exceptions, the halides of mercury, cadmium, and lead are the most notable. Because salts are completely ionized, they have no biological properties other than those of the individual ions of which they are composed. Thus calcium chloride can have no conceivable physiological effects other than those peculiar to calcium ions and to chloride ions. This simple conception needs modification when a salt is derived from either a weak acid or a weak base, because some of the uncharged species is liberated by hydrolysis (see below), thus adding its own biological effect to those of the constituent ions of the salt.

In general the physiological properties of a salt can be neither more nor less than the sum of those of its ions. For example, Hata (1932) examined the toxicity for the mouse of 3,6-diamino-10-methylacridinium (6.4) chloride and the corresponding iodide, and found the iodide half as active, weight for weight. He then compared the ability of these substances to save mice infected with streptococci; once again the iodide was half as active. Now, as both of the anions are biologically inert at the dilutions tested, the biological activities must be proportional to the amount of cations in these substances which are completely ionized in neutral solutions (Albert, 1966). The formula-weights are respectively 260 and 351, so that the iodide would have 74 per cent of the potency of the chloride. The biological results are in as good agreement with this calculation as could reasonably be expected from the serial dilutions that were used. Hence these experiments amount only to a biological comparison of the diaminomethylacridinium cation with itself. The antibacterial properties of a number of other acridine salts have been tested as their sulphates, nitrates, hydrochlorides, and hydriodides. As expected, no effect attributable to the anion was found (Browning *et al.*, 1922).

Acids and bases. Unlike salts, acids and bases need not be completely ionized in solution. Strong acids (e.g. hydrochloric acid) and strong bases (e.g. sodium hydroxide) are completely ionized in the pH range of 0–14, but weak acids or bases show variable ionization within this pH range. Even small variations in pH on either side of the neutral point (pH 7) make considerable changes in the proportions of drug ionized in such cases as barbiturates, alkaloids, local anaesthetics, and antihistaminics. Several examples will be given later.

Salts which are formed from a weak acid (or from a weak base) hydrolyse partly, in solution, to the acid (or base) from which they are derived and which are incompletely ioinzed. This situation is simpler than it may seem, because the degree of ionization in solution depends on only two factors, the pH and the pK_a. The latter (which will be defined below) is a constant for any acid or base. Hence, if the pH is controlled, the degree of ionization depends only on the nature of the acid (or base) added, *regardless of whether or not it has previously been neutralized.* Thus the same ratio of atropine ions to atropine molecules will result from the addition of atropine hydrochloride, atropine sulphate, or free atropine to a bath that has been buffered at pH 7. If the pH of the bath is raised, the proportion of atropine ions to atropine molecules will decrease, but the new ratio will again be independent of the form in which the atropine was added. Because it is confusing to speak of 'free' or 'non-ionized' acids and bases, the term 'molecule', or 'neutral species' is customarily used for all uncharged forms.

In 1944, some American bacteriologists (who shall be nameless, here) published a paper in which they found that 9-aminoacridine (*10.7*) was 64 times more bactericidal than its hydrochloride (against *Pneumococcus* type III in glucose-broth). The authors did not say whether their medium was buffered. If it was buffered, the same result should have been obtained in both cases, and hence the technique was at fault. If the medium was not buffered, the results could have no quantitative significance because of the greatly increased pH of a solution of a strong base (pK_a 10.0 in this case) compared to that of solutions of its salts. As it happened, the striking increase in the antibacterial action of acridines, when the pH rises, had long been on record (Graham-Smith, 1919; Browning, Gulbransen and Kennaway, 1919.

For further reading on acids, bases, and ionization, see Bell (1973).

10.1 The ionization constant (K_a)

As essential part of Arrhenius's theory of ionization was the application of the *law of mass action* to describe the state of ionic equilibrium. Thus, acetic acid (CH_3COOH) is a weak acid which ionizes in water to give some hydrogen ions (H^+) and some acetate anions (CH_3COO^-). The product of the concentration of the ions (which is $[H^+]$ $[CH_3COO^-]$) always bears a fixed ratio to the concentration of the neutral molecules $[CH_3COOH]$. This ratio is called the acidic ionization constant (K_a), or more simply the ionization constant. Thus:

$$K_a = \frac{[H^+][CH_3COO^-]}{[CH_3COOH]} \qquad \text{(i)}$$

and this has been found, experimentally, to be 1.75×10^{-5} (at $25°C$).

Sometimes the expression 'dissociation constant' is used for ionization constant, but the latter term is more precise. Many complexes, such as enzyme systems, 'dissociate' into their components, and micelles into their monomers: the relevant equilibria are expressed as dissociation constants similarly derived from the law of mass action. Nevertheless, such constants are not ionization constants.

The state of ionization of weak bases also can be described by acidic ionization constants. For example, ammonia is a weak base which can take up hydrogen ions to form ammonium ions. This is, of course, equivalent to thinking of the ammonium ion (NH_4^+) as a weak acid which ionizes in water to give some hydrogen ions (H^+) and some molecules of ammonia (NH_3). Thus:

$$K_a = \frac{[H^+][NH_3]}{[NH_4^+]} \qquad \text{(ii)}$$

and this has been found, experimentally, to be 5.5×10^{-10} (at $25°C$).

The use of acidic constants to describe the ionization of bases was introduced in 1929 by Brönsted in order to record the ionization of both bases and acids on the *same* scale, just as a single pH scale serves to measure both acidity and alkalinity.

Earlier workers had toyed with a separate scale for bases, writing:

$$K_b = \frac{[OH^-][NH_4^+]}{[NH_4OH]} \qquad \text{(iii)}$$

and the value of K_b (the basic dissociation constant) was found to be 1.8×10^{-5} (at $25°C$). Equation (iii) is unreal because no substance with pentacovalent nitrogen, such as NH_4OH, is capable of existence. Equations (i) and (ii) show that an acid produces hydrogen ions and a base receives them. Thus both acid and base can be related in terms of a single quantity, their affinity for the hydrogen ion. This relationship allows the use of the acidic ionization constant for both acids and bases.

The definition of pK_a. Ionization constants are small and inconvenient, but their negative logarithms (known as pK_a values) are convenient to say and to write. Thus the pK_a of acetic acid is 4.76 and of ammonia, 9.26. When the older literature offers only pK_b values for bases (e.g. 4.74 for ammonia), these can be converted to pK_a values by subtraction from the negative logarithm of the ionic product of water (K_w) at the temperature of determination. (The value of pK_w is 14.16 at 20°C, 14.00 at 25°C, and 13.58 at 37°C.)

It is evident that pK_a values provide a very convenient way of comparing the strengths of acids (or of bases). The stronger an acid is, the lower its pK_a (the stronger a base is, the higher its pK_a). The pH at which an acid or base is half ionized is equal to its pK_a. When the pH is one unit below the pK_a, an acid is 9 per cent ionized, and a base is 91 per cent ionized (see Appendix 1).

Any acid or base, if partly neutralized, is an effective buffer within the range from one unit below the pK_a value to one unit above it. Biologists use initiative in selecting buffers suitable for particular experiments. They do not use anionic buffers (such as citrate and phosphate, which form complexes) if metal cations are essential to the system under study. To give just one example, phosphate buffers inhibit the action of *iso*citric dehydrogenase (in pig's heart) by removing manganese (Lotspeich and Peters, 1951). In place of these anionic buffers, cationic buffers such as *N*-ethylmorpholine (pH range 7.0–8.2) and 'Tris' (aminotrishydroxymethylmethane) (7.5–8.7), and the zwitterionic buffers such as 'Hepes' and 'Tes' (6.9–8.1) (Good, *et al.*, 1966) are well established. For a useful book on buffers, see Perrin and Dempsey (1974).

How to locate pK_a *values.* The commoner pK_a values may be obtained from ionization constant manuals (e.g. Albert and Serjeant, 1971). Others are easily located through the International Union of Pure and Applied Chemistry's two compilations (acids by Kortüm, Vogel, and Andrusson, 1961, and bases by Perrin, 1965a). New values are listed in *Chemical Abstracts* under 'Ionization, electrolytic'. Table 10.1 gives the relative strengths of some common acids and bases; this table should be committed to memory because it provides a comparison for new pK_a values encountered in reading. Acids and bases of equivalent strength have been placed opposite one another.

A pK_a value of about 5 (cf. acetic acid) is typical of a great many monocarboxylic acids, both aliphatic and aromatic. The value of 10 is typical of a phenol. Acids with pK_a values greater than 7 scarcely affect neutral indicator paper and, if greater than 10, do not even taste acidic.

The value of 11 for ethylamine is representative of aliphatic bases; that of 5 for aniline is typical of aromatic bases which are much weaker. As pK_a figures are logarithms, there is a difference of one millionfold (i.e. antilog 6) between the strengths of ethylamine and aniline. Many alkaloids and other biologically active bases have pK_a values about 8. Bases with pK_a values less than 7 scarcely affect neutral indicator paper.

Electron-releasing groups (e.g. $-CH_3$) strengthen bases and weaken acids, whereas electron-attracting groups (e.g. $-NO_2$) weaken bases and strengthen acids. The electronic properties of various substituents are summarized in Appendix III. Understanding of these influences is now so complete that an acid or base of any desired strength can be synthesized in any series (Clark and Perrin, 1964; Perrin, 1965b; Barlin and Perrin, 1966).

For detailed practical instruction in the determination of ionization constants in the laboratory, see Albert and Serjeant (1971).

Table 10.1

RELATIVE STRENGTHS OF SOME COMMON ACIDS AND BASES

Acids	pK_a	Bases	pK_a
Hydrochloric acid	< 0	Sodium hydroxide	<14
Phosphoric acid (first proton lost)	2		12
	3	Ehylamine	11
	4		10
Acetic acid	5	Ammonia	9
Carbonic acid	6	Quinine, strychnine	8
Phosphoric acid (second proton lost)	7		7
	8		6
Hydrocyanic acid, boric acid	9	Aniline, pyridine	5
Phenol	10		4
	11		3
Phosphoric acid (third proton lost)	12		2
Glucose	13	p-Nitroaniline	1

Calculation of the percentage ionized. The degree of ionization of any base, in aqueous solution, can be calculated from the following equation, provided that two things are known, the pH of the solution and the pK_a of the substance:

$$\% \text{ ionized} = \frac{100}{1 + \text{antilog} (pH - pK_a)} \tag{iv}$$

This equation shows that the degree of ionization varies with pH, but that it does not bear a straight-line relationship to the extent of the change. On the contrary, a sigmoid curve is followed, as shown in Fig. 10.1. It will be seen from this figure that a small change in pH can make a large change in ionization, particularly if the pH of the solution is numerically close to the pK_a of the substance investigated. This is readily seen from Table 10.2. By way of example: if one were working at pH 7 with a nitro-phenol of $pK_a = 7$, half of the substance would be in the ionized state. If the pH were allowed to rise to 8, the phenol would be nearly all ionized; but if it fell to 6, almost all of the phenol would be in the non-ionized condition.

Table 10.3 may be regarded as a magnification of the central part of Table 10.2.

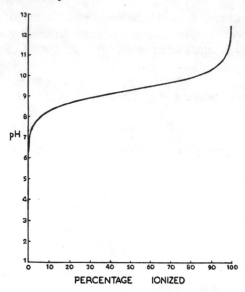

FIG. 10.1 Typical curve obtained in the potentiometric titration of an acid (boric acid, $pK_a = 9.21$ at 20°C).

Table 10.2*

CALCULATION OF THE EXTENT OF
IONIZATION, GIVEN pK_a AND pH

pK_a –pH	Per cent ionized (if anion)	Per cent ionized (if cation)
−4	99.99	0.01
−3	99.94	0.10
−2	99.01	0.99
−1	90.91	9.09
0	50.00	50.00
1	9.09	90.91
2	0.99	99.01
3	0.10	99.94
4	0.01	99.99

* An extended form of this table will be found as Appendix I at the end of this book.

Polyelectrolytes. These are molecules with a large number of ionizing groups which may have the same charge, as in polyacrylic acid, or both charges may be present, as in proteins. The titration curves of polyelectrolytes have a rather indefinite ('smeared-out') appearance. Contrary to

Table 10.3

CALCULATION OF THE EXTENT OF
IONIZATION WHERE pK_a IS CLOSE TO pH

pK_a −pH	Per cent ionized (if anion)	Per cent ionized (if cation)
− 0.5	75.97	24.03
− 0.4	71.53	28.47
− 0.3	66.61	33.39
− 0.2	61.32	38.68
− 0.1	55.73	44.27
0	50.00	50.00
+ 0.1	44.27	55.73
+ 0.2	38.68	61.32
+ 0.3	33.39	66.61
+ 0.4	28.47	71.53
+ 0.5	24.03	75.97

what happens with mono- and di-ions, a polyion retains a large fraction of the oppositely charged counterions close to it. For further reading, see Albert and Serjeant (1971).

Zwitterions. So far, no mention has been made of zwitterions, i.e. ionic forms which carry both positive and negative charges. In discussing whether a substance is zwitterionic or not, the pH range in which the information is required must be specified, because a sufficiently alkaline solution will change the zwitterion to an anion, and a sufficiently acid solution will change it to a cation.

For example, the acidic group in glycine has a pK_a of 2.2, and the basic group has a pK_a of 9.9. It is evident from Table 10.2 that at pH 3.2, only 90 per cent of the acidic groups (but *all* of the basic groups) will be ionized; hence at this pH, about 90 per cent of the substance will be present as zwitterion and 10 per cent as cation. Glycine is almost entirely zwitterionic between pH 3.2 and 8.9.

Not all substances with an acidic and a basic group are zwitterions (internal salts), because there may be no pH at which both groups are ionized. The pH of the solution is another factor. Thus a substance is 90 per cent or more in the zwitterionic state when the pH is at least one unit above the acidic pK_a and at least one unit below the basic pK_a. If this rule is applied to p-aminobenzoic acid (acidic pK_a 4.8; basic pK_a 2.7), it will at once be seen that this substance unlike glycine, is exclusively anionic in neutral and alkaline solutions. For other tests to distinguish between zwitterionic and merely amphoteric substances (e.g. glycine and p-aminobenzoic acid respectively), see Albert and Serjeant (1971).

Although noradrenaline and its N-alkyl homologues exist mainly in the form of cation between pH 6 and 8, the presence of acidic and basic groups in the one molecule gives rise to a complex pattern of minor ionic species. This arises from the fact that the pK_a values of both amino- and the first phenolic group fall in the narrow range of 8.9 to 10.3 (the ionization of the second phenolic group is repressed by Coulomb's principle). By methods similar to those used for tyrosine (Edsall, Martin and Hollingworth, 1958), the four microscopic ionization constants were obtained from the two apparent constants. The microscopic constants arise from the circumstance that when two constants (for groups of opposite charge) lie within 2 pK units of one another, each group has *two* distinct values, depending on whether the other is ionized or not. However, it was found that the constants of noradrenaline and its N-methyl-, ethyl-, *iso*propyl-, *n*-butyl-, *sec*-butyl-, *tert*-butyl-, and *iso*butyl-derivatives varied so little with the nature of the alkyl-group that the great variation in physiological properties between members of this series could not be explained by the presence of specified minor ionic species in particular members (Sinistri and Villa, 1962).

10.2　Differences in ionization that can bring about selectivity

Students often ask, 'How can the degree of ionization be relevant where biological action is concerned? Surely poorly ionizing substances produce at least a few ions and, as these are removed, fresh ones are generated from the neutral molecules according to the mass-action law, as in Equation (i)?'

This objection is intelligently argued, but it must be remembered that ions are not bound to their receptors by *covalent* bonds, and hence they can easily leave the receptors. In short, to keep a receptor saturated with a given ion, there must be an excess of this ion in the solution bathing the receptor. For example, crystal violet* is bacteriostatic to *E. coli* at a dilution of 1 in 10 000, but not at 1 in 20 000, although both solutions are intensely violet. The violet colour denotes the presence of the cations, which are the active form of this antibacterial drug (the neutral species is colourless).

Equations (v) and (vi) help to explain this phenomenon. Equation (v) shows that the magnitude of K_a the (ionization constant) governs the proportion of cation (BH^+) to neutral species (B) at any given hydrogen ion concentration $[H^+]$. Equation (vi) similarly deals with the magnitude of K_s which is the stability constant of the ion-pair (ABH) formed by combination of the cation (BH^+) of the drug with the vulnerable anionic group $[A^-]$ of the bacterium. This complex is maintained by an ionic bond supplemented usually by a hydrogen bond or several van der Waals bonds.

---

* Crystal violet is the N, N′,N″-hexamethyl derivative of (*10.4*).

$$K_a = \frac{[\text{B}][\text{H}^+]}{[\text{BH}^+]} \text{ (ionization constant)} \qquad \text{(v)}$$

$$K_s = \frac{[\text{ABH}]}{[\text{A}^-][\text{BH}^+]} \text{ (stability constant)} \qquad \text{(vi)}$$

If K_a and K_s are of comparable magnitudes, then any deficiency of cations in the solution will be replenished from the drug-bacterium complex (ABH) as well as from the non-ionized drug (B). Under these circumstances the ionization constant of the drug becomes the limiting factor governing its use: not only must ions be present, but they must be present abundantly. It is not to be supposed from this reasoning that the acids in receptors are necessarily weak. Rather, the dwell-time of an adsorbed cation, unless its ionic bond is reinforced by hydrogen bonding or van der Waals forces, is very short because of exchange with sodium cations (from the sodium chloride solution that bathes the area).

Many bacteria are much more sensitive than *E. coli* to crystal violet. Thus *Streptococcus pyogenes* is inhibited by a dilution of 1 in 320 000 (though not by 1 in 640 000); and *Staphylococcus aureus* is killed by 1 in 2 000 000. Although these differences may be partly due to differences in sites of loss, there are different K_s values for different species and (in the hosts) for different tissues in the one species. This affords a basis for the selective action of cationic drugs.

Other types of selectivity depend not on the relative adsorbability of a given ion but on properties in which ions, as a class, differ from molecules. These differences will now be discussed under three headings: covalent reactivity (used here to mean the making and breaking of covalent bonds), adsorption at surfaces, and penetration of membranes.

Covalent reactivity.   Nitration of the neutral species of aniline occurs in the *ortho-* and *para-*positions, whereas its cation becomes nitrated mainly in the *meta-*position. Thus by changing the acidity of the nitration mixture, the proportions of the isomers can be controlled. An example of greater biochemical interest is ascorbic acid (*10.1*), which is readily oxidized by air when present as the di-anion, whereas the mono-anion and the molecule (either of which can be made the principal species present, by a change in pH) are quite stable (Weissberger and LuValle, 1944).

Ascorbic acid
(*10.1*)

Table 10.4

AUTOXIDATION OF ASCORBIC ACID

pH	Di-anion %	Mono-anion %	Molecule %	Velocity constant min^{-1} × 10^3	
9.21	0.5	99.5	—	22	No metallic ions
8.71	0.2	99.8	—	11	,, ,, ,,
7.61	0.01	99.99	—	0.7	,, ,, ,,
5.80	—	97.8	2.2	0.1	,, ,, ,,
4.70	—	79.4	20.6	0.03	,, ,, ,,
9.31	0.6	99.4	—	101	Copper-catalysed
7.49	0.01	99.99	—	170	,,
6.12	—	99.0	1.0	134	,,
5.08	—	90.1	9.9	91	,,
3.87	—	36.0	64.0	26	,,
2.59	—	2.9	97.1	2	,,

(Weissberger and Lu Valle, 1944.)

This is shown in the top half of Table 10.4, where a decrease in alkalinity is seen to slow the rate of oxidation in proportion as the concentration of di-anion is lowered, even though the proportions of the other two species are therby increased. In the presence of cupric ions, the autoxidation of ascorbic acid goes much faster; but the mechanism is obviously different, for here the rate is proportional not to the concentrations of the di-anion or of the molecule, but to that of mono-anion (Table 10.4, lower half).

The breaking of covalent bonds, by enzymes, greatly influences the metabolism of selectively toxic agents. Each may become changed to a more active or to an inert substance. However, because ion and molecule must react at very different rates, variations in pK_a among members of a series will produce marked differences.

Adsorption at surfaces. There are two kinds of adsorption, the *indiscriminate* and the *specific.* Indiscriminate adsorption is shown by amphiphilic substances, i.e. those having a water-attracting end-group attached to a comparatively large residue that has little affinity for water. Ordinary soap is an example of this class of substances. It will be recalled that water molecules are extensively hydrogen-bonded to one another and that substances dissolve in water only by virtue of their ability to break some of these bonds and form new bonds with water molecules. Amphiphilic molecules, dissolved in water, are in a state of uneasy equilibrium, because the hydrocarbon portion is constantly being squeezed out by the water molecules in their endeavour to unite with one another.

This property of water gives rise to indiscriminate adsorption because such substances become deposited on any surface that presents itself, regardless of its chemical nature. Soap, for instance, is thus caused to accumulate not only at the air-water interface of a vessel in which its solution is stored, but also at the glass-water interface. Furthermore if various objects are immersed in the soapy solution, soap will be found to accumulate on them also. This is typical indiscriminate adsorption, in which molecules tend to be adsorbed more strongly than ions, e.g. oleic acid is more strongly adsorbed than (sodium) oleate. This happens because an ion is more strongly hydrated than the corresponding neutral species, so that the latter has the greater tendency to undergo expulsion.

Specific adsorption is often shown by hydrophilic substances which tend to leave water when they can accumulate on a surface that has a chemically complementary character. Among the commonest cases of complementarity is that of an anion attracted to a positively charged portion of a surface or, conversely, a cation attracted to a negatively charged portion. In such cases, an ion is obviously adsorbed much more strongly than the corresponding molecule. [Many ingenious applications of specific ionic adsorption have been worked out in mineral flotation (cf. Sutherland and Wark, 1955).] Some examples of this phenomenon among selectively toxic agents occur later in this chapter (e.g. the aminoacridines). Perhaps even more striking examples are the phosphorylated vitamins B which, water-soluble as they are and occurring in food at immense dilution, nevertheless become concentrated on their complementary surfaces in enzyme systems, with astonishing speed and efficiency.

Penetration of membranes. Every living cell is surrounded by a semi-permeable membrane which is about four molecules in thickness. Such a membrane, usually lipoprotein in nature, is strongly charged, and its interior is almost inaccessible to ions. The difficulties in the way of the penetration of ions are (a) their relatively greater size, due to hydration, and (b) their charge, which is either *similar* to the portion of protein surface which they approach (resulting in repulsion) or is *opposite* (resulting in fixation).

However, neutral molecules, provided they have no more than three water-attracting groups and a molecular weight of not more than 150, usually penetrate membranes readily (see Section 3.1). A good example of the control that ionization exerts over penetration is illustrated in Fig. 10.12 (p. 377). (This difference between molecules and ions is reminiscent of the ease of penetration of atoms by neutrons, which are uncharged, whereas electrons and protons, because of their charge, penetrate only with the greatest difficulty.)

It must not be supposed, however, that no ions ever penetrate natural membranes. In the first place, specific mechanisms exist for the uptake of each ion for which the cell has a need. Thus cholinium ions are taken up by a 'Type 2' mechanism (see p. 62), and Na^+ and K^+ ions by an energy-consuming 'Type 3' mechanism (p. 62). The human gut is readily permeable to sodium and chloride ions, and fairly permeable to citrate and acetate ions; but for Ca^{2+}, Mg^{2+}, Fe^{2+}, and phosphate, it has evolved specific, easily saturated intake mechanisms, which reject all but the traces of these ions essential for the body's needs, and sulphate and tartrate anions pass through the intestines largely unabsorbed. In the second place (and this refers specially to synthetic agents) a non-penetrating ion can often be made penetrating by the addition of a lipophilic-group; the chloro- and other lipophilic-groups of the antimalarials mepacrine ('Atebrin') and chloroquine may assist in the necessary penetration of red blood cells.

A further effect of ionization upon penetration must now be considered. The action of a drug obviously depends upon ability to reach its receptor. Now an agent with a pK_a between 6 and 8 is in the position that, at the physiologically interesting pH of 7, it is always in equilibrium with at least 10 per cent of its more poorly represented ionic species (see Table 10.2). Such an agent will encounter membranes through which only the non-ionic species can pass. Yet this species, when it has penetrated, is likely to encounter an aqueous medium of similar pH value, and in this it is obliged to re-form ions until the same degree of ionization exists on both sides of the membrane. Quite a large number of agents have pK_a values between 6 and 8: but some have pK_a values which lie entirely outside this range and hence they have a different pattern of distribution and different types of action.

Pseudo-bases. The time taken for ionic equilibria to occur, in solution, is so exceedingly small (e.g. 10^{-7} s) that ionic reactions may be regarded as instantaneous. However, there are a few kinds of cation which slowly combine *covalently* with hydroxyl ions to give non-ionized substances known as 'pseudo-bases' from which the original cation can be regenerated by acid. In different examples, any time from a minute to a week may be needed for equilibrium to be achieved. The two most common examples of pseudo-bases are heteroaromatic quaternary compounds and triphenyl-methane dyes. Suitable methods for calculating the equilibrium ionization constants (expressed as pK_a^{Eq}), and the velocity constant at which equilibrium is attained, are available, e.g. Goldacre and Phillips (1949), Cigén (1958).

Because pseudo-base formation can assist permeability, the relevant

(10.2)   (10.3)

(10.4)   (10.5)

chemistry will now be discussed. Formula (*10.2*) shows the 5-methyl-phenanthridinium cation, such as exists in phenanthridine methochloride. This substance will serve to represent all quaternary amines which have a double-bond attached to a ring-nitrogen atom (the cations of the related *tertiary* amines do not form pseudo-bases). Because tetracovalency, as in (*10.2*), is the maximal valency of nitrogen, and because a methyl-group is not mobile like a hydrogen ion, there can be no neutral species corresponding to structure (*10.2*). Thus one might suppose that it would remain ionized at every pH. However, this ion undergoes a slow, reversible reaction with a hydroxyl ion which, by the formation of a new covalent bond, produces the neutral molecule (*10.3*) (Magrath and Phillips, 1949). This secondary alcohol is the pseudo-base of (*10.2*). Pseudo-bases have a much greater liposolubility than the cations from which they are derived, and it is probably in the form of the pseudo-bases that these ions enter cells. No explanation of the action of the trypanocidal quaternary heterocycles (see Section 10.3d) can be complete without considering both the equilibrium, e.g. (*10.2*) ⇌ (*10.3*), and the time of half conversion ($t_{\frac{1}{2}}$).

This tendency to pseudo-base formation increases with the complexity of the heterocyclic nucleus. Thus, whereas pseudo-base formation does not occur for the 1-methylpyridinium cation, and only at a very high pH for the 1-methylquinolinium and 2-methylisoquinolinium ions, the reaction takes place much more readily upon further annelation (as in 10-methylacridinium). The insertion of an electron-attracting substituent (such as $-NO_2$), or a second doubly-bound ring-nitrogen atom, as in quinoxalinium and quinazolinium, has the same effect. Some examples are listed in Table 10.5, in which pK_{ROH} is the pH at which the pseudo-base and the quaternary cation are present in equal concentrations. Formally pK_{ROH} is similar to a pK_a value, but the equilibrium is only slowly achieved.

Formula (*10.4*) shows the cation of parafuchsin, a typical triphenylmethane dye, which reacts slowly with hydroxyl ions to give the pseudo-base (*10.5*). Pseudo-bases of both types (*10.3*) and (*10.5*) react rapidly with alcohols to give colourless ethers; hence alcoholic extraction must be avoided in colorimetric estimation of the amount of dye taken up by a biological specimen.

Table 10.5

EQUILIBRIUM BETWEEN QUATERNARY CATIONS
AND THEIR PSEUDO-BASES

Quaternary cations	pK_{ROH}
1-Methylquinolinium	~ 16
2-Methylisoquinolium	~ 15
10-Methylacridinium	9.9
5-Methylphenanthridinium (10.2)	10.4
1-Methyl-3-nitroquinolinium	6.7
2-Methyl-4-nitroisoquinolinium	5.0
1-Methylquinoxalinium	8.6
3-Methylquinazolinium	< 7

(Bunting and Meathrel, 1972)

Zwitterions are usually rather inert pharmacologically. For example histidine, which is a zwitterion, has none of the marked physiological properties shown by the closely related cationic substance, histamine. Again the vinyl group of quinine can be oxidized to a carboxylic acid, thereby converting the cation to a zwitterion: concomitantly, the anti-malarial properties disappear. When this acid (quitenine) is esterified, the substance of necessity becomes cationic again and this ester is strongly antimalarial (Goodson, Henry, and MacFie, 1930). Similar examples have been found in the acridine series (see Section 10.3a).

10.3 Substances that are more biologically active when ionized

It is now known that many kinds of organic cations are antibacterial, but this knowledge came only in the second quarter of this century. It had been found earlier that aliphatic amines (which exist mainly as cations at pH 7) were bactericidal, and aromatic amines (which exist mainly as molecules at pH 7) were not. However, no early worker sensed a connection between antisepsis and organic cations; antibacterial activity was supposed to be due 'to the presence of hydroxyl ions liberated through ionization of the alkylammonium hydroxides which are formed through the combination of the amines with water' (Morgan and Cooper, 1912). In other words, the effect was ascribed to alkalinity: yet the same bases, tested in the form of salts or in a neutral buffer solution, show the same bactericidal properties. The problem began to be better understood in 1924 when Stearn and Stearn suggested that triphenylmethane dyes owe their anti-bacterial activity to a reaction of the *cation* with some anionic groups of bacteria to give feebly dissociated complexes of the type discussed in Section 10.2 [cf. Equation (vi)]. Although the Stearns did not know the percentage ionization of their dyes,* they predicted that the salts of many strong bases would be found to be antibacterial because these would provide a sufficient supply of cations in the physiological pH range. They also showed that increasing the pH of the medium increased the antibacterial activity by bringing about increased (anionic) ionization of the receptors of the bacterium. They pointed out that this alkalization of the medium must not be carried to the point where it begins to suppress the ionization of the antiseptic itself.

The first rigorous proof of a positive correlation between ionization and biological action was made 17 years later (Albert, Rubbo, and Goldacre, 1941). This work showed that a quantitative relationship existed between antibacterial action and the percentage ionized as cations in the amino-acridine series. This correlation was then confirmed and extended (Albert et al., 1945).

Proflavine
(3,6-diaminoacridine)
(10.6)

Aminacrine
(9-aminoacridine)
(10.7)

(a) *The antibacterial aminoacridines*

Acridine (2.15) is a planar, feebly basic molecule. However, two of the five possible mono-aminoacridines are rather strong bases, namely the 3- and 9-amino isomers; this strength comes from the resonance immanent in their cations as explained in Section 2.2 (p. 31). For reasons of valency there can be no extra resonance in 2- or 4-aminoacridine, and there is little in the 1-isomer because an *ortho*quinonoid disposition of bonds (which it would require) is energetically unfavoured (Albert and Goldacre, 1946; Albert, Goldacre and Phillips, 1948).

The aminoacridines were introduced by the Scottish pathologist Carl Browning in 1913 as antibacterials for use in wounds. One of these, pro-flavine (10.6) (3,6-diaminoacridine), was shown to be toxic to a wide range of Gram-positive and -negative organisms without injurious effect on human tissues (Browning and Gilmour, 1913; Browning et al., 1917; War Office, 1922). The quaternized acridines, such as euflavine, are more toxic to mammals yet no more active as antibacterials than the non-quaternized acridines, such as proflavine. Apart from these quaternized acridines, no source of pseudo-bases is encountered in the acridine series; thus the difficulties encountered in working with triphenylmethane dyes were easily avoided.

---

* The ionizations could not be measured at that time because of technical difficulties with pseudo-bases, since overcome (Goldacre and Phillips, 1949; Bunting and Meathrel, 1972).

Preliminary experiments in 1939 had convinced my colleagues and myself that acridines became more antibacterial in proportion as they became more ionized, i.e. as cations (Albert, *et al.*, 1941). These results were extended to 101 acridines and 22 species of bacteria (Albert, Rubbo and Goldacre, 1945; Albert and Goldacre, 1948). Some typical results are given in Table 10.6, which is an expansion of Table 2.2, in terms of derivatives tested. For comparison of 100 derivatives, see Albert (1966, p. 437).

Of the five possible mono-aminoacridines, two are well ionized at pH 7,

Table 10.6

DEPENDENCE OF BACTERIOSTASIS ON IONIZATION IN THE ACRIDINE SERIES

Acridine	Minimal bacteriostatic concentration for Strept. pyogenes (48 *hours* incubation in 10 *per cent* serum broth at 37°C; pH 7.3)	Per cent ionized as cation (pH 7.3, 37°C)
(unsubstituted)	1 in 5000	1
4-Amino-	5000	< 1
2-Amino-	10 000	2
1-Amino-	10 000	2
4,5-Diamino-	< 5000	< 1
2,7-Diamino-	20 000	4
3-Amino-	80 000	72
9-Amino- (aminacrine) (*10.7*)	160 000	99
3,9-Diamino-	160 000	100
3,7-Diamino-	160 000	76
3,6-Diamino- (proflavine) (*10.6*)	160 000	99
2-Amino-9-methyl-	20 000	3
1-Amino-4-methyl-	20 000	1
4-Amino-5-methyl-	< 5000	< 1
2-Amino-6-chloro-	< 5000	< 1
3-Amino-9-chloro-	< 5000	11
3-Amino-7-chloro-	40 000	20
3-Amino-6-chloro-	40 000	24
9-Amino-1-methyl	160 000	99
9-Amino-2-methyl	160 000	99
9-Amino-3-methyl	160 000	99
9-Amino-4-methyl-	320 000	99
9-Amino-1-chloro-	160 000	86
9-Amino-2-chloro-	160 000	94
9-Amino-3-choloro-	160 000	98
9-Amino-4-chloro-	80 000	83

(Albert, Rubbo, Goldacre, Davey, and Stone, 1945.)

whereas the remainder are poorly ionized. (The chemical reason for this difference was given in Section 2.2, p. 31.) It can be seen from Table 10.6 that the two isomers which are well ionized have a powerful antibacterial action, whereas the three that are poorly ionized have only a feeble action.

Table 10.7

COMPARATIVE SENSITIVITY OF 22 SPECIES OF BACTERIA TOWARD AMINOACRIDINES
Highest dilutions completely preventing visible growth
in 48 hours at 37°C
(Medium: 10 per cent serum broth, pH 7.3)
All substances were completely ionized under the conditions of the test

Organism		A	B	C	D	E
Gram-positive species:						
Cl. welchii	1 in	320 000	640 000	160 000	1 280 000	320 000
Cl. sporogenes		160 000	320 000	160 000	640 000	160 000
B. subtilis		80 000	160 000	80 000	320 000	80 000
B. anthracis		160 000	320 000	80 000	640 000	80 000
Strep. pneumoniae		320 000	320 000	160 000	640 000	160 000
Strept. pyogenes A		160 000	320 000	160 000	640 000	160 000
Strept. viridans		160 000	640 000	160 000	640 000	160 000
Staph. aureus		40 000	80 000	40 000	160 000	40 000
Lactobacillus		320 000	320 000	160 000	640 000	160 000
C. diphtheriae		160 000	320 000	40 000	320 000	160 000
Mycobact. phlei		160 000	320 000	160 000	640 000	160 000
Average inhibitory dilution		160 000	300 000	110 000	540 000	140 000
Gram-negative species:						
E. Coli		40 000	40 000	20 000	40 000	40 000
Proteus vulgaris		40 000	40 000	10 000	20 000	40 000
Ps. pyocyanea				(completely inactive)		
B. Friedlanderi		80 000	80 000	20 000	160 000	80 000
Eberthella typhosum		80 000	160 000	80 000	80 000	80 000
Shigella dysenteriae		320 000	320 000	160 000	320 000	320 000
Vibrio cholarae		160 000	160 000	160 000	320 000	160 000
Pastuerella		160 000	160 000	40 000	160 000	160 000
Brucella		640 000	640 000	320 000	1 280 000	320 000
Haem. influenzae		320 000	640 000	320 000	640 000	160 000
Neiss. meningitidis		320 000	640 000	320 000	2 560 000	320 000
Average inhibitory dilution		100 000	130 000	60 000	150 000	100 000

A 9-Aminoacridine (10.7) (aminacrine).   B 4-Methyl-9-aminoacridine.
C 3,6-Diaminoacridine (10.6) (proflavine).   D 3,6-Diamino-4,5-dimethylacridine.
E 3,7-Diaminoacridine.
(Albert et al., 1945).

The same correlation is seen in the remaining parts of Table 10.6 (compare the *well* ionized methyl-aminoacridines with the *poorly* ionized methyl-aminoacridines, and the well ionized chloro-aminoacridines with their poorly ionized isomers). In all cases ionization has brought about a large increase in activity: usually eight- to sixteen-fold. Plainly, structure is relatively unimportant in this series except in so far as it influences ionization. This is true for a wide variety of bacterial species (see Table 10.7 which extends Table 2.6 in terms of species, both Gram-positive and -negative).

For a further extension of Table 10.6 to include many more acridines and species of bacteria (anaerobes and aerobes, Gram-positive and -negative), all supporting the correlation of bacteriostasis with ionization, see Albert (1966).

The ionization which governs the antibacterial action of acridines must be *cationic* in character. By inserting acidic groups into the nucleus of a strongly basic acridine, it is easy to make a substance which is zwitterionic, and hence no longer cationic. Such a substance is 9-aminoacridine-2-carboxylic acid (Table 10.8). It is seen that this has lost its antibacterial action, but regains it upon esterification which restores the cationic condition. By inserting acidic groups into the nucleus of a weekly basic acridine, an anionic substance is formed. Such a substance is acridine-9-carboxylic acid (Table 10.8). It is seen that this substance, like its ester and like acridine itself (none of them cationic), has no appreciable antibacterial action.

Much more has been learnt about the mode of action of acridines by

Table 10.8

IMPORTANCE OF CATIONIC IONIZATION FOR BACTERIOSTASIS
IN THE ACRIDINE SERIES

Substance	Min. bacteriostatic concentration for Strept. pyog. after 48 hours' incubation at 37°C (Medium 10 per cent serum broth; pH = 7.3)	Per cent ionized (pH 7.3; 37°C)			
		Cation	Anion	Zwitter-ion	Neutral molecule
9-Aminoacridine (*10.7*)	1 in 160 000	99	0	0	0
9-Aminoacridine-2-carboxylic acid	< 5000	0	0.2	99.8	0
Methyl ester of above	160 000	89	0	0	11
Acridine	5000	0.3	0	0	99.7
Acridine-9-carboxylic acid	< 5000	0	99.3	0.7	0
Methyl ester of above	< 5000	0	0	0	100

(Albert, Rubbo, Goldacre, Davey, and Stone, 1945.)

using a test-organism that withstands both acid and alkaline media (*E. coli*). In Fig. 10.2, the logarithms of the minimal bacteriostatic concentrations of four acridines have been plotted against a range of pH values from 5.5 to 8.5.

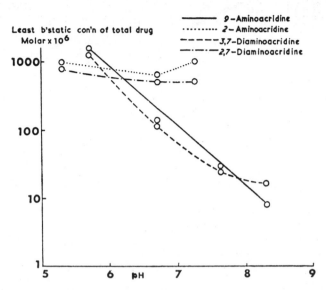

FIG. 10.2 Competition between hydrogen ions and acridines (cations + molecules). Organism: *E. coli*.

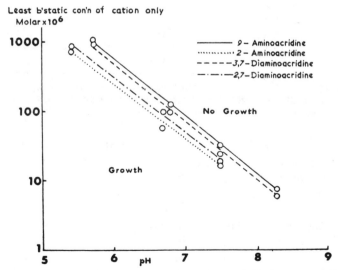

FIG. 10.3 Competition between hydrogen ions and acridine cations. Organism: *E. coli*.

One of these acridines is a strong enough base to be ionized throughout this pH range, the others are not. It will be seen that the result is a
rather disorderly set of curves. However, when the amount of actual
cation (instead of the total amount of substance) is plotted on the ordinate,
an orderly set is obtained (Fig. 10.3). These curves make a family of parallel
straight lines, and they lead to some interesting conclusions.

Firstly, it is evident that the most important factor governing bacteriostasis at any pH is the amount of the acridine *present as cation* (this
depends on both the pH of the medium and the pK_a of the acridine; see
Table 10.2) and not the total amount of the acridine (cation + neutral
species). Secondly, the slope of the curve shows that there is direct competition between acridine cations and hydrogen ions. The simplest interpretation is that acridine cations compete with hydrogen ions for a vitally
important anionic group on the bacterium. The location of this site is
discussed below. That cations of the same size and flatness as those under
discussion can liberate hydrogen ions from bacteria is evident from
Table 10.9.

Table 10.9

LIBERATION OF HYDROGEN IONS FROM *BACILLUS BELLUS*,
CAUSED BY ADSORPTION OF CRYSTAL VIOLET CATIONS*

(1) pH *of bacterial suspension*	(2) pH *of crystal violet solution*	(3) pH *of mixture of* 1 *and* 2	Fall in pH *caused by adsorption*
8.5	8.5	6.6	1.9
6.5	6.3	4.8	1.7
5.5	5.5	3.8	1.7
5.0	5.1	3.5	1.6
4.1	4.2	3.0	1.1

(McCalla, 1941.)
*pH was measured with a glass electrode. Crystal violet is the *NN'N''*-hexamethyl-
derivative of parafuchsin (6.54).

Fig. 10.3 also suggested that a smaller amount of an aminoacridine would
be effective in wounds if these were prevented from becoming acid. Some
very interesting work along these lines was carried out during the Second
World War by the Australian Army, who had adopted 9-aminoacridine
hydrochloride as the best of the aminoacridines. They recommended
that sodium bicarbonate lavage should precede treatment with this acridine
(*10.7*). The excellent results of this therapy established it as a valuable
measure for the prevention and treatment of sepsis in war wounds, even
deep, ramifying, purulent, and neglected wounds. As a result of the laboratory tests, summarized in Tables 10.6 and 10.7, and the clinical success

in treatment of severe war wounds (Poate, 1944; Turnbull, 1944), this acridine was made official in the British Pharmacopoeia, under the name Aminacrine.

The four steps that led to the discovery of the exact site of action of aminoacridines were, (i) the discovery that only *flat* molecules were effective (Albert, Rubbo, and Burvill, 1949), (ii) finding that aminoacridines stain only the DNA and RNA of vertebrate cells (Strugger, 1940), (iii) discovery that aminoacridines are intercalated into DNA, (Lerman, 1961), and (iv) finding that aminoacridines inhibited bacterial DNA polymerase by binding to the DNA starter (Hurwitz *et al.*, 1962). Evidence relevant to (ii) and (iv) will be considered now, whilst that relevant to (i) and (iii) is deferred to Section 10.3b because evidence from larger and smaller nuclei also is concerned.

Vital staining. It is firmly established that living mammalian cells, including those of the brain (Manifold, 1941) are not easily harmed by aminoacridines (Russell and Falconer, 1941, 1943; Selbie and McIntosh, 1943). In 1940, two independent laboratories showed that aminoacridines accumulate in the nucleic acids of living vertebrate cells without harming them in any way. The RNA in the nucleolus and cytoplasm was seen to fluoresce fiery red and the DNA in the nucleus green, when viewed under the fluorescence microscope (Strugger, 1940; Bukatsch and Haitinger, 1940). Even the delicate germ cells were unharmed by the application of these stains, and subsequent reproduction took place normally. In this way, the technique of vital staining, which Ehrlich had discovered, was refined further and a clear demonstration given that *nucleic acids selectively accumulate aminoacridines* in the living cell.

The following mammalian (rat, mouse, rabbit) cells have been observed to take up aminoacridines and concentrate them in the nucleus: lung, heart, liver, bone-marrow, spleen, tongue, kidney, and small intestines (De Bruyn, Robertson, and Farr, 1950). That aminoacridines are not accumulated by the cell's protein is not surprising because their antibacterial action, *in vitro*, is not lowered by serum protein (Browning and Gilmour, 1913). Nucleic acids, on the other hand, strongly inhibit bacteriostasis by proflavine and acriflavine (McIlwain, 1941). The maximal amount of dye which dissolved DNA can bind follows an order for the mono-amino-acridines that is the same as the order of their antibacterial action, namely; 9- > 3- > 1- > 2- > 4- (Jackson and Mason, 1971).

Inhibition of polymerases. Two pieces of evidence point to the outside of the bacterial plasma membrane as the site of action of the aminoacridines. Firstly, there was no loss of antibacterial action when ionization (as cation) was increased from 70% to 100%, thus removing the more readily penetrating neutral species. Secondly, there was a great loss of activity when the aminoacridines were made more lipophilic (Albert, *et al.*, 1945).

In bacteria, a single, ring-shaped chromosome contains most of the

DNA of the cell, and it is externalized at one point of the cytoplasmic membrane (Ryter and Jacob, 1964). RNA also occurs in the cytoplasmic membrane (Yudkin and Davis, 1965) and in the ribosomes.

It has been shown, *in vitro*, that proflavine (30 µM) inhibits bacterial DNA polymerase by 85 per cent and RNA polymerase by 30 per cent (Hurwitz *et al.*, 1962). Some typical data are shown in Fig. 10.4. The inset graph (of the reciprocal of the velocity plotted against the reciprocal of the DNA-starter concentration) points to the site of action of proflavine as being mainly on this starter, thus inhibiting DNA (or RNA) synthesis in the living bacterium. The intercalating mechanism by which amino-acridines combine with DNA helices and impede strand separation is outlined in the next Section (10.3b).

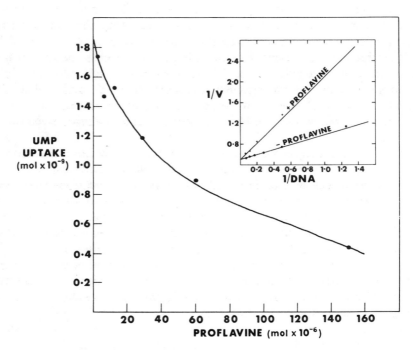

FIG. 10.4 Inhibition of RNA-polymerase by proflavine (excess of DNA, ATP, GTP, and CTP are present). (Hurwitz, *et al.*, 1962.)

It has been considered whether acridines exert some of their antibacterial action by inhibiting other enzymes. However, the known inhibitions do not seem to be very serious and usually require high concentrations, whereas quite low concentrations of aminoacridines upset the synthesis and functioning of nucleic acids (see Chapter 22 in Albert, 1966).

Ingenious attempts have been made to link the antibacterial action of aminoacridines to their oxidation-reduction potentials (Breyer, Buchanan, and Duewell, 1944), or to the stability of the free radicals produced upon reduction (Kaye, 1950). Thus E'_0 of the first step in reduction at pH 7.3 lies between -0.47 and -0.92 V for the highly antibacterial substances 3-amino-, 9-amino-, and 3,6-diamino-acridine whereas the corresponding E'_0 for the poorly antibacterial acridine and 1-, 2-, and 4-aminoacridine lies between -0.31 and -0.39 V.* Thus the small difference between a potential of -0.47 and -0.39 V would have to determine whether an acridine is antibacterial or not. That this is not the case is clearly shown in Fig. 10.3. Those acridines (e.g. 2-aminoacridine) which are feebly antibacterial at pH 7.3 (where they are poorly ionized) become as active as those that are highly antibacterial at pH 7.3 when the pH is lowered to a value (say 5.4) where both kinds of acridine are well ionized. Because this fall in pH does not lessen the difference in reduction potential between 2- and 3-aminoacridine, it must be concluded that reduction potentials do not affect antibacterial activity in the acridine series.

The free radical hypothesis also is incorrect, because the free radicals in question are the product of the first step in the reduction of *all* these acridines. Completely unreducible substances such as 2-anthrylguanidine (Table 10.10) can possess a typical acridine-type antibacterial action. [Anthracenes show no reductive step even at -2.0 V (Zanker and Schnith, 1959)].

The action of acridines on fungi will be briefly mentioned here, leaving the actions on protozoa for Section 10.3d. Although, in common with most cationic substances, aminoacridines have very little effect on fungi, a few of them have a strong transforming action on yeasts, in which they combine with the DNA occurring in the mitochondria, thus causing an inherited change (namely loss of all oxidative phosphorylation) without affecting the nucleus. The most active of these acridines is euflavine (3,6-diamino-10-methylacridinium chloride) (*6.4*) (Ephrussi and Hottinguer, 1950; Marcovich, 1953). However, the two aminoacridines found least toxic to human tissues and most useful in surgery (9-aminoacridine and 3,6-diaminoacridine) do not act in this way on yeast.

(b) *Cationic antibacterials that have the aminoacridine type of action*
The relationship between cationic ionization and antibacterial activity, as demonstrated above in the acridine series, is valid also for at least seven other series, namely the three series of benzoacridines (*10.8*) to (*10.10*) of which 16 examples were studied, the phenanthridines (*10.11*), six examples, and the three series of benzoquinolines (*10.12*) to (*10.14*) of which 21 examples were studied (Albert, Rubbo, and Burvill, 1949). Some of these examples are given in the first half of Table 10.10 (p. 359).

---

* These potentials refer to the normal hydrogen electrode. E_0 is defined in Section 11.4, and the above E'_0 values are adjusted to pH 7.3.

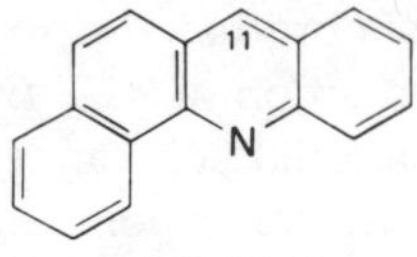

Benzo[h]acridine
(10.8)

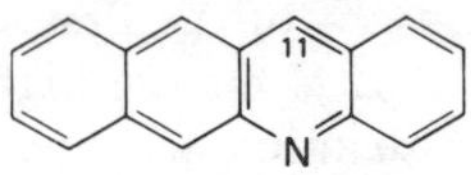

Benzo[i]acridine
(10.9)

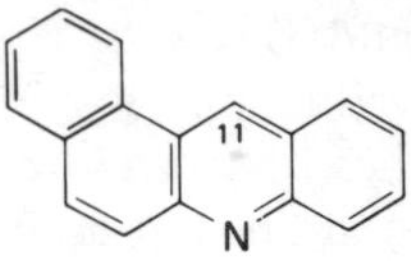

Benzo[j]acridine
(10.10)

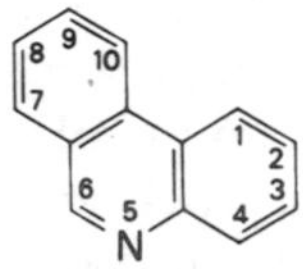

Phenanthridine
(International Union numbering)
(10.11)

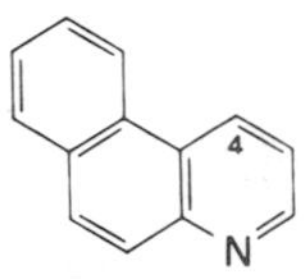

Benzo [f] quinoline
(10.12)

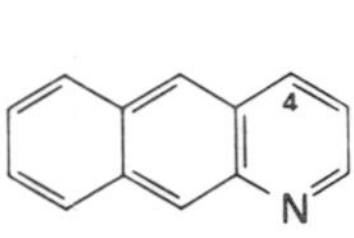

Benzo[g]quinoline
(10.13)

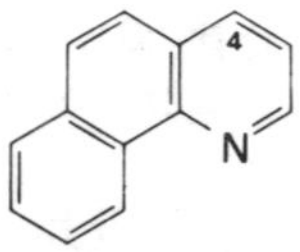

Benzo[h]quinoline
(10.14)

The requirement for flatness. My colleagues and I found that removal of one or two rings from 9-aminoacridine (10.15) produced molecules which had no antibacterial action, even though they remained completely ionized. This may be seen in Table 10.10 by comparing 9-aminoacridine (10.15) with the structurally analogous 4-aminoquinoline (10.16) and 4-amino-pyridine (10.17). The lack of antibacterial properties in the last two sub-stances has been correlated with an insufficient area of flatness in these molecules (Albert, Rubbo, and Burvill, 1949). If an envelope (as shown in Fig. 10.5) is drawn around the various nuclei, an area of only 28 Å² is obtained for quinoline and 17 Å² for pyridine, whereas acridine has an area of 38 Å².

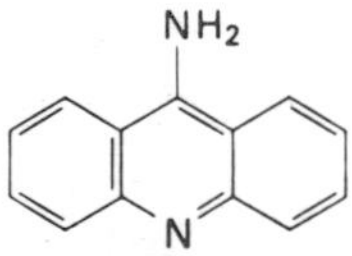

9-Aminoacridine
(1 : 160 000)
(10.15)

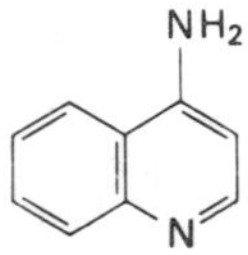

4-Aminoquinoline
(< 1 : 5000)
(10.16)

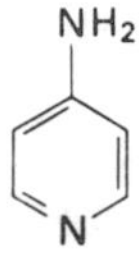

4-Aminopyridine
(< 1 : 5000)
(10.17)

NH₂

9-Aminotetrahydrocridine
(1 : 5000)
(*10.18*)

NH₂

4-Amino-2-styryl-quinoline
(1 : 80 000)
(*10.19*)

1 : 160 000 (etc) = minimal bacteriostatic concentration, as in Table 10.10

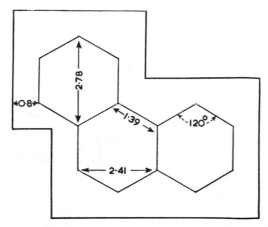

FIG. 10.5 Minimal rectangular envelope, drawn at a distance of 0.8 Å from the carbon and nitrogen atoms.

All the heterocyclic nuclei discussed so far are perfectly flat, because they are conjugated throughout (i.e. every second bond is a double-bond). However, when 9-aminoacridine (*10.15*) is hydrogenated in one ring, to give 9-aminotetrahydroacridine (*10.18*), only 28 Å² of flat surface remain, because hydrogenated rings are always three-dimensionally voluminous. Coincident with this change in flat area, the antibacterial activity almost completely vanishes.

This insight into the planarity required for activity at once suggested that it should be possible to create highly antibacterial quinolines and pyridines by the insertion of a group to increase the total area of flatness of the molecule. It is known, from X-ray diffraction studies, that stilbene is a perfectly flat molecule*, hence it was thought that the addition of a styryl-group to 4-aminoquinoline [giving (*10.19*)] would produce a highly antibacterial compound. This indeed proved to be the case (see Table 9.10), and the addition of two styryl-groups to 4-aminopyridine was similarly successful (Albert *et al.*, 1949).

* Diphenyl, on the contrary, is not flat (Karle and Brockway, 1944).

It should be pointed out that all the substances under discussion, (*10.15*) to (*10.19*), are completely ionized at pH 7. Analogues of (*10.19*) which were not well ionized were not antibacterial. In the larger nuclei with a sufficient area of flatness (such as the acridine nucleus), cationic ionization is the only important limiting factor; but in the smaller nuclei (such as quinoline and pyridine), the minimal flat area of the molecule becomes another limiting factor.

Representations of the cations of 9-aminoacridine (*10.15*) and its tetrahydro-derivative (*10.18*) are shown in Plate 4. These have been built from space-filling models which produce the correct interatomic and van der Waals distances. The non-coplanarity of the tetrahydro-derivative is clearly seen, especially in the side view.

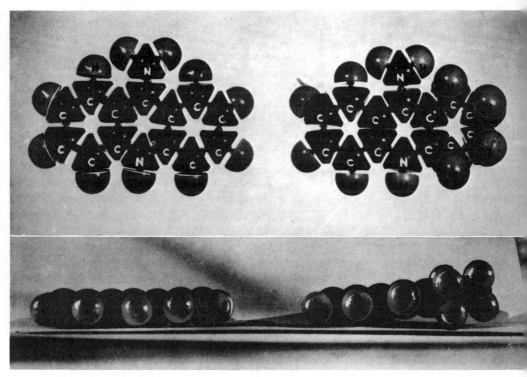

PLATE 4 Accurate space models of the ions of 9-aminoacridine (left-hand figures) and tetrahydro-9-aminoacridine (right-hand figures) (see p. 355.)

Why is the size of the flat area of these cations so important? Obviously, increasing the number of atoms in a molecule can increase its chances of adsorption. This is because the small van der Waals forces, each of which unites an atom of the agent to an atom of the receptor, become collectively a really strong force when a larger number of atoms are concerned on each side. This force is opposed by the molecule's kinetic energy of translation, which does not increase as the size of the molecule increases. The ion-pair formed by the cation (drug) and an anion (on the receptor) would be very short-lived without supplementary bonds of this kind (Section 8.0). The special requirement of the present series, namely that the atoms in the drug should all lie *in one plane*, revealed that the atoms in the biological surface with which they had to make effective contact also lay in one plane.

It may be asked whether one may expect to obtain powerful antibacterials of the acridine type (i.e. acting at great dilution against both Gram-positive and -negative species, an action not decreased by the presence of protein) from *all* molecules having sufficient cationic ionization and area of flatness. The answer is 'yes', so long as the substance is chemically stable. A typical unstable substance is methylene blue, flat and highly ionized, but with a reduction potential so large that the cations are reduced by the metabolic products of most bacteria, such as *E. coli*; it is toxic to a related strain *Aerobacter aerogenes*, which cannot reduce it (the product of reduction is not ionized at pH 7). However, there are very definite limitations to the number of flat heteroaromatic nuclei which can yield highly ionizing amino-derivatives, because heteroatoms, in excess of one, tend drastically to reduce basic strength (Albert, Goldacre, and Phillips, 1948; Albert, 1968).

We found that this difficulty can be overcome by building a short, highly basic side-chain on to a flat aromatic 38 Å^2 nucleus, so long as side-chain and nucleus are conjugated with one another. A guanidine or diguanide side-chain is suitable. In such a case, the nucleus need not be heteroaromatic: an aromatic hydrocarbon nucleus of the appropriate dimensions (e.g. anthracene) will do. Using this hypothesis, we soon found substances having a true 'acridine-type' antibacterial activity without any heterocyclic nucleus; the two anthracene derivatives in Table 10.10 are examples (Albert *et al.*, 1949).

It is surprising how closely the biochemical action of acridine analogues follows that of the acridines. Thus homidium bromide ('Ethidium'*) (*10.22*) inhibits the same two DNA-dependent polymerases as proflavine does, namely the one which synthesizes DNA and (although less strongly) the one that synthesizes RNA, by combining in each case with the DNA template (Elliott, 1963; Waring, 1965).

How acridines, and their analogues, are bound to nucleic acids. It has been shown, *in vitro*, that proflavine (*10.6*) (3,6-diaminoacridine) is bound to DNA by two mechanisms, (a) a first-order reaction that reaches equilibrium at one proflavine per four or five nucleotides, and (b) a weaker,

---

* Protozoologists, if inclined to molecular biology, often use this name, although it is a registered trade mark.

2-Anthrylguanidine
(*10.20*)

2-Anthryldiguanide
(*10.21*)

Homidium bromide ('Ethidium')
(*10.22*)

higher-order process that leads to the fixation of one proflavine molecule per nucleotide (Peacocke and Skerrett, 1956). The latter process apparently consists of an adsorption of further acridine molecules, very loosely, on to the outside of the DNA helix.

In 1961, Lerman suggested that the stronger attachment was caused by the *intercalation** of a 3,6-diaminoacridine molecule between two layers of base-pairs in such a way that the primary amino-groups were held in ionic linkage by two phosphoric acid residues of the Watson-Crick spiral, and the flat skeleton of the acridine ring rested on the purine and pyrimidine molecules to which it was held by van der Waals forces (Lerman, 1964a).

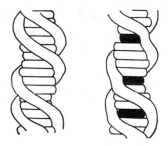

FIG. 10.6 Sketches representing the secondary structure of normal DNA (left) and DNA containing intercalated proflavine molecules (right). The helix is drawn as viewed from a remote point, so that the base-pairs and the intercalated proflavine appear only in edgewise projection, and the phosphate deoxyribose backbone appears as a smooth coil. (After Lerman, 1964b.)

* A word whose meaning had been confined to the insertion of February 29th into the leap-year calendar.

Table 10.10

DEPENDENCE OF BACTERIOSTASIS ON (a) IONIZATION, AND
(b) FLAT AREA OF MOLECULE, IN A SERIES OF CATIONIC AGENTS
(For other examples and other bacteria, *see* Albert, *et al.*, 1949)

Substance	Min. bacteriostatic concentration for Strept. pyog. after 48 hours' incubation at 37°C. (*Medium*: 10 per cent serum broth; pH = 7.3)	Per cent ionized (pH 7.3; 37°C)	Flat area estimated as in Fig. 9.5 (sq. Å)
Acridine	1 in 5000	1	38.5
9-Amino (*10.15*)	160 000	100	38.5
Benzo [*h*] acridine	< 5000	< 1	48.7
11-Amino	160 000	97	48.7
Benzo[*i*] acridine (*10.9*)	10 000	< 1	48.9
11-Amino	320 000	100	48.9
Benzo[*j*] acridine	< 5000	< 1	48.7
11-Amino	160 000	98	48.7
Phenanthridine (*10.11*)	10 000	< 1	38.3
6-Amino	40 000	50	38.3
3,6,8-Triamino	80 000	98	38.3
Benzo [*f*] quinoline (*10.12*)	5000	< 1	38.3
4-Amino	20 000	98	38.3
Benzo[*g*] quinoline	10 000	< 1	
4-Amino	40 000	100	38.3
Benzo[*h*] quinoline	< 5000	< 1	
4-Amino	80 000	96	
Quinoline	< 5000	< 1	27.9
4-Amino (*10.16*)	< 5000	98	27.9
4-Amino-2-styryl (*10.19*)	80 000	99	49.9
Pyridine	< 5000	< 1	17.4
4-Amino (*10.17*)	< 5000	98	17.4
4-Amino-2,6-distyryl	80 000	95	61.6
9-Amino-5,6,7,8-tetrahydro acridine (*10.18*)	5000	100	27.9
Phenylguanidine	< 5000	100	17
2-Anthrylguanidine (*10.20*)	40 000	100	38.5
Phenyl-N_1-diguanide	< 5000	100	17
2-Anthryl-N_1- diguanide (*10.21*)	40 000	100	38.5

(Albert, Rubbo, and Burvill, 1949.)

An edgewise view of this arrangement is shown in Fig. 10.6 (p. 358). The need a large flat area in the antibacterial molecules, as discussed above, was now explained, and so was the requirement for ionization.

It is evident from X-ray diffraction data that the base layers of DNA are, normally, making van der Waals contact with one another above and below, and that the distance between the centres of the atoms, in adjacent pairs on a strand, is 3.36 Å. This means that another 3.36 Å of space (6.72 Å in all) must be provided to admit the aminoacridine molecules, which have exactly the same thickness as those of the purine and pyrimidine bases. This space could be provided, if the helix untwisted slightly,* and that turned out to be exactly what happened.

The steps by which Lerman reached this picture of intercalation will now be given. The interaction between proflavine and DNA gave a three-fold increase in *viscosity*. This change was attributed to the helix being not only extended, but also stiffened and straightened by the intercalated molecules. The DNA-proflavine complex was found to have a lower *sedimentation coefficient* than free DNA. This was attributed to loss of mass per unit length (a proflavine molecule has less than half the mass of the same volume of DNA). The above results were obtained in dilute aqueous solution. It was also found that fibres drawn from the complex gave much simpler *X-ray diffraction patterns* than those given by pure DNA. The meridional spot, corresponding to the 3.4 Å separation between stacked layers, was retained but the new positions of the first equatorial reflections suggested that each DNA molecule was now more closely packed than pure DNA and hence had a smaller diameter (Lerman, 1961). In 1963, Lerman showed that the ratio of the fluorescence intensities of *flowing and stationary solutions* were compatible with perpendicularity of the acridine molecules to the helical axis. He next reported that the *rates of diazotization* of the primary amino-groups of proflavine were so much diminished in the presence of DNA as to suggest that it protected them from attack by the nitrous acid (Lerman, 1964). It was noted that an increased temperature was required to denature DNA after it had formed a complex with 9-amino-acridine (Lerman, 1964b) (cf. Chambron, below).

Meanwhile powerful support for the idea of intercalation began to arrive from other laboratories. *Autoradiography* of DNA molecules (containing ^{3}H-thymine), obtained from T2 coliphage, was performed before and after immersion in a dilute solution of proflavine. It was found that the aminoacridine had expanded the DNA strands from about 45 to 70 µm (Cairns, 1962). Equally convincing evidence came from the fact that the *melting-temperature* (T_m) of DNA was increased 20°C by proflavine, and that most of the bound proflavine was suddenly released when the

* This unwinding angle is somewhat variable, depending on the substance. For homidium ('Ethidium') it is 26°, as found from a high precision buoyant-density gradient titration (Wang, 1974); for proflavine and the alkaloid ellipticine, it is rather less (Kohn *et al.*, 1975).

complex 'melted' (i.e. the strands of the double-helix parted) (Chambron, Daune, and Sadron, 1966). This phenomenon was confirmed by Kleinwächter, Bakarova, and Bohacek (1969).

An X-ray *diffraction* study of the proflavine-DNA complex gave direct evidence of intercalation, by showing one molecule of the aminoacridine stacked parallel to the base pairs in a 1:3 ratio (Neville and Davies, 1966). *Linear and circular dichroism* studies of flowing solutions of all five mono-aminoacridines (complexed to DNA) confirm that the acridine cations lie in planes parallel to those of the base-pairs (Jackson and Mason, 1971). Finally, the *free-energy* of binding of aminoacridines to DNA was determined and found to be of the order expected for intercalation, but far too high for any form of binding on the exterior of the DNA strands (Jordan, 1968).

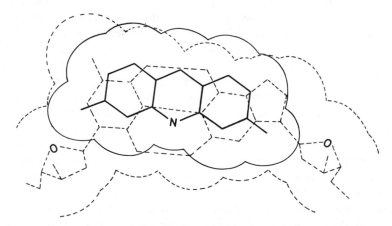

FIG. 10.7 Intercalation of 3,6-diaminoacridine into the base-pair layers of DNA. The left-hand ring of the acridine is almost superposed over cytosine, and the right-hand ring of the acridine is almost superposed over the pyrimidine ring of guanine. The van der Waals boundary of the acridine molecule is shown as an unbroken line. (After Lerman, 1964b.)

Details of intercalation, finer than those indicated in Fig. 10.6, are shown in Fig. 10.7. More recently, it was found that denatured DNA binds aminoacridines almost as well as double-stranded DNA at room temperature (Pritchard, Blake, and Peacocke, 1966). This is certainly not the case at higher temperatures; at 84°C double-stranded DNA binds much 9-aminoacridine but single-stranded DNA binds very little (at all temperatures DNA binds proflavine a little less firmly than 9-amino-acridine, but the same differences are shown between single and double strands) (Jordan and Sansom, 1971). There are, of course, numerous helical areas in cold, denatured DNA (i.e. it is not entirely single-stranded) and the presence of an aminoacridine is likely to increase their number. The flat area of an average base-pair in a DNA or RNA spiral has been calculated as about 50 Å², which is larger than the 38.5 Å² calculated for acridine by the method of Fig. 10.5. However, in any one-strand model, a little of each acridine molecule would be protruding.

One acridine proved unsuitable for investigation of intercalation: acridine orange (3,6-*bis*dimethylaminoacridine), the four methyl-groups of which caused the molecules to associate with one another on the outside of the DNA fibre.

Other substances which intercalate. As often happens with new ideas, the hypothesis of intercalation was at first held to be unlikely. However (and this, too, is usual), no sooner had it become established than the action of all kinds of drugs began to be ascribed to it. To test these claims, a standard test for intercalation became desirable. This was achieved by observing if the suspected drug causes local uncoiling of the double-helix of a supercoil of circular DNA, such as that from coliphage (Waring, 1970). During the first additions of an aminoacridine, the number of right-handed supercoils steadily decreases; at a critical ratio of added molecules, the supercoils are all removed and the DNA molecule behaves as an un-twisted open circle, of greater perimeter than before thanks to the inter-calation. As further additions of the agent are made, the accumulated stretching of the DNA ring re-introduces supercoiling, but this time it is left-handed. Because supercoils are more compact than the open circles from which they are derived, they sediment more rapidly: hence the whole process is easily observed by changes in the sedimentation coefficient, which passes through a minimum (Waring, 1970).

Using this method, intercalation was demonstrated for some amino-phenanthridines, including (*10.22*), for the antimalarial drug chloroquine (*10.28*), for three carcinostatic antibiotics: nogalomycin, daunorubicin, and actinomycin D (*4.21*) (see Section 4.0). However, chlorpromazine and lysergic acid diethylamide (LSD), for which an action by intercalation had been suggested, gave no evidence of it. The following substances were found to interact strongly with DNA without any tendency to inter-calate: spermine, streptomycin, diminazene and mithramycin (Waring, 1970).

Other important examples of intercalation have been established. The red triphenylmethane dye parafuchsin (*6.54*) intercalates with DNA, but less tightly than proflavine does (Armstrong and Panzer, 1972). The anti-leukaemic alkaloid ellipticine, which comes from a tropical evergreen tree, and which intercalates, has the planar ring structure: 5,11-dimethyl-pyrido[4,3-*b*] carbazole (Woodward, Iacobucci, and Hochstein, 1959).

Bifunctional types exist. Canellakis *et al.*, (1976) inserted an acridine nucleus into either end of the putrescine and spermine molecules, and found that the products produced a higher T_m in DNA than did single acridine intercalators, and were more strongly carcinostatic. The site of action was traced to DNA-directed RNA polymerase. Echinomycin, an antibiotic with two widely-spaced quinoxaline rings, intercalates them simultaneously into different sites of DNA, as a result of which it doubles the unwinding and extends the helix twice as far, compared to the usual amino- acridines and phenanthridines (Waring and Wakelin, 1974).

By far the most clinically useful of the newer intercalators is doxorubicin (*10.23*) (adriamycin), an antibiotic isolated from *Streptomyces peucetius* after separation from the less valuable daunorubicin (daunomycin) which has $-COCH_3$ in place of $-COCH_2OH$, and is much less selective (Arcamone *et al.*, 1969).

Doxorubicin (Adriamycin)
(*10.23*)

Adriamycin has an astonishingly higher chemotherapeutic index against solid tumours than anything known previously. It is used in the wards, quite effectively, in a wide range of sarcomas, in adenocarcinoma of the breast, carcinoma of the bladder, bronchogenic carcinoma, neuro-blastoma, and metastatic thyroid carcinoma (Blum and Carter, 1974; Gottlieb and Hill, 1974). Its chief drawback is a toxic action on the heart which, it seems, can be avoided by chelation with iron (see Section 11.5).

Daunorubicin had been shown by X-ray crystallography to intercalate into DNA (Pigram, Fuller, and Hamilton, 1972), and hence there was every reason to expect adriamycin to do so also. This has been confirmed by the rise in T_m, decrease in buoyant density, decrease in sedimentation constant, and increased viscosity of native double-stranded DNA when adriamycin is added. Moreover, the visible spectrum, fluorescence, and ease of reduction of adriamycin were altered by DNA in the directions expected for an intercalated substance. In a set of derivatives, carcinostatic activity fell off with decreasing intercalation, and also with decrease in basic strength. From these data, it was concluded that the highly basic amino-group in the sugar-residue forms an ionic bond with a phosphate group of the DNA (just as can be seen in the X-ray diagram obtained for dauno-mycin), and the flat anthraquinone skeleton lies between a layer of purine and pyrimidine bases (di Marco and Arcamone, 1975). Adriamycin inhibits DNA-directed RNA-polymerase and DNA-polymerase; the latter is inhibited 50% at 7.4 ug/ml. Probably it is a matter of distribution, but nothing has yet emerged at the molecular level, to suggest why adriamycin is so much more selective an anticancer drug than, say, the aminoacridines.

In closing this section, it is necessary to ask why aminoacridines, and cognate intercalating drugs, are so selective against bacteria and sparing of mammalian cells. It is established that intercalation, antibacterial proper-ties, and percentage-ionization are three properties that run parallel in the acridine series (Jackson and Mason, 1971). The selectivity against bacteria seems to be due to two factors, the exposed situation of the solitary chromosome in bacteria (Section 5.3), and the preference shown by inter-calating drugs for *circular* DNA (Waring, 1970). Apart from their selective action on bacteria, aminoacridines also act selectively on the following examples of circular DNA: they eliminate bacterial plasmids (Bouanchaud, Scavizzi, and Chabbert, 1968); and they produce a heritable change in yeast by suppressing replication of DNA in mitochondria without affecting that of the nucleus (see end of Section 10.3a, also Hollenberg *et al.*, 1970).

Further, aminoacridines and aminophenanthridines can either suppress the kinetoplast in trypanosomes, or (in lower concentrations) distort its circular DNA (Riou and Delain, 1969). It has been calculated that, so long as these agents are removing superhelical turns from circular DNA, a negative free-energy change is occurring which increases the affinity for the agent; whereas the same DNA, once it is nicked and becomes a strand, has a decreased affinity (Bauer and Vinograd, 1970). It looks as though this is another example of selectivity by accumulation, the type discussed in Chapter 3.

(c)   *Cationic and anionic antibacterials with other types of action*
Many other antibacterials act in the form of cations but do not have the aminoacridine type of activity, the typical features of which were given on p. 351.

The *triphenylmethane dyes*, e.g. parafuchsin (6.54), crystal violet, brilliant green, and malachite green, are cationic antibacterials of a special chemical type (p. 343). The equilibrium between the cation and its base (actually a pseudo-base) is only slowly established. Thus there are both equilibrium and ionization constants to be taken into account. These have been deter-mined by Goldacre and Phillips (1949). It can be seen from Table 2.6 that antibacterial action is linked with ionization in this series. However, unlike the aminoacridines, they have little activity against Gram-negative bacteria, and their activity against Gram-positive species is seriously depressed by serum protein (Goldacre and Phillips, 1949). The triphenyl-

methane pseudo-bases are liposoluble and penetrate cells easily. They
have non-rigid structures whereas their cations are rigid and completely
flat. The cations readily form covalent bonds with all kinds of nucleophilic
reagents.

Chlorhexidine   (*10.24*),   1,6-*bis*-(*N*-*p*-chlorophenyldiguanido)hexane,
is used as the gluconate for the disinfection of skin and mucous membranes.
It is effective in high dilutions against Gram-positive and -negative organisms, and remains bactericidal in the presence of blood. See further Section
14.2.

Aliphatic amines (including the *quaternary amines*) are also antibacterial,
but are in no way acridine-like. They cause lysis of the cell membrane
(see Section 14.2) and hence acheive a rapid bactericidal action, whereas
the acridines, which are only slowly bactericidal, are used mainly for their
bacteriostatic properties. Aliphatic amines with side-chains of C_{12} (or
longer) have this lytic action well developed. They are completely non-
rigid molecules which become easily adsorbed on the acidic groups of
serum proteins: this wasteful effect is decreased if they are quaternized
with at least one bulky substituent, such as a benzyl-group, as in Domagk's
benzalkonium chloride ('Zephiran'). Cetyl trimethylammonium bromide
is another well-known example of this class of quaternary amine. In this
series, also, the activity increases as the pH is raised, although the drug
remains completely ionized throughout (Blubaugh, Botts, and Gerwe,
1940; Gershenfeld and Milanick, 1941).

Salts of aliphatic sulphonic acids and ethereal sulphates are mildly
antibacterial if the chain has 12 or more carbon atoms (e.g. sodium tetra-
decylsulphate). These function as the anion (Gershenfeld and Milanick,
1941; Putnam and Neurath, 1944).

$$Cl-\bigcirc-NH\cdot\overset{NH}{\underset{\overset{..}{N}H}{C}}\cdot NH\cdot\overset{..}{C}\cdot NH\cdot(CH_2)_6\cdot NH\cdot\overset{NH}{\underset{\overset{..}{N}H}{C}}\cdot NH\cdot\overset{..}{C}\cdot NH-\bigcirc-Cl$$

Chlorhexidine
(*10.24*)

(d) *Antiprotozoal examples*

Many effective biocides, selective against protozoa, are the salts of strong
organic bases, and one important trypanocide is the salt of a strong organic
acid.

Flagellates.   Attention has already been drawn to the collossal consumption of food by trypanosomes, as necessitated by their constant movement
(Section 4.9). This Achilles' heel is attacked by the arsenical trypanocides:
tryparsamide (*6.6*) and melarsoprol (*12.4*), but their principal use is in a
late stage of the disease. Another site for selective attack was indicated at the
end of Section 10.3b, namely the ability of amino-acridines and -phen-

anthridines, by combining with its circular DNA, to distort and eventually suppress the kinetoplast in these flagellates. The kinetoplast carries information to make mitochondria in that alternative form of the parasite which exists in the insect vector (a fly). Although drugs which injure the kinetoplast effectively prevent transmission to this secondary host, and hence can break an epidemic, they give no help to the infected patient. Rather, the curative effect of cationic drugs depends on their injury of nucleolus, ribosomes, and lysosomes (Williamson, Macadam, and Dixon, 1975).

Because pathogenic trypanosomes are difficult to grow in culture, much work has been done on a related, easily grown, protozoon, *Crithidia oncopelti* (also known as *Strigomonas*). Recently, these difficulties have been mastered, and more relevant tests have been done with highly pathogenic trypanosomes (*Tr. rhodesiense*). This organism was examined *in vitro*, in the presence of drugs, for (a) loss of mobility as an index of injury to energy yielding metabolism, and (b) infectivity for mice as an index of injury to cell-division. In a third test, an infection sustained in mice by this strain was treated with the same drugs. It was found that suramin (6.7) first injured the structure of ribosomes and then suppressed cell division. Homidium (*10.22*) ('Ethidium') and quinapyramine (*10.26*) ('Antrycide') injured the kinetoplast and suppressed cell-division. Pentamidine (*10.25*) primarily inhibited glycolysis, but also injured the kinetoplast (DNA) and nucleolus (RNA) (Williamson, Macadam, and Dixon, 1975).

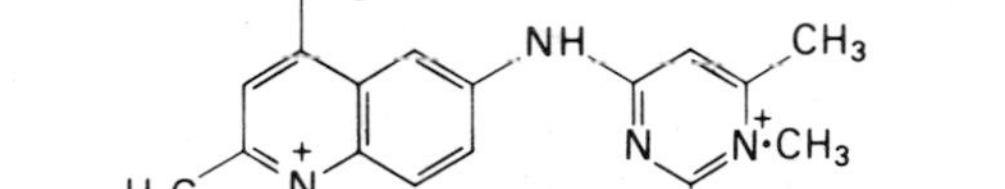

Pentamidine
(*10.25*)

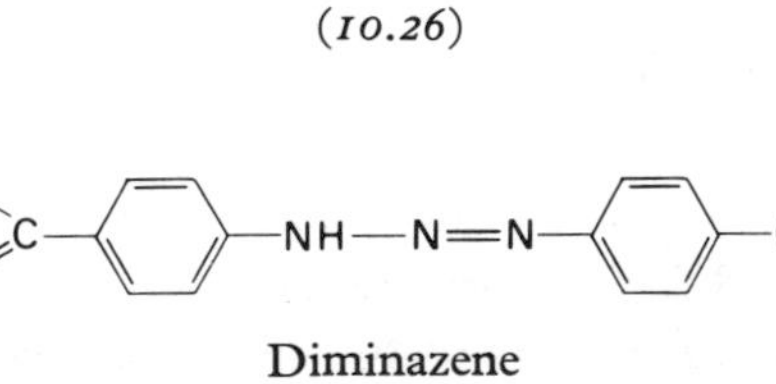

Quinapyramine (di-cation)
(*10.26*)

Diminazene
(*10.27*)

It is common practice to protect residents in tropical Africa against trypanosomiasis by injecting pentamidine (*10.25*) or suramin (*6.7*) every
three months. Pentamidine and diminazene (*10.27*) are used in the treatment of established infections. Neither of these drugs intercalates (Waring,
1970), but each of them binds across the small groove of the DNA helix-
ring in the kinetoplast, cross-linking by attachment of each amidine-group
to a phosphate anion (Festy, Sturm, and Daune 1975). However their
selective damping down of carbohydrate metabolism by inhibiting
α-glycerophosphate oxidase, even at a dilution of 2 μM (Fairlamb and
Bowman, 1975) plays a more important role in treatment, and the molecular
basis for this is not known. Homidium acts similarly.

Pentamidine is rapidly absorbed by trypanosomes and at once exerts
a trypanostatic effect on them, both *in vitro* and *in vivo* (Hawking, 1944).
The parasites are finally killed by the body's defensive forces, some days
later. [For the distribution of these and other amines in trypanosomes,
see Williamson and Macadam (1965).] One indirect factor that helps a cure
is the following. Those parasites that survive the direct effect of the drug
remain infective, but they show a large number of drug-containing granules.
When the first of these parasites die, they liberate the drug, and also an
antigen which causes the host to make an adequate amount of antibody.
This indirect process is believed to explain the slow onset of the curative
action of the diamidine drugs, and their prolonged prophylactic effect
(Fulton and Grant, 1956). When the immune response of a rat was blocked
by splenectomy, or by injecting copper, trypanosomiasis could no longer
be cured by stilbamidine, suramin, or quinapyramine (Ormerod, 1961).

It is relevant to the action of diamidines on DNA that spermine (*11.4*),
so widely present in Nature (Cohen, 1971), has been shown by X-ray
diffraction to combine with DNA by spanning the double-helix across the
minor groove, and forming ionic linkages with the phosphate anions
(Suwalsky *et al.*, 1969). The interval between phosphate groups is 10 Å
across the minor groove, and 20 Å across the major. The exceptionally
strong and durable nature of the ionic linkages given by amidines has
already been indicated (*8.4*). Diminazene (*10.27*), 4,4′diamidino-diazamino-
benzene ('Berenil'), is a more recently introduced trypanocide which
selectively binds to the circular DNA of the kinetoplast without affecting
the parasites' nuclear DNA.

Two types of cationic trypanocides are used exclusively for treating
the disease in cattle, horses, and camels, namely the phenanthridines,
[particularly homidium (*10.22*) ('Ethidium')] and quinapyramine (*10.26*),
whereas diminazene is used for both humans and stock. Quinapyramine and
the phenanthridines are quaternary amines in equilibria with their pseudo-
bases, the section on which (p. 342) may be useful here too. The aromatic
diamidines, however, are uncomplicated strong bases of pK_a 11.

Few anionic drugs are used in human medicine, and of these suramin

(6.7) is one of the most important. Weekly injection with this drug is still considered a very acceptable alternative to treatment with pentamidine or diminazene. The human body retains suramin, bound to protein, as a depot. The structure of this drug is remarkably specific in that the removal of the two methyl groups abolishes activity completely. Nevertheless, quite unrelated polyanions, such as dextran sulphate have strong, if not quite medically useful, trypanocidal action. It has long been known that suramin abolishes the infectivity of trypanosomes without affecting their mobility (Roehl, 1926b). The electron microscope shows that this drug strikes hard and specifically at the parasite's ribosomes which lose their polysomal character and form the 'cytoplasmic granules' described by the light microscopists. Fundamentally their attack seems to be on RNA polymerase; the nucleus, nucleolus, and kinetoplast remain unaffected and the synthesis of DNA continues (Macadam and Williamson, 1974).

The aromatic diamidines are also effective in treating leishmaniasis, another disease caused by flagellates. Suramin is also much used for treating onchocerciasis, caused by guinea worms (Section 6.3e).

Sporozoa.   Compared to flagellates, these protozoa lead a placid existence, but they have a more complicated life cycle. The genus *Plasmodium* causes the various types of malaria.

Acridines become strongly antimalarial if substituted with a basic side-chain in the 9-position, but are inactive if quaternized. Mepacrine (Fig. 10.8) (quinacrine, 'Atebrin') was the first antimalarial acridine, and the first synthetic antimalarial to achieve widespread use. For further information, on connections between structure and action in the acridine antimalarials, see Albert (1966).

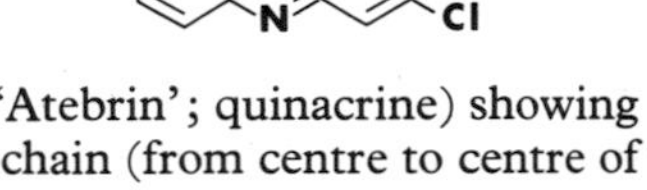

FIG. 10.8 Mepacrine ('Atebrin'; quinacrine) showing distance between nitrogens of side-chain (from centre to centre of the atoms).

Simplification of mepacrine led to the colourless analogue chloroquine (*10.28*) (7-chloro-4-δ-diethylamino-α-methylbutylaminoquinoline), another effective schizontocide much used in the treatment of malaria. It stays a little longer in the body than mepacrine does, but a larger dose is needed. Clinical studies with dabechin, a 4-aminobenzo[g]quinoline, are giving promising results in the USSR. These antimalarials are not trypanocidal, and trypanocides are not antimalarial.

Whereas the antimalarials that interfere with folic acid metabolism (pyrimethamine, sulphadiazine, chloroguanide, see Section 9.3) injure the schizonts only at the time of their division, the nucleic acid combining drugs (especially mepacrine, chloroquine) and quinine injure the schizonts at all times (Josephson *et al.*, 1953) provided that they are in erythrocytes. Thanks to their high selectivity, mepacrine and chloroquine are harmless to the mammalian and avian hosts in doses which are highly injurious to the intra-erythrocytic schizonts (trophozoites), and yet are harmless to exoerythrocytic schizonts, also to the mosquito-borne sporogenic (gamete, or sexual) stages. The clue to this differentiation seems to lie in the fact that parasitized erythrocytes concentrate these drugs about one thousand-fold. Thus a patient under chloroquine treatment may have only 10^{-6} M of this drug in his blood-stream, but as much as 10^{-3} M inside the erythrocytes (cf. Macomber, O'Brien and Hahn, 1966).

Chloroquine
(*10.28*)

Quinine
(*10.29*)

It is generally thought that mepacrine and chloroquine act by combining with DNA in the parasite, the flat aromatic ring (in each example) undergoing intercalation, and the basic group forming an ionic link with a phosphate group on the DNA (O'Brien, Olenick and Hahn, 1966). Lerman (1963) had shown that mepacrine readily became intercalated into DNA, just as the simpler acridines described in Section 10.3b. That chloroquine was similarly intercalated was shown by decreases in sedimentation rate, enhancement of viscosity, and elevation of the melting profile. It reacted very little with single-stranded DNA (Allison, O'Brien, and Hahn, 1965). Also chloroquine was shown to inhibit bacterial DNA polymerase by combining with the DNA starter (Cohen and Yielding 1965). Naturally it would have been more interesting if these tests had been done also with nucleic acid from *Plasmodia*. These three antimalarials inhibited incorporation of phosphate (^{32}P) into the DNA and RNA of *Pl. gallinaceum* at 10^{-5} M in chicks and in parasitized whole blood; *Pl. berghei* behaved similarly (Schellenberg and Coatney, 1961). It is noteworthy that the gametocidal 8-aminoquinolines do not inhibit phosphorus incorporation.

Another action has been proposed for chloroquine, in which this drug, by blocking a haemoglobin protease, halts degradation of haemoglobin by the parasite which is then assumed to succumb to aminoacid starvation (Howells *et al.*, 1970). It is possible that, like pentamidine in trypanosomiasis, chloroquine has two sites of action.

The side-chain, which is such an important feature of the molecules of mepacrine and chloroquine, will now be discussed. It is currently thought to bind two vertically adjacent phosphate anions on the *same* strand of DNA. Much simpler diamines, such as ethylenediamine, firmly bind to (and rigidify) single-stranded polynucleotides as well as helical DNA. The dication of ethylenediamine is just long enough to bind adjacent anions (7 Å apart), but it is too short to reach across the minor groove (10 Å) of the DNA double-helix and bind two strands together (Gabbay, 1968).

The approximate distance between the two basic groups of the side-chain of mepacrine (Fig. 10.8) can be worked out as follows. Inspection of tables of interatomic distances (Sutton, 1947, 1955, 1965) showed that butanediamine, which would have been the best model, had not been examined. In its place, recorded data for *meso*-erythritol was used (X-ray diffraction work). For this molecule, the distance between the two oxygen atoms (as shown in Fig. 10.9) was found to be 6.2 Å (Sutton, 1965). The distance between the two nitrogen atoms of the mepacrine side-chain may be assigned a similar value, because the CCN angle and the C−N bond in diethylamine, as found by electron diffraction in the gas phase (Sutton, 1958), are almost identical with those for similarly placed components in *meso*-erythritol. Better still, the N−N distance in the side chain of chloroquine diphosphate has been directly measured and found to be 5.54 Å by X-ray diffraction (Preston and Stewart, 1970): that of mepracine could hardly differ from this.

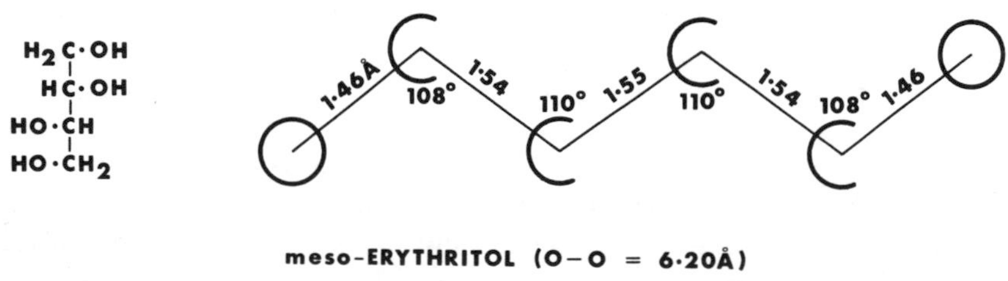

DIETHYLAMINE

meso-ERYTHRITOL (O−O = 6·20Å)

FIG. 10.9 Interatomic distances (from centre to centre of the atoms).

The ionization properties of the side-chain of mepacrine are also relevant to its activity. The pK_a of the nitrogen atom at the free end of the chain is 10.48, but only 7.92 at the fixed end (at 20°C, cf. 10.1 and 7.0 for ethylenediamine). Both ends of this side-chain are ionized at pH 7 (see Table 10.3), but the lower pK_a is greatly decreased by any shortening of the side-chain, with the result that both the ionization and the antimalarial action fall steeply away (Albert, 1966). This drop is caused by the coulombic effect (repulsion between like charges varies inversely with the square of the distance).

Quinine (*10.29*) has been the mainstay in treating chloroquine-resistant cases of malaria. It intercalates into DNA very little and acts on the parasites in some quite different, but as yet unknown, way from chloroquine. (Estensen, Krey and Hahn, 1969). Quinine is a wasteful drug because a high proportion of each dose is oxidized, in the 2-position, by the patient's liver and the product is inactive. This defect was overcome by the insertion of non-oxidizable substituents into that position. A particularly successful drug of this kind is mefloquine (*10.30*) which, in a single dose, can produce clinical cure in patients whose life is threatened by chloroquine-resistant strains of *Plasmodium falciparum*. This drug does not react in any way with DNA (Davidson *et al.*, 1977).

This, and much related work, largely concerning the quinolyl -carbinols, has been supported by the Walter Reed Army Institute of Research, in Washington, D.C. The piperidine ring in mefloquine, by replacing the quinuclidine ring in quinine, greatly simplifies the synthesis. In other (chemically related) substances, the piperidine ring has been opened up to give a dialkylaminomethyl-group, with good retention of antimalarial powers. The latent flexibility of these structure-action relationships is illustrated by the drug WR 30090, in which the piperidyl ring has been replaced by a dibutylaminomethyl-group, and the 2-trifluoromethyl- by a dichlorophenyl- group, plus one further change, but still retaining excellent clinical activity against chloroquine-resistant strains.

Similar side-chains can convert a non-heterocyclic nucleus into a good antimalarial. Excellent results against *Pl. falciparum* infections were obtained, in laboratory and field, with the phenanthrene drugs WR 33063 (*10.31*) (Canfield and Rozman, 1974), and WR 122455 which is 3,6-*bis*(trifluoromethyl-α,2-piperidyl-9-phenanthrenemethanol (Rinehart, Arnold, and Canfield, 1976).

Mefloquine
(*10.30*)

'Walter Reed 33063'
(*10.31*)

(e) *Pharmacodynamic examples*
Acetylcholine (*7.4*), important transmitter of the nervous impulse between cells, is an aliphatic quaternary amine and hence completely ionized in all circumstances. The active form of nicotine (*7.18*), which mimics the action of acetylcholine at several sites, must be the cation because its methiodide (quaternized on the pyrrolidine nitrogen atom) is no less active (Barlow and Hamilton, 1962). The arecoline (*13.57*) cation, too, has potent acetyl-choline-like properties (see Section 13.6). However, in experiments made (over the pH range 6.05 to 9.36) on the guinea-pig ileum, the neutral species of arecoline was found to have only 2 per cent of the activity of the cation (Burgen, 1965).

The great majority of alkaloids, local anaesthetics, antihistaminics, and ionizable depressants have pK_a values between 6 and 8, so that both ionic and neutral species are present, in equilibrium, at physiological pH values. These substances will be considered in Sections 10.4 and 10.5. Among the alkaloids, atropine (pK_a 10) (*7.14*) and tubocurarine (*2.6*) are untypical in having a higher degree of ionization. Tubocurarine is a quaternary amine and hence completely ionized at all pH values. Other quaternary amines used in medicine are: carbachol (*2.11*), neostigmine (*7.26*), decamethonium salts (*7.20*), suxamethonium salts (*7.21*), and gallamine (*7.23*)*. For a study of the ionization of noradrenaline (*7.5*) and its *N*-alkyl homologues, see Section 10.1 (under zwitterions).

Few pharmacodynamic agents are known which function totally as anions, but the potent uricosuric (anti-gout) activity of phenylbutazone (*10.32a*) ('Butazolidin') is due to the anion and can be increased by enhancing the acid-strength of the molecule (to pK_a 3, or even to 2) by appropriate substitution (Burns *et al.*, 1960). These drugs block the resorption of uric acid by the renal tubular cells (the pH of urine is 4.8 or higher). Establishment of this correlation between anionic ionization and uricosuric activity led to the discovery of the clinically useful uricosuric drug, sulphinpyrazone ('Anturan') (*10.32b*).

(a) Phenylbutazone (R = $-(CH_2)_3 \cdot CH_3$)
(b) Sulfinpyrazone (R = $-(CH_2)_2 \cdot SO \cdot C_6H_5$)
(*10.32*)

Ledakrin
(*10.33*)

---

* These are all 'ammonium' type quaternaries, and hence are fully ionized under all conditions. Some trypanocides which are the 'immonium' type (i.e. the quaternized nitrogen carries a double-bond) give pseudo-bases, see Section 10.3d.

(f)   *Cationics and cancer* (see also Adriamycin, p. 363)
Mepacrine (Fig. 10.8) has long been used to diminish the serous exudation
that is such a troublesome side-effect of the growth of solid tumours
in the patient. Nitracrin ('Ledacrin') (*10.33*) [1-nitro-9(dimethylamino-
propylamino)acridine] is a much more active and selective acridine with
strong carcinostatic properties. It has proved particularly useful in colonic
cancer, after surgery: a series of 30 patients showed no recurrence after
5 years (Bratkowska-Seniów *et al.*, 1976). Nitracrin has basic pK_a values
of 6.2 (nuclear) and 9.7 (side-chain) (cf. 7.9 and 10.5 for mepacrine). It
is thought that the drug functions through reduction of the nitro-group
to a hydroxylamino-group, which covalently unites with DNA (Ledóchowski, 1976).

   Although lacking any ionization in the 9-substituent, the 9-anilino-
acridines made by Cain and his associates in New Zealand, are ionized
(pK_a about 7.5) and have high activity against the L1210 strain of leukaemia
in the mouse (cf. Cain, Atwell, and Denny, 1976).

10.4 Substances that appear to be less active when ionized

In 1921, Vermast suggested that many weak acids exhibit their biological
activity most fully at pH values where they were least ionized. An interesting
example is the inhibition of cell-division in echinoderm eggs by salicylic
acid (H. Smith, 1925). It can be seen from Fig. 10.10 that this acid is more
active at pH 5 than at any other pH tested. At pH 5, a larger proportion
of this acid (pK_a = 3.0) is in the form of molecules than at any higher pH,
namely 0.99 per cent (see Appendix I). The only simple explanation is
that the molecules, but not the anions, of salicylic acid inhibit the division
of these eggs. It would be expected that at still lower pH values salicylic
acid would be a more powerful inhibitor, because it would contain a higher
ratio of molecules to anions; one wonders why this region was not explored.
However, complications often occur when such changes are attempted.
Firstly, the organism may not continue to show indifference to pH. Secondly, the receptor for salicylic acid may undergo a change in ionization as the
pH falls and would then hardly be likely to have the same affinity as before
(see Section 10.6).

   Similarly, it has been found (Clowes, Keltch, and Krahl, 1940) that all
members of a series of 30 barbiturates enter both eggs and larvae of the
sea-urchin *Arbacia* exclusively as molecules. Moreover, the resulting
depressions of cell division and of respiration were shown to be entirely
due to molecules. Again, it has been shown for theophylline that the
non-ionized form (as distinct from the anion) is the species causing stimulation of the turtle's heart (Hardman, 1962).

   At present, there is anxiety that nitrous acid, which people consume in
cigarette smoke and in preserved meats, may be uniting with secondary

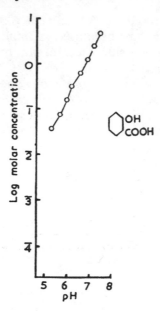

FIG. 10.10 The effect of pH on the concentrations of salicylic acid required to stop the cell division of *Echinarachnius parva*. Curve: total drug (= ions + neutral molecules) (Smith, 1925.)

amines in the stomach, to form nitrosamine carcinogens (see Section 12.4). In this connection, it is interesting that the molecular form is the species of secondary amines that reacts fastest with nitrous acid, so that amines that are only feebly ionized at pH 2 would be the most susceptible to nitrosamine formation (Sander, Schweinsberg, and Menz, 1968). These weak amines seem to be quite uncommon in the stomach-contents.

When observing the effect of a weaker acid on biological material, it is usual to find that a constant amount of the substance is required, regardless of the pH of the medium, provided that the pH is at least one unit lower than the pK_a, thus ensuring that there is no ionization of the toxic agent. This is well illustrated in Fig. 10.11, which shows the effect of pH on the concentrations of phenol and acetic acid required to prevent the growth of various common moulds. Within the pH range of the experiment (2 to 6) it is seen that a constant amount of phenol is required, but a decreasing amount of acetic acid suffices as the pH drops. This is so because the pK_a of phenol is 9.9, and hence it is non-ionized within the pH range of the experiments, whereas the pK_a of acetic acid is 4.8, and hence it is 90 per cent ionized at pH 5.8, but only 9 per cent ionized at pH 3.8, and so on.

All such experiments are unsatisfactory unless controls are set up to establish if the change of pH has had an effect on the test-organism, as is often the case. This precaution was taken in experiments, summarized in

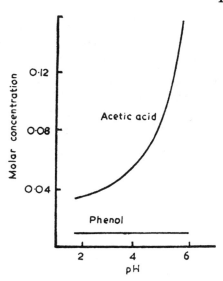

FIG. 10.11 The effect of pH on the concentration of phenol ($pK_a = 9.9$) and acetic acid ($pK_a = 4.8$) required to prevent the growth of common moulds. (Hoffman, *et al.*, 1940 and 1941.)

Table 10.11, which deal with the narcotizing action of various substances on the worm *Arenicola* (Clowes and Keltch, 1931). It can be seen that the effect on non-electrolytes such as chloroform is independent of pH. These non-ionizing substances show that the changes of pH do not affect the worms. The weak bases, such as cocaine, behave differently. They become more effective as the pH is increased, i.e. in proportion as their ionization is suppressed. Similarly, the weak acids (four isomeric barbiturates) are more effective as the pH is decreased; again this corresponds to the suppression of their ionization. By washing the worms with sea-water, the narcotic action is readily reversed in each case. Actually (although the authors did not do so), it is easily calculated that the ions make a small contribution to the toxic action in this series (see next section).

The above studies of *Arenicola* were simplified by the fact of the pH change having no effect on the test-organism. Less fortunate were some (better unnamed) workers who investigated the action of quinine derivatives on bacteria. They thought that they had shown that the neutral molecules were more active than the ions because these drugs became more effective as the alkalinity rose [*Z. Immunitäts.* (1922), **34**, 194]. Unfortunately they had overlooked the ionizing effect of alkali on the bacterial receptors (see Section 10.6).

The 'parabens', esters of *p*-hydroxybenzoic acid, especially the methyl, ethyl, propyl, and heptyl esters, are much used as food preservatives. Their high pK (8.5) ensures their non-ionized character in neutral foods.

Table 10.11

THE CONNECTION BETWEEN IONIZATION AND THE
NARCOSIS OF *ARENICOLA*

(Minimal anaesthetic doses, in g per 100 ml of sea-water,
rendering this worm immobile after 5 min)

	pH 7.0	pH 8.0	pH 9.0
Non-electrolytes			
*iso*Propyl alcohol	2.5	2.5	2.5
*iso*Amyl alcohol	0.1	0.1	0.1
Chloroform	0.012	0.012	0.025
Chlorbutol	0.025	0.025	0.025
Weak bases (pK_a about 8.5)			
Coacine	0.01	0.005	0.0025
Procaine	0.002	0.001	0.0005
Butacaine ('Butyn')	0.001	0.0002	0.0002
Barbituric acids (pK_a about 8.0)			
*iso*Amyl, ethyl ('Amytal')	0.006	0.025	0.05
Propylmethylcarbinyl, ethyl			
('Nembutal')	0.003	0.006	0.012
Diethylcarbinyl, ethyl	0.006	0.012	0.05
n-Amyl, ethyl	0.006	0.012	0.05

(Clowes and Keltch, 1931.)

They are thought to act by preventing passage, through the plasma membrane, of aminoacids, other organic acids, and phosphates (Freese, Sheu, and Galliers, 1973).

10.5 Substances of which both ion and molecule play a part in the biological action

It is reasonably certain that many substances, particularly those whose pK_a lies in the range 6–8, penetrate into cells as molecules, even though they exert their biological action as ions (see Section 10.2). Fig. 10.12 illustrates this effect: it shows that the penetration of benzoic acid into yeast is inversely proportional to the percentage ionized.

Many agents are known in which (a) biological activity depends mainly on the proportion of neutral molecule present, and yet (b) the proportion which is ionized contributes also to the activity. Several examples of this behaviour will now be discussed.

When submitting a weak acid to biological test, it is usually found that a constant amount of the substance is required to produce a standard response at *all* pH values one unit or more below the pK_a. Under such conditions the ionization of the acid is slight (see Section 10.1), and hence

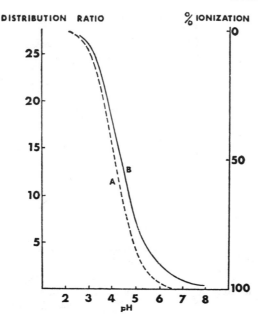

FIG. 10.12 The uptake of benzoic acid by bakers' yeast at various pH values. The uptake is inversely proportional to the percentage ionized. (A) Ratio of distribution of total substance (cell/fluid). (B) Percentage ionization. (Bosund, 1960.)

the biological effect is due, in the first place, to the molecule. This effect is illustrated on the left-hand side of Fig. 10.13. However, if the pH is allowed to rise above the pK_a, an ever-increasing amount of the substance will be required to give the same response. When this response is analysed, one of two results is obtained, (a) a constant amount of the molecule is still required (cf. Section 10.4), or (b) an ever-decreasing amount of the molecule is required because the anion seemingly exhibits, although to a limited extent, the biological action of the molecule. Result (b), which is illustrated by the action of benzoic acid on the mould *Mucor* (Fig. 10.13), is by far the more common.

This method of plotting ionic data was developed in Oxford by Simon (1950), who found that the vast majority of those substances that are most active when least ionized nevertheless have ions which exert some of the activity.

Biological actions involving phenols are known in which the molecule is apparently far more active than the ion, but in which the ion does show some activity. Fig. 10.14 illustrates this kind of activity. It will be seen that these substances are most economical in use at a pH value where they are almost entirely non-ionized. It is not surprising that, in less acidic solutions, more of the substance must be used to get the standard biological response:

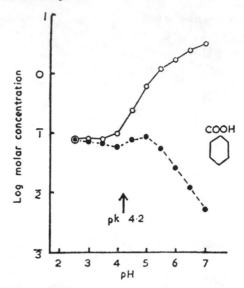

FIG. 10.13 The effect of pH on the concentrations of benzoic acid required to
prevent the growth of the fungus *Mucor*. Upper curve: total substance (ions + neutral molecules). Lower curve: neutral molecules,
(Cruess and Richert, 1929.)

what is surprising is that this extra amount need not be so large as to maintain a standard amount of neutral molecules. Thus the ions of this substance have at least a fraction of the biological activity of the molecules.
This forms a contrast with the results summarized in Fig. 10.10.

That pH has, of itself, very little effect on the fungus *Trichoderma* may
be seen from Fig. 10.15, where the action of two (weakly toxic) phenolic
ethers is shown. These ethers are closely related to the phenol shown in
Fig. 10.14, but they are incapable of ionization.

The ultimate site of action of nitrophenols, when used as weed killers,
is unknown, although presumably they act as uncouplers of mitochondrial
phosphorylation (see Section 4.4). Blackman (1951) pointed out that
when high concentrations are used, precipitation of cell proteins and the
rupture of cell membrane are likely as well.

Many nitrogen heterocycles having five-membered rings and an
(an)ionizable −NH group (of which the N forms part of the ring) are
potent inhibitors of the Hill reaction in photosynthesis (Section 4.5).
However, activity is lost if the percentage ionized is too high [examples
of substances that penetrate as the molecule but act as the ion, (Büchel
and Draber, 1969)]. Suitable ring systems are imidazoles, benzimidazoles,
pyrido-imidazoles, purines, pyrazoles, indazoles, 1,2,3-triazoles, 1,2,4-
triazoles, and benzotriazoles. The 2-trifluoromethylbenzimidazoles, which
are active only when the molecule is so substituted that the pK_a falls in

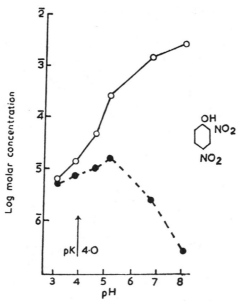

FIG. 10.14 Effect of pH on the antifungal action of dinitrophenol (pK_a 4.0) on *Trichoderma viride*. Upper curve: total substance (ions + neutral molecules). Lower curve: neutral molecules. (Simon and Beevers, 1952.)

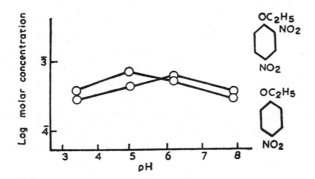

FIG. 10.15 Comparatively small effect of pH on the antifungal action of some phenolic ethers on *Trichoderma viride*. (Simon and Blackman, 1949.)

the range 5–8 (Jones and Watson, 1965), are commercially used, but rather expensive.

Similar results have been obtained with bases. Thus, pyrimethamine (4.7) which has pK_a 7.2, is best absorbed by bacteria from solutions alkaline enough to have a high proportion of neutral species. But the critical internal enzyme (dihydrofolate reductase) is inhibited only by the cation (Wood, Ferone, and Hitchings, 1961).

Local anaesthetics are very dependent on a high proportion of molecules for transportation to the site of action, and this requirement confines clinically useful examples to the weak bases (Trevan and Boock, 1927). However, the cation is the active species at the receptor site. Thus, when the sheath is stripped from mammalian nerve-trunks, anaesthesia becomes directly proportional to ionization (Ritchie and Greengard, 1966). Desheathed rabbit vagus nerves, first exposed to cinchocaine or ametho-caine, and then immersed in plain buffer solutions, remained anaesthetized at pH 7, but rapidly lost the anaesthetic at pH 9.6, evidence of an ionic link between drug and nerve (Ritchie and Greengard, 1961). That lignocaine (7.13) similarly acts as the cation was shown in Section 7.6b. Even quatern-ary analogues of local anaesthetics are active if injected inside the nerve membrane (Narahashi and Frazier, 1968) and, when the quaternization of cocaine, procaine, and cinchocaine was effected with a benzyl-group (to help lipophilicity), local anaesthetic action could be demonstrated by external application (Nador et al., 1953). It will be appreciated that these quaternary amines are completely ionized under all conditions.

Very many alkaloids, local anaesthetics, and antihistaminics have pK_a values about 8, so that they are about 16 per cent non-ionized at pH 7.3. It is almost certain that these penetrate as molecules and act biologically as cations. The H_2-type histamine antagonists, like cimetidine (9.43) need to be largely ionized at pH 7, to exert their action, but if totally ionized at this pH, they cannot penetrate to their receptor (Black et al., 1974).

The ionization as anions of many commonly used anti-inflammatory agents is positively correlated with their biological action provided that ionization is not complete and that they are sufficiently lipophilic to reach their prostaglandin-inhibiting site of action. Examples include indomethacin and the salicylates (Whitehouse and Dean, 1965). In the phenylindanedione (9.29) series, observation of the effect of varying the pK (on the anti-inflammatory action) pointed to a need for more accurate determina-tions of pK in the ortho-substituted aryl derivatives, which are by far the most biologically active (van der Berg et al., 1975).

The first four editions of this book carried a table of examples of increased biological effects of a weak acid brought about by repressing ionization in the test medium. This effect was demonstrated for aliphatic acids (from formic to stearic), aromatic acids (including salicylic acid), phenols, barbiturates, and the following inorganic acids: hydrofluoric, sulphurous, and arsenious, as well as phenylarsenoxides. The test material ranged from bacteria, through fungi (including yeasts), to inhibition of fertilization (or, alternatively, division) of echinoderm eggs, and to killing insects as larvae or in the egg. This material has historical interest and demonstrates the scope of the topic. However, the treatment was non-quantitative, because ionization constants were not used; hence these data have been omitted in favour of work based on pK_a values.

A strong decrease in antibacterial action was noted quite early with derivatives of sulphapyridine and sulphathiazole in which the $SO_2.NH$-group had been replaced by $SO_2.NMe$- group, so that no anion could be formed (Shepherd, Bratton, and Blanchard, 1942), and again for sulpha-guanidine (*10.34*) which has no acidic group. The relationship of ionization to activity was explored in depth by Bell and Roblin (1942), and their results are epitomized in Fig. 10.16. The fact that the optimal pK, for the ionization of the sulphonamide group as an acid, lies between 6 and 8, suggests (just as with the other examples cited in this Section) that penetration depends on the non-ionized species (Cowles, 1942).

That sulphonamides act as the anion but penetrate into the bacterial cell as the neutral species was later confirmed by comparing their behaviour in (a) a cell-free folate-synthesizing preparation of *E. coli* and (b) the intact cells of *E. coli*. The antibacterial action was directly proportional to per-centage ionized in (a), but became dependent on lipophilicity, as well, in (b) (Miller, Doukos, and Seydel, 1972). Although as many as 46 examples were used to obtain the curve shown in Fig. 10.16, an extension of this series by Seydel produced several aberrant points because of secondary effects and, for a while, Seydel, relying on infrared studies of the SO_2 group, doubted the role of ionization and polarization. (Seydel, Krüger-Thiemer, and Wempe, 1960; Seydel, 1966).

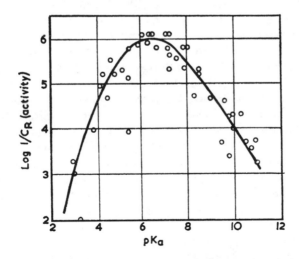

FIG. 10.16 Effect, on bacteriostatic action, of variation in the pK_a of a series of sulphonamides. Organism: *E. coli*. The substances on the left are the most highly ionized (as anions) at the pH of the test (pH 7, synthetic medium). (Bell and Roblin, 1942.)

H₂N—⟨benzene⟩—SO₂NH·C·NH₂
                            ‖
                            NH

Sulphaguanidine
(*10.34*)

5,5-Dimethyloxazolidin-2,4-dione
(*10.35*)

10.6 The ionization of receptors

The pK_a values of receptors cannot be predicted in advance of experiment because their chemical nature is largely unknown. Obviously cationic drugs combine with anionic receptors which may have pK_a values of 2 or 7 (presence of phosphoric acid groups), 2-6 (carboxylic acid groups), 10 (tyrosine-, pyrimidine-, cysteine- residues). Cationic receptors could have pK_a values of 4 (adenine), 7 (histidine), 10 (lysine), 13 (arginine).

Receptors outside cells. By no means are all receptors within cells. For example, the frog's heart is affected (in opposite ways) by acetylcholine and methylene blue without penetration of the cells taking place (Clark, 1933). These and many similar observations are in harmony with current knowledge that the outside of the plasma membrane is rich in enzymes, including permeases. For example, yeast is known to have adenosinetriphosphatase and several hydrolases on the outer surface (Rothstein and Meier, 1948).

The pK_a of a receptor on the outside of cells can often be studied by measuring the response to drugs over a range of pH values, provided that (a) the cell is known not to be injured by the pH changes and (b) that the ionization of the drug does not change within this range. For the application of this approach to learning something of the site of action of aminoacridine antibacterials on *E. coli*, see Section 10.3a.

Not all workers have realized that the degree of ionization of a receptor can alter as the pH is changed. For example, the respiration of avian red blood cells (whole or haemolysed) was found to be inhibited 2.5 times as strongly by quinine at pH 10 as at pH 5. Because quinine has a pK_a of 8.4, it was concluded that the inhibition was caused by the molecule and not by the ion. The likelihood that an acidic receptor became more ionized at the higher pH (whereupon it could bind more quinine cations) was not mentioned [*Biochem. Zeitschr.* (1922), **128**, 169].

Receptors inside cells. A receptor may be supposed to be intracellular if (a) agents with lipophilic groups are more effective than examples without those groups, and (b) agents which yield only 70 per cent of the active ionic species (at the pH of the test) are more active than those which are present completely as this species. Ionization studies then become more difficult, because the pH close to the receptor is the one of prime importance.

In the Waddell and Butler (1959) method for determining intracellular pH, three measurements are required: the external pH, and the extracellular and intracellular concentrations of an indicator *ion* to which the membrane is impermeable (it must be freely permeable to the neutral species). These authors used a colourless, fluorescent indicator 5,5-dimethyloxazolidin-2,4-dione, DMO (*10.35*), a weak acid of pK_a 6.13 at 37°C. By this method, the pH inside resting muscle (dog) was found to be 7.04, but inhalation of carbon dioxide brought it down to 6.6. Using a radioactive form of this indicator, Addanki, Cahill, and Sotos (1967) found pH 7.74 inside resting mitochondria. The indicator is considered to be safe to use in patients.

Another method for measuring the pH inside cells is to observe the ^{31}P phosphate shift in n.m.r.; this procedure has an accuracy of ±0.02 unit of pH (Navon *et al.*, 1977). It is also possible to use recessed-tip microelectrodes inside cells, useful for recording continuously during several hours (Thomas, 1974).

Work with indicators suggests that the pH of animal and plant cytoplasm is 6.8 ± 0.2, and that these fluids are well buffered. Nucleoplasm was found to be 7.6 ± 0.2 (Chambers and Chambers, 1961). The external surfaces of organelles, if anionic (e.g. protein surfaces), can be richer in hydrogen ions than the cytoplasm because of a zeta potential effect. The cytoplasm of amoebae was found to be 6.7. The pH of plant vacuoles averaged 5.2, but was much lower in some species. The pH of cancerous tissues in mammals is often lower than that of the surrounding organ, a circumstance with a possible application in therapy (Section 4.6, p. 142). This low pH, which is connected with the high rate of anaerobic respiration, has led to more careful selection of pK_a values in designing carcinostatic drugs of the nitrogen mustard type (Ross, 1961).

That the pH within bacterial cells may vary with those of buffers in which they are placed is suggested by the following experiment. The tyrosine-decarboxylase of *Strept. faecalis* has its maximal activity *in vitro* at pH 5.5. In the intact bacterium, it is only moderately active when the external environment is neutral or alkaline, but it becomes most active when placed in buffer at pH 5.0–5.5 (Gale, 1946). Again, in the turtle's heart, a linear relationship exists between the pH of extracellular water and intracellular water (ventricular tissue) in the range 6.5–9.5. Thus pH$_{int}$ = pH$_{ext}$ + 2.98 (Waddell and Hardman, 1960). For further reading on cell pH, see Bittar (1964).

It is desirable in pharmacology to work with a buffer, even when the receptor is known to be an internal one. The external buffer brings about uniform conditions by (a) presenting the drug to the cell in a standard state of ionization, regardless of the form in which it was supplied, and (b) maintaining in a standard state the chemical groups responsible for the adsorption of the drug to the cell surface and its penetration into the cell.

The success of buffering depends on the proportion of cells with which the buffers come into contact. In bulky tissue-preparations, this proportion may be very small, and the drugs can reach their receptors only after passage through other cells or intercellular fluids. The results from such experiments are not comparable with those obtained from experiments in which all the cells are in direct contact with the drug at a known pH (Simon and Beevers, 1951).

10.7 Conclusions

Consideration of the principles discussed in this chapter makes it clear that it is highly advantageous to know the ionization constants of all substances which are being examined biologically.

The next step is to discover which is the most effective, the ion or the molecule. This may be done in two ways, which are not alternative but complementary. In the first approach, the pK_a of the drug should be varied by appropriate substitution, taking full advantage of the chemist's ability to produce substances of any desired pK_a in almost any series (see Appendix III). The advantage of this approach is that the ionization of the receptor is not interfered with, and the living cells are not removed from their optimal pH. The disadvantage is that the chemical change in the molecule may, of itself, be responsible for a changed biological response; this difficulty can be avoided by working with *two* analogues at each desired pK_a, and accepting the results only if they agree. In the second approach, the composition of the drug should be kept constant, but the pH of the medium varied. This has the advantage that the living cells are exposed to only one drug, but the effect of pH changes on the receptor and on the viability of the cell itself must be independently examined.

Because ionization, one of the commonest of variables, is brought under control by these methods, studies of this kind can greatly assist in the design of more meaningful experiments.

11 Metal-binding substances

Heavy metals, in traces, are essential for all forms of life. They are taken up by the living cell as cations, and their uptake is strictly regulated because most (or all) of them are toxic in excess. A remarkable specificity has been found: seldom can an excess of one essential metal prevent the damage caused by deficiency of another. In fact, such an excess often increases the injurious effect of the deficiency.

Metal-binding substances, many of which function by chelation,* have furnished many useful drugs and other substances of value in selective toxicity. They are manufactured in huge quantities for this purpose, particularly those that are used in agriculture as fungicides. They function by upsetting the delicate balance that exists between the cations of heavy metals in nature. Some of them withdraw metals from living tissues, but many others reinforce the natural toxicity of a heavy metal.

* A substance which binds metals is called a *ligand*. When a metal is gripped, in a ligand, between any two of the elements, N, O, or S, a *chelate* ring is formed, and the metal is more tightly bound than when it is not a chelate, i.e. when it is not part of a ring. The term, coined by Morgan and Drew (1920) to describe this phenomenon, is derived from *chela*, the crab's claw, and the 'ch' is pronounced 'k'.

Apart from their use as agricultural fungicides, metal-binding substances have found three types of use in veterinary and human medicine. Some which differentiate between vertebrates and their parasites make a valuable contribution to the fight against fungi, bacteria, and viruses (see Sections 11.7–11.9). Others, which may be described as antidotes, are used to distinguish between essential and poisonous metals (see Section 11.6). The third type favours normal over pathological processes, e.g. in rheumatic diseases, cardiovascular disease, and cancer (see Sections 11.9 and 11.11).

11.0 Metals in the living cell

Man, and other vertebrates, require cations of the following metals to facilitate a great many essential life processes. Moreover, many of these metals are essential for all other forms of life:

(a) The heavy metals: cobalt, copper, iron, manganese, molybdenum, and zinc, and in still smaller amounts: chromium, vanadium, nickel, and tin.

(b) The lighter, and usually more abundant, metals: calcium, magnesium, potassium, and sodium.

Of these, copper, iron, molybdenum, cobalt, and occasionally manganese, assist oxidation-reduction equilibria; zinc, magnesium and manganese are concerned with hydrolysis and with group-transfer; calcium plays its most important part in creating structures, flexible or rigid, but also it (and sometimes magnesium) can trigger a reaction, possibly by effecting a structural change. Sodium and potassium, because of their abundance, function as charge-carriers; they are only weakly bound and hence can exchange rapidly. Some examples of the biological functions of heavy metals will now be given [in the order of (a) and (b), above].

Cobalt is necessary for activity of a carboxypeptidase which destroys various kinins (inflammation-causing peptides that circulate in mammals) and plays a role in the digestion of polypeptides (Davies and Lowe, 1966). Cobalt is strongly bound in the large tetrapyrrole ring of the cobamide family of coenzymes. Two substances used for replacement therapy in pernicious anaemia, hydroxycobalamine and cyanocobalamine (vitamin B_{12}), are formed by the breakdown of these coenzymes during isolation from yeast or liver. These coenzymes catalyse the reduction of ribose nucleotides to deoxyribose nucleotides, the interconversion of β-methyl-aspartate and glutamate anions (Barker *et al.*, 1960), the interconversion of methylmalonate and succinate anions, and the methylation of homocysteine to methionine.

In 1935, two groups of workers in Australia found that the vast, lush pastures that produced severe anaemia in sheep in that country and New

Zealand, did so through lack of cobalt, an element which is not required by plants. When the cobalt content of grass was less than 0.2 of a part per million, the sheep became weak and died. This debility was traced to a failure of microflora in the sheep's rumen to synthesize the cobalt-containing coenzymes (Marston, Allen and Smith, 1961). Addition of cobalt to the sheep's diet is now used to prevent this condition, and the productivity of the land has increased almost unbelievably.

In the human, as little as one microgram of vitamin B_{12} (intramuscularly) is sufficient daily therapy for pernicious anaemia. In a man weighing 70 kg, this represents only 0.000 002 p.p.m. of his weight.

Copper is an essential constituent of many enzymes. The effects of traces of copper on oat-seedlings, grown in a copper-deficient medium, is shown in Plate 5 (p. 395). Plainly, too little copper is bad for growth, and so is too much. Until recognized as such, copper-deficiency was the cause of many a crop failure in the reclaimed areas of Holland and Denmark. Copper-deficiency in farm animals leads to anaemia, demyelination of the spinal cord, and loss of pigmentation. Excessive copper-storage in the liver of sheep leads to haemolysis and death (Albiston, *et al.*, 1940).

Copper is essential for the action of many oxidases, such as phenolase (tyrosinase) which plays an important metabolic role in plants (including fungi) and in mammalian pigment cells, and also in providing the protein-tanning agent that hardens insect integument. Copper in the closely related laccase has been shown by electron spin resonance spectroscopy to be bivalent in the resting state but to become univalent (Cu^+) while the enzyme is in use. Cytochrome oxidase contains two iron and two copper atoms per molecule; although the iron is porphyrin-bound, copper never is in Nature. Copper is also essential for the action of dopamine hydroxylase (a key enzyme in the synthesis of the catecholamine hormones), monoamine oxidase, and ascorbic oxidase.

Electron spin resonance has also shown that the copper in the mammalian blood protein, caeruloplasmin, is partly cuprous and partly cupric. A bright blue copper-containing pigment, called plastocyanin, is involved in photo-synthetic electron transport of plants. Copper takes the place of iron in the blue respiratory pigment (haemocyanin) of certain molluscs and crustaceans. This element is essential for the production of haemoglobin in man. Copper is known to be concentrated several-fold (relative to other metals) in sympathetic nerve-endings, and in the synaptic vesicles of brain and other nerve tissue. There it seems to assist in storing noradrenaline in a ternary complex with ATP (Colburn and Maas, 1965), and 5-hydroxy-tryptamine is similarly stored (Roberts, 1966). Cupric ions, adenosine triphosphate, and noradrenaline form a tightly bound ternary complex (1:1:1) with a log K value of 12.15 [without the ATP, the (1:1) log K value is 10.25]. Adrenaline is bound a little more firmly, and dopamine rather less. The medicinally used analogues, such as amphetamine, and phenylephrine were relatively weakly bound. It is evident that both oxygen atoms of the catechol moiety play an important part in the binding. These adrenergic transmitters and drugs bind to the granules of synaptosomes in the ranking order of their stability constants (Rajan, Davis, and Colburn, 1974).

Absence of caeruloplasmin, the copper-scavanging globulin, is the basis of Wilson's disease, which runs in families: the destructive effect of free copper ions on the nervous system causes death if untreated.

The green-coloured enzyme superoxide-dismutase, present in every tissue of all eukaryotes, contains both copper and iron linked to the same imidazole nucleus (His-61) in the apoenzyme. The copper undergoes a cycle of oxidation and reduction as it destroys highly toxic superoxide radicals ($\cdot O_2^-$) which arise from reactions using atmospheric oxygen. Analogous enzymes in mitochondria and bacteria have either manganese or iron, but never zinc or copper (Fridovich, 1975). Other examples where analogous enzymes differ in their supporting metals, have been given in Section 4.6.

Iron is a vital constituent of the porphyrin enzymes: catalase, peroxidases, and the various cytochromes which are essential for all living cells. Haemoglobin is the respiratory pigment in the red blood corpuscles not only of mammals but of birds, reptiles, amphibians, and fish. It is also found free in the plasma of some molluscs and annelid worms (some annelids have a green iron respiratory pigment, chlorocruorin). Myoglobin, the oxygen-transfer pigment of muscle, closely resembles haemoglobin.

Transferrin, a glycopeptide of mol. wt. 86 000, binds ferric ions firmly between imidazole and tyrosine residues. It occurs in blood serum, where it masks ferric ions which, if free, would damage the heart. Transferrin is the only form of iron acceptable to reticulocytes for making haemoglobin. Like a similar β-globulin in hen's eggs (conalbumin), transferrin can so lower the concentration of ferric ions in a medium that bacteria can no longer grow in it. A similar polypeptide, lactoferrin, is found in sweat, tears, milk, and nasal and bronchial secretions. It is thought that the ability of these substances to prevent uptake of iron by bacteria can constitute an important defence against bacterial infections, especially as iron enhances the lethality of many bacteria, even as much as 100 000-fold (Bullen and Rogers, 1969).

The principal iron-storage compounds of vertebrates are the proteins ferritin, found mainly in liver, and haemosiderin, found in spleen and muscles.

Iron is also an essential constituent of several non-porphyrin enzymes, e.g. aconitase, aldolase and succinic hydrogenase. Inhibition of the synthesis of glucose by tryptophan in animal cells depends on chelation. The tryptophan is metabolized to pyridine-2,3-dicarboxylic acid, which complexes the divalent iron necessary for the action of phosphoenolpyruvic-carboxykinase (a key enzyme in the neogenesis of glucose) (Veneziale *et al.*, 1967).

Bacteria and fungi use the siderochromes, a remarkable series of phenols and hydroxamic acids, to forage for iron (more in Section 11.1).

Ferredoxins are proteins containing equal numbers of iron and sulphur atoms in each active centre. They transfer electrons below the potential of the hydrogen electrode. The 8Fe-8S ferredoxins are associated with the most primitive organisms (obligate anaerobic fermenters and photo-synthesizers) where they are used for electron-transfer in the pyruvate phosphoroclastic system; the 4Fe-4S types probably came next in evolution and are found in sulphate- and nitrate-reducing bacteria. The later 2Fe-2S ferredoxins are found in plants and animals where they are essential for oxidative phosphorylation in mitochondria, for photosynthetic phospho-rylation in chloroplasts, and for the synthesis of catecholamine hormones. The individual types are distinguished by e.s.r. and Mössbauer spectra. For a review, see Hall and Evans (1969).

Iron-deficiency in fruit trees (citrus and pomes) causes poor crops. A soil may be rich in iron, and yet so basic that the iron is not available to the rootlets. Ethylenediaminetetracetic acid (EDTA), sprayed on such soil, extracts iron by forming the EDTA-ferric complex, which is absorbed by the rootlets. Experiments with tomato plants, grown in an iron-EDTA medium labelled with ^{59}Fe, and with ^{14}C in the 2-position of the acetate-group, showed that the plant absorbs the intact complex, which is trans-located. Later, the organic part is broken down by metabolism which leaves the inorganic iron (Hill-Cottingham and Lloyd-Jones, 1961). When soil is poor in iron, ferric EDTA is sprayed on the ground with the same result.

Manganese, although a metal of variable valence, is rarely involved in biological oxidations. It is essential for the activity of many degradative enzymes such as oxaloacetic decarboxylase, arginase, and prolidase, as well as other enzymes where large groups, such as sugar residues, are exchanged. (See above, under *Copper*, and below, under *Cation antagonism*.)

It seems that manganese is an essential component of that part of the Hill reaction which cleaves a hydroxyl ion to liberate molecular oxygen, in the course of photosynthesis.

Molybdenum has an essential function in the following enzymes: xanthine oxidase, aldehyde oxidase, nitrate reductase, and nitrogenase. In all of these it seems, on the basis of the electron spin resonance spectrum, to be bound to sulphur and to undergo the valency change $Mo^{5+} \rightleftharpoons Mo^{6+}$; iron is usually present as well. Molybdenum is essential for nitrogen fixation, by the various species of *Rhizobium* and *Azotobacter* in plant root nodules.

Formate dehydrogenase, in the plasma membrane of *E. coli*, is a versatile enzyme which contains functional molybdenum, iron, and (tightly bound) selenium (Enoch and Lester, 1975).

Zinc is essential for the functioning of at least twenty different enzymes, and their functions are widely varied. They include the alcohol dehydrogenases of yeast and mammalian liver, glyceraldehyde phosphate dehydrogenase, phosphoglycomutase of yeast, DNA and RNA polymerases (at least in bacteria), alkaline phosphatase in bacteria, mammalian carboxypeptidase, carbonic anhydrase, AMP hydrolase, pyruvate carboxylase (yeast), and aldolase (yeast and bacteria). The alkaline phosphatase of *E. coli* has, in each molecule, four atoms of zinc: the two which maintain structure can be replaced by Mn^{2+}, Co^{2+}, or Cu^{2+}, whereas the other two atoms are essential for enzyme action (Trotman and Greenwood, 1971).

Reverse transcriptase, isolated from several viruses, contains zinc in the proportion of one atom per molecule of enzyme (Poiesz, Battula, and Loeb, 1974; Vallee, 1975). One example, the RNA-dependent RNA polymerase of influenza B virus, is inactivated *in vitro* by o-phenanthrolines, selenocystamine, and other chelating agents (Oxford and Perrin, 1974).

The over-refined food of highly industrialized countries seems to produce zinc deficiency in the elderly, characterized by loss of acuity in taste and slow healing of cuts and abrasions. The mammalian kidney has a protein, metallothionein, which binds excess of zinc, cadmium, or mercury (Rupp, Voelter, and Weser, 1974).

A deficiency of zinc causes serious disease in apple and citrus trees and grape vines. Lack of zinc in the soil causes poor yields of cereals. In the 1930s, the uneconomic sparse scrub in the Ninety Mile Plain in South Australia was converted to lush grasslands by regular aerial spraying with zinc salts; it now supports a large population of sheep.

Chromium (Cr^{3+}), present in yeast as a complex with nicotinic acid and aliphatic aminoacids, is considered to be the 'glucose tolerance factor' essential for normal carbohydrate metabolism in man and acting by increasing the hypoglycaemic properties of insulin (Mertz, 1975). In highly-industrialized countries where the food is plentiful but too refined, and again in developing countries, chromium deficiency is quite common (Gurson and Saner, 1971; Levine, Streeten, and Doisy, 1968).

Vanadium, essential for vertebrate nutrition (Lambert *et al.*, 1970), seems to be a natural inhibitor of $Na^+ K^+$-ATPase (Cantley *et al.*, 1978). In the urochordates (sea-squirts), animals which stand just below vertebrates in the phylogenetic tree, vanadium takes the place of iron in the oxygen-transport pigment of the blood.

Other heavy metals : nickel (Nielsen and Ollerich, 1974), and *tin* (Schwarz, Milne, and Vinard, 1970) are claimed as essential for animal nutrition. Modern refinements in analytical technique, such as neutron activation analysis, were needed to establish these recent claims, because the quantities present are so much smaller than with the earlier discovered essential metals. The enzyme urease seems to be nickel-dependent (Dixon *et al.*, 1975).

For further reading on newer trace elements in nutrition, see Mertz and Cornatzer (1971).

Calcium is generously distributed in most living organisms (not much, however, in bacteria). The grosser accumulations of calcium include teeth, bones, shells, and the oxalate crystals of plants. Nature's use of calcium to rigidify load-bearing tissues is exemplified by tendons which are fragmented into fine collagen fibrils when their calcium is withdrawn, e.g. by a solution of EDTA, cf. (*11.22*). Replacement of the lost calcium largely reverses this process. Cartilage is turned to bone by incorporating calcium and phosphate ions, a process which magnesium ions competitively reverse.

In mammals, both a thyroid and a parathyroid hormone exist to regulate the level of circulating calcium. One of the most important functions of calcium is to control the permeability of semi-permeable membranes which maintain their integrity in its presence and become porous and leaky in its absence. This control follows from the abundance of this ion, its divalent character, and the presence of phosphate anions in the membranes (Ames, Tsukada, and Nesbett, 1967).

Another important role that calcium ions play is as a 'second messenger'. They can couple a chemical stimulus to a secretion, as in releasing neuro-transmitters after receipt of a nervous impulse, whether at synapses or at a neuromuscular junction (Miledi and Slater, 1966), or in the release of adrenaline from the adrenal medulla at the instance of acetylcholine (Douglas, 1968). Likewise calcium is needed to couple the release of a neurotransmitter to a muscular contraction. Calcium seems also to initiate proliferation in many kinds of cells, such as muscle cells, lymphocytes, and fibroblasts. It also plays a role in phagocytosis. Those ionophores (Section 14.1) that transport calcium into cells can initiate many of these effects. Some think that, at the molecular level, calcium functions by giving ATPase access to its substrate (ATP), thus providing the energy for these various actions.

Calcium plays a vitally important part in possibly as many as three sequences of the contraction-relaxation cycle of vertebrate muscle (Taylor, Lymn, and Moll, 1970). The important role of calcium in bringing about blood clotting has long been known. In some tissues, particularly in the lower animals, calcium can partly or completely replace sodium in carrying the inward current during nerve conduction.

The mitochondria of mammals (only) accumulate calcium and give it up again on demand, possibly controlling the calcification of tissues in this way (Lehinger, 1970). The endoplasmic reticulum is also a calcium accumulator (Moore *et al.*, 1975).

Biochemists make much use of aequorin to locate and measure traces of calcium in the various situations described above. This protein, respon-sible for the blue glow of the jellyfish *Aequorea*, fluoresces specifically in response to calcium (Shimomura and Johnson, 1969).

Magnesium is the second commonest intracellular cation, just as calcium is the second commonest extracellularly. It is the irreplaceable link that keeps ribosomes intact, and attaches mRNA to ribosomes. It is a cofactor of all the enzymes that utilize ATP in phosphate transfer, and in many other enzymes concerned with group transfer or hydrolysis. It inhibits release of acetylcholine at the motor end-plate, and in many other ways acts as a reversible antagonist to calcium. In bacteria, magnesium is the most abundant bivalent metal. The essential central atom of the chlorophyll molecule is magnesium. The higher incidence of death from heart disease in soft-water areas seems to arise from lack of Mg^{2+}.

Potassium and sodium, two ions apparently so similar physically, differ quantitatively in ability to penetrate cell membranes at rest and during excitation, in their affinities for active transport mechanisms, and in their ability to activate enzymes. For example, resting nerve membrane is about 30 times more permeable to K^+ than to Na^+ but, when active, it becomes 10 times more permeable to Na^+ than to K^+ (cf. Section 7.5a). The size of the cations, hydrated or anhydrous, plays little part in this selectivity, which is governed by the free energy difference:

$$\triangle F_{a,\,site} - \triangle F_{b,\,site} - \triangle F_{a,\,water} + \triangle F_{b,\,water}$$

where $\triangle F_{site}$ is the free energy of attraction between the cation and the negatively charged site, and $\triangle F_{water}$ is the free energy of hydration of the cation. The principal variable governing Na^+/K^+ selectivity is the strength of the negative charges on the membrane as reflected in the pK_a values; Na^+ favours the stronger acids, and the crossover point occurs near pK_a 3 (Diamond and Wright, 1969).

Potassium is the essential intracellular ion of all living matter, and there is little sodium *inside* most cells except at the moment of stimulation. Terrestrial plants have little sodium anywhere.

Even univalent ions can be sequestered, and part of the Na^+ in living animal tissue is in an osmotically inactive form. It is held by polymers whose repeating units carry at least one acidic group (examples: nucleic acids, mucopolysaccharides). These sequestered sodium ions can instantly be liberated by ions of a higher valency, and the concentration measured with a sodium-responsive electrode (Palaty, 1966).

In recent years many experimentally useful agents have been found for altering permeability of membranes to these ions. Tetrodotoxin (Section 7.5a) decreases permeability to sodium ions, and valinomycin (Section 14.1) promotes the uptake of potassium (Moore and Pressman, 1964). By forming a complex with the potassium ion, sodium tetraphenylborate ($NaBPh_4$) can dissociate tissues into single cells (Rappaport and Howze, 1966).

The healthy kidney secretes sodium while retaining potassium. Diuretics are the more valued the less they disturb this pattern (see Section 14.1).

Lithium is not a normal cell constituent but, unlike any other known ion, it can replace sodium in facilitating nervous transmission although not efficiently. Also it is transported across isolated frog skin by the mechanism normally reserved for sodium (Schou, 1957). Its successful use in the treatment of chronic mania was initiated in Australia (Cade, 1949) and developed by Schou to the point where it has become the corner-stone of therapy for chronic mania. No lethargy accompanies its use.

Cation antagonism. Many diseases of plants and animals are traceable to maladjustments in the balance between metals. Soybean plants, treated with an excess of manganese, quickly develop signs of iron-deficiency which has to be corrected by dosing them with iron. If, on the contrary, they are grown in soil that is too rich in iron, they develop manganese-deficiency (Somers and Shive, 1942). In Britain, various pastures cause the economically serious disease in lambs called swayback. This is relieved by copper, and is associated with the presence of excessive amounts of zinc or lead in the grass. Other pastures, rich in molybdenum, cause signs of copper-deficiency in sheep (teart), relieved by the feeding of copper. Excess of zinc in the diet of rats causes an anaemia relieved by copper (Smith and Larson, 1946). Land in Holland which had been dressed with copper to prevent 'reclamation disease' (copper-deficiency) often produced crops with a marked deficiency of manganese, although the soil had the normal content of manganese. These antagonisms are reminiscent of the simple antagonism (calcium versus potassium) which is responsible for regulating the beat of the heart, as Ringer showed in 1883. A similar antagonism between magnesium and calcium governs the contractility of muscle.

Many of these antagonisms present a picture that is the inorganic equivalent of the metabolite analogues discussed in Chapter 9.

The poisoning effects of foreign metals are often traceable to cation antagonism. Thus lead, a well-known neurotoxin, displaces calcium from several parts of the nervous system, thus hindering release of neuro-transmitters (Kober and Cooper, 1976). The widespread contamination by cadmium on the West Coast of Toyama Prefecture in Japan, coupled with a low calcium intake and overcast skies, caused the painful disease 'itai itai', a form of osteomalacia, around 1960. This turned out to be a straight-forward case of cadmium-calcium antagonism (Friberg, Piscator, and Nordberg, 1971).

The biphasic response. The response of organisms to heavy metals is known to be biphasic: given too little, the organism suffers severely; this is understandable from our knowledge of the large number of enzymes which cannot function without the appropriate trace-metal. But if the organism is given too much metal, a second phase of injury is seen, due to the toxic action of the excess.

This biphasic response is well illustrated by the action of copper on oats

(Piper, 1942). Plate 5 shows graphically that too much copper is as injurious as too little. These oat plants are seen growing in a series of vessels in which concentrations of copper vary from 0 to 3000 µg per litre: growth is seen to reach a maximum at 500 µg, and to fall away on either side of this figure. The growth of micro-organisms is often critically dependent on the concentration of one or more metal cations in the nutrient medium: too little and too much must be avoided to secure growth. In recent years, it has become the practice to keep the concentration of *free* cation constant by including an organic ligand (with an appropriate stability constant) in the medium.

Metal-depleted media. Newcomers to the trace-metal field are often surprised that it is necessary to deplete the medium before beginning experiments. Unfortunately 'chemically pure' and 'analytical grade' reagents are rich sources of the heavy metals. This is inevitably so, because a substance that is 99.99 per cent pure would have 600 000 000 000 000 000 foreign molecules in each gram. This figure was calculated from the Avogadro number (6×10^{23} particles per mole of any substance) and assumes an average molecular weight of 100. Actually the makers of analytical reagents do not usually claim their products to be even as pure as 99.99 per cent. Moreover, the metallic content of bacteriological media is normally high. A typical example of contamination was revealed by the algal flagellate *Euglena gracilis*. This cell requires only 4800 atoms (5×10^{-19} g) of cobalt for the formation of a new organism. In a preliminary experiment the 'analytically pure' iron salt used for making the culture medium was found to contain enough cobalt to furnish 33 times this amount (Hutner, 1949).

Metal-depleted medium, used in the work depicted in Plate 5, was conveniently made as follows. The required nutrient salts were dissolved in water. This solution was shaken out with a solution of dithizone in chloroform. This operation was repeated many times, and finally the solution was shaken out with chloroform (to remove the dithizone) and finally aerated (to remove the chloroform) (Piper, 1942). Other substances with a high avidity for metals have been used similarly, e.g. 8-hydroxyquinoline for depleting bacteriological media (Rubbo, Albert, and Gibson, 1950). Thirty-eight methods of metal depletion have been compared by Donald, Passey, and Swaby (1952).

Non-metallic trace nutrients include boron (for plants only), iodine and fluorine (for vertebrates), selenium, and silicon. Selenium forms an essential part of the important mammalian enzyme glutathione peroxidase which prevents the oxidation of unsaturated fats and is one of the microbiocidal enzymes in phagocytes. A selenium, iron, and molybdenum enzyme was described above under 'molybdenum'. Silicon is thought to contribute to the architecture and resiliance of connective tissues of vertebrates. In rats, silicon is essential for growth and development. It seems to be present

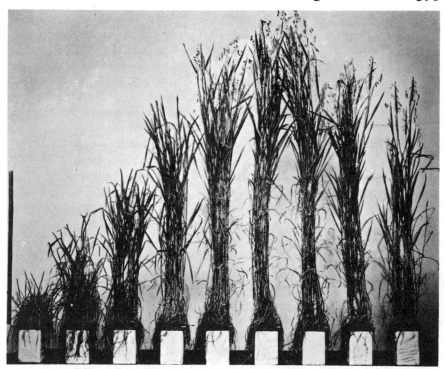

PLATE 5   Effect of copper on the height of oat-seedlings grown in nutrient
copper-deficient medium. From left to right the quantities of copper
present are nil, 3, 6, 10, 20, 100, 500, 2000, and 3000 μg per litre
(see p. 387). (Piper, 1942.)

as a silanolate, with Si-O-R bridges to such polysaccharides as heparin and
hyaluronic acid (Schwarz, 1973).

For further reading on trace elements in nutrition, see Underwood (1977),
and Prasad (1976); and for the inorganic chemistry of biological processes,
see Hughes (1972), and Williams (1976).

11.1 Biochemical differences that can assist selectivity

Every biological system can be seen as an arena where a constant struggle
is in progress for traces of heavy metal cations. Some of the strategies
are ingenious. Vertebrate hosts, when invaded by micro-organisms,
promptly decrease their level of plasma iron and zinc. Of all biologically
essential heavy metals, iron is the most critical for bacterial welfare, as
is zinc for yeasts and other fungi. Mammals decrease plasma iron by
transferring it to the liver, at the same time decreasing intestinal absorption
(Weinberg, 1974). In acute chronic infections, the level of plasma

copper rises by 50 to 90% (Weinberg, 1972) and this hypercupraemia is often assumed to be antiparasitic.

Hosts with tumours behave similarly. They have a decreased plasma level of iron (Konka and Matsuoka, 1967) whereas that of copper is elevated (Mortazani, *et al.*, 1972). Some malignant tumours cause plasma zinc to fall (Davies, Musa, and Dormandy, 1968), and this may be the host's doing, for many animal tumours are inhibited by a dietary deficiency of zinc (De Wys and Pories, 1972).

These observations lead to the question, 'What substances do living cells use for binding heavy metal cations?' There is quite a formidable array, of which the aminoacids form a useful point of reference. Most of the aminoacids which make up protein have almost exactly the same binding constants as glycine (*11.1*). Exceptionally, two common aminoacids have outstandingly high binding affinity, namely histidine (*11.2*) through its imidazole ring and cysteine (*11.3*) through the thiol group (Albert, 1952). To these two examples must be added cystine, an intense, specific binding agent for copper (Hawkins and Perrin, 1963). It is currently understood that metals are bound to proteins mainly by histidine and cysteine residues in the protein. For example, the X-ray diffraction diagram of myoglobin shows a strong link between the iron and an imidazole nitrogen atom of histidine.

Computer analysis of 160 potentiometrically determined equilibria of Cu^{2+}, Zn^{2+}, and 17 aminoacids (all simultaneously present) showed that 85 per cent of the copper was present as a single complex (1:1:1 histidine-copper-cystine), and 67 per cent of the zinc was bound by cysteine and histidine (Hallman, Perrin, and Watt, 1971). This may reflect the situation in the blood-stream. The ternary complex histidine-copper-threonine (1:1:1) has been isolated from serum by thin layer chromatography, a method conducive to re-equilibration and hence not necessarily indicative of the picture in the blood-stream (Sarkar and Kruck, 1966).

Peptides and proteins may be expected to have less avidity for metals than aminoacids, because the $-CO \cdot NH-$ group does not ionize at all readily (Datta and Rabin, 1956; Dobbie and Kermack, 1955), and the metal is usually bound between this group and a terminal NH_2. However, by *specific* folding of the peptide chain, the metal can become much more firmly held. For example, most of the copper in the blood-stream is bound to a protein, caeruloplasmin, so tightly that no exchange can be demonstrated. About 5% of the copper, however, is bound to serum albumin and about the same amount is held by single aminoacids: however albumin readily loses its copper to histidine (Neumann and Sass-Kortsak, 1967).

About 12 per cent of all known enzymes need a metal co-factor (Commission on Enzymes, 1971). How does the metal help? Metals seem often to act as a bridge between the substrate and the protein, which can activate the metal by withdrawing electrons from it. The excess positive charge,

$H_2N\cdot CH_2\cdot CO_2H$

Glycine

(11.1)

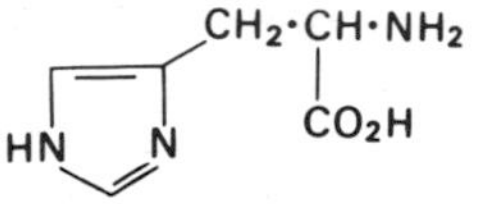

$CH_2\cdot CH\cdot NH_2$

CO_2H

Histidine

(11.2)

$HS\cdot CH_2\cdot CH(NH_2)CO_2H$

Cysteine

(11.3)

thus created on the metal, is well placed to withdraw electrons from the substrate. Thus the lowering of the free energy of activation is attributed to electronic deformation (in the substrate) mediated by the metal (Smith, 1949). A somewhat similar picture has been obtained by electron spin resonance studies of two manganese-containing enzymes: creatine kinase and muscle enolase. In the former, manganese was shown to form a bond to the coenzyme (adenosine diphosphate) and to the substrate, but not to the protein; in the latter, manganese seemed to act as a bridge between substrate and protein (Cohn and Leigh, 1962).

In some other cases, the sole role of the metal seems to be to ensure the correct tertiary folding of the protein, similar in effect to the S−S bond. This folding often brings together two or three aminoacid residues that are situated far from one another in the extended polypeptide chain, but which can form the active site when assembled in this way. An example is zinc in the alkaline phosphatase of *E. coli*: when deprived of zinc, its circular-dichroism spectrum was radically changed by 6M urea, as the

Table 11.1

SOME METALLOENZYMES

Enzyme	Catalyses	Metal
Alcohol dehydrogenase	Dehydrogenations	Zn
Aldolase	The aldol reaction	Zn
Alkaline phosphatase	Hydrolysis of phosphate esters	Zn
Carbonic anhydrase	Hydration of CO_2	Zn
Carboxypeptidase	Hydrolysis of peptides	Zn
Carboxytransphosphorylase	Transfer of phosphate group	Co
Glycol dehydrase	Rearrangement	Co
Cytochrome oxidase	Terminal oxidation	Cu, Fe
Phenol oxidase(s)	Oxidation	Cu
Cytochrome *c*	Electron transfer	Fe
Ferredoxin	Electron transfer	Fe
Xanthine oxidase	Oxidation	Mo, Fe
Pyruvate oxidase	Oxidation	Mn
ATPases*	Phosphate transfer	Mg or Ca
Enolases*	Dehydration	Mg
Oxalacetate decarboxylase*	Decarboxylation	Mg

* These three enzymes, when isolated, have no combined metal; but those shown in the third column are necessary for their activation.

native conformation gave way to a random coil (Trotman and Greenwood, 1971). For more about this enzyme see Section 11.0, under *Zinc*. Some typical metalloenzymes are shown in Table 11.1.

Although many enzymes (e.g. trypsin) function without the aid of a metal, those enzymes which require heavy metals usually hold them very tightly. In many cases, dialysis does not remove the metal; also, powerful chelating agents can enter the cells of micro-organisms without causing harm (see Section 11.7a below). This inaccessibility is more likely to be due to tertiary folding than to unusually high stability constants (see above).

Apart from aminoacids, peptides and proteins, many other metal-binding substances play essential roles in all living cells. Firstly, there are the pteridines (including folic acid) and purines, whose stability constants have been determined (Albert, 1953; Albert and Serjeant, 1960). Riboflavine is most avid in the partly reduced state (Hemmerich, Veeger and Wood, 1965). Spermine (*11.4*), and the simpler diamines such as spermidine and cadaverine, are widely distributed metal-binders.

$$H_2N(CH_2)_3NH(CH_2)_4NH(CH_2)_3NH_2$$

Spermine

(*11.4*)

All kinds of phosphates bind metals in living cells. Starting with inorganic phosphates, it is useful to note that the stability constants of orthophosphates (Ca, Mg, Zn, Cu^{2+}) have been re-determined recently, and a tendency was noted for $1:1$ complexes, like $CaHPO_4$, to dimerize, e.g. to $Ca_2H_2(PO_4)_2$ (Childs, 1970). For similar pyrophosphate data, see Wolhoff and Overbeck (1959). The stability constants of adenosine triphosphate complexes of Mg^{2+}, Ca^{2+}, Mn^{2+}, Co^{2+}, Ni^{2+}, Zn^{2+}, and Cu^{2+} have been re-determined (Perrin and Sharma, 1966), also values for AMP, ADP, UTP, GTP, CTP, and ITP (Phillips, 1966; Walaas, 1958). Magnesium ions are tightly bound by the phosphate groups of ATP as shown by potentiometric titration and ^{31}P n.m.r. (Tuck and Baker, 1973). The stability constants of Cu^{2+}, Cd^{2+}, and Fe^{3+} with DNA have been found to be of the same order as those of AMP, which has far less avidity for cations than ATP (Bryan and Frieden, 1967; Goldshtein and Gerasimova, 1966; Zakharenko and Moshkovski, 1966). Some of the heavier metal cations are associated with nucleic acids in Nature, and it has been suggested that zinc ions are co-ordinated to purine bases when reversible winding and unwinding of DNA is taking place (Shin and Eichhorn, 1968). Acids of the citric acid cycle also bind cations.

As far as is known, most of the above substances have stability constants similar in magnitude to those of the aminoacids (Table 11.2, p.408). Only the porphyrins exceed these figures: they hold iron so firmly that no exchange with radioactive iron can be detected (Hahn *et al.*, 1940).

It will be realized, from the above, that experiments involving trace-metals have no meaning if performed in the presence of phosphate or citrate buffers. N-ethyl morpholine (b.p. 138–9°C) is a useful, non-chelating buffer for the pH range 7.0–8.2 (for other buffers, see Perrin and Dempsey (1974).

Chelating agents characteristic of particular classes of organism. Studies in comparative biochemistry are constantly bringing to light new species differences in the binding and use of metals, some of which have been mentioned in Sections 4.6 and 11.0. Again, the crystalline aldolase of yeast requires iron (Warburg and Christian, 1943), whereas that of mammals does not (Taylor, Green, and Corgi, 1948).

The bacterial cell, living aerobically, is faced with the problem of fulfilling its biological need for iron from an environment where most of the iron is in the form of highly insoluble ferric oxide (the solubility product is only 10^{-39}M). This plight led to the evolution of sequestering agents to dissolve and transport the iron, and make it biologically available. These siderochromes, as they are called, are confined to bacteria, yeasts and other fungi. The two commonest types are the phenolates, such as enterochelin (*11.5*), and the hydroxamates, like desferrioxamine B (*11.6*). Both types are weak acids with a pK_a about 9, and bind ferric iron very strongly.

The most important member of the phenolate class of siderochromes, enterochelin, is a cyclic triester of 2,3-dihydroxyl-N-benzoyl-L-serine. It was isolated from *E. coli* by O'Brien and Gibson (1970), and its mode of action established by Gibson (in Australia) and Nielands (in the United States), using a series of mutants, each one of which reliably failed to carry out one of the biochemical steps. X-ray diffraction analysis showed that each ferric cation was bound to the six oxygen atoms supplied by the three catechol dianion moieties, giving the purple complex (Anderson *et al.*, 1976). The bacterium excretes enterochelin which then forms the ferric complex from environmental iron; the complex is then absorbed by the bacterium, and hydrolysed with a specific enzyme to obtain the iron (O'Brien, Cox, and Gibson, 1971).

Enterochelin
(*11.5*)

The desferrioxamines, e.g. (*11.6*), of which eight varieties are known, are hexapeptides formed by linking the amino and hydroxylamino groups (of aliphatic metabolites) by succinyl residues. X-ray diffraction showed a ferric iron held octahedrally by the six oxygen atoms of three hydroxamic acid groups. The log K_1, which is (31), greatly exceeds that of ethylenediamine tetracetic acid (24) (Table 11.2).

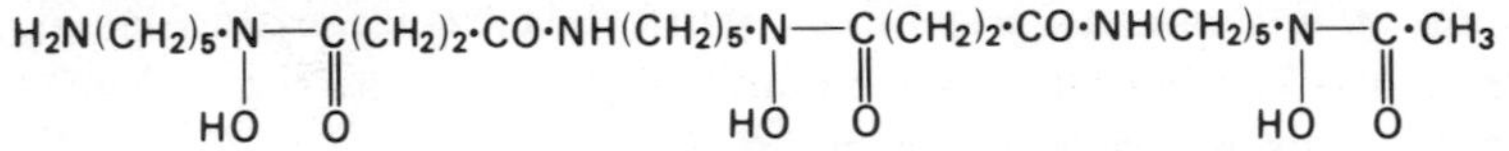
H₂N(CH₂)₅·N—C(CH₂)₂·CO·NH(CH₂)₅·N—C(CH₂)₂·CO·NH(CH₂)₅·N—C·CH₃
HO O HO O HO O

Desferrioxamine B
(*11.6*)

Mycobactin T (*11.7*) is the siderochrome of the bacterium that causes human tuberculosis. Eight other mycobactins have been obtained from other species of *Mycobacteria*, a genus to which they are confined. They have only two hydroxamate-groups, but another group is present to aid the three-centre binding of ferric iron as strongly as in other siderochromes (Snow, 1970). Pyrimine (*11.8*), 5-(2-pyridyl)- △′-pyrroline-5-carboxylic acid, was isolated from the bacterium *Pseudomonas* and, unlike the examples mentioned above, it binds ferr*ous* iron.

Interesting chemotherapeutic possibilities are suggested by this knowledge that the iron-foraging of bacteria is very different from that of mammals. For information on the use of siderochromes as antidotes in iron poisoning, see Section 11.6.

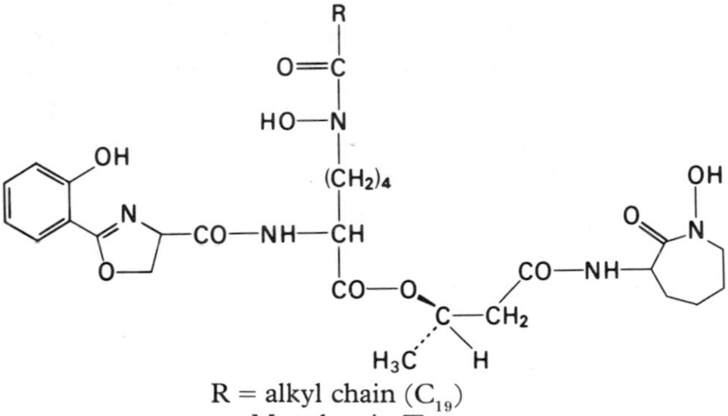
R
O=C
HO—N
OH
(CH₂)₄
OH
N
O
N
CO—NH—CH
O
CO—NH
CO—O
C—CH₂
H₃C
H

R = alkyl chain (C_{19})
Mycobactin T
(*11.7*)

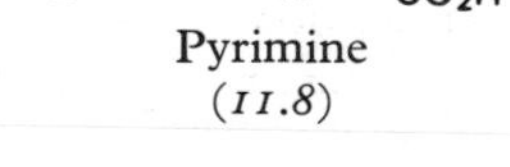
N
N
CO₂H

Pyrimine
(*11.8*)

Many fungi, such as *Aspergillus aerogenes*, excrete enterochelin whereas others (including *Aspergillus niger* and *Penicillium reticulosum*) angle for their iron with ferrichrome, a cyclic hexapeptide in which the iron is firmly held between three hydroxamate groups. Fungi contain many strongly chelating pyrones, such as kojic acid (*11.9*) which has the cumulative log stability constant (β_3) of 25 for ferric iron (McBryde and Atkinson, 1961), but their biological role is unknown, and this is also the case with the many polyhydroxyanthraquinones that fungi contain. All yeasts release the hydroxamic derivative rhodotorulic acid (*11.10*) to bring iron into the cell.

For a review of microbial iron metabolism, see Nielands (1974).

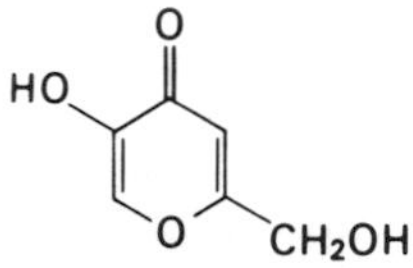

Kojic acid
(*11.9*)

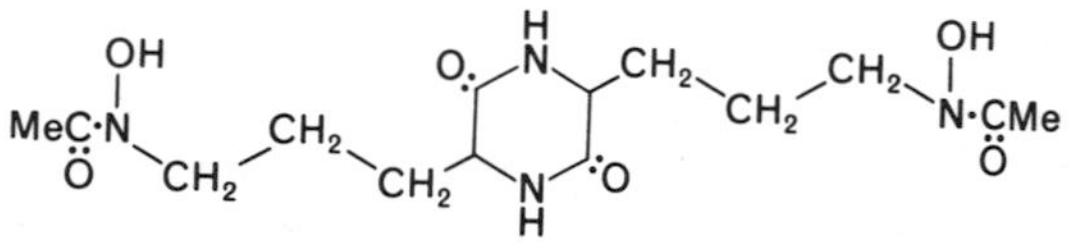

Rhodotorulic acid
(*11.10*)

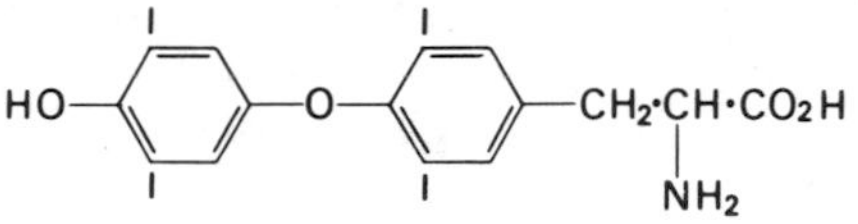

Thyroxine
(*11.11*)

Several mammalian hormones are metal-binding, e.g. thyroxine (*11.11*), histamine (*7.6*), and noradrenaline (*7.5*). The accumulation of calcium by mitochondria (mammalian only) was discussed in Section 11.0.

11.2 The chemistry of chelation

Biochemists who work with enzymes, many of which are specific for a particular metal, must regret that selectivity is quite rare among the man-made reagents for metals. In fact, most chelating agents show approximately the same order of preference for metals, which goes as follows:

Fe^{3+}, Hg^{2+} greatest avidity
Cu^{2+}, Al^{3+}
Ni^{2+}, Pb^{2+}
Co^{2+}, Zn^{2+}
Fe^{2+}, Cd^{2+}
Mn^{2+}
Mg^{2+}
Ca^{2+}
Li^+
Na^+
K^+ least avidity

The first recognition of a general trend of this kind was made by Mellor
and Maley (1947). Several of the bivalent metals, in the above scheme,
follow one another sequentially in the periodic table, thus (atomic numbers
in parentheses): (Mn (25), Fe (26), Co (27), Ni (28), Cu (29), Zn (30).
This is known as the first transition series and, in it, avidity steadily rises
to a peak for Cu^{2+}. The increase in avidity follows the decline in ionic
radius as the series is ascended (Irving and Williams, 1953). This relationship provides a rough clue to the above scheme. Because increasing the
valence of a metal tends to diminish its radius, it is not surprising to find
Fe^{3+} more avid than Fe^{2+}, or the tervalent ions at the top of the scheme and
the univalent ions at the bottom (see Table 11.4). However, many secondary
factors interfere with the operation of so simple a rule. The important
conclusion, though, is that most ligands cannot depart very far from the
order of avidities shown in the above scheme.

Fortunately there are some exceptions and special attention will be
given to those chelating agents, few in number, which depart from the
above order. Before discussing such irregular examples, the principles of
normal chelating behaviour will be reviewed. The chemical significance
of heavy metals in biology arises from their ability to form bonds that are
tighter than ordinary ionic bonds through being partly coordinate (Section 8.0).

A few ligands (known as *multi*dentate ligands, EDTA is an example)
form more than one chelate ring with a metal ion when making a 1:1-
complex. However, to simplify discussion, it is more convenient to deal
first with the three principal kinds of *bi*dentate ligands, i.e. those forming
a single ring in the 1:1-complex. These may have two electron-releasing
groups (as in ethylenediamine and 2,2′-bipyridyl), in which case the charge
on the metal cation is unaffected by chelation; or there can be one electron-
releasing and one anionic group as in glycine, in which case the charge
on the metal is diminished by one unit; or there can be two anionic groups
as in oxalic acid, in which case the charge on the metal is decreased by two
units. In general, chelation through oxygen or nitrogen takes place only
when five- or six-membered rings can be formed, and of these, five-membered rings are much more stable. [However, chelation through sulphur
enables stable four-membered rings to be formed (Peyronel, 1940; Deskin,
1958)]. The three main types of chelation are illustrated in Fig. 11.1. The
arrows in the ring imply that a normally unshared electron-pair is released
from O, N, or S to the metal.

In the presence of excess ligand, 2:1-complexes can be formed. Ligands
of the oxalic acid type use up their charge in forming 1:1-complexes, but
these can unite further with the ethylenediamine type, forming a mixed
complex (e.g. Watters and De Witt, 1960). A 1:1-complex of the glycine
type can combine with another glycine-type ligand. An ethylenediamine
type 1:1-complex can combine with any one of the three types of ligands.

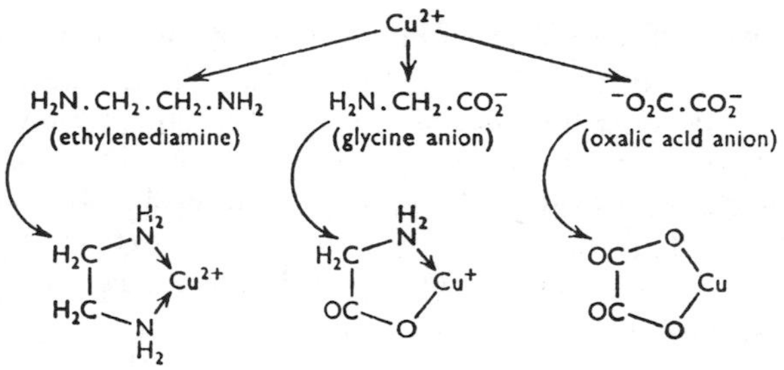
Cu2+
H2N.CH2.CH2.NH2
(ethylenediamine)
H2N.CH2.CO2−
(glycine anion)
−O2C.CO2−
(oxalic acid anion)
H2
N
H2C
Cu2+
H2C
N
H2
H2
N
H2C
Cu+
OC
O
OC
O
Cu
OC
O

FIG. 11.1 Three main types of 1 : 1 complexes.

In general, bivalent copper is quadricovalent and is usually saturated when it has combined with two ligand molecules (whether the same or different). The same is usually true for bivalent calcium, magnesium, and manganese. But bivalent iron, cobalt, and zinc are sexacovalent towards ligands of the ethylenediamine type, and tervalent ions are sexacovalent towards the glycine types as well. The ligands are gathered around the metal in configurations which depend on the direction of the valence lines proceeding from the metal cation. Most of the above metals have usually been found to give tetrahedral complexes with the main types of ligand of Fig. 11.1, but Cu^{2+} prefers planar complexes, and Fe^{2+} and Fe^{3+} prefer octahedral complexes.

It should be carefully noted that the term 'ligand' does not apply to all of the organic material present, but only to that part of it which is in the *appropriate ionic form* for combining with the metal cation. For ethylenediamine, glycine, and oxalic acid, the ligands are the molecule, the mono-anion, and the di-anion, respectively. Hence, when stability constants are used to compare the relative avidity of ligands under physiological conditions, the pK_a values of the ligands must also be considered (see Section 11.3).

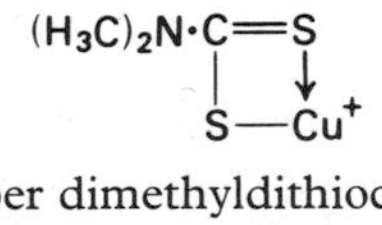
(H3C)2N·C=S
S—Cu+

Copper dimethyldithiocarbamate complex
(*11.12*)

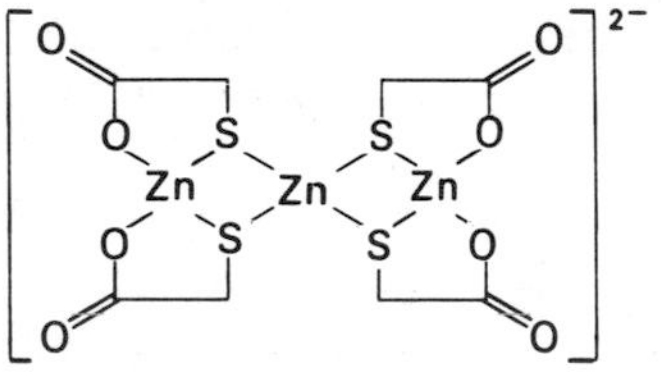
2−
O
S
Zn
Zn
Zn
S
O

Zinc mercaptoacetic acid complex
(*11.13*)

Although sulphur can take part in simple four-membered rings such as in cupric dimethyldithiocarbamate (*11.12*), which is formed from cupric ions and dimethyldithiocarbamic acid (*3.41*), sulphur-containing ligands form an equilibrium mixture of many complexes. Thus zinc and mercaptoacetic acid (L^{2-}) form the series:

$$ZnL, ZnL_2^{2-}, ZnL_3^{4-}, Zn_2L_3^{2-}, Zn_3L_4^{2-}$$

The last of these ($Zn_3L_4^{2-}$) is one of the most stable and is shown as (*11.13*). Information about the above series was derived from computer analysis of titration data, a procedure which gave the following series for cysteine (L^{2-}) (Perrin and Sayce, 1968):

$$ZnHL_2^-, ZnH_2L_2, ZnL_2^{2-}, Zn_3L_4^{2-}$$

In more acidic solutions, protonated forms of the zinc-cysteine complex are present also (Shindo and Brown, 1965). It is evident that sulphur-containing ligands give a more complicated pattern of complexes than the simple patterns produced by oxygen- and nitrogen-containing ligands, which are more common and to which the next section will be devoted.

For detailed discussion of conformation and absolute configuration of chelated complexes, see Hawkins (1971). For books on principles and applications of metal chelation, see Bell (1976); Perrin (1964, 1970); for a periodical series of books, see Sigel (1973 <).

11.3 Quantitative treatment of metal-binding

In order to quantify the various degrees of tightness in binding (which vary between wide limits), stability constants are used. These are the constants governing the mass-action equilibrium between the ligand(s) and one ion of the metal. Thus for the 1:1-complex of glycine and cupric ion, the equilibrium is:

$$K_1 = \frac{[H_2N \cdot CH_2 \cdot CO_2Cu^+]}{[Cu^{2+}][H_2N \cdot CH_2 \cdot CO_2^-]}$$

and for the 2:1-complex,

$$K_2 = \frac{[H_2N \cdot CH_2 \cdot CO_2CuO_2C \cdot CH_2 \cdot NH_2]}{[H_2N \cdot CH_2 \cdot CO_2Cu^+][H_2N \cdot CH_2 \cdot CO_2^-]}$$

where K_1 is the stability constant for the 1 : 1-complex, and K_2 is that for the 2 : 1-complex. In each case the product is in the top line, and the substances from which it is formed are in the lower line.

For many purposes the *cumulative stability constant* (β) is required; this is the product of the individual constants. If there are two individual constants, the product is designated β_2; if there are three constants, β_3. Stability constants are usually determined by potentiometric (glass electrode) titration of the ligand, in the presence and absence of the metal, and the results are processed by a set of rather complex calculations for which a computer programme can conveniently be used.

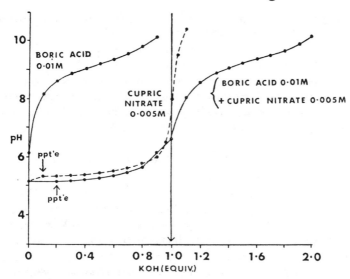

FIG. 11.2 Example of the use of potentiometry to see if a substance can chelate. The above curves show plainly that boric acid does not chelate. Contrast this with Fig. 11.3.

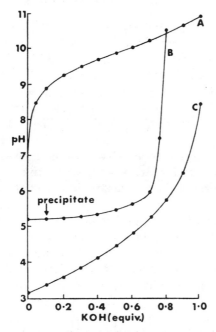

FIG. 11.3 The above curves show that glycine is a strong chelating agent. A, glycine (0.01 M); B, cupric nitrate (0.005 M); C, glycine (0.01 M) plus cupric nitrate (0.005 M).

In brief, the acidic group of the suspected chelating agent is titrated with alkali, and the pH is recorded after each tenth of an equivalent is added. Then a 1:1-mixture of the substance and a salt (e.g. copper perchlorate or nitrate) is titrated. If there is no complex formed, the new curve follows, in turn, the individual curves for the two components (see Fig. 11.2). But when chelation occurs, the hydrogen cations liberated by the chelation of the cupric cations displace the whole curve to lower pH values (see Fig. 11.3). Non-acidic substances, in the form of their salts with acids, may be similarly titrated with alkali.

Potentiometry can be used even for dilute solutions of sparingly soluble substances if unusual care is taken; e.g. 0.1 mM adenine, titrated in the presence of 8 μM cupric ions (in water), readily gave a precise constant (Albert and Serjeant, 1960). Solvents other than water should never be used if results of biological significance are required. Mixtures of water and an organic solvent give particularly misleading results (Albert and Serjeant, 1971).

The glass electrode, in potentiometric titration, can sometimes be advantageously replaced by a copper electrode (e.g. Dobbie and Kermack, 1955) when this is the metal of principal interest. For excessively insoluble complexes, potentiometry is replaced by exchange methods. Thus two ligands may be allowed to compete for one metal, or two metals for one ligand; the result is conveniently measured if one of the two components is isotopic (Schubert, 1956). Partition methods are useful when the constants are so high that the free $[H^+]$ is large in comparison with total $[H^+]$ (free and bound): in these circumstances, potentiometry is inaccurate. The method, in brief, is to shake a solution of the ligand (of known concentration in a water-immiscible solvent) with an aqueous solution of the metal cation (of known concentration in an aqueous buffer). The concentration of the ligand is then measured spectroscopically in the non-aqueous solution (McBryde, 1967). Of its own, ultraviolet spectrometry is not very useful (for an example, see Ågren, 1954). Other methods used in special circumstances are: potentiometry with cation-selective electrodes, infrared spectroscopy in deuterium oxide, magnetic resonance spectroscopy (both e.s.r. and n.m.r.), optical rotatory dispersion, conductimetry, thermal relaxation (temperature jump), and polarography. For general purposes, straight potentiometry is superior to any of these.

It was not possible to calculate stability constants from titration data until Bjerrum (1941) showed that they are related to two variables ($\bar{n}$) and $[L]$ by the following equation:

$$K_1 = \frac{\bar{n}}{(1 - \bar{n})[L]}$$

where $\bar{n}$ (pronounced 'enbar') is the average number of complex-forming molecules bound by one atom of metal and $[L]$ is the concentration of the free chelating species of the ligand. Both $\bar{n}$ and $[L]$ depend on the ionization constant of the ligand and on the pH, but each is related to these factors differently. The net result is that an increase in acidity leads to less metal being bound.

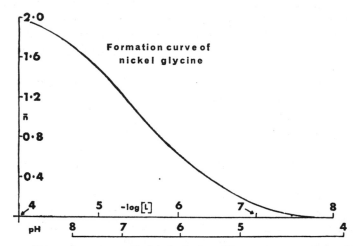

FIG. 11.4 Formation curve of nickel-glycine. The average number of molecules ($\bar{n}$) of glycine which are united to one atom of metal is plotted against the concentration of the negative logarithm of the chelating species (L) of glycine.

Fig. 11.4 illustrates a typical formation curve (the plot of $\bar{n}$ against $-\log$ $[L]$. It will be observed how $\bar{n}$ decreases with falling pH. But the stability constant does not vary with pH, and the use of the above equation will give the same value for K_1 anywhere between $\bar{n} = 0$ and $\bar{n} = 1$, above which a related equation for K_2 is applicable. When, as is usual, K_1 and K_2 differ by less than a hundredfold, these equations need a least-squares treatment to deal with mutual interference, especially in the $\bar{n}$ 0.8 to 1.2 region. For this reason, and to refine the results to the utmost, the use of computers has become universal in converting potentiometric readings to stability constants. A suitable programme is available (Sayce, 1968 and 1971) which can even deal with two metals and two ligands, simultaneously present. This programme is called 'Stability Constants of Generalized Species' (or SCOGS for short) and it is written in Fortran IV. It also reports any polynuclear, hydrolysed, or protonated species provided that data from several titrations (covering a range of metal and ligand concentrations) are inserted. It also reports mixed complexes. A different programme exists for reporting the equilibria produced by 10 metals and 10 ligands simultaneously present (Perrin and Sayce, 1967).

Many titrations of one metal and two different ligands, present together in the solution, have been quite simply dealt with (Perrin, Sayce, and

Table 11.2

STABILITY CONSTANTS (LOGARITHMIC) OF SOME COMPLEXING AGENTS (IN WATER AT 20°C)

Constants are reported as log β. To save space, the order is given as a pre-index; thus manganese forms a 2 : 1-complex with bipyridyl (log β = 6), reported as $^{2}6$; whereas it forms only a 1 : 1-complex with EDTA (log β = 13), reported as 13.

Ligand	Fe^{3+}	Cu^{2+}	Ni^{2+}	Zn^{2+}	Co^{2+}	Fe^{2+}	Mn^{2+}	Mg^{2+}
Glycine (11.1)	10	$8.5; {}^{2}15$	$6; {}^{2}11$	$5; {}^{2}9$	$5; {}^{2}9$	$4; {}^{2}8$	$3; {}^{2}5.5$	$2; {}^{2}4$
Cysteine (11.3)	*	*	$10; {}^{2}19$	$10; {}^{2}18$	$^{3}16$	6	4	<4
Histidine (11.2)	?	$10.5; {}^{2}19$	$9; {}^{2}16$	$7; {}^{2}12$	$7; {}^{2}13$	$5; {}^{2}9$	3.5	<4
Histamine (7.6)	?	$10; {}^{2}16$	$7; {}^{2}11$	$5; {}^{2}9$	$5; {}^{2}9$	4	?	?
Ethylenediamine (Fig. 11.1)	?	$11; {}^{2}20**$	$8; {}^{3}18$	$6; {}^{3}12$	$6; {}^{3}14$	$4; {}^{3}9.5$	$3; {}^{2}5$	0.4
Ethylenediaminetetracetic acid (EDTA) (cf. 11.22)	24	19	18	16	16	14	13	9
Pteroylglutamic acid (folic acid) (cf. 2.14)	?	$^{2}8$	$^{2}9$	$^{2}7.5$	$^{2}8$	$^{2}8$	$^{2}6$	?
Hypoxanthine	?	6	5	?	4	4	2	?
Guanosine	?	6	4	4.5	3	4	3	?
Adenine (4.3)	?	$^{2}14$	4	?	$4; {}^{2}8$	?	?	?
8-Hydroxyquinoline (oxine) (11.24)	$12; {}^{2}24; {}^{3}36$	$12; {}^{2}23$	$10; {}^{2}18$	$8.5; {}^{2}16$	$9; {}^{2}17$	$8; {}^{2}15$	$7; {}^{2}12$	4.5
o-Phenanthroline (11.15)	$^{3}14$	$^{2}20$	$^{3}24$	$^{3}17$	$^{3}20$	$^{3}21$	$^{3}10$	?
Bipyridyl	?	$^{3}17$	$^{3}20$	$^{3}13$	$^{3}16$	$^{3}17.5$	$^{2}6$	?
Oxalic acid	10	6	5.5	5	4.5	4.5	4	3***
Salicylic acid	$16; {}^{2}28$	$11; {}^{2}19$	$7; {}^{2}12$	7	$7; {}^{2}11$	$6; {}^{2}11$	$6; {}^{2}10$	?
Tetracycline (11.30)	$10; {}^{3}25$	$8; {}^{3}13$	$6; {}^{2}11$	$5; {}^{2}9$	$5; {}^{2}10$	$5; {}^{2}9$	$4; {}^{2}8$	4
Isonicotinic hydrazide (isoniazid) (11.31)	?	8	5.5	5	5	?	?	?
Dimethyldithiocarbamic acid (3.41)	?	$11; {}^{2}22$	?	?	?	?	?	?

* Cysteine is oxidized by this cation.   ** cf. $^{2}11$ for Cu^{+}.   *** Ca^{2+} is also ~3.

Tetracycline (Albert and Rees, 1956), isoniazid (Albert, 1956), salicylic acid (Perrin, 1958), bipyridyl and o-phenanthroline (Irving and Mellor, 1962), dimethyldithiocarbamic acid (Janssen, 1958), aminoacids (Albert, 1950, 1952), other values (Sillén and Marrell, 1964).

Sharma, 1967; Perrin and Sharma, 1968, 1969). When two ligands, A and B, are equally avid for a metal M, the mixed complex AMB is statistically favoured by a factor of 2 over simple complexes such as AMA. Similarly when three such ligands (A, B, and C) are present, the complex MABC is favoured by a factor of 6 (Watters and DeWitt, 1960).

The constants of a number of substances of interest to biological workers are given in Table 11.2. For other constants see the compilation edited by Sillén and Martell (1964, 1971).

There is no certain way of predicting the stability constants of a substance in advance of synthesizing it, and making the measurements. The most useful guides in the prediction of approximate stability constants are as follows. In any one series, the more tightly a ligand combines with hydrogen ions (as measured by the pK values) the more tightly will it bind metals. [Present-day knowledge of inductive constants makes it easy to forecast ionization constants (as pK_a values) in advance of synthesis (see Appendix III).] This rule, which it must be emphasized holds only for a series of *related* substances, breaks down if bulky groups cause steric hindrance (see below).

When we have to compare members from *different* series, the most common disturbing factor, in the $pK_a : \log K_1$ relationship, is resonance in a chelated ring. Here the most useful clue is to examine the double-bond composition of the ring: factors which lower double-bond character usually also decrease stability (Calvin and Wilson, 1945). Thus in the copper chelate of acetylacetone, the chelate ring contains two full double-bonds and the metal is more tightly bound than in the salicylaldehyde chelate where, on account of the resonance of the benzene ring, one of the double-bonds is virtually only half present. Similar considerations show that in 2-hydroxy-1-naphthaldehyde and 2-hydroxy-3-naphthaldehyde, the shared double-bond is virtually present about two-thirds and one-third of the time respectively. It was found that the stabilities of the copper-derivatives varied accordingly (Calvin and Wilson, 1945).

Help in the prediction of stability constants is expected to come from developments of ligand field theory. The core of this treatment is crystal field theory which postulates that the five d orbitals of heavy metals, although normally equal in energy, become differentiated when lying in the electrostatic field of the ligand. In particular, those d orbitals lying *in* the direction of the ligands are raised in energy, and those lying *away* from the ligands are lowered in energy. The donor electrons on the ligands repel the d electrons of the metal: this repulsion is reduced by the movement of d electrons into those d orbitals which are further from the ligands. The energy liberated by this effect is called the crystal field stabilization energy. It varies with the ligand and the number of d electrons, and it can be calculated in simple cases. Although evolved for crystals, this theory is applicable to complexes in solution. For aromatic ligands and certain

metals (notably iron, nickel, and cobalt) allowance must be made for
π-bonding. With this modification, crystal field theory has been combined
with molecular orbital theory to give what is called ligand field theory.
For further reading, see Basolo and Pearson (1967).

Ranking order at a fixed pH. When members of a series of chelating
agents have much the same ionization constants, the relative stability
constants place the members in order of their ability to segregate the metal
cations at any given pH value. However, when chelating agents of very
different ionization constants have to be compared, stability constants
do not give a good estimate of the relative competing value for cations.
The reason is that, at the pH at which information is desired, these agents
are likely to be ionized to different extents. The one which has the less
affinity for metals (as shown by the lower stability constant) may, through
a difference in pK_a, produce enormously more anion than the other agent.
In this case, the substance with the less affinity for the metal may well be
the one that gets most of it. This is so because chelation requires not only
an affinity between ligand and metal, but also a ready supply of ligand
anions from the agent (or of ligand molecules, if the agent is a base). This
type of competition between stability constant and ionizing constant is
illustrated in Table 11.3.

Table 11.3

DISTRIBUTION OF CATIONS AMONG SOME LIGANDS IN NEUTRAL SOLUTION

Figures in italics: proportional parts
Figures in brackets: log 1 : 1 stability constants
(columns to be read vertically)

Ligand	Cu^2	Fe^{2+}	Fe^{3+}
Glycine	*45* (8.5)	*30* (4.3)	*1* (10.0)
Salicylic acid	*1* (10.6)	*1* (6.6)	*400* (16.4)
Oxine	*200 000* (12.2)	*150 000* (8.0)	*200* (12.3)

(Perrin, 1958.)

A statisfactory solution is to calculate the percentage of metal bound at
the given pH, and to use this percentage for ranking. The necessary calculation is as follows:

$$\text{Per cent metal bound as 1 : 1-complex} = \frac{100K_1WA}{1 + K_1WA + K_1K_2W^2A^2}$$

$$\text{Per cent metal bound as 2 : 1-complex} = \frac{100K_1K_2W^2A^2}{1 + K_1WA + K_1K_2W^2A^2}$$

Here A is the concentration of *un*complexed ligand. When the ligand is in great excess, the concentration of total ligand may be used in place of A; if otherwise, A may be calculated by successive approximations;

W is the factor: $1/(1 + 10^{(pK_{a_1} - pH)} + 10^{(pK_{a_1} + pK_{a_2} - 2pH)})$.

For further data on the use of ligands to mask and unmask reactions catalysed by metal cations, see Perrin (1970).

11.4 Chemical differences that can assist selectivity

Now that the regular features of affinity for metals have been reviewed, some interesting *irregular* features can be discussed. Selectivity for particular ions is dependent on such irregularities. The strong tendency of cupric ions to form planar complexes means that copper is uniquely sensitive to a type of steric effect imposed by bulky groups. Thus, in Table 11.2, the stability constants for the cupric complexes of bipyridyl, phenanthroline, and folic acid lie below those of the corresponding nickel complexes, which is contrary to the natural order discussed in Section 11.2.

Another type of steric effect arises when a bulky group is inserted near to the chelating groups. This prevents two ligands from approaching close enough to form a strong 2 : 1-complex, and, in the case of metallic cations of small diameter, the cation cannot be gripped. Thus, 2-methyl-oxine (*11.14*) binds all cations less strongly than oxine does, but the difference is greatest for aluminium (Irving and Rossotti, 1956), which has the smallest crystal radius (0.50 Å) of any common metal (see Table 11.4). Again, two molecules of 2,9-dimethyl-*o*-phenanthroline (*11.15*, R = CH_3) hinder one another too much to retain the ferrous ion. In this case the two ligand molecules push one another into planes where the nitrogen atoms can no longer form the octahedral complex required by Fe^{2+}; even the planar complex preferred by Cu^{2+} is formed only with difficulty. Yet the new planes are highly suitable for binding Cu^+ (which prefers tetrahedral complexes); the high stability of the cuprous complex forms the basis for the use of this substance in analysis.

Let us return to those ligands that are too bulky to approach one another closely and hence cannot form a strongly held 2 : 1-complex with a cation

2-Methyl-oxine
(*11.14*)

o-Phenanthroline (R = H)
(*11.15*)

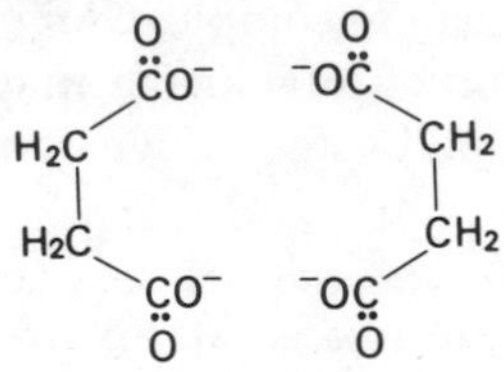

Succinate anions
(*11.16*)

of small diameter. The radius of the magnesium ions is 0.34 Å smaller than that of calcium (Table 11.4). Normally Mg^{2+} is more tightly held than Ca^{2+}, but this order is reversed by ligands that are too bulky for a pair of them to grip the metal. All dicarboxylic acids show this effect, e.g. succinic acid in (*11.16*) (note oxalic acid in Fig. 11.5), but tartaric acid is outstanding in its preference for Ca^{2+} over Mg^{2+} (Williams, 1952). Some relevant radii are given in Table 11.4. It should be noted that Fe^{2+}, Co^{2+}, Ni^{2+}, and Zn^{2+} have such similar diameters that they could not be separated through this steric effect.

Table 11.4

CRYSTAL RADII OF CATIONS (IN Å)

Li^+	0.60	Be^{2+}	0.31	Al^{3+}	0.50
Na^+	0.95	Mg^{2+}	0.65	Fe^{3+}	0.64
K^+	1.33	Ca^{2+}	0.99	Ga^{3+}	0.62
Rb^+	1.49	Sr^{2+}	1.13	Tl^{3+}	0.95
Cs^+	1.69	Ba^{2+}	1.35	Co^{3+}	0.63
Cu^+	0.96	Mn^{2+}	0.80		
Tl^+	1.40	Fe^{2+}	0.76		
Ag^+	1.26	Co^{2+}	0.74		
		Ni^{2+}	0.72		
		Cu^{2+}	~0.72		
		Zn^{2+}	0.74		
		Cd^{2+}	0.97		
		Hg^{2+}	1.10	U^{4+}	0.97
		Pb^{2+}	1.20	Pb^{4+}	0.84

(Pauling, 1960.)

The dimensions of the radii of anhydrous cations are constantly under revision (Ladd, 1968). All methods depend on inferences and assumptions. The data in Table 11.4 remain the most comprehensive and widely used. It will be appreciated that anhydrous radii are the relevant ones in chelation chemistry.

See Section 14.1 for ionophores that are specific for transporting univalent ions, e.g. Na^+, through natural membranes (this is not chelation).

All of the above are *equilibrium* steric effects; for some *kinetic* steric effects, see Wilkins (1962). Some non-steric effects that change the natural order of avidities will now be described.

A selective enhancement of the bonding of iron is found in heteroaromatic ligands. This is caused by *back double-bonding*, i.e. a π-bonding in which unused electrons in a suitably placed 3*d* orbital are contributed by the iron to empty molecular orbitals in the ligand. The result is that electrons flow in the direction shown in (*11.17*), instead of the normal direction, as in (*11.18*). In consequence, the ligand-metal bonds are reinforced and the complex gains extra stability. Ferrous iron usually gives complexes which are paramagnetic and almost colourless; but with heteroaromatic ligands, containing doubly bound nitrogen, Fe^{2+} forms deeply-coloured complexes (usually red) with loss of paramagnetism. The effect is seen (in Table 11.2) for bipyridyl, folic acid, and *o*-phenanthroline, where the constants for ferrous iron greatly exceed those for zinc. Nickel and cobalt are also capable of back double-bonding, but to a smaller extent.

(*11.17*)   (*11.18*)

Examination of the log K values for *o*-phenanthroline and 2,2′-bipyridyl (in Table 11.2) reveals the action of *two* principles which have been described above. The preference of Cu^{2+} for a planar structure does not readily admit a third molecule of ligand. Hence Cu^{2+} takes an unusually low place in the table, below Ni^{2+}. Remarkably high values β are seen for Fe^{2+}. These arise from the outstandingly high third partial constant (K_3), where a spin-paired complex admits of back double-bonding. The net result is that Fe^{2+} takes an unusually high place above Zn^{2+} and Co^{2+}. The extraordinary result of the combination of these two principles is that Fe^{2+} is bound as strongly as Cu^{2+} (Irving and Mellor, 1962).

Another kind of differentiation is illustrated in the plot of stability constants against atomic number in the series: calcium, magnesium, manganese, iron, cobalt, nickel, copper, and zinc (Fig. 11.5). This curve rises most steeply for ligands that use two nitrogen atoms for chelation (e.g. ethylenediamine), less steeply for those that chelate with one nitrogen and one oxygen atom (e.g. glycine), and least steeply for those which use two oxygen atoms (e.g. oxalic acid) (Irving and Williams, 1953). The curves for substances of these different classes cross one another between Mn^{2+} and Fe^{2+} in Fig. 11.5. Not only Mg^{2+} and Ca^{2+}, but also Fe^{3+}, Tl^{3+}, Mo^{5+}, and V^{5+} show a preference for combining with oxygen rather than nitrogen.

Most metals prefer combination with oxygen to sulphur, but Cu^+, Ag^+,

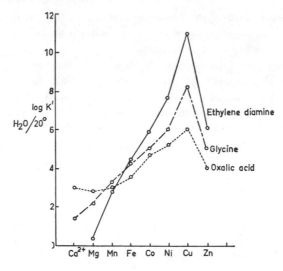

FIG. 11.5 The relative affinities of bivalent cations for oxygen and nitrogen types of chelating agent. The logarithms of the first stability constants are plotted against rising atomic numbers.

Au^+, Hg^{2+}, As^{3+}, and Sb^{3+} prefer sulphur to oxygen, thus explaining the successful use of dimercaprol (*11.19*) as an antidote for poisoning by several of these cations. Three other cations, Cu^{2+}, Ni^{2+}, and Co^{2+}, slightly prefer sulphur to oxygen if the sulphur is non-ionic, as in an organic sulphide.

Another factor, which can cause the relative affinities of a series of metals to change, is the reduction-oxidation potential* of a metal, which is always altered by chelation in a metal of variable valency (e.g. Cu, Fe, Co, Mn, Mo, V). It can even result that the metal quickly changes, after chelation, to a valency higher or lower than the one originally chosen. The scope can be gleaned from Table 11.5. (It should be borne in mind that the scale of potentials ranges from about + 2 V for the most powerful oxidizing agents to about −2 V for the most powerful reducing agents.) Cobalt provides an interesting example of this effect. Normally cobaltous salts are stable in aqueous solution whereas a cobaltic salt is instantly decomposed by water with the evolution of oxygen. However, upon chelation with ethyl-

---

* E_o is the oxidation-reduction potential, a constant calculated at pH o by the following expression:

$$E_o = E_H - \frac{RT}{nF} \ln \frac{[ox]}{[red]}$$

where E_H is the measured potential, R is the gas constant, T the absolute temperature, F the faraday, n the number of electrons concerned, and ln is the natural logarithm. At any other pH than o, the symbol E' is used, and the pH specified. Potentials obtained by polarography are often quoted 'versus the saturated calomel electrode', and need the addition of 0.246 V to put them on the above (normal hydrogen electrode) scale.

enediamine the potential falls so drastically that the cobaltous complex becomes readily oxidized to the more stable cobaltic state.

The potential of a complex is determined by (a) the ionic charge on the ligand, (b) back-bonding of metal to ligand, and (c) the crystal field effect (Perrin, 1959). For example, concerning (a) it is known that when the ligand is anionic the higher valence state of the metal is favoured; concerning (b) it is known that back-bonding from iron favours the lower valences; and concerning (c) it is known that the crystal field effect favours Cu^{2+} and Fe^{2+} to other valences of these metals. Unfortunately, these factors cannot yet be integrated to predict the potential of a complex in advance of measurement.

It is evident from Table 11.5 that some complexes are more powerful

Table 11.5

THE EFFECT OF LIGANDS ON REDUCTION-OXIDATION POTENTIALS

(Mainly at 20°C)

Simple ion	E_0 (potential in volts)	Complexes* with :		E_0
$Fe(H_2O)_6^{2+} = Fe(H_2O)_6^{3+}$	+ 0.77	[1]EDTA		+ 0.14
		[1,2]Salicylic acid	+ 0.20	− 0.22
		[6]Cyanide ion		+ 0.36
		[1]Glycine		+ 0.38
		[1,2]8-Hydroxyquinoline	+ 0.52	+ 0.27
		[1,2]Oxytetracyline	+ 0.57	+ 0.43
		[3]Bipyridyl		+ 1.06
		[3]o-Phenanthroline		+ 1.06
$Co(H_2O)_6^{2+} = Co(H_2O)_6^{3+}$	+ 1.84	[6]Cyanide ion		− 0.83
		[3]Ethylenediamine		− 0.22
		[6]Ammonia		+ 0.14
$Cu(H_2O)_x^+ = Cu(H_2O)_4^{2+}$	+ 0.17	[2]Ethylenediamine		− 0.38
		[2]Glycine		− 0.16
		[2]Bipyridyl		+ 0.12
		[2]o-Phenanthroline		+ 0.17
		[1,2]Methylthio-ethylamine	+ 0.19	+ 0.24
		[1,2]Pyridine	+ 0.20	+ 0.27
		[2]4-Methylpyridine		+ 0.30
		[2]Ammonia		+ 0.34
		[1,2]Imidazole	+ 0.26	+ 0.35
		[2]Benzimidazole		+ 0.36

* The pre-indexes have the same meaning as in Table 11.2 (e.g. [3]Bipyridyl means the 3 : 1-complex of bipyridyl). Data taken principally from Perrin (1959), and Hawkins and Perrin (1962).

oxidizing agents than the free metal cations. Such complexes could cause the destruction of vital metabolites, e.g. the copper diethyldithiocarbamate chelate destroys thioctic acid (2.25) (Sijpesteijn and Janssen, 1959).

A more subtle aspect of ligand-metal interaction is that the bound metal may change the selectivity of the organic ligand by : (a) changing the electron distribution in the ligand, (b) masking a chemically active centre of the ligand, (c) forcing the ligand molecules into a particular conformational form, (d) providing a conducting pathway for electron-addition or -removal, (e) increasing the liposolubility of the ligand, and hence helping it to penetrate into a living cell.

11.5 The various modes of biological action of chelating agents (an introduction)

The biphasic response of organisms to metals, so neatly illustrated by Piper's oats (Plate 5, p. 395), suggests two distinct mechanisms for the action of a chelating agent in biology : (i) the removal of metals from the cell, or the masking of metals within the cell, and (ii) the imposition on the cell of metals in greater quantity (or at a higher oxidation potential) than normal. Further sub-divisions can be made, depending on whether the metals in question are essential or toxic.

Mechanism (i).   Most of the chelating agents that have achieved a biological use by this mechanism are antidotes, designed to mask or remove toxic metals that have accidentally been ingested by higher mammals. They are dealt with further in Section 11.6.

Few cases are known where a metal-binding agent is, of itself, highly injurious to an organism. Thus oxine (*11.24*) can enter the cells of bacteria and fungi without apparent injury (see Section 11.7a). Such freedom from damage arises from the normal steric and affinity factors which allowed the active site to accumulate and retain the metal.

The most throughly investigated example of injury by masking is that caused by hydrogen cyanide. This agent binds the free valencies of the iron in cytochrome oxidase without detaching it from its four-bond contact with the porphyrin nucleus. Thus, this enzyme is prevented from uniting with its substrate, and respiration comes to a standstill. In many species this causes immediate death of the organism.

Mechanism (ii).   How this mechanism has been used to supply iron to trees has been recounted in Section 11.0. Another example is the injection into lime-deficient patients of the calcium gluconic acid complex, which slowly breaks down and liberates ionic calcium. The best investigated examples of mechanism (ii) are found among the chelating bactericides and fungicides (see Section 11.7). Data necessary for the understanding of mechanism (ii) will now be discussed under two headings, '*the co-operative effect*' and '*the partition effect*'.

The co-operative effect.   That a metal can become much more chemically active after chelation is evident enough in the oxygen-binding properties of haemoglobin and the oxidizing powers of the heme enzymes. Inorganic salts of iron have catalase- and peroxidase-like properties, but these are enormously increased upon incorporation in the porphyrin nucleus attached to a specific protein. Similarly, cuprous ions catalyse the aerial oxidation of ascorbic acid, but this effect is immensely magnified in the enzyme ascorbic oxidase (Table 10.4).

Proteins are not always necessary to elicit this co-operative effect. In fact it often happens that, by adding metal-binding substances to sequester a metal, the very metal-catalysed effect that it is desired to suppress becomes aggravated. The offending metals are usually those which can undergo a change of valency, particularly copper and iron. The co-operative effect is most likely to be encountered if insufficient metal-binding agent is added, so that the complex is unsaturated. Some examples will now be given.

The oxidative blackening of dihydroxyphenylalanine in the presence of cupric sulphate is greatly accelerated if *o*-phenanthroline (*11.15*) is added (Isaka, 1957). The auto-oxidation of glutathione in an extract of ocular lens tissue (catalysed by trace of iron in the extract) is accelerated by EDTA (Pirie and van Heyningen, 1954). Both *o*-phenanthroline and bipyridyl increase the rate of iron-catalysed decomposition of hydrogen peroxide by a hundredfold: these are, in fact, models for haemo-protein enzymes. The copper-catalysed hydrolysis of di*iso*propyl fluorophosphate is much accelerated by aminoacids, ethylenediamine, *o*-phenanthroline, and bipyridyl. The best proportions are those which give a 1 : 1-complex (Wagner-Jauregg *et al.*, 1955). EDTA does not assist this hydrolysis, indeed EDTA is not a co-operator with copper, and can prevent oxine from acting as one (Byrde and Woodcock, 1957).

The mode of action of many selectively toxic agents is due to this co-operative effects, as will be demonstrated in Section 11.7a. Metals usually have more specificity in the chelated state than when free as inorganic salts.

The partition effect.   It is known that cell membranes carefully regulate the intake of heavy-metal cations, and even cations essential in traces for nutrition are toxic in excess.* But uncharged complexes are liposoluble and hence should readily penetrate cell membranes in a way which the cell cannot regulate. Fig. 11.1 shows that, for a divalent metal, the complexes of the oxalic acid type, and 2 : 1-complexes of the glycine type, are uncharged and hence should penetrate cells readily. (Complexes of polydentate substances like EDTA, cf. (*11.22*), often have hydrophilic groups in excess

---

* Iron is more toxic than is commonly believed; large oral doses of ferrous sulphate cause hepatic necrosis in man within 48 hours (Luongo and Bjornson, 1954). The toxic action of encephalomyelitis virus, which is rich in iron, has been ascribed to viral transport of this metal across the blood-brain barrier which is normally impervious to it (Racker and Krimsky, 1947).

of those with which the metal can combine, and such complexes are not expected to penetrate ordinary cell membranes.) The liposoluble complexes enable the chelating agent to transport the metal into the cells in quantities larger than would normally occur. (Conversely, the metal may be thought of as transporting the chelating agent.)

Metal chelates may sometimes act on the *outside* of micro-organisms, whose characteristic negative charge would cause them to attract, and accumulate, positively charged complexes such as (a) the glycine type of chelating agent furnishes when unsaturated (e.g. 1 : 1-complexes of divalent metals) and (b) the ethylenediamine type furnishes at all degress of saturation (see Fig. 11.1).

A novel use of chelation is to suppress host-toxic effects in a potentially useful drug by *masking* the offending group with a metal. This has been done for adriamycin (*10.23*) whose highly selective action against cancers, including the otherwise difficult to control solid tumours, was outlined in Section 10.3b. Unfortunately, adriamycin exerts a toxic effect on the patient's heart by withdrawing iron necessary for the cardiac ATPase. This has been lessened by converting adriamycin to the (water-soluble) triferric complex which is free from cardiotoxicity while maintaining unimpared its curative intercalating action on the tumour DNA (Gosálvez, 1976; Gosálvez et al., 1978; Cortés et al., 1978). The complex is marketed under the name 'Quelamycin'.

11.6 Diminution by chelation of the toxic effect of a metal

Several chelating agents are regularly used in hospitals as antidotes for occupational poisoning by metals, for chronic metal intoxication arising from therapy or household contamination, or to hasten the excretion of radioactive elements. They have been used in this way only since 1945. These antidotes circulate in the blood-stream without causing much depletion of the body's essential heavy metals; this is, of course, a matter of dosage. To ensure that little of the antidote enters cells, and that it is rapidly excreted, the molecules of antidotes are provided with polar (preferably ionizable) groups such as $-OH$, $-CO_2H$, $-SH$, $-NH_2$. These are present in such excess that at least one remains free after the agent is saturated with metals. In addition to these considerations, an antidote is usually so designed that its chelated complexes cannot penetrate from the blood-stream into cells and are easily excreted by the kidneys.

The first of these antidotes, dimercaprol (*11.19*), was invented to counter poisoning by an arsenical war gas (Peters, Stocken, and Thompson, 1945), and hence was at first called British antilewisite (or BAL). Today it is much used to treat poisoning by compounds of gold, mercury (in inorganic or organic combination), antimony, and arsenic. Binding occurs as shown in (*11.20*). This antidote is given intramuscularly (2 or 3 mg per kg of body-weight) every four hours during the first day, and then in accordance with the patient's needs. Not only is the toxic nature of these elements masked by the dimercaprol, but they are excreted still bound to it. (Dimercaprol is rather toxic if the above dose is exceeded).

$$
\begin{array}{ll}
\begin{array}{l}
CH_2\!-\!SH \\
| \\
CH\ \ \!-\!SH \\
| \\
CH_2\!-\!OH
\end{array}
&
\begin{array}{l}
CH_2\!-\!S \\
| \qquad\qquad\diagdown Hg \\
CH\ \ \!-\!S\diagup \\
| \\
CH_2\!-\!OH
\end{array}
\\[6pt]
\quad\text{Dimercaprol} & \qquad (11.20) \\
\qquad (11.19) &
\end{array}
$$

D-penicillamine (11.21), similarly used in copper poisoning, is non-toxic. It is employed in Wilson's disease, an inherited error of metabolism in which dietary copper is stored in brain, kidneys, and liver in such quantities that death occurs in the early years of life. Oral administration of penicill-amine prevents this and can even reverse the pathological lesions produced by the copper ions. The copper-penicillamine complex is readily voided in the urine (Walshe, 1968). Penicillamine, being effective orally, is con-venient to use in the later stages of treating chronic lead poisoning with intravenous EDTA, as follows.

Calcium ethylenediaminetetracetic acid (11.22) injected as its sodium salt, sodium calcium edetate, is a most effective remedy for lead poisoning (Bessman, Rubin, and Leikin, 1954). Sodium edetate (the same substance minus the calcium) was used in an attempt to decalcify stenosed valves in the heart; even though it also caused a fall in blood calcium, the patients were none the worse after long courses of injections, e.g. 3 g (as a 0.5 per cent solution) every 24 hours for 5 days a week, and 3 weeks per month. However, adverse symptoms were encountered if this dosage scheme was exceeded (Seven, 1960). Sodium edetate has been used successfully for treating lime burns of the cornea (Gundorova et al., 1967), and to overcome digitalis-induced cardiac arrythmia by restoring K^+/Ca^{2+} balance (Szekely and Wynne, 1963).

Contamination by plutonium of atomic-energy workers can be effectively overcome by daily injections of diethylenetriaminepentacetic acid (Smith, Chapman, and Marlow, 1969). More powerful, related substances are now on trial.

Beryllium poisoning is treated with large doses of sodium salicylate, or smaller doses of aurine tricarboxylic acid. The latter, which has three salicyl-ate moieties linked to a central carbon atom, does not assist the excretion of this metal, as salicylate does, but keeps it, in the tissues, as a very insoluble complex.

Better antidotes are required for treating chronic iron poisoning, which is common after the repeated blood transfusions used in treating two genetically-determined diseases, thalassaemia (Cooley's anaemia) and

$$\begin{array}{c} CH_3 \\ | \\ H_3C-C-SH \\ | \\ CH-NH_2 \\ | \\ CO_2H \end{array}$$

Penicillamine
(11.21)

Calcium edetate
(11.22)

$$\begin{array}{c} CH_2-SH \\ | \\ CH_2-NH_2 \end{array}$$

Cysteamine
(11.23)

sickle-cell anaemia. In thalassaemia, the beta chain of the haemoglobin molecule is produced in an inadequate amount, so that the blood transports oxygen inefficiently. Patients do not survive childhood without repeated transfusions, yet frequently die in mid-teens or early twenties from the excess of inorganic iron that accumulates in kidneys, liver, and heart from these transfusions. This disease is most common among populations bordering the Mediterranean Sea, and in Southeast Asia. In some parts of Nigeria, as many as 30% of the population carries the gene for sickle-cell anaemia, a disease in which haemoglobin is not deficient but much of it is chemically different. About 0.15% of black children in the United States have the disease and, although the childhood mortality used to be high, some now live to have children of their own. In this disease, blood transfusions are needed only during the painful hypoxic crises.

The standard antidote for iron poisoning is desferrioxamine B (11.6) (deferoxamine) (Keberle, 1964), which must be injected. Other iron-chelating agents undergoing trial are rhodotorulic acid (11.10), cheaply made from yeast but still requiring injection, 2,3-dihydroxybenzoic acid which is part of the enterochelin molecule (11.5) and is active orally, and ethylenediamine-bis(2-hydroxyphenylacetic acid) which is related to EDTA.

2-Mercaptoethylamine (11.23) (cysteamine) effectively prevents radiation injury. It has been shown that, in a mouse irradiated with 750 rad (whole-body single dose), significant increases of iron and copper occur in the bone-marrow, adrenals, spleen, liver, lungs, and thymus, and of iron in muscle and kidney (Yendell, Tupper, and Wills, 1967). One school of thought assigns the radio-protective properties of cysteamine to its ability to sequester the heavy-metal cations released from cells by irradiation (Jones, 1960). Other hypotheses are summarized by P. Brown (1967). One very interesting and plausible hypothesis of radiation injury is as follows. Ionizing radiation produces hydroperoxides of the pyrimidines in DNA such as 5,6-dihydro-6-hydroperoxy-6-hydroxythymine. The hypothesis supposes that these hydroperoxides react with transition metal ions to from free radicals which chemically change neighbouring bases, and this leads to misparing during replication (Thomas et al., 1976).

It is clear that effective masking of iron and copper ions would break any destructive chain reaction (oxidative) which they may catalyse. Many other substances, all modelled on cysteamine, are available for preventing radiation sickness. An example is 2-mercaptoethylguanidine, generated in the body from S-(2-aminoethyl)*iso*thiuronium salts (Doherty, Shapira, and Burnett, 1957).

Radioactive cations can, in some cases, be removed from the body by exchange dilution: the same cation (*not* radioactive) is injected as a complex of moderate stability. Thus zirconium citrate has been used to remove radioactive zirconium (Schubert, 1957).

Hydroxyurea exerts its valued anticancer action by diminishing a biological (*not* a toxic) effect of a metal in the uneconomic species. There it sequesters the iron required by the hydrogenase that converts ribosides to deoxyribosides (see Section 4.0, p. 116).

For a book on the use of chelating agents in heavy-metal poisoning, see Levine (1978).

11.7 Augmentation, by chelation, of the toxic effect of a metal

8-hydroxyquinoline (*11.24*) has a similar antibacterial spectrum to penicillin. Although by no means so selective, it and its derivatives have been in regular use, since about 1895, for topical application in wounds. It has the advantage over many other antibacterials of acting quickly and of being fungicidal as well; but it is not very active against Gram-negative bacteria. Ointments containing 8-hydroxyquinoline are used in dermatology, e.g. in rashes due to resistant staphylococci, in secondarily infected eczemas, and also as a fungicide. The complex which 8-hydroxyquinoline forms with copper is much used for proofing structural materials, including tents, against fungal attack.

When it was found in 1944 that 8-hydroxyquinoline exerts its destructive effect on micro-organisms through chelation (Albert, 1944; Albert, Rubbo, Goldacre, and Balfour, 1947), a new prospect was opened up that many other antibacterial and antifungal substances might be found to act in this way. It was soon shown that *oxine* (as 8-hydroxyquinoline had long been called by analytical chemists) had little activity in media depleted of heavy metals (Rubbo, Albert, and Gibson, 1950; Albert, Gibson, and Rubbo, 1953). Thus it acts, not by removing a metal essential for life, but by forming a lethal complex with a metal accidentally present (see Section 11.7a). Several substances chemically related to oxine (see 11.7b), and others chemically unrelated (see 11.7c), were subsequently shown to act against micro-organisms by this mechanism, which is the 'co-operative effect' discussed in Section 11.5. It seems that only metals of variable valence can activate these agents.

(a) *Mode of action of 8-hydroxyquinoline (oxine)*
That the antibacterial action of oxine (*11.24*) is due to chelation was shown as follows (Albert *et al.*, 1947). Oxine has long been used in chemical

analysis as a chelating agent, and it has outstanding chelating properties (Table 11.2). The other six hydroxyquinolines, all isomers of oxine, did not chelate at all when tested, and they were without antibacterial action. Yet even two parts per million (M/100 000) of oxine prevented the growth of staphylococci and streptococci. Further, the *O*- and the *N*-methyl-derivatives (*11.25*) and (*11.26*) of oxine were found to be without chelating action (as expected, because –CH₃, unlike H, cannot exchange with a metal), and neither of them was antibacterial. Thus the connection between chelation and antibacterial action was established.

8-Hydroxyquinoline (oxine)   8-Methoxyquinoline   Oxine methochloride
(*11.24*)   (*11.25*)   (*11.26*)

It remained to be shown whether the toxic action of oxine was due to the withdrawal of essential metals, as had been suggested (Zentmyer, 1944), or whether it actually increased the toxic action of metals normally present

Table 11.6

THE EFFECT OF INCREASING CONCENTRATION ON
THE BACTERICIDAL ACTION OF OXINE IN BROTH
('CONCENTRATION QUENCHING')

Staph. aureus in meat broth at pH 7.0–7.3 (20°C)

Concentration of oxine 1/M	Growth after exposure			
	0	1 h	3 h	24 h
800	+ + +	+ + +	+ + +	+
1600	+ + +	+ + +	+ + +	+
3200	+ + +	+ + +	+	+
6400	+ + +	+ + +	+	−
12 000	+ + +	+	+	−
25 000	+ + +	+	−	−
50 000	+ + +	+	−	−
100 000	+ + +	−	−	−
200 000	+ + +	+ + +	+ + +	+ + +

The bactericidal test in this, and the following tables, is based on that of Miles and Misra (1938). At the end of the given time, samples were withdrawn, diluted, and inoculated on a dried blood-agar plate. The plates were read after forty-eight hours at 37°C. Symbols: —, no growth; +, up to 50 colonies; + +, 50–150 colonies; + + +, uncountable. (Albert, Gibson and Rubbo, 1953.)

in the medium. The latter proved to be the case for both the bacteriostatic and bactericidal actions (Rubbo *et al.*, 1950; Albert *et al.*, 1953). As was indicated in the outline of this work presented in Section 2.2 (p. 35), the first clue came from concentration quenching.

Concentration quenching.   It is highly unusual for the effect of a bio-logically active substance to decrease as the concentration is increased. However, oxine shows this phenomenon to an unprecedented degree. As will be seen from Table 11.6, staphylococci which are killed in an hour by M/100 000 oxine are not killed (even in 3 hours) by M/1600 oxine (in fact, even a saturated solution, which is M/200, will not kill them). There was, however, a degree of toxicity after 24 hours (Albert *et al.*, 1953). Streptococci behaved similarly. The meaning of this concentration quenching became evident when it was found that it occurred in broth, but not in distilled water.

Experiments with oxine in distilled water.   The viability of staphylococci for at least 24 hours in distilled water permits some decisive tests to be made. It will be seen, from the distilled water experiments in Table 2.3 (p. 36), that oxine (M/100000) is not bactericidal on its own, but becomes so in the presence of a similar quantity of iron, although the iron alone is not toxic. Clearly, the toxic agent is not oxine, but an oxine iron complex.

Experiments with oxine in broth.   When broth is used instead of water, no added iron is necessary (Table 2.3), because a sufficient amount has been introduced from the meat. When the concentration of oxine was increased to M/800, the bactericidal action disappeared (concentration quenching). It seemed evident to us that the toxic action was caused by the 1 : 1-complex (*2.22*) (if fer*rous*) but not by the saturated 2 : 1-complex (*11.27*) which must be the only form present when oxine is in excess. Therefore we added iron in sufficient amount (M/800) to equal that of the oxine, and thus restore the unsaturated 1 : 1-complex. As expected, this combination proved just as highly bactericidal as the earlier one (see Table 2.3). It should be noted that M/800 iron is not toxic on its own, but the oxine has made it so.

The 2 : 1 oxine ferrous
complex (saturated)
(*11.27*)

The metals co-toxic with oxine.   In the absence of added heavy metals, oxine enters the bacterial cell (*Staph. aureus*) without harming it (Beckett, Vahora, and Robinson, 1958). Similarly, it enters the fungal cell (*Aspergillus niger*) without causing any harm (Greathouse *et al.*, 1954). (The latter investigation was done with two varieties of radioactive oxine, one from ^{14}C aniline, and the other from ^{14}C glycerol, labelled in the benzene and the pyridine ring, respectively). Yet when a suitable metal was made available at the same time, these organisms were severely injured.

Damage to Gram-positive bacteria has been observed only when one of the following cations was present in the medium : Cu^{2+}, Fe^{2+}, or Fe^{3+}, and of these, iron seemed the more important. In aerobic cultures ferrous oxine enters into rapid equilibrium with the ferric form. Oxine has only a feeble action on most Gram-negative bacteria and shows no clear requirement for a particular metal (Rubbo *et al.*, 1950). Oxine damages mycelial fungi only when cupric ions are present in the medium, and iron cannot release copper for this purpose (Anderson and Swaby, 1951; Block, 1956); this is true also for yeasts (Nordbring-Hertz, 1955).

Antagonism by cobalt of the toxic action of oxine-iron.   It is evident that

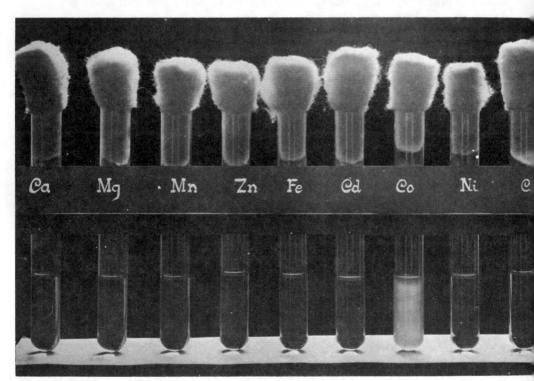

PLATE 6   The antagonism between oxine and traces of cobalt. *Staph. aureus* in nutrient broth at pH 7.2.

the addition of a large excess (say, 200 equivalents) of an inert metal could prevent the toxic action of oxine-iron, if the stability constant of the new complex was greater than, or not much less than, that of oxine-iron; thus, by the law of mass action, the oxine should almost entirely combine with the inert metal. As expected, experiments showed that cadmium, cobalt, zinc, and nickel were protective under these conditions, and manganese, magnesium, and calcium were ineffective (see Table 11.2 for stability constants).

Cobalt, however, has a unique position. Not only is it protective in large amounts, but in traces also. As little as M/25 000 cobaltous sulphate completely prevents the *bacteriostatic* effect of M/100 000 oxine (Rubbo *et al.*, 1950): this antagonism is illustrated in Plate 6. Table 11.7 shows how effective cobalt is in preventing the bactericidal action of oxine-iron. It is only a little less effective against oxine-copper.

Cobalt also protects yeasts against oxine-copper (Nordbring-Hertz, 1955), but mycelial fungi are not protected, apparently because of their slow rate of growth (Anderson and Swaby, 1951). However, see the protective effects of cobalt on DMDC (p. 426). Cobalt uniquely protects trypanosomes against the lethal action of oxine, as shown in Table 11.8 (Williamson, 1959).

What is the explanation of this protective action of cobalt? At first it might seem that the cobalt combined with the oxine and thus denied it to the iron. But if this were so, nickel would be still more effective because the stability constant of nickel-oxine is much higher than that of cobalt-oxine (Table 11.2, also Albert, 1953). Yet nickel has no protective action at low concentrations.

Table 11.7

PROTECTIVE ACTION OF COBALT AGAINST THE BACTERICIDAL
ACTION OF OXINE-IRON AND OXINE-COPPER

Staph. aureus in metal-depleted broth at pH 7.3 (20°C)
M/25 000 oxine present in every tube

Tube	Conc. of metal added, 1/M			Growth after exposure			
	$FeSO_4$	$CuSO_4$	$CoSO_4$	0	2 h	4 h	24 h
1	nil	nil	nil	+ + +	+ + +	+ + +	+ + +
2	50 000	nil	nil	+ + +	−	−	−
3	50 000	nil	50 000	+ + +	+ +	+ +	+ + +
4	nil	50 000	nil	+ + +	−	−	−
5	nil	50 000	50 000	+ + +	−	−	−
6	nil	50 000	10 000	+ + +	+ + +	+ + +	+ + +

(Albert, *et al.*, 1953.)

Table 11.8

PROTECTIVE EFFECT OF COBALT AGAINST THE TRYPANOCIDAL
ACTION OF OXINE

T. rhodesiense in horse-serum glucose saline at 37°C,
incubated for 4 hours

Tube	Concentration $1/M$		Any one of the following: $Cu^{2+}, Ni^{2+}, Zn^{2+}$ $Fe^{2+}, Mn^{2+}, Mg^{2+}$	No. of trypanosomes surviving (per cent of control)
	Oxine	Co^{2+}		
1	nil	nil	nil	100
2	800 000	nil	nil	< 1
3	800 000	400 000	nil	117
4–9	800 000	nil	400 000	< 1

(Williamson, 1959.)

A better clue comes from knowledge that several vital cell constituents, particularly mercapto-compounds (such as thioctic acid, see Section 11.7c) and ascorbic acid, are easily oxidized by atmospheric oxygen if traces of iron or copper are present. These oxidations lead to the formation of hydrogen peroxide and superoxide radicals ($\cdot O_2^-$) which, in the presence of the metal cations, produce a fulminating chain reaction so that a very small amount of metal can catalyse widespread destruction. In some model reactions of this kind, traces of cobalt have been found to act as a chainbreaker which greatly moderates the destruction (see Fig. 11.6)*.

Oxine is a co-operative chelating agent (as defined in Section 11.5). Thus a mixture of inorganic iron and oxine catalyses the aerial oxidation of the – SH groups in nucleoproteins from rat liver and from fish eggs, whereas inorganic iron is ineffective on its own (Bernheim and Bernheim, 1939). The superior catalytic powers of oxine-iron probably spring from the rearrangement of the orbitals of the ferric cation caused by chelation (the unusual colours, red for ferrous-oxine and green for ferric-oxine, are evidence of rearrangement).

It is reasonable to assume that the toxic species of oxine is the 1 : 1-ferrous complex because it is unsaturated; in other words it has the unused combining power that is necessary in a catalyst. The 2 : 1-complex (*11.27*), on the other hand, is saturated and unlikely to be catalytic. (In aerobic systems, both ferr*ous* and ferr*ic* species are present in equilibrium; it follows that the 1 : 1- and 2 : 1- ferr*ic* complexes are unsaturated and presumably catalyti-

* For information on chain reactions, see Dainton (1966).

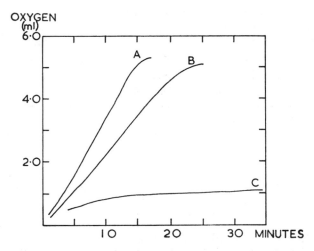

FIG. 11.6 The protective action of cobalt upon the copper-catalysed oxidation (by O_2) of cysteine (M/40) (20°C). A, M/10 000 cupric sulphate; B, M/100 000 cupric sulphate; C, as B, but with M/500 cobaltous sulphate. (Baur and Preis, 1936.)

cally active, whereas the 3 : 1-complex is saturated and likely to be inert.) This concept reinforces a similar conclusion made on the basis of concentration quenching (p. 36).

The site of action of oxine-iron in bacteria is unknown, but a strong clue is afforded by the site in fungi, namely the oxidative destruction of thioctic acid (see p. 431). More general information on the site is afforded by data on liposolubility. Derivatives of oxine having a low oil/water partition coefficient are not antibacterial. Thus although oxine-5-sulphonic acid has the same stability constants as oxine (Albert, 1953), unlike oxine, it has no tendency to pass from water into lipids; also, it has no antibacterial properties whatsoever. To find if the high partition coefficient of oxine was essential for its antibacterial action, a series of uncharged derivatives of oxine having low partition coefficients were synthesized (Albert and Hampton, 1952, 1954) and tested (Albert, et al., 1954). These aza-oxines, which are dealt with in Section 11.7b, showed that antibacterial action fell and rose, as partition coefficients fell and rose in response to small changes in molecular structure. Thus a high partition coefficient plays a very important part in determining the action of oxine and related substances. This is evidence that the action of oxine take place *inside* the cell, or at least within the cytoplasmic membrane.

Halogenated derivatives of oxine. Halogenation of oxine improves the performance against Gram-negative bacteria, and many such derivatives are in use. Halquinol (a mixture of 5-chloro- and 5,7-dichloro-oxine) and chlorquinaldol (5,7-dichloro-2-methyloxine), which are also issued as

'Quinolor' and 'Steroxin' ointments, respectively, are used in dermatology. 5,7-Di-iodo-oxine (diiodohydroxyquin, 'Diodoquin'), found in many pharmacopoeias, and 5-chloro-7-iodo-oxine (clioquinol, chinoform, iodochlorhydroxyquin, 'Vioform') are used for bacterial dysentery. Between 1955 and 1970, some 10 000 Japanese people suffered from subacute myelooptic neuropathy (SMON), a painful, disabling, and sometimes fatal disease, thought to have been brought on by clioquinol. The outbreak led to suspension of sales in Japan, and protracted litigation. However Meade (1975) found the data correlated poorly. In July 1977, the British Government's Committee on Safety of Medicines reviewed the evidence and concluded that the hazard of SMON was insignificant at the dosage approved for travellers' diarrhoea. For further discussion on potential hazards of halogenated oxines, see Goodman and Gilman (1975, p. 1074).

(b) Substances chemically related to oxine

It was found that a pyridine or benzene ring can be annelated to the oxine molecule without loss of activity; however, annelation to the 2,3-face introduced steric hindrance to chelation (Albert et al., 1947).

Increasing the partition coefficient of oxine fourfold, by inserting lipophilic substituents, did not appreciably improve the in vitro action: this physical property must already be maximal in oxine (Albert, Rees, and Tomlinson, 1956). It is therefore more interesting to know what happens when the partition coefficient is lowered. In oxine, this is suitably managed by synthesizing analogues where one or more =CH-group is replaced by the far more hydrophilic =N-atom (Albert and Hampton, 1952, 1954). Although these substances also have trivial names, such as 8-hydroxy-cinnoline, -quinazoline, and -quinoxaline, they can properly (and for the present purposes most conveniently) be termed 2-aza-oxine, 3-aza-oxine (11.28), and so forth.

Nitrogen and oxygen atoms lower (and halogens and alkyl-groups raise) partition coefficients. It can be seem from Table 11.9 that (as expected) the substitution of =N— for =CH— lowered the partition coefficient. With this lowering, the antibacterial action fell, often to vanishing point. Next, without removing the extra nitrogen atom, the partition coefficient was raised (by inserting a small alkyl-group, never exceeding three carbon atoms in length) until it reached, and even exceeded, that of oxine. When this was done, the antibacterial action also rose until it reached a maximum, as shown in Table 11.9 (Albert, et al., 1954).

3-Aza-oxine
(11.28)

(11.29)

Table 11.9

THE FALL AND RISE OF BACTERIOSTATIC ACTION WITH
FALL AND RISE OF PARTITION COEFFICIENT

Strept. pyogenes in meat broth at pH 7.3 (37°C)

Substance	Partition coefficient oleyl alcohol/water	Lowest inhibitory dilution 1/M	log first stability constant (Ni^{2+})
Oxine	67	200 000	9.8
5-Aza-oxine	< 0.02	< 800	5.8
7-Aza-oxine	0.1	< 800	6.7
6-Aza-oxine	1	< 800	5.9
3-Aza-oxine	5	13 000	7.6
2-Aza-oxine	6	13 000	7.8
4-Aza-oxine	8	6400	7.6
4-Methyl-2-aza-oxine	16	25 000	8.1
4-Methyl-3-aza-oxine	17	50 000	7.9
4-Propyl-3-aza-oxine	135	100 000	7.9
7-Allyl-3-aza-oxine	310	100 000	7.9

(Albert, Hampton, Selbie, and Simon, 1954.)

Because of the inductive effect of the second nitrogen atom, neither the high stability constant nor the high antibacterial action of oxine is quite reached (the latter falls short by only one twofold serial dilution). However, the last seven substances in Table 11.9 all have stability constants of the same order. For these seven substances, the antibacterial action runs parallel to the partition coefficient, which establishes the correlation.

(c) *Substance acting like oxine but not chemically related*
The *N*-oxides of pyridine, quinoline, and benzoquinoline are antibacterial provided that an ionizable group is present in the 2-position to make chelation possible. A mercapto-group has been found best for this purpose. Thus 2-mercaptopyridine-*N*-oxide (1-hydroxypyridine-2-thione) (*2.23*) (pyrithione, 'Omadine') is as intensely antibacterial as oxine. Although the chelated complex, e.g. (*11.29*), has an entirely different structure from that of oxine, e.g. (*2.22*), the mode of action is judged to be the same by the three following criteria: both substances are bactericidal only in the presence of iron, this action is prevented by cobalt, and also by an excess of the substance itself (Albert *et al.*, 1956). Its innocuousness in the absence of iron is shown in Table 11.10. It is much used as a fungicide in ointments and soaps. In a shampoo base, it has proved very effective against *Pityrosporum ovale*, one of the commonest causes of dandruff. It is also much used as an industrial fungicide (textiles, cooling systems, cutting oils).
Dimethyldithiocarbamic acid, or DMDC (*2.24*), is a potent fungicide

Table 11.10

THE INNOCUOUSNESS OF 2-MERCAPTOPYRIDINE-*N*-OXIDE
IN THE ABSENCE OF IRON
(BACTERICIDAL TEST, IN GLASS-DISTILLED WATER)

Staph. aureus: pH 6–7 (20°C)

2-Mercaptopyridine-N-oxide (pyrithione) 1/M	Fe³	Growth (plated out after 1 hour)
80 000	nil	+ + +
nil	80 000	+ + +
80 000	80 000	−

+ + + means prolific growth with uncountable colonies.
  −   means no detectable growth.
(Albert, Rees, and Tomlinson, 1956.)

much used in agriculture as the sodium ('NaDDC'), iron ('Fermate' or 'Ferbam'), and zinc ('Zerlate' or 'Ziram') salts. Formula (*11.12*) shows the 1 : 1-copper complex. The Australian work on oxine, described above, led to a parallel study on DMDC in Denmark in which this substance was shown to act antifungally only as its copper complex (Goksøyr, 1955). This work was taken up and extended in Holland (Sijpesteijn, *et al.*, 1957). Table 11.11 shows some typical results from the latter workers.

Table 11.11, which contains evidence of concentration quenching, reveals the necessity of a metal ion (copper) for the action of DMDC on

Table 11.11

EFFECT OF COPPER ON GROWTH INHIBITION IN
ASPERGILLUS NIGER
BY SODIUM DIMETHYLDITHIOCARBAMATE

(3 days at 24°C)
Medium: Glucose, salts, and vitamins in glass-distilled water at pH 7

Cu²⁺ 1/M	Sodium DMDC 1/M							
	nil	700 000	280 000	140 000	70 000	28 000	14 000	7000
nil	+	+	+	+	+	+	+	+
83 000	+	+	+	+	+	+	+	+
25 000	+	+	−	−	−	±	+	+

(Sijpestejin and Janssen, 1959.)

Aspergillus niger. Iron is ineffective. Several other moulds behave similarly (Sijpesteijn and Janssen, 1959). It will be evident from Table 11.11 that the effective proportions of metal and chelating agent are critical, as in oxine (Table 2.3, and Albert *et al.*, 1956). The Dutch workers attribute the zone of no inhibition (which lies between 10 and 50 parts per million of DMDC) to the extraordinary insolubility of the 2 : 1-copper complex. (The 2 : 1-copper complex of DMDC is soluble in water only 0.01 p.p.m., and this restricts the supply of agent to the cell). The third zone, a toxic one, appearing in concentrations higher than 50 p.p.m., has been attributed to an intrinsic toxic effect of DMDC, unconnected with metal-binding (Sijpesteijn *et al.*, 1957). ·

Cobalt antagonizes the action of sodium dimethyldithiocarbamate on *Aspergillus niger* just as it does that of oxine (copper-catalysed) on yeast (p. 425) (Dr A. Kaars Sijpesteijn, personal communication, 1969). [For the copper-activated bactericidal properties of DMDC, see Liebermeister (1950).]

The accumulation of pyruvic acid in treated *Aspergillus* points to the molecular site of action of DMDC, oxine, and pyrithione, namely catalysis of the oxidative destruction of lipoic acid [thioctic acid (*2.25*)] (Sijpesteijn and Janseen, 1959). This is the essential coenzyme for oxidative decarboxylation of pyruvic acid by lipoate acetyltransferase, a component of the multienzyme complex known as pyruvate dehydrogenase (Danson and Perham, 1976).

For further reading on the dimethyldithiocarbamates, see Thorn and Ludwig (1962). Some agriculturalists prefer to use the zinc and iron complexes of DMDC, principally because of the excellent adhesion to plants which enables the complexes to resist long periods of rain. Others prefer tetramethylthiuram disulphide, which is the disulphide obtained by oxidizing DMDC, and which is slowly reduced to DMDC under field conditions.

11.8 The tetracyclines

Tetracycline (*11.30*) and its derivatives are octahydro-napthacenes which are among the most used of all drugs in treating systemic bacterial infections. They do not act like oxine because their action on bacteria is slow and is not promoted by iron (Albert and Rees, 1956). They have very little action on fungi. [See Section 4.1 (p. 125) for historical material on tetracyclines.]

Tetracycline
(*11.30*)

That tetracycline and its derivatives such as chlorotetracycline and oxytetracycline were chelating agents was found by determination of their stability constants (Albert and Rees, 1956), which showed that their avidity for divalent metals was similar to that of glycine. Stability constants of tetracycline are given in Table 11.2.

Tetracycline is a zwitterion in which the hydroxy-group shown at position 3 has pK_a 3.3 (it is actually part of a tricarbonylmethane system formed from the oxygen atoms in positions 1, 2, and 3). The remaining pK_a values (7.8 and 9.6) represent simultaneous ionizations from both (a) the dimethylamino-group, and (b) the phenolic β-diketone system which embraces positions 10, 11, and 12 (Leeson, Krueger, and Nash, 1963; Rigler et al., 1965; Kalnins and Belen'ski, 1964). The simultaneous dissociation of two groups, whose pK_a values are separated by less than two pK units, is well known from work on cysteine (Edsall, Martin, and Hollingworth, 1958).

Studies of the structure-activity relationships of tetracyclines show that many changes can be made at positions 5, 6 and 7 without harming the antibacterial action (McCormick et al., 1960; Blackwood, 1970). The following details are more critical. The tricarbonylmethane area, as defined above, plays a prominent part in metal binding and is essential for antibacterial activity. ^{1}H n.m.r. spectra show line-broadening in this area when Ca^{2+}, Cu^{2+}, Mn^{2+}, and Co^{2+}, are added to a solution of tetracycline; but Mg^{2+} gave such an anomalous signal as to suggest that it, uniquely, caused a conformational change before binding (Williamson and Everett, 1975). It is known that the phenol-diketone area (based on positions 10, 11, 12) must be present and free for Mg^{2+} and Ca^{2+} to be bound (Mitscher, Bonacci, and Sokoloski, 1968; Doluizio and Martin, 1963). It is also known that the stereochemistry of the 4a–12a fold [defined as the junction between the third and fourth rings, reading (11.30) from left to right] must be as in Nature (Caswell and Hitchison, 1971). (These last three correlations, taken together, define the locus of magnesium cations in the chelated complex.) Finally, the dimethylamino-group is essential for in vivo (but not for in vitro) antibacterial properties.

As was pointed out in the introduction to Chapter 3, the selectivity of tetracyclines rests on their being accumulated far more by bacteria than by mammalian cells. There is evidence that these drugs form a liposoluble complex with magnesium in the bacterial plasma membrane, and that this leads to their availability to the cytoplasm (Franklin, 1971; Dockter and Magnuson, 1973; Franklin and Snow, 1975). The decisive site of action in bacteria is on the ribosomes, which are also rich in magnesium, and whose protein-synthesizing activity is brought to a halt by these antibiotics. Although nickel, cobalt, and zinc ions (which bind tetracyclines much more tightly than magnesium) do not reverse the action of these drugs, magnesium does so (Weinberg, 1954), and fluorescence studies have shown that chelation of Mg^{2+} in bacterial ribosomes precedes the inhibition of protein synthesis by tetracyclines (White and Cantor, 1971).

Because of their chelating action, tetracycline drugs are inactivated in the patient's bowel by any dietary calcium or magnesium ions, whether from milk or from antacid medication. Through such mishaps, many patients have lost the potential benefit of these antibiotics.

11.9 Substances whose biological action is at least partly due to chelation

Many other chelating agents have found widespread employment in medicine. Although, because of their constitution, they could not fail to combine with heavy metals in the tissues, enough is not always known of their mode of action to decide whether they act by chelation alone. Yet, no matter how much or little their chelating properties may govern the mode of action, these properties deserve study because of their role in adsorption and the causation of side-effects.

Isoniazid (11.31).   This substance, the hydrazide of isonicotinic acid, is the keystone of the modern treatment of tuberculosis. It has an affinity for the ions of heavy metals of the same order as that of glycine. The complexes *(11.33)* of isoniazid are formed through the anion *(11.32)*. No anion can be formed by the methyl-derivative *N*-methyl-*N*-isonicotinoylhydrazine *(11.34)*, and this substance has virtually no antitubercular activity (Cymerman-Craig and Willis, 1955; Cymerman-Craig *et al.*, 1955). Thus isoniazid inhibited *Mycobacterium tuberculosis* H_{37} Rv. (*in vitro*, in the presence of 10 per cent of serum) at M/5 000 000, but substance *(11.34)* was inactive.

Isoniazid   *(11.32)*   *(11.33)*   *(11.34)*
(11.31)

In the presence of cupric ions, isoniazid is taken up much more rapidly by *M. tuberculosis* H_{37} Rv., in culture (Youatt, 1962). Blood serum copper averages 115 µg/100 ml which should be adequate to convert a therapeutic concentration of the drug into its chelate. However, the action of isoniazid cannot be due entirely to chelation, because neither of its two isomers has any notable action against *M. tuberculosis*, even *in vitro*, although their stability constants are as high, or even higher (Albert, 1956). This is shown in Table 11.12. It is known that isoniazid enters the cells of non-resistant tubercle bacteria, and does not penetrate the cells of resistant strains; also the common bacterial species such as *Staph. aureus* and *E. coli*, which are never affected by isoniazid, do not absorb it (Youatt, 1958).

Table 11.12

PHYSICAL AND ANTITUBERCULAR PROPERTIES OF HYDRAZIDES

Hydrazide	pK_a hydrazide group	log stability constant** 1 : 1				Relative activity on M. tuberculosis H_{37} Rv.	
		Cu^{2+}	Ni^{2+}	Co^{2+}	Zn^{2+}	In vitro	In vivo
Isonicotinic*	10.77	8.0	5.5	4.8	5.4	1	1
Nicotinic*	11.47	8.7	6.0	5.4	?	0.001	—
Picolinic*	12.27	12.4	10.7	9.6	8.4	0.017	—
Benzoic	12.45	9.0	6.3	?	?	0.002	—
Cyanoacetic	11.17	8.5	6.0	5.3	?	0.008	0.2

* These three substances are isomers. They have the hydrazide group in the 4-, 3-, and 2-position respectively.
** For some 2 : 1-stability constants, *see* Albert (1956).
(Albert, 1956.)

It seems fairly certain that chelation with trace copper makes the drug liposoluble enough to penetrate the most lipophilic of all bacterial integuments, but the question remains: what happens next? The answer was first outlined two decades ago (Krüger-Thiemer, 1957), and has since become more firmly supported (Seydel, *et al.*, 1976a). In this explanation, isoniazide is seen as the transport form (pro-drug) of the true drug isonicotinic acid which, it is supposed, is *N*-methylated and built into an analogue of nicotinamide adenine dinucleotide (NAD). The replacement of NAD by this analogue is held to disturb lipid metabolism. Undoubtedly, isoniazid at a therapeutically effective concentration, causes a decrease in mycobacterial NAD leading to a breakdown in the synthesis of mycolic acid (the typical waxy material that forms a protective coating around the H_{37} strain of the bacterium (Winder and Collins, 1970).

Seydel and his colleagues (1976b) synthesized the isonicotinic analogue and found it identical with material isolated from the H_{37} strain of *M. tuberculosis*. They presented the following additional evidence: only those strains of *M. tuberculosis* which contain peroxidase are susceptible to injury by isoniazid (the highly pathogenic strains, if not drug-resistant, contain abundant peroxidase). Peroxidase turns isoniazid to isonicotinic acid *in vitro* (cell-free experiment) and, during isoniazid therapy, isonicotinic acid accumulates in the bacterial cells. Nicotinic acid and nicotinic hydrazide can antagonize the bactericidal action of isoniazid *in vitro*.

It was once thought that isoniazid acted on *Mycobacteria* by combining with pyridoxal. This was soon disproved, but some side-effects on the patient have been traced to this reaction.

Other chelating antituberculous drugs. Thiacetazone (*p*-acetamido-benzaldehyde thiosemicarbazone) (*11.35*), also known as 'Tibione', is (like isoniazid) specific for the tuberculosis bacterium. The thiosemi-carbazone-group chelates metal cations strongly and the antitubercular action of thiacetazone is enhanced by copper [blood-serum contains enough copper to show this effect (Liebermeister, 1950)]. Presumably, as with isoniazid, the absorption of the drug depends on chelation. Strains of *M. Tuberculosis* that have become highly resistant to isoniazid are still fully sensitive to thiacetazone (Barry, 1954). This argues a different mode of action.

Thiacetazone (150 mg) and isoniazid (300 mg), combined in one daily dose, is a much favoured contemporary treatment of tuberculosis. This combination has less toxicity to the patient than a higher dose of isoniazid alone, and staves off the drug resistance that so often develops when treatment depends on one single drug. One year's therapy seldom fails to cure, and six months usually suffice. Thiacetazone is also used a little in treating leprosy. A serious drawback is a tendency to cause agranulocytosis.

$$CH_3CO \cdot HN \text{—} \bigcirc \text{—} CH{:}N \cdot N \cdot \overset{\overset{\displaystyle S}{\|}}{\underset{}{C}} \cdot NH_2$$

Thiacetazone
(*11.35*)

$$\underset{C_2H_5}{\underset{|}{\overset{OH \cdot CH_2}{\overset{|}{CH}}}} \cdot NH \cdot CH_2 \cdot CH_2 \cdot NH \cdot \underset{C_2H_5}{\underset{|}{\overset{CH_2OH}{\overset{|}{CH}}}}$$

Ethambutol
(*11.36*)

Other metal-binding drugs used in treating tuberculosis will now be mentioned. Ethambutol (*11.36*) chelates metals in the same way as ethylene-diamine (Fig. 11.1 and Table 11.2) of which it is a simple hydroxy-alkyl-derivative. It is highly active against *M. tuberculosis*, and, although expensive, is used clinically against infections resistant to isoniazid and streptomycin. A troublesome side-effect is a reversible blurring of vision. It is almost inactive against other species of bacteria and against fungi. Its selectivity is attributed to steric hindrance arising from the α-branching of the alkyl-chains (Shepherd and Wilkinson, 1962).

p-aminosalicylic acid, though capable of binding metals, can act as a metabolite analogue for *p*-aminobenzoic acid (see Section 9.3b), also for salicylic acid which is a constituent of *M. tuberculosis*. *p*-Aminosalicylic acid is converted by some enterobacteria to an analogue of folic acid in which *p*AS replaces *p*AB. This analogue is non-functional, and hence injures the bacteria by wasting the pteridine fragment (Wacker, Kirschfeld, and Weinblum, 1954).

Streptomycin has a complex action on bacteria; the general background is given in Section 4.1 (p. 126), and the unusual penetration of the plasma membrane is described in Section 14.2. What is of interest here is that streptomycin displaces magnesium from ribosomes, as shown in Fig. 11.7. This effect seems to be a case of competition among cations rather than a metal-binding effect.

Other chelating antibacterial drugs. Hexachlorophane (*11.37*) and related phenols have antibacterial properties dependent on a one-atom bridge (methylene, oxygen, or sulphur) located in the 2,2′-position relative to two hydroxyl-groups. Potentiometric titration, which shows that these substances bind Fe^{2+}, Fe^{3+}, and Cu^{2+}, suggests that part of the action of these *bis*phenol antibacterials is derived from their metal-binding properties (Adams, 1958). A related substance, dichlorophen (*6.28*), is used against tapeworm in humans.

Salicylic acid is a strong chelating agent (Tables 11.2, 11.3), the ligand of which is the dianion (*11.38*) (Perrin, 1958a). Derivatives, such as salicyl-anilide (*6.20*), salicylamide, and salicylic aldehyde, which cannot produce a carboxy ion, are much weaker chelating agents. Stability constants for salicylic acid and many derivatives are available (Perrin, 1958). Aspirin, where the phenolic group (only) is blocked, has no chelating power, but is fairly rapidly hydrolysed in the body to salicylic acid which Sih and Takeguchi (1973) think may chelate the copper in prostaglandin synthetase in the therapy of rheumatic diseases. The antibiotic antimycin has a 3-formamido-salicylamide structure, and strongly binds ferric iron (Farley, Strong, and Bydalek, 1965).

Hexachlorophane
(*11.37*)

Salicylic acid (di-anion)
(*11.38*)

Sodium diethyldithiocarbamate, cf. (*2.24*) has been introduced as a new treatment of leprosy. The tyrosinase of *M. leprae*, which is copper containing, is an analogous enzyme compared to that in the host, and much more sensitive to this drug (Prabhakaran, 1973).

Mycoplasmas, humblest, cell-wall deficient members of the prokaryotes, and usually hard to kill selectively, are susceptible to derivatives of 2,2′-bipyridyl and 1,10-phenanthroline provided a trace of copper is

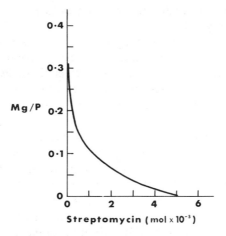

FIG. 11.7 Loss of magnesium from ribosomes (*E. coli*) in presence of streptomycin (pH 7.4). (Choi and Carr, 1968.)

present. The most active derivative is 2,9-dimethyl-1, 10-phenanthroline
which is used by analysts specifically to chelate cupr*ous* copper (Nauta,
1977). 1,10-phenanthroline (*11.15*) and its *C*-methyl-derivatives have
general antibacterial properties. The metal complexes are also antibacterial,
but the speed of action becomes greater when metals of decreased binding
power (see Table 11.2) are used. Bactericidal action was greatly enhanced
by the addition of six methyl-groups (Shulman, 1964; Butler *et al.*, 1969).

Nalidixic acid (*4.14*) should be able to bind metals between the carboxylic-
and the oxo-groups. It is not known if this plays a part in its biological
action, which is inhibition of the synthesis of DNA (Section 4.0, p. 114).
The antibacterial action of kojic acid (*11.9*), a pyrone extracted from certain
fungi, is enhanced by metallic cations (Weinberg, 1957). Bacitracin, a
polypeptide antibiotic (Section 12.2), loses its antibacterial action against
Staph. aureus in the presence of EDTA; the action is restored by bivalent
cations (Adler and Snoke, 1962).

Antiviral drugs. It is thought that methisazone (*6.16*) and its analogues
owe their antiviral action (see Section 6.3b) to chelation in which the metal
is held between the oxygen atom and the second nitrogen of the side-chain
(O'Sullivan and Sadler, 1961).

Methisazone inactivates a wide spectrum of tumour-causing viruses
(RNA types) is tissue-culture (Levinson, Woodson, and Jackson, 1971). A
simpler analogue, 5-hydroxy-2-formylpyridine thiosemicarbazone, was
found to be highly active against several types of experimental cancer in
mice, when given intraperitoneally (Blanz and French, 1968).

Antifungal examples. Apart from the powerful antifungals mentioned
in Section 11.7, and salicylic acid (this section, p. 410), special economic

value is attached to simple derivatives of tropolone (*11.39*) which occur in the heartwood of several species of conifers. These substances combine with copper, often accidentally present, and the complex confers several decades of protection against fungal attack, justifying the erection of unpainted buildings. Mono*iso*propyl derivatives of (*11.39*), the thujaplicins, are common examples, and the site of action is thought to be inhibition of the formation of acetyl-coenzyme A from acetate ions (Raa and Goksøyr, 1966).

Anticancer examples.   Thiosemicarbazones have been mentioned above in connexion with their antiviral and antitubercular properties. They also have anticancer activity, as already mentioned for 5-hydroxypicolinic aldehyde thiosemicarbazone (*4.18*), in Section 4.0. Such substances powerfully inhibit ribonucleoside diphosphate reductase, the enzyme which converts ribo- to deoxyribo- nucleotides, leading to inhibition of DNA synthesis. Interaction with the enzymatically-required iron by these drugs in thought to lie at the root of their action (Agrawal, *et al.*, 1972).

Dimethylglyoxime (*11.40*), which showed no activity against Ehrlich's carcinoma and Crocker sarcoma mouse test-systems, did so when a minute, non-toxic amount of Cu^{2+} ions was added to the system (Takamiya, 1960). Cupric ions are able to transport the anticancer compound 3-ethoxy-2-oxobutyraldehyde *bis*thiosemicarbazone into the living cell (Sartorelli and Creasey, 1969). For the carcinolytic effect of dichlorodiammine-platinum (*11.41*), see Section 11.10.

Concanavalin A, a protein (isolated from jack-beans) which binds carbohydrates and has the general properties of a 'lectin', agglutinates and inhibits growth of malignant cells (Sharon and Lis, 1972), but it also agglutinates erythrocytes. Each monomeric unit of concanavalin A has one site that binds calcium ions and another that binds Zn^{2+}, Co^{2+}, or Mn^{2+}, and *both* sites must be occupied by the appropriate metal for biological activity to occur.

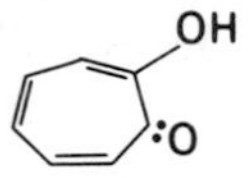

Tropolone
(*11.39*)

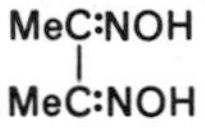

Dimethylglyoxime
(*11.40*)

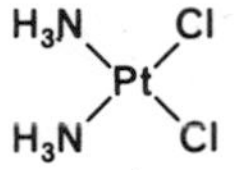

Dichlorodiammine
platinum
(*11.41*)

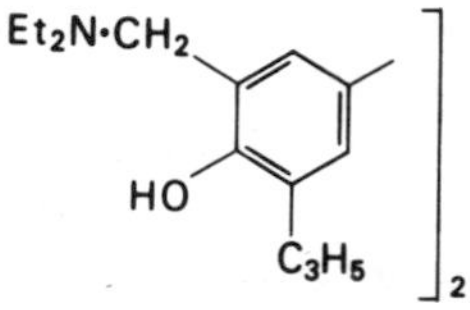

Biallylamicol
(*11.42*)

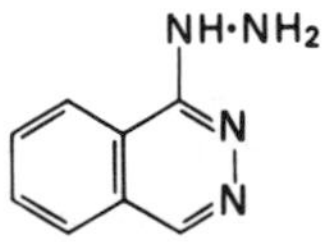

Hydrallazine
(*11.43*)

Anti-protozoal and anthelmintic examples.   Biallylamicol ('Camoform') (*11.42*), which has proved a successful drug in amoebiasis, has chelating properties (Thompson *et al.*, 1955; Dill *et al.*, 1957).

It is noteworthy that several quite simple N,N' chelating agents have anthelmintic properties, e.g. 2,2'-bipyridyl and *o*-phenanthroline (*11.15*) (Baldwin, 1948a; Dwyer *et al.*, 1952). The much-used vermicide, thiabendazole (*6.32*), strongly chelates transition metals between the two nitrogen atoms (Kowala *et al.*, 1971).

Hormone examples.   The metal-binding properties of adrenaline, thyroxine, and histamine were mentioned in Section 11.1.

Those polypeptide hormones that have a bisulphide $(-S \cdot S-)$ group are potentiated by bivalent metal cations. Thus the contractile effect of oxytocin on the uterus is potentiated by Co^{2+}, Mn^{2+}, and Ni^{2+}, but less by Ca^{2+} and Cu^{2+}. It is thought that the metal forms a ternary complex with the hormone and its receptor (Schild, 1969).

Cortisone is sometimes credited with chelating power; but, from inspection of the formula, this seems unlikely, and no proof has been produced. The suggestion that indole-3-acetic acid exerts plant-growth regulating effects through chelation has been discounted by showing that it lacks chelating properties (Perrin, 1961).

Pharmacodynamic examples.   Many metal-binding agents have been found to reduce high blood-pressure in man without, apparently, acting through the nervous system. These agents include sodium azide, sodium thiocyanate (e.g. from sodium nitroprusside), dimercaptopropanol (*11.43*), and hydrallazine. When sodium nitroprusside is injected intravenously in severe hypertensive crises, the blood-pressure falls to a safe level immediately. Hydrallazine is one of the most frequently prescribed drugs for patients with moderately severe hyperpiesia. It acts by relaxing the smooth muscle of the arterioles (Goodman and Gilman, 1975, p. 722).

11.10 The special case of robust complexes

In aqueous solution, the complexes of most metal cations exist in dynamic equilibrium with their components. If we disturb this equilibrium, another one is instantly formed. It is quite otherwise with *robust complexes* which persist for hours (or even days) under conditions favourable to their decomposition; any biological properties that they may have are strikingly different from those of their components. Robust complexes are formed where metal ions have 3,4 (low spin), 5, or 6 d electrons provided that formation of the complex involves large values of ligand-field stabilization energy. Metals most prone to form robust complexes are the transition metals: platinum, iridium, osmium, palladium, rhodium, ruthenium, also (but not so frequently) nickel, cobalt, and iron. The halide and, particularly, the cyanide anions most readily form robust complexes with these transition metals, then come other nitrogen anions, whereas oxygen-presenting types show the effect least.

The curariform action of some robust chelates was discovered by Beccari (1938) who found that a doubly-charged co-ordination complex of ferrous iron and three molecules of 2,2′-bipyridyl caused mild paralysis and respiratory failure in rabbits. Later he showed that rabbits, as well as frogs, excreted this complex unchanged (Beccari, 1941). Extending this work, Dwyer, Gyarfas and O'Dwyer (1951) examined complexes of iron, nickel, cobalt, ruthenium, and osmium and found that their most active example was the 2,2′,2″-terpyridyl complex of ruthenium which had one tenth the activity of tubocurarine. Only positively charged complexes were active. Working with the isolated rat diphragm, or the whole mouse, they found that the paralysed muscles responded to direct electrical stimulation and the paralysis was reversed by physostigmine, just as with tubocurarine. In these complexes there are no chemically-active groups exposed, and the redox-potentials are out of the biological range. It has to be concluded that the geometry and the charge of these robust complexes is responsible for their biological effects, and that the role of the metal is no more than that of holding the remaining atoms together in a configuration complementary to that of the receptor (Shulman and Dwyer, 1964). Examples more active than tubocurarine have since been made by arranging for *two* positive charges to be present at the same distance apart as in tubocurarine (Taylor, Callahan, and Shaikh, 1975).

In 1970, it was shown that *cis*-dichlorodiammine platinum (II) (*11.41*) could effect regression of large, solid sarcoma-180 tumours (Rosenberg and van Camp, 1970). The type of action resembled that of the bifunctional alkylating agents such as nitrogen mustard (Section 12.4); it seems that intra-chain linking of DNA guanine bases is occurring (Shooter *et al.*, 1972). Clinical trials (Wittes, *et al.*, 1977; Hill *et al.*, 1975) have shown promise in squamous cell carcinoma of the head, and in bladder and gonad cancer, but been marred by the nephrotoxicity caused by a metabolite of the drug. The corresponding *trans* isomer has little activity. When molecules of cyclohexylamine replace the two ammonia molecules in the drug, a better chemotherapeutic index is found in laboratory trials (Connors *et al.*, 1972).

11.11 Fundamental considerations in designing new chelating agents. Promising avenues of application

The starting-point for these considerations must be the hard fact that the majority of chelating agents have no biological action. For example, very few of the metal-binding agents commonly used in analytical work are antibacterial (Albert, *et al.*, 1947; Schraufstätter, 1950).

No chelating agent can be expected to be active, in a biological environment, unless its stability constants are at least as high as those of the common aminoacids, e.g. glycine in Table 11.2. However, no good purpose may be served by flying to the other extreme and producing agents with very high stability constants: such substances are liable to become lost by saturation before reaching the desired site of action. For some applications, at least, moderate ease of cation exchange is necessary (Schubert, 1957).

At some stage in the design it must be decided whether penetration into cells is to be desired or to be avoided. If desirable, lipophilic groups should be added to the molecule. For this purpose carbon, halogens, hydrogen, and sulphur are considered as lipophilic, and nitrogen and oxygen as hydrophilic; the effect can be followed by determining oil/water partition coefficients. The effect of adding first hydrophilic, and then lipophilic, groups to oxine is illustrated in Table 11.9. Complexes of the ethylene-diamine type (see Fig. 11.1), which preserve the original charge on the metal, need to be supplied with lipophilic groups to acquire ease of penetration; in fact they need more of this help than would be necessary for an uncharged complex.

Very small changes in a molecule can produce large changes in partition coefficients. Thus, the insertion of an extra ring-nitrogen into oxine to give 3-aza-oxine (8-hydroxyquinazoline) makes the molecule much more hydrophilic and it lowers the oil/water partition coefficient from 67 to 5 (see Table 11.9). The addition of a side-chain of only three carbon atoms (the propyl-group) restores the partition coefficient.

Apart from this use of partition coefficients, uptake of an agent by cells can be forced in another way: by using ligands which resemble natural substrates such as aminoacids and carbohydrates.

Steric and other chemical differences which can assist selectivity were discussed in Section 11.4.

Many biologically active chelating agents are unsuited for internal therapy in man simply because they are not selective enough. One must always proceed cautiously with metal-binding substances because some of them, such as sodium dimethyldithiocarbamate (Kadota and Midorikawa, 1951), injure the islets of Langerhans and thus cause diabetes in experimental animals. The 5-amino-, also the 2-methyl-derivatives of oxine act similarly (Kadota and Abe, 1954).

Chelating agents can sometimes be used for overcoming drug-resistance in bacteria. For example, EDTA restored susceptibility in polymyxin-resistant strains of *Pseudomonas*, presumably by removing calcium and magnesium from the plasma membrane (Brown and Richards, 1965). EDTA also resotred susceptibility in hospital strains of penicillin-resistant *Staphylococcus aureus* (Rawal, 1969). Oxytetracycline, a known chelating agent (Section 11.8), also renders penicillin-resistant *Staph. aureus* susceptible to the latter drug (Michael, Michael, and Massell, 1967).

Current topics in chelation research include the search for new methods of detoxification and decontamination of tissues injured by chemically toxic or radioactive metals, attempts to combat the element of chelation in dental caries, and to prevent the loss of calcium from bones that occurs in old age, the cause of so much precocious senility.

12 The covalent bond in selective toxicity

Although the majority of biologically active substances combine only loosely with receptors and are easily released by washing, a few agents combine by covalent bonds which are of a more durable character (see Section 8.0). Covalent bonds involving carbon can be broken by great heat and also by powerful chemicals, but few can be ruptured by mild reagents at temperatures compatible with life.

One aspect of covalent bond formation has already been adequately treated, namely the degradation of a pro-drug to the true active agent (see Section 3.5). Also, many covalent bonds are made and broken by enzymes in the normal metabolic reactions of the cell, and also in disposing of foreign materials (see Section 3.4). However, the present chapter is concerned solely with the formation of a covalent bond between an agent and its receptor, i.e. the chemical group with which it reacts to produce its biological response. Consideration will first be given to metalloids like arsenic which forms bonds with the sulphur of mercapto-groups. The discussion will then move on to acylating and alkylating agents, in that order, followed by those agents which become built into vitally active constituents of cells.

12.0 Arsenicals, antimonials, and mercurials

The arsenicals were the first drugs to be recognized as acting through formation of covalent bonds. Ehrlich (1909) suggested that some arsenicals combine with essential mercapto-groups (also called sulphydryl-groups, thiol-groups, or SH groups) in the parasite. This suggestion arose from the fact that arsenoxides very readily gave the reaction shown in (12.1), even in the presence of a great excess of water. What makes this reaction so relevant is that it is the only one available to arsenoxides under biological conditions. The three levels of oxidation of arsenic are exemplified in (*12.2*), (*6.3*) and (*6.2*), which are respectively the pentavalent and the two trivalent (arsenoxide and arsenobenzene) states. It is noteworthy that the arsenobenzene state is at a lower level of oxidation than the arsenoxide state, but the arsenic atom is trivalent in both. X-ray diffraction studies have shown that arsenobenzenes are trimeric in the solid state, as (*11.3*) (Hedberg, Hughes, and Waser, 1961).

Although Ehrlich had found that pentavalent arsenicals did not act in the body until reduced to arsenoxides, it had not occurred to him that arsenobenzenes acted only after oxidation to arsenoxides. This was established between 1920 and 1925 by Swiss-born Carl Voegtlin and his co-workers in the United States Public Health Service (for a review, see Voegtlin, 1925).

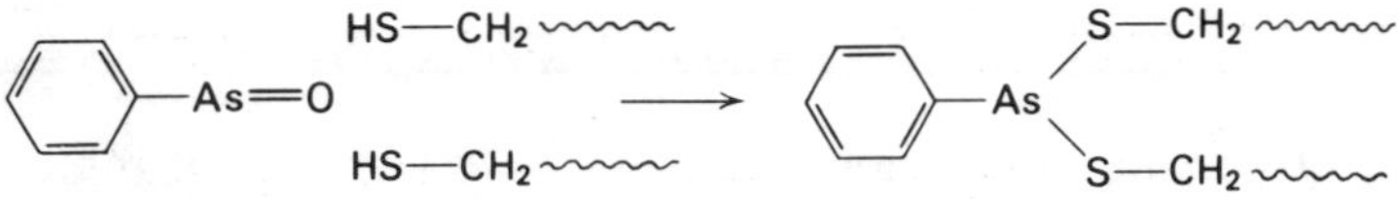

(*12.1*)

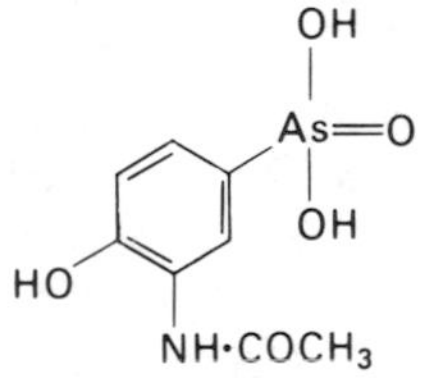

Acetarsol
(*12.2*)

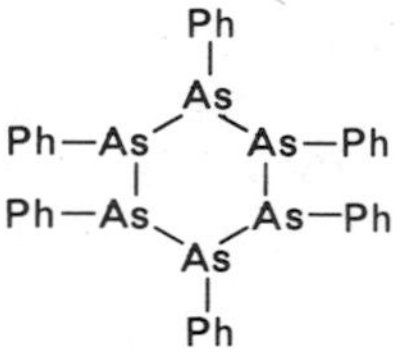

(*12.3*)

Voegtlin showed that the arsenoxide level is the only one at which organic arsenicals are therapeutically active. In Fig. 12.1 it can be seen that oxophenarsine (*6.3*) brings about a dramatic lowering of the trypanosome population in the rat's blood-stream within half an hour of administration, but arsphenamine (*6.2*), which is the corresponding arsenobenzene, requires more than 5 hours to accomplish the same result. This indicates that arsphenamine has to be changed to a more active substance before it can act. Voegtlin found that, when arsphenamine was shaken with air for a few minutes, it was converted to its arsenoxide (oxophenarsine) which then exerted the typical rapid action. The same result was obtained when arsphenamine was incubated with oxidizing tissues, such as fresh liver.

Fig. 12.1 also illustrates how the action of arsenoxides is antagonized by substances containing thiol-groups (such as glutathione, cysteine, or sodium thioglycollate). This effect is not durable if the amount of thiol is small, because the complex can hydrolyse to its original components. With larger amounts of thiols, the effect is prolonged because of the mass-action law effect. Voegtlin demonstrated that trypanosomes gave the nitroprusside reaction and other tests showing that free thiol-groups were present.

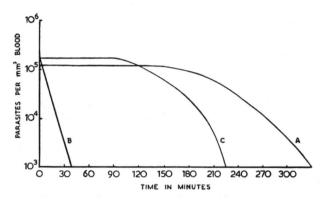

FIG. 12.1 The parasiticidal effect in trypanosome-infected rats of (A) arsphen-amine ('Salvarsan'), (B) oxophenarsine ('Mapharside'), and (C) oxo-phenarsine plus reduced glutathione. (Redrawn from Voegtlin, 1925.)

The reaction of arsenoxides with thiol-groups is reversible, and parasites that have been treated with several lethal doses of arsenic can be saved if subsequently treated with many equivalents of a thiol-compound.

It is now accepted that death of the parasite, because it occurs so quickly, often in less than 30 minutes, must be derived from the drug's interference with respiration and glycolysis, and not from any attack on nucleic acids or protein synthesis (Macadam and Williamson, 1974). This leads to the question, To what are the vital thiol-groups of the parasite attached? At first Voegtlin suspected glutathione, later, the thiol-groups of proteins (Rosenthal and Voegtlin, 1930). Current opinion favours enzymic thiol-groups, many of which have been shown, in pure isolated enzymes, to be strongly inhibited by arsenoxides and protected by thiols (Dixon and Webb, 1964). The most arsenic-sensitive of known enzymes are (a) lipoic acid dehydrogenase, and (b) the α-oxidases (e.g. pyruvate oxidase) which use lipoic acid (thioctic acid) as a coenzyme. Lipoic acid dehydrogenase has two cysteine residues on different chains of protein which are kept adjacent by tertiary folding (Massey, Hofmann, and Palmer, 1962). Arsenicals can bind these cysteine thiol-groups as in (*12.1*). In (b), the lipoic acid (6,8-dimercapto-octanoic acid) (*2.25*) is easily bridged by arsenicals as in (*12.1*) (Peters, 1963).

However, the question remains, how do organic arsenicals injure the parasite without harm to the host? It was pointed out in the introduction to Chapter 3 that the parasites have a relatively higher abundance of free SH-groups than the host's cells, but additional selectivity is derived from analogous enzymes and from favourable distribution, as follows. It has been observed that several enzymes in trypanosomes, e.g. phosphopyruvate kinease, are highly sensitive to arsenicals, whereas the corresponding mammalian enzyme is much less affected (Grant and Sargent, 1960). In addition, much selectivity is conferred by the aromatic-ring structure of the drug. Inorganic and aliphatic arsenicals are no less toxic to trypanosomes than are the aromatic arsenicals; but only the aromatic arsenicals are selective, and they are most selective if substituted as in (6.3). This conclusion is supported by drug-resistance studies (see Section 6.5) which point to selective adsorption.

Voegtlin's studies, extended by his colleagues Rosenthal (1932) and Eagle (1939), have shown that arsenical drugs act on spirochaetes by the same mechanism as on trypanosomes. No matter at what level of oxidation the drug may be, it has first to be converted to the arsenoxide level and then it combines with essential thiol-groups in the parasite. For a review of the connection between constitution and selective action in arsenicals designed for treating syphilis, *see* Eagle (1951).

Why is the arsenic-sulphur bond so readily split by mercaptans? The arsenic atom, quite unlike those of nitrogen, carbon, and oxygen, has a vacant *d* orbital, into which can go a lone pair of electrons from the sulphur atom of cysteine. This leads to a higher-valency transition-complex having three* sulphur atoms united to one arsenic atom. Such a complex is unstable, and each As – S bond has a roughly equal chance of breaking. Thus there is a one in three chance that the newly formed bond will survive. If an excess of cysteine is present and this process is allowed to continue, there would soon be very little of the arsenical drug bonded to the receptor (a simple mass-action effect). A well-known analogue of this situation is the hydrolysis of silicon tetrachloride, which is rapidly decomposed by water because silicon has a vacant *d* orbital. But carbon tetrachloride is stable because carbon has no vacant *d* orbital.

Lewisite (ClCH : CH · AsCl$_2$), the most vesicant of the arsenical war gases, produces lesions in man that are not reversed or even averted by any mono-thiol. The work done by Peters and his colleagues at Oxford from 1923 onwards led to the discovery that lewisite injures the skin and exerts widespread toxicity by blocking – SH – groups of pyruvate oxidase (Peters, 1936, 1948). Injuries caused by lewisite can be completely reversed by those dithiols which have two – SH – groups close together (Peters, Stocken,

---

* Two sulphur atoms are supplied by the receptor, as in (*12.1*), and the third comes from the attacking thiol (e.g. cysteine).

and Thompson, 1945). Thus an unusually firm combination with $-SH-$ groups can be reversed by an unusually potent antidote. The great virtue of having two mercapto-groups in the one molecule is that one bond will always hold when the other is temporarily broken by thermal agitation. The best of these dithiols (2,3-dimercaptopropanol (*11.19*); dimercaprol) has since proved to be an excellent hospital antidote for poisoning (see Section 11.6).

Until 1944, it was generally supposed that arsenicals had no effect on common pathogenic bacteria. This misconception arose from failure to test the substances at the various levels of oxidation. When this was done, it was found that arsenicals are capable of strong antibacterial activity (Albert, Falk, and Rubbo, 1944). The results, in Table 12.1, show that the active level for bacteriostasis is the arsenoxide level, and that the conditions can convert a little material to this from the arsenobenzene level, but

Table 12.1

THE EFFECT OF ORGANIC ARSENICALS ON BACTERIA

Greatest dilutions completely inhibiting visible growth in 48 hours at 37°C. (*Medium*: Peptone broth, containing 10 per cent serum; pH 7.2)

Substance	Organism				
	Cl. welchii	Strept. haem. A	Staph. aureus	B. coli	Proteus
Acetarsol (*11.2*) (*m*-acetamido-*p*-hydroxyphenyl arsonic acid)	*	*	*	*	*
Oxophenarsine (*11.3*) (*m*-amino-*p*-hydroxyphenyl arsenoxide)	1 : 160 000	1 : 80 000	1 : 160 000	1 : 10 000	1 : 10 000
Neoarsphenamine (*m*-amino-*p*-hydroxy-arsenobenzene-*N*-methylenesulph-oxylate)	1 : 10 000	1 : 10 000	1 : 10 000	*	*
Oxophenarsine in 0.1 per cent thioglycollate broth	1 : 5000	1 : 10 000	*	*	*
Mercuric chloride (for comparison)	1 : 40 000	1 : 160 000	1 : 40 000	1 : 80 000	1 : 80 000

* Signifies not inhibitory, even at a concentration of 1 : 5000.
(Albert, Falk, and Rubbo, 1944.)

none from the pentavalent level. The antibacterial action of the arsenoxide is seen to be neutralized by a mercaptan (sodium thioglycollate).

Because Ehrlich had thought that arsenoxides were too toxic for human use, syphilis was treated for a quarter of a century with unnecessarily large doses of arsenic, in the form of arsphenamine ('Salvarsan') and neoarsphenamine ('Neo-salvarsan'). A small portion of those massive doses was converted to the potent arsenoxides in the body; the greater part engaged in side-reactions, dangerous for the patient. Eventually, Tatum and Cooper (1934) showed that oxophenarsine, the arsenoxide corresponding to arsphenamine, was a safer drug than 'Salvarsan' because, although it was more toxic to the host, it was even more toxic to the parasite and hence smaller doses were effective. This substance (*m*-amino-*p*-hydroxyphenylarsenoxide) (6.3) ('Mapharsen') made it possible to cure syphilis with small, safe doses of arsenic. Penicillin has now taken the place of arsenic in treating this disease.

Arsenicals in comtemporary medical practice.   The clinical use of organic arsenicals is now confined to the treatment of advanced cases of sleeping sickness (trypanosomiasis) where the brain has become infected. Tryparasamide (6.6) is used because it can penetrate into the central nervous system, presumably as an analogue of phosphoric acid. For cases that resist this drug, melarsoprol (12.4) has been found useful. It is the condensation product of an arsenoxide with 1,2-dimercaptoethane, and is split into its components after passing the blood-brain barrier (Friedheim, 1951).

Melarsoprol
(*12.4*)

Antimony potassium
tartrate
(*12.5*)

Antimonials.   Pentavalent antimonials, such as sodium stibogluconate, are widely used in the treatment of the protozoal disease leishmaniasis. The drug has no action on the parasites *in vitro*, but reduction *in vivo* has not been reported, so that a mode of action parallel to those of tryparsamide, although likely, has not been demonstrated. Trivalent antimonials are much used in management of the severe worm infestation shistosomiasis. The favoured drugs are antimony potassium tartrate (*12.5*) which was introduced in 1918, antimony sodium dimercaptosuccinate, and stibophen (*4.37*). All of them work through selective inhibition of phosphofructokinase, of which the worm's analogue is more susceptible than the mammalian analogue (see Table 4.4). It is generally assumed that the antimony acts on an important SH-group. Yet this inhibition of the worm enzyme is not overcome by mercaptoethanol (Mansour and Bueding, 1954). Whether it could be overcome by a dimercaptan, such as (*11.19*), remains to be seen.

Mercurials.   Mercurials, such as mercuric chloride and phenyl mercuric nitrate, exert their antiseptic action on bacteria by combining with essential SH groups (Fildes, 1940b). The bacteria appear to be dead, but are easily revived by treatment with a thiol such as thioglycollic acid or even hydrogen sulphide (Chick, 1908).

All the organo-mercurial diuretics are broken down by acidity in the kidney to give a small yield of mercuric ions, and it is generally agreed that mercurial diuresis depends on the blockade of a mercapto-group in the enzyme responsible for resorption of sodium chloride.

12.1 The penicillins

Bacteria stand in sharp contrast to vertebrate cells by having a cell wall, and this wall is of a unique chemical character (see Section 5.1). The most vulnerable component of this wall is acetylmuramic acid (*5.2*) linked to polypeptides such as (*5.3*). Penicillin (*12.6a*) acts on bacteria by blocking the incorporation of these acetylmuramic peptides into new cell wall (Rogers and Mandelstam, 1962). It was found that the concentration of drug required to inhibit cell wall synthesis and that required to inhibit growth in the same organism agree within a two- to three-fold range for both Gram-positive and -negative bacteria.

Bacteria are somewhat unusual in having a high internal pressure. Penicillin kills *growing* bacteria by causing them to burst because of this high pressure which a defective wall can no longer sustain. However, they do not burst if placed in a non-absorbable medium of high osmotic pressure (e.g. 0.3M-sucrose solution). Lederberg (1957) worked out these details (of the lysis of bacteria by penicillin) using *E. coli*, and they have been confirmed in other species. The bursting of bacterial cells by penicillin is apparently assisted by an enzyme known as mucopeptidase which is present in almost all bacteria. When the biosynthesis of this enzyme is halted by chloramphenicol, penicillin is much less effective (Rogers, 1967). Penicillin does not affect protein synthesis at the concentrations reached in therapy.

Cycloserine (*5.4*) (see Section 9.4), vancomycin (Chatterjee and Park, 1964), and bacitracin (Abraham, 1957) also lyse bacteria by interfering with the synthesis of wall materials. The last two antibiotics are discussed in Section 12.2.

Many penicillins have been isolated from the liquor in which active strains of *Pencillium notatum* are growing (see Section 6.3). They have the general structure (*12.6*), differing only in the nature of the side-chain. The variety known as benzylpenicillin (*5.8*) soon became the standard, and is always to be understood when 'pencillin' is specified.

The early workers with penicillin were inconvenienced by its proneness

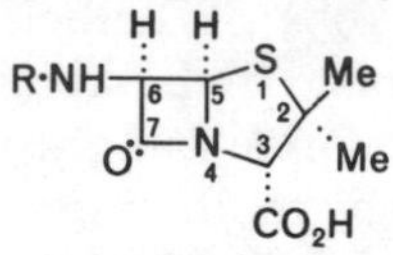

H H
R·NH─┬─┬─S Me
    6│5 1│2
  O⁼─N─3─ ̈Me
      4
     CO₂H

(a) 6-Aminopenicillanic acid (R = H—)
(b) Benzylpencillin (R = C₆H₅CH₂CO—)
(12.6)

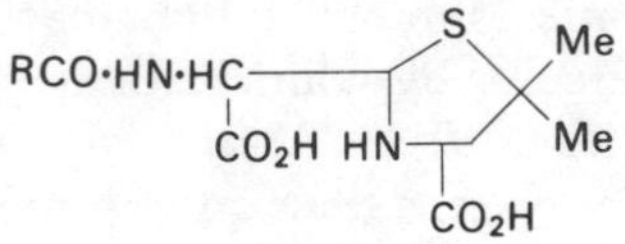

RCO·HN·HC──┬─S Me
           │
       CO₂H HN─┴ Me
              CO₂H

Penicilloic acids
(12.7)

O⁼─⌐NH ⟷ O⁻─⌐=NH⁺

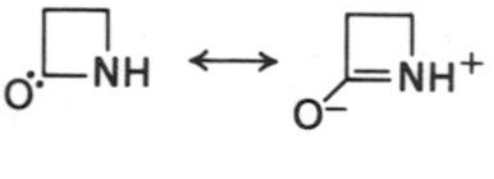

(12.8)

to hydrolysis. This is greater than that of β-lactams, generally due to the suppression of the expected stabilizing resonance (12.8), thanks to a tetrahedral geometry enforced by the five-membered ring to which it is fused (Woodward, Neuberger, and Trenner, 1949; Butler, Freeman, and Wright, 1977; Sweet and Dahl, 1970). X-ray diffraction studies show the two rings almost at right-angles to one another.

Benzylpenicillin is hydrolysed, to the corresponding penicilloic acid (12.7), by alkali, cupric ions, or β-lactamase (usually called penicillinase), and to penillic acid, and penicillamine (11.21). In natural biosynthesis it is formed by the condensation of 6-penicillamine, D-valine, and phenylacetic acid. The presence of the highly strained four-membered lactam ring in penicillin makes it a powerful, but specific, acylating agent. This ring readily opens between C-7 and the nitrogen atom.

Studies on the inactivation of benzylpenicillin have shown that this substance has a strong preference for acylating β-aminomercaptans, much less affinity for other amines, and none for other mercaptans. The product [e.g. (12.9) from β-mercaptoethylamine] is acylated on the amino-group. The function of the mercapto-groups seems to be to form a hydrogen bond with the oxygen atom of the lactam and hence increase the polarization of the C=O bond in the penicillin.

Experiments with ^{35}S penicillin show that resistant strains of staphyl-

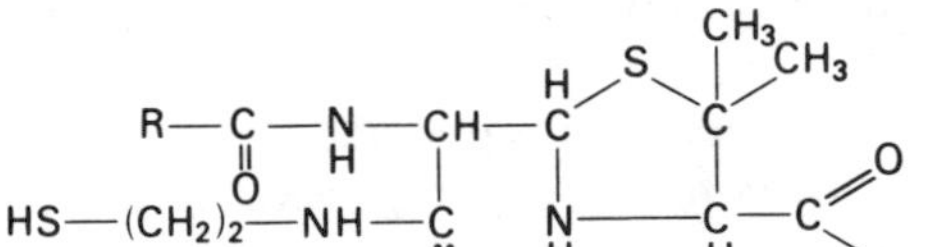

Product from β-mercaptoethylamine
and a penicillin
(12.9)

ococci, even those that produce no penicillinase, take up no penicillin from solution, but susceptible strains of various species combine with from 200 to 750 molecules per cell. This amount is held tightly, cannot be washed away, and does not exchange with non-radioactive penicillin (Rowley, *et al.*, 1950; Maass and Johnson, 1949). The first molecules of penicillin are bound by inert material but, when this is saturated, the penicillin combines covalently with a receptor playing a key role in the biosynthesis of cell wall. Mammalian cells do not take up penicillin, but the bacterial cell binds it in less than 2 minutes. The penicillin-binding component is on the exterior, in the cytoplasmic membrane where the cell wall is synthesized. This component occurs in a phospholipid-containing fraction of staphylococci (Cooper, 1956).

In finer detail, penicillin acts by stopping cross-linkage between the peptide portions of the material being polymerized (Section 5.1) to make new cell wall (Martin, 1964). In recent years, several hypotheses have been put forward linking the first stage in the action of penicillin to its structural resemblance to a portion of the relevant acetylmuramic peptide. The most plausible of these hypotheses will be given first, but it must be borne in mind that variation in the composition of these peptides may make one of the alternatives equally, or even more, valid for a particular bacterial species.

Comparison of molecular models of penicillin and D-alanyl-D-alanine showed that the former could effectively function as a metabolite analogue of the latter. Thus the N' to N'' distances in these molecules, shown as projections of molecular models in (*12.10*) and (*12.11*), are identical, namely 3.3 Å. Also the N'' to C' distances are similar in both models, namely 2.5 Å. From N' to C' is 5.4 Å in the penicillins and 5.7 Å in alanylalanine, distances which are not identical but still quite similar. The D-configuration of the penicillin is maintained by the sulphur atom in conjunction with the carbon atom that is common to both rings (Tipper and Strominger, 1965). [Epimerization at the 6-position, see (*12.6*), causes loss of all antibacterial activity.] The most reactive bond in the penicillin molecule (the β-lactam bond) corresponds in position to the peptide bond joining the two D-alanine residues. Admittedly, there are second-order discrepancies; the bond linking the two alanine residues is about 25% longer than the lactam bond; moreover the C-CO-N angle in D-ala-D-ala is $117°$, but only $91°$ in penicillin. Rather more serious evidence against this structural analogue hypothesis is that 6-methyl benzylpenicillin (cf. *12.6*), although an even better structural analogue of D-ala-D-ala, is completely inactive against bacteria (Boehme *et al.*, 1971). This seems at variance with the Strominger hypothesis of penicillin action, but no better hypothesis has emerged.

The main site of action of the penicillins is apparently a membrane-bound enzyme like the peptidoglycan transpeptidase isolated from *E. coli*.

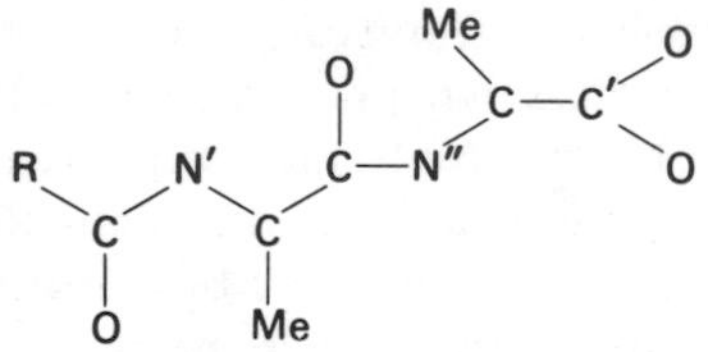

(Acyl)-D-alanyl-D-alanine
(12.10)

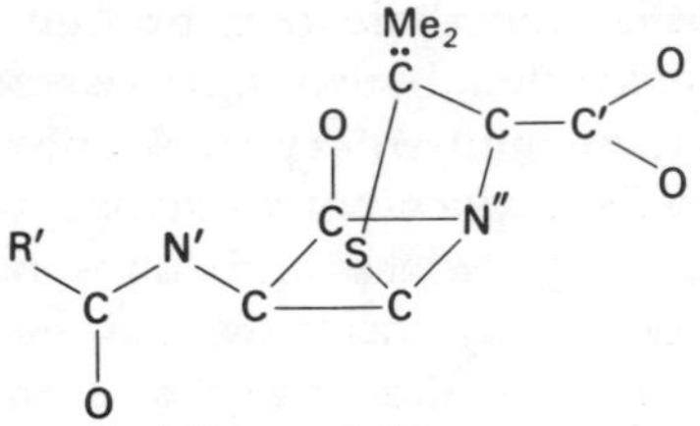

The penicillins
(projection from molecular models)
(12.11)

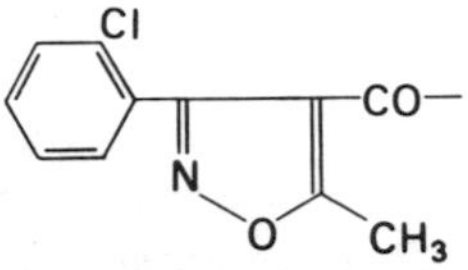

Cloxacillin
[insert, as R, into (11.7)]
(12.12)

It catalyses the cross-linking reaction in cell-wall biosynthesis. In this final polymerization, two strands of peptidoglycan (i.e. muropeptide units polymerized through their carbohydrate components, see Section 5.0) are joined by union between a penultimate D-alnine residue and the chain of four glycine residues attached to lysine (slight variants of this linkage occur in different bacterial species). This cell-free transpeptidase is inhibited irreversibly by penicillin at a concentration lethal to the intact bacterial cell (Izaki, Matsuhashi, and Strominger, 1966). It is supposed, by this group of workers, that penicillin is taken up on the transpeptidating site of the enzyme and that it acylates this site irreversibly, using the β-lactam ring as the acylating agent (Izaki, Matsuhashi, and Strominger, 1968).

The transpeptidase of *B. subtilis*, after rigorous purification, has four SH-groups, one of which is inactivated by penicillin. The covalently-bound penicillin molecule can be removed with either ethanethiol or hydroxylamine, and this operation restores the enzyme's activity (Lawrence and Strominger, 1970).

The Belgian school, using the soluble transpeptidase-polymerase secreted by a *Streptomyces*, found that the penicillin site is near, but not identical with, the substrate-acceptor site. When this enzyme binds penicillin, the configuration of the active site is distorted, and locked in a non-operable conformation (Ghuysen *et al.*, 1974). This may, of course, be only a peculiarity of this prokaryote, so far removed in type from pathogenic bacteria.

Benzylpenicillin (Penicillin G) is still the most generally useful of all antibiotics employed in daily medical practice, and is still the most used form of injectable penicillin, just as Penicillin V, i.e. phenoxymethyl-penicillin (*12.6*), R = C$_6$H$_5$OCH$_2$CO−), is the most prescribed form of oral penicillin. In 1957, 6-aminopenicillanic acid (6-APA) was isolated from the fermentation liquors of *Pencillium chrysogenum* (Batchelor et· al., 1961) and proved to be an ideal starting material for the production of many semi-synthetic analogues of penicillin. In many of these, 6-APA, is acylated with a group similar to that of the phenylacetyl-group in benzylpenicillin (*12.6b*), but carrying at least one extra substituent in the methylene (CH$_2$) group. These analogues, less susceptible to acid hydrolysis in the stomach than benzylpenicillin, were the forerunners of the contemporary specialized penicillins. It was found that the introduction of steric hindrance into an acyl-group enabled the molecule to resist acid hydrolysis. One of these products, ampicillin (6-α-aminophenylacetamidopenicillanic acid) ('Penbritin', 'Omnipen'), besides killing Gram-positive bacteria at a great dilution as benzylpenicillin does, is active against many Gram-negative bacteria. Unfortunately it is readily inactivated by penicillinase. Carbenicillin (6-α-carboxyphenylacetamidopenicillanic acid) ('Pyopen') is also active against Gram-negative bacteria but, unlike ampicillin, is inactive orally. Activity against Gram-negative organisms has followed introduction of an ionizing group (either anionic or cationic) into the methylene (CH$_2$) of (*12.6b*).

Some related products are quite resistant to penicillinase. For example, methicillin ('Celbenin', 'Staphcillin') (6-2′,6′-dimethoxybenzamido-penicillanic acid) which, although having a narrower range and intensity of action than benzylpenicillin, is highly effective in treating patients infected with staphylococci resistant to benzylpenicillin. Unfortunately methicillin is hydrolysed by acid and so must be injected. Two more recently introduced oral penicillins can withstand both acid and penicillinase: cloxacillin ('Orbenin') (R = *12.12*), and oxacillin ('Prostaphlin') which is cloxacillin minus the chlorine atom.

From the above account, it is evident that the therapeutic range of penicillins has been considerably extended, although the new products tend to be costly. All penicillins which have been clinically successful have an aromatic ring fairly near to the acylating group (7-CO). This requirement, present also in the cephalosporins, suggests that a corresponding flat area is present in the receptor.

For further reading on the relationship of structure to activity in penicillins, see Hou and Poole (1971).

12.2 Cephalosporins, bacitracin, and other inhibitors of the formation of new cell walls.

From Brotzu's fungus *Cephalosporium* (Section 6.3), the antibiotic cephalosporin C, isolated in Oxford, was found by Newton and Abraham (1956) to be a derivative of what is now called 7-aminocephalosporanic acid (*12.13*), whose close chemical relationship to 6-aminopenicillanic acid (*12.6a*) was seen at once. The action of cephalosporin C was weak, but interesting. As a result, semi-synthetic cephalosporins were made by attaching new side-chains to 7-aminocephalosporanic acid; concomitant alteration of the side-chain in the 3-position was found advantageous. Finally a useful drug emerged: Cephalothin ('Keflin'), but it is not absorbed from the gut and has to be injected four times a day. Finally an orally active analogue was obtained, cephalexin (*12.14*) ('Keflex', 'Ceporex'). The resemblance to ampicillin (p. 453) is striking.

7-Aminocephalosporanic acid
(*12.13*)

Cephalexin
(*12.14*)

Cephalosporin derivatives are expensive, but useful for organisms that are resistant to penicillins, and they may be given (but cautiously!) to patients who have become sensitized to the penicillins. They are more active than benzylpenicillin against Gram-negative bacteria, and specially effective in the respiratory and urinary tracts where they tend to concentrate. Although cephalosporins are not sensitive to penicillinase, resistant bacteria have been found to harbour a parallel β-lactamase called cephalosporase.

The antibacterial action of this family is exerted on the synthesis of new cell wall, and by acylating the same enzyme site attacked by the penicillins (Abraham, 1962). The double-bond in the six-membered ring of cephalosporin-derivatives activates the β-lactam group in the same way as the torsional effect of the 5-membered ring in penicillin does (Sweet and Dahl, 1970). The sulphur atom of cephalosporins may be replaced by oxygen or methylene substituents without loss of antibacterial activity (Cama and Christensen, 1974).

For further reading on cephalosporins, see Abraham (1967).

Vancomycin is a chlorinated polyphenyl ether antibiotic, with sugar and aminoacid residues, obtained from *Streptomyces orientalis*. It specifically and strongly binds to the disaccharide peptides that are the raw material from which bacteria build new cell wall. It is still sometimes used clinically for penicillin-resistant organisms. Its action resembles that of penicillin in that the synthesis of new cell wall is prevented, so that growing cells quickly die by rupture of the plasma membrane (Anderson *et al.*, 1965).

Bacitracin, extracted from *B. subtilis*, is a decapeptide containing four

D-aminoacid residues and a thiazoline nucleus. Its point of attack is the formation of a complex with the sugar-transporting undecaprenyl pyrophosphate in the plasma membrane, an early stage in cell-wall synthesis briefly referred to in Section 5.1 (Stone and Strominger, 1971).

The above two antibiotics, quite unlike penicillin and oxamycin, also slowly increase the permeability of the cytoplasmic membrane (Reynolds, 1966). The need of bacitracin for a divalent metal, mentioned in Section 11.9, is apparently connected with this secondary site of attack.

12.3 Organic phosphates and carbamates

The substances discussed in this Section have become both interesting and important because of their property of acylating esterases, particularly acetylcholinesterase. The toxicity of the organic phosphorus derivatives to mammals is directly proportional to the inhibition of the host's acetylcholinesterase (Aldridge and Barnes, 1952). These phosphorus compounds were originally developed in Germany, first as chemical defence agents ('nerve gases') during the Second World War, and after that as agricultural insecticides, with which G. Schrader and the Bayer laboratories are identified. The organic phosphorus insecticides first used in the field were insufficiently selective, and there were many casualties among birds, and even men. Later, products of quite remarkable selectivity were marketed.

The phosphorus insecticides act by acylating their target enzyme, but this is a phosphorylation and not a carbonylation as with penicillin and the carbamates. Kinetic studies on the enzymes chymotrypsin and acetylcholinesterase showed that ^{32}P-di*iso*propyl phosphorofluoridate* (Dyflos) (*12.15*) di*iso*propylphosphorylated the hydroxy-group of serine in each enzyme, splitting off hydrofluoric acid as it did so (Schaffer, May, and Summerson, 1954). The strong β-emission of ^{32}P, and its half-life of 14 days, makes isotopic phosphorus very convenient for following the behaviour of the phosphorus insecticides in tissues. Similarly, paraoxon (*12.16*), which Gage (1953) showed to be the active form of Schrader's parathion (*12.17*), diethylphosphorylates this hydroxy-group, at the same time liberating *p*-nitrophenol (Hartley and Kilby, 1952). Tetraethyl pyrophosphate acts similarly. Electron-withdrawing groups, which weaken the P−O−P bonds and the P−F bond, increase, the activity up to a maximum, beyond which further weakening of the bonds leads to wasteful hydrolysis by water (Aldridge and Barnes, 1952; Aldridge and Davison, 1952). Thus, below this maximum, there is a linear relationship between (a) *log* hydrolysis constant and (b) the *log* bimolecular rate constant for the reaction between the enzyme and the organic phosphate.

The essentials of enzyme phosphorylation are shown in Scheme 12.1.

---

* Formerly described as a 'fluorophosphonate'.

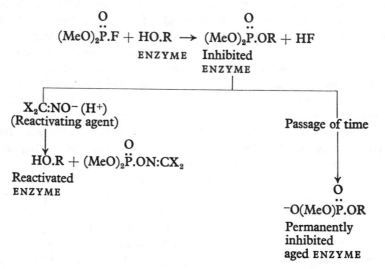

$(CH_3)_2CHO$, F
P
$(CH_3)_2CHO$, O

Dyflos
(12.15)

EtO, $O·C_6H_4NO_2(p)$
P
EtO, O

Paraoxon
(12.16)

EtO, $O·C_6H_4·NO_2(p)$
P
EtO, S

Parathion
(12.17)

If the inhibited enzyme has not 'aged', it can be reactivated by the anionic group of a hydroxylamine (see below). The phenomenon of ageing was discovered by Hobbiger (1955), who noted that esters of secondary alcohols evoke this phenomenon faster than those of primary alcohols. The correct interpretation, namely that ageing is proportional to the hydrolysis of an alkoxy-group to an anion, came later (Berends, *et al.*, 1959). Coulombic repulsion prevents the response of the aged, inactivated enzyme to the antidote.

$$(MeO)_2\overset{O}{\overset{..}{P}}.F + HO.R \rightarrow (MeO)_2\overset{O}{\overset{..}{P}}.OR + HF$$

ENZYME   Inhibited
ENZYME

$X_2C:NO^- (H^+)$
(Reactivating agent)

$$HO.R + (MeO)_2\overset{O}{\overset{..}{P}}.ON:CX_2$$

Reactivated
ENZYME

Passage of time

$$^-O(MeO)\overset{O}{\overset{..}{P}}.OR$$

Permanently
inhibited
aged ENZYME

SCHEME 12.1   Inactivation of an enzyme by phosphorylation and its reactivation if not 'aged'.

In insects poisoned by organic phosphorus compounds, assays for acetylcholinesterase show that this enzyme becomes increasingly inhibited during the first hour and the levels of free acetylcholine rise sharply (Smallman and Fisher, 1958). This rise causes a great increase in spontaneous nerve activity (neuronal hyperexcitation), both autonomic and somatic. This state brings about liberation of tissue toxins, ion imbalance, with eventual paralysis, dehydration, and death; this sequence is reminiscent of that caused by the chlorinated insecticides (see Section 7.6e for this comparison and for general information on biochemistry of the insect nervous system).

Acetylcholinesterases isolated from various insect species differ greatly in their susceptibility to phosphorus insecticides (R. O'Brien, 1967). Access to this enzyme is more difficult in insects than in mammals; hence it is understandable that ionized analogues of (*12.15*), etc., have proved not to be insecticidal because foreign ions do not readily penetrate membranes (Section 3.1).

The insecticide industry realized that, to achieve selectivity, new kinds of organic phosphorus compounds must be found, ones that would be differently metabolized in insects and vertebrates, i.e. they must either be inert substances which only insects can activate, or they must be active substances which only mammals can detoxify. A step in the right direction was made by Schrader with parathion (*12.17*) (*OO*-diethyl *O*-*p*-nitrophenyl phosphorothionate), introduced in 1944. This had a wider, though insufficient, margin of safety which depended upon the presence in the insect of an enzyme that changed P : S to P : O, thus producing paraoxon (*12.16*) which is the true toxicant. This change, which occurred to a smaller degree in vertebrates, provided a small margin of selectivity. It was later found that the margin of safety could be much improved by replacing the two ethoxy-groups in parathion by two methoxy-groups, giving 'parathion-methyl' which was introduced in 1954. Meanwhile, success had crowned attempts to introduce two different safety mechanisms into the one molecule. This was achieved by the discovery of malathion (*12.18*) (*S*-[1,2-di-(ethoxycarbonyl)ethyl] *OO*-dimethyl phosphorodithionate). The actual toxicant is malaoxon in which P : S is replaced by P : O. Malathion is rapidly de-esterified in mammals by carboxyesterases and the resultant acid is quickly eliminated; whereas the insects perform the P : S to P : O change, but carry out very little de-esterification. Thus two metabolic changes which lead to favourable selectivity take place in the one substrate (Krueger and O'Brien, 1959). The P : S to P : O change in insects is effected by microsomes in the gut, nerve cord, and fat body. Insect microsomes can be isolated and used as experimental aids (Nakatsugawa and Dahm, 1965). The detoxifying enzymes in mammals are carboxyesterases, microsomal oxidases, and (for amides) carboxyamidases. Analogous enzymes occur in insects, but are much less effective. It should be borne in mind, too, that an insect receives a much higher dose (w/w) than any vertebrate is likely to.

It can be seen from Fig. 12.2 that the mouse converts only a small pro-

Malathion
(*12.18*)

Diazinon
(*12.19*)

portion of a dose of malathion into the toxic malaoxon, whereas the cockroach not only converts much more but retains the toxin longer. This graph needs to be read in conjunction with Table 12.2 which shows that the mouse can withstand a huge dose of malathion because it does not readily convert it to the toxic derivative malaoxon, whereas the cockroach, and particularly the housefly, are excellent converters. Similarly mammalian carboxyamidases are capable of removing amide-groups which insects are almost unable to hydrolyse (see dimethoate, below).

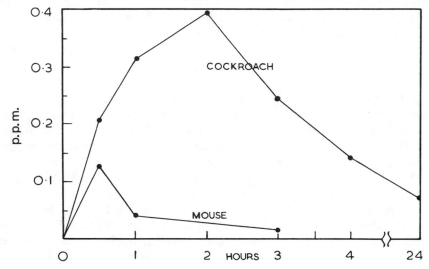

FIG. 12.2 Malaoxon level after injecting 30 p.p.m. of ^{32}P-Malathion. (Krueger and O'Brien, 1959.)

Table 12.2

TOXICITY OF PHOSPHORUS INSECTICIDES TO MAMMALS AND INSECTS

$(LD_{50}$ in p.p.m. w/w)

Species	Malathion	Malaoxon
Mouse (i/p)	1590	75
House fly	30	15
Cockroach	120	15

(Krueger and O'Brien, 1959.)

At this stage, the quest began to move in two directions. One of these was to increase the selectivity of the comparatively inexpensive agent parathion-methyl, and the other was to seek new agents which, like malathion, placed trust also in preferential mammalian destruction. Introducing a methyl-group into the 3-position of the benzene ring of parathion-methyl, gave the remarkably selective fenitrothion of which the oxygen analogue* strongly inhibited the acetylcholinesterase (AChE) of houseflies at concentrations that had little effect on the analogous enzymes in bovine erythrocytes and mouse brain (Hollingworth, Fukuto, and Metcalf, 1967). Next, it was found that the OO-diisopropyl-analogue of paraoxon (*12.16*) inhibited the AChE of flies but not that of honeybees, apparently for steric reasons (Camp, Fukuto, and Metcalf, 1969).

Simultaneous movement of the quest in the other direction produced diazinon (*12.19*), menazon, and dimethoate. Diazinon [OO-diethyl O-(2-isopropyl-6-methyl-4-pyrimidinyl) phosphorothionate], discovered in 1952, has the same two built-in safeguards as malathion: mammals quickly C-hydroxylate the isopropyl-group, leading to rapid elimination in the urine, whereas insects cannot do this readily but convert $P:S$ to $P:O$, resulting in excellent selectivity (Miyazaki et al., 1970); Krueger, O'Brien, and Dauterman, 1960). Diazinon has proved extraordinarily successful, when sprayed on the hindquarters of sheep, in ridding them of the maggots of blowflies which cause intense irritation and subsequent loss of condition.

Menazon
(*12.20*)

Dimethoate
(*12.21*)

Menazon (*12.20*), a somewhat similar compound, but based on the triazine ring, caused a pleasant surprise because, when applied to the soil, it was taken up by roots and translocated to all parts of the plant. This gave protection from aphids and other sucking insects for up to six weeks. It is still used as a seed-dressing for the 'early protection' of crops (Sherlock, 1962). In horticulture, these *systemic insecticides* are valuable because no insects can be killed except those that bite the plant, which, lacking a nervous system, escapes all injury. Dimethoate (*12.21*) is now much used for this purpose. Unselective agents which kill all insects are avoided because they interfere with pollination and contribute to the starvation of field birds.

That component of the selectivity of dimethoate that favoured mammals was found, surprisingly, to depend little on differences in $:S \to :O$ conversion (as in malathion and diazinon), but to rely mainly on preferential operation of mammalian amidase (Krueger, O'Brien, and Dauterman,

---

* OO-Dimethyl O-3-methyl-4-nitrophenyl phosphorothionate.

1960). From this point onwards, research began to concentrate on detoxication mechanisms that did not require a : S → : O change.

Substances with P : O bonds were found that had the requisite ability to differentiate between insects and mammals. Usually these incorporated a short aliphatic side-chain with two or more electron-attracting features such as a double-bond and a halogen atom. For example, dichlorvos (*12.22*) ('Vapona') is a highly volatile organic phosphate introduced in 1955, and used as a domestic fly-killer. Chemically, it is dimethyl 2,2-dichlorovinyl-phosphate. When inhaled by mammals, or absorbed through the skin, it is rapidly hydrolysed to dichlorovinylphosphoric acid (of which 50 per cent is excreted in 6–12 hours) and some is oxidized to 2,2-dichloroethanol, both of which are harmless. Mammalian liver tissues and plasma (rat, rabbit) hydrolyse it rapidly to dimethyl phosphate and monomethyl 2,2-dichlorovinylphosphate; the latter is then quickly hydrolysed, first to dichlorovinylphosphoric acid, then to inorganic phosphate (Casida, McBryde and Niedermeir, 1962). To insects, however, its toxicity is cumulative (Hodgson and Casida, 1962). The American Conference of Government Industrial Hygienists set a human threshold limit value, for dichlorvos in air, of 1 µg per litre (Ashe, 1964). 'Vapona' slow-release strips, when used as directed (one strip per 1000 ft³), give off this concentration initially, but for the major part of the life of the strip, the concentration is about 0.1 µg per litre. Although dichlorvos pest-strips went through a period of public suspicion, current opinion is that they are safe to use, even in households and kitchens.

A variation on the dichlorvos molecule produced chlorfenvinphos (*12.23a*) [2-chloro-1-(2,4-dichlorophenyl)vinyl diethyl phosphate] used under the name 'Birlane' to kill a wide range of insect pests on major crops; one application lasts about 3 weeks on foliage, or 2 months on the soil. Under the name 'Supona', it is used as a dip for sheep and cattle to give long-lasting freedom from ecto-parasites (flies, lice, keds, ticks, and mites). Much less toxic to mammals, but not so long-lasting, is tetrachlorvinphos (*12.23b*), known as 'Gardona' when used in agriculture and 'Rabond' for ecto-parasites.

Some mammalian and insect toxicites of organic phosphates are

Dichlorvos
(*12.22*)

(a) Chlorfenvinphos   (R = Et, X = H)
(b) Tetrachlorvinphos (R = Me, X = Cl)
(*12.23*)

Trichlorophon
(*12.24*)

Table 12.3

COMPARATIVE TOXICITY OF ORGANOPHOSPHORUS INSECTICIDES

(LD_{50} is the dose lethal to 50 per cent of the animals)

Substance	LD_{50} for rat (mg/kg)		LD_{50} for insects				
	Oral (acute)	Dermal	Megoura viciae (vetch aphid) in p.p.m.	Tetranychus telarius (mite) in p.p.m. Adults	Eggs	Pieris brassicae (larvae) (cabbage butterfly) in lb/acre	Musca domestica (adult housefly) (female) in mg/ft²
Tetraethyl pyrophosphate	0.5	20	2	75	—	—	—
Parathion	3	50	2	65	—	—	—
Schradan	5	50	—	—	—	—	—
Dichlorvos	25	75	30	35	550	< 0.016	< 0.1
Dimethoate	200	750	3	2	60	0.7	1.8
Diazinon	300	> 1200	12	14	175	0.04	34
Trichlorophon	650	> 2800	—	—	—	—	—
Menazon	1200	> 500	4	90	50	> 10	—
Malathion	1400	> 4000	18	125	175	0.44	8.9
Haloxon	(900–2000)	?	—	—	—	—	—

(Partly from Edson, et al., 1964, also personal communication from Dr E. F. Edson.)

compared in Table 12.3. It can be seen that the lowering of mammalian toxicity, achieved in recent years, has not been at the expense of insect toxicity. For further data, see Tolkmith (1966); Edson, Sanderson, and Noakes 1964, 1966).

Some organic phosphates have been made so selective that they may be taken by mouth. Thus, trichlorophon (*12.24*) is given orally (as a single dose) to cattle to protect them against the hide-piercing warble fly. This substance, also known as metriphonate and 'Dyvon', is dimethyl 2,2,2-trichloro-1-hydroxyethylphosphonate.

In 1978, WHO announced that it was extensively using chlorpyriphos and fenthion to control the *Culex* mosquito vector of filariasis; these are respectively *O,O'* -diethyl *O"* -(3,5,6-trichloropyrid-2-yl) phosphorothioate and *O,O'*-dimethyl *O"*-(3-methyl-4-methylthiophenyl) phosphorothioate. Against *Aedes* mosquitoes, carriers of dengue and yellow fever viruses, they were using temephos: *O,O'*-(thiodi-4,1-phenylene) *O,O,O',O'*-tetramethyl phosphorothioate. To supplement their control of anopheline mosquitoes (vectors of the malarial parasites) they had introduced bromophos, iodfenphos, and pirimiphos-methyl, which are respectively: *O*-(4-bromo-2,5-dichlorophenyl)   *O',O"*-dimethyl   phosphorothioate; *O*-(2,5-dichloro-4-iodophenyl) *O',O"*-dimethyl phosphorothioate; and *O*-(2-diethylamino-6-methylpyrimid-4-yl)   *O',O"*-dimethyl   phosphorothioate.

Phosphorus anthelmintics.   Dichlorvos (*12.22*) is administered orally as a broad spectrum anthelmintic for swine (as 'Atgard'), horses ('Equigard'), and dogs ('Canogard'). Haloxon, another orally administered anthelmintic, kills nematode worms in cattle and sheep, oxyurid and ascarid worms in horses, and several species of worms in pigs and poultry. It is *OO*-di-(2-chloroethyl) *O*-3-chloro-4-methylcoumarin-7-yl phosphate (*12.25*). The chloroethyl group, present in haloxon, is known to be generally detoxifying to mammals (and to insects) but not to worms. The selectivity of haloxon, at its receptor (acetylcholinesterase), rests on the principle of analogous enzymes. The agent irreversibly inhibits the acetylcholinesterase of the worm *Haemonchus contortus*, but the corresponding enzyme in sheep erythrocytes is only temporarily blocked, and recovery is rapid (Lee and Hodsden, 1963). Replacement of the chloroethyl- by ethyl-groups causes toxic anticholinesterase effects in the host (N. Brown, *et al.*, 1962).

For the use of metriphonate (*12.24*) in human schistosomiasis, see Section 6.3e.

Phosphorus fungicides.   These are a relatively new development. Kitazin P (*12.26*) (*S*-benzyl *OO*-di*iso*propyl phosphorothionate) causes accumulation of UDP-*N*-acetylglucosamine in fungal mycelia, even at 50 p.p.m. It is thought that a late step in the synthesis of cell-wall chitin is being prevented (Maeda *et al.*, 1970). It is used systemically in rice-fields.

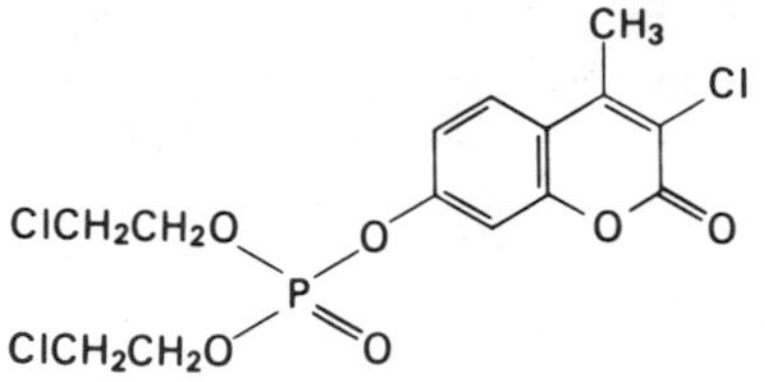

CH₃ ... (chemical structures)

Haloxon
(12.25)

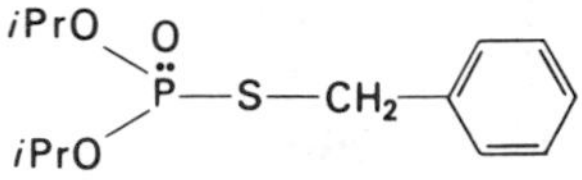

Kitazin P
(12.26)

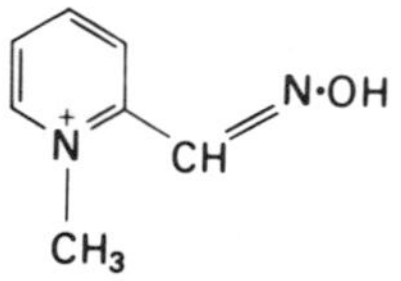

Pralidoxime
cation
(12.27)

Antidotes.   Because the acute toxicity to man of many of the phosphorus insecticides is high, first-aid remedies are kept on hand. The most useful of these is an injection of atropine (which acts primarily on muscarinic sites) followed by an oxime specific for nicotinic sites. These oximes reactivate phosphorylated acetylcholinesterase in patients (Holmes and Robins, 1955) just as with the isolated enzyme (Wilson and Meislich, 1953). This reaction involves a competition, between the hydroxyl-groups of serine and of the hydroxylamine, for the phsphoryl-group. The covalent bond with the serine is broken, and simultaneously a new covalent bond formed with the hydroxylamine (see Scheme 12.1). One of the best reactivators is pralidoxime (12.27) (2-PAM), which is the *anti* form of pyridine-2-aldoxime methochloride. Widely differing doses of antidote are required, depending on the strength of the phosphate-enzyme bond, which varies with the nature of the insecticide.

Medicinal use.   A dilute solution of dyflos (12.15) in oil is used in the human eye to lower intraocular tension in glaucoma; an aqueous solution of echothiophate (*OO*-diethyl *S*-trimethylammonioethyl phosphorothionate) is used similarly. These drugs achieve an increased local concentration of acetylcholine by inhibiting its esterase.

For further reading on organic phosphorus agents, see Eto (1974); Kosolapoff and Maier (1972); and Schrader (1963).

Carbamates (urethanes).   From 1947 onwards, carbamate insecticides have been brought very much to the fore on the grounds that they are less toxic to humans and more selective among insect species. These substances act by acylating serine residues in acetylcholinesterase (the $R_2N \cdot CO-$ group is transferred to the hydroxyl-group of serine, thus forming a carbamyl-derivative of the enzyme) (Hobbiger, 1954; Wilson, Harrison and Ginsburg, 1961). Carbamylated enzymes become hydrolysed faster than their phosphorylated analogues provided that the *N*-alkyl-group is kept small (Davies, Campbell and Kearns, 1970), and hence the human recovery rate is, on the average, faster.

Carbamate insecticides tend to be, on average, more hydrophilic than phosphorus insecticides and have proved excellent for systemic use, because avoidance of solubility extremes favours a good uptake by plant tissues as well as insect nerves. (Ionic carbamates, such as those used in human medicine, do not penetrate into insect nerves.) A typical and much used carbamate insecticide is carbaryl (*12.28*) (1-naphthyl *N*-methyl-carbamate; 'Sevin'). The mammalian toxicity is low (LD$_{50}$ 540 mg/kg, oral, rat). Carbaryl is destroyed in the mammal by ring-hydroxylation followed by conjugation of the phenolic group (Fukuto, 1972). It is used systemically in plants to kill leaf-eating caterpillars. Propoxur ('Baygon') (*12.29*), a simplified carbaryl, is recommended by WHO as a self-degrading outdoor spray against the malaria-spreading anopheline mosquitos. Chemically it is 2-*iso*propoxyphenyl *N*-methylcarbamate. Aldicarb (*12.30*) is another much-used insecticide. It is 2-methyl-2-methylthiopropionalde-hyde *O*-methylcarbamoyl oxime.

Carbamate insecticides are often used in conjunction with the synergists commonly employed with pyrethrum (Section 3.4). For further reading on carbamate inseticides, see Street (1975); Weiden and Moorefield (1964). For the carbamate fungicides, see Section 6.4 (p. 218).

In human medicine, carbachol (carbamoylcholine chloride) (*2.11*), which is isosteric with acetylcholine (*2.8*), is used to block acetylcholine-sterase and is slowly hydrolysed by it. It exhibits both the muscarinic and nicotinic actions of acetylcholine in a more prolonged and intense form. Other examples used in human medicine (Section 7.6c) include physostig-mine (*2.7*) and neostigmine (*2.10*) for myasthenia and glaucoma. Carbaryl does excellently in pediculosis.

MeS·CMe$_2$·CH:NO·CO·NHMe

Aldicarb
(*12.30*)

Carbaryl
(*12.28*)

Propoxur
(*12.29*)

12.4 Alkylating agents

All alkylating agents (e.g. methyl sulphate, diazomethane) are toxic to mammals, but several examples with *two* alkylating groups show a selective toxicity towards mammalian tumours. The chemical nature of alkylating agents is to esterify the anions of phosphoric and carboxylic acids, etherify the anions of phenols and mercaptans, and the more powerful of them also alkylate neutral amino-groups (primary, secondary, and even tertiary) (Boyland, 1947). Alkylating agents can react with these nucleophilic groups (Y^- or HY) by one of two mechanisms, either S_N1 or S_N2 (Ross, 1962).

The S_N1 mechanism is a first-order nucleophilic substitution whose rate depends only on the concentration of the alkylating agent. Chlormethinum (mustine, mechlorethamine) (*4.19*) and all other agents reacting in this way have an inbuilt tendency to ionize, although very slightly and very slowly. The course of the alkylating reaction is:

$$RX \xrightarrow{slow} R^+ + X^-$$
$$R^+ + Y^- \xrightarrow{fast} RY$$
or
$$R^+ + HY \xrightarrow{fast} RY + H^+$$

The S_N2 mechanism is a second-order nucleophilic substitution whose rate depends on the concentrations of both the alkylating agent and the nucleophilic site. Busulphan (*12.31*), which is one of the few agents reacting by this mechanism, achieves this result by a propinquity effect without prior ionization, thus:

$$RX + Y^- \xrightarrow{slow} RY + X^-$$
or
$$RX + HY \xrightarrow{slow} RY + HX$$

Most of the carcinostatic alkylating agents used in medicine are 2-*bis*-(chlorethyl)amines, a class of substances often referred to as 'nitrogen mustards'. How these were discovered is related in Section 6.3f. The first example, chlormethinum (*4.19*), is still in clinical use, particularly for treating lymphadenoma (Hodgkin's disease). It is used intravenously. In contact with water, it soon cyclizes to the aziridinium cation (*12.32*), the true drug. Although much of the dose of mustine becomes hydrolysed or fixed on sites of loss, enough reaches the cancerous cells to produce a powerful anti-proliferative effect. The toxic effect of the nitrogen mustards shows a small but definitely favourable selectivity, largely confined to the bone-marrow, blood-stream, and lymphatics (Ross, 1962). For *solid* tumours, which these drugs do not massively influence, their use must be preceded by surgical excision of the core.

$$CH_3SO_2 - O - (CH_2)_4 - O - SO_2CH_3$$

Busulphan
(*12.31*)

$$HO_2C - (CH_2)_3 - \langle\bigcirc\rangle - N(CH_2 - CH_2Cl)_2$$

Chlorambucil
(*12.33*)

$$H_3C·\overset{+}{N}\overset{CH_2}{\underset{CH_2·CH_2Cl}{\diagup|}}CH_2$$

Intermediate in action
(*12.32*)

$$HO_2C—(CH_2)_3—\langle\!\!\!\bigcirc\!\!\!\rangle—N(CH_2—CH_2Cl)_2$$

Melphalan
(12.34)

Chlorambucil (12.33) [p-bis-2-(chloroethyl)aminophenylbutyric acid], discovered in 1953 (Everett, Roberts, and Ross), exemplifies the 'aromatic nitrogen mustards'. These, because of the low basic strength of the aniline-type nitrogen atom, can form aziridinium salts only very slowly. The result is that they reach their target sites before becoming dissipated by side-reactions. Actually, chlorambucil is an extreme case: it is the slowest acting and least toxic of the nitrogen mustards in clinical use. It has proved highly suppressive in chronic lymphocytic leukaemia, and useful in Hodgkin's disease, lymphomas, and ovarian carcinoma. Treatments are often begun with the more powerful mustine, and then continued (often at home) with oral chlorambucil.

The related drug, melphalan (12.34) (L-sarcolysin), a derivative of phenylalanine, was designed in the hope that its aminoacid structure might lead to activated passage through membranes (see Section 3.1, p. 64). This apparently occurs, because the D-stereoisomer is inactive (Bergel and Stock, 1954). It is intermediate in activity between mustine and chloram-bucil. Mannomustine [1,6-bis-(2-chloroethyl)amino-1,6-dideoxymannitol] represents a similar attempt to secure activated uptake, in this case with reference to glucose (Vargha et al., 1957). Although effective, it seems to offer no special advantage.

A clinically valuable alkylating agent of quite another kind is busulphan (12.31) ('Myleran') (1,4-dimethanesulphonyloxobutane), discovered by G. Timmis. It is highly effective in, and almost specific for, chronic myelo-cytic leukaemia, and has few side-effects (Haddow and Timmis, 1953; Galton, 1956). Its mode of action is apparently the alkylation of, and eventual stripping of sulphur from, cysteine residues of proteins and peptides (Parham and Wilbur, 1961; Roberts and Warwick, 1961).

Chlormethinum (4.19) is not in circulation long enough to be fully effective. The Japanese drug 'Nitromin' (12.35) was introduced to overcome this disadvantage: the slow reduction of the N-oxide function gradually liberates the true drug (Druckrey, 1955). It is as effective orally as parente-rally. Its action is mild and it is in regular clinical use for the more easily controlled conditions.

Nitromin is an example of chemical change as a step in the activation of a drug which, until activation occurs, exists in a stable and beneficial depot (a principle discussed in Section 3.5). Cyclophosphamide (3.28) ('Endoxan', 'Cytoxan') is another pro-drug of this kind. This substance cannot form an aziridinium cation, like (12.32), until the phosphonolactone ring is opened, as happens in the liver. It can be given orally, and produces very good

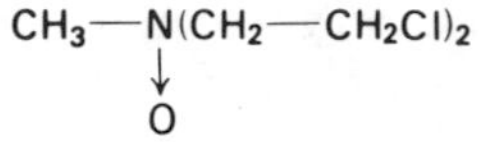

$$CH_3 \!-\! N(CH_2 \!-\! CH_2Cl)_2$$
$$\downarrow$$
$$O$$

'Nitromin'
(*12.35*)

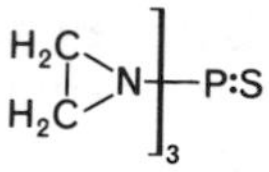

$$\begin{matrix} H_2C \\ | \\ H_2C \end{matrix} \! N \! - \! P\!:\!S \Big]_3$$

Thiotepa
(*12.36*)

clinical results in several malignant conditions (Gerhartz, 1960). It is the most often prescribed of all alkylating agents. Like methotrexate (Section 9.3c), cyclophosphamide has effected many radical cures of Burkitt's lymphoma in children (Burkitt, Hutt, and Wright, 1965). For further information on cyclophosphamide, see Fairley and Simister (1965).

At therapeutic dose levels, nitrogen mustards (mustine and cyclophospha-mide were used) have been found to inhibit DNA synthesis (Wheeler and Alexander, 1969). To explain the need for *two* alkylating groups in the anti-cancer alkylating agents, it is generally assumed that these agents act by cross-linking twin strands of DNA (joining guanine to guanine), thus preventing them from replicating. This is shown in Scheme 12.2. It has long been recognized that, to have anti-cancer action, a drug requires two alkylating functions (e.g. −Cl), separated by about five atoms, as in sub-stances (*12.31*) to (*12.35*) (Haddow, Harris, Kon and Roe, 1948). These alkylating functions must not be so reactive that they can be hydrolysed by water, and yet they must not be so firmly attached that they fail to alkylate the biological receptors. The idea that bifunctional molecules of this kind act by forming cross-linkages in the chromosomes is consistent with this critical distance of separation of the functions and the frequent mitotic irregularities seen under the microscope (Goldacre, Loveless and Ross, 1949). This may not seem a mode of action that could lead to high

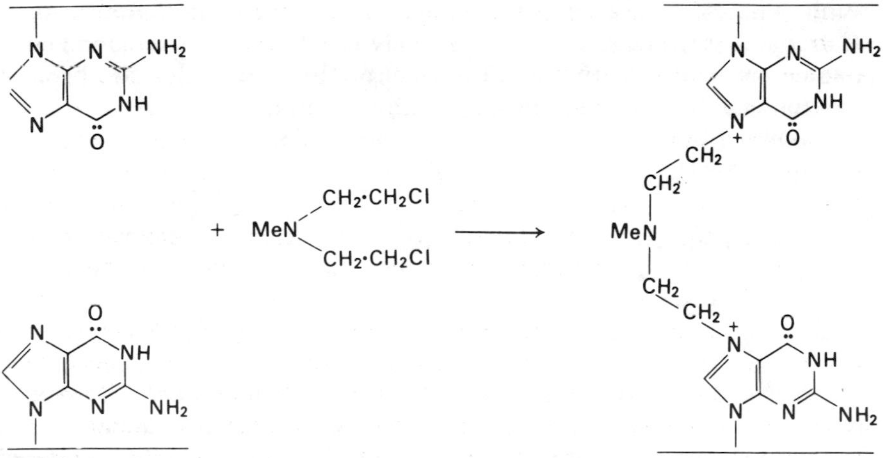

SCHEME 12.2

selectivity, but the nitrogen mustards are not very selective. The isolation of di-(guanin-7-ylethyl) sulphide from a hydrolysate of DNA alkylated with di-(2-chlorethyl) sulphide provided the first evidence of cross-linking by a bifunctional alkylating agent. RNA was much less affected (Lawley and Brookes, 1967).

Many *bis*-azirane drugs have a similar action, e.g. tretamin (triethylene melamine) and triethylenephosphonamide (tepa). Because of irregularity of action, their clinical use has been virtually abandoned. However, thiotepa (*12.36*), which is *tris*-(1-aziridinyl)phosphine sulphide, is a very mild agent which is infiltrated directly into solid tumours (Bateman, 1958). Some antibiotics, notably porfiromycin and mitomycin C, become bifunctional alkylating agents when acted upon by the mammalian metabolism. They irreversibly unite two complementary strands of DNA, thus causing the death of cells (Iyer and Szybalski, 1964). These antibiotics, tested clinically in cancer, have proved rather disappointing.

Most bifunctional alkylating agents mimic the action of ionizing radiations, but there are difference of detail.

In the present decade, the search for new types of alkylating agents led to the alkyl nitrosoureas, such as CCNU (lomustine) (*12.37*) which is chemically 1-(2-chloroethyl)-3-*cyclo*hexyl-1-nitrosourea. The nitrosoureas, unlike the mustards, can penetrate the blood-brain barrier and are giving good clinical results with brain tumours. Their action has been shown to be partly by alkylation of macromolecules, but to an even greater degree by carbamoylation after intermediate formation of an isocyanate species (Cheng *et al.*, 1972; Connors and Hare, 1974).

Another surprising drug is dacarbazine (*12,38*) ('OTIC') whose chemical nature is 5-(3,3-dimethyl-1-triazeno)imidazole-4-carboxamide, first synthesized by Shealy and Krauth (1966). It has given very good clinical results with melanoma, a tumour for which there is no other effective drug (Carter and Friedman, 1972). In the body it is twice demethylated giving 5-aminoimidazole-4-carboxamide plus the methyl radical (detected by mass spectroscopy); this radical ends by methylating guanine in the 7-position (Nagasawa *et al.*, 1974).

Lomustine
(*12.37*)

Dacarbazine
(*12.38*)

Some fungicides were described in Section 6.4 that alkylate – SH groups in essential enzymes, namely captan (*6.40*) and chlorothalonil (*6.42*).

It has been shown in the above how selective uptake can be facilitated by incorporating aminoacid and carbohydrate residues, or in the special ways outline for cyclophosphamide and 'Nitromin'. Those who design new carcinolytic nitrogen mustards are using knowledge of reaction rates (Ross, 1953). The choice and insertion of groups to lower the electron densities can decrease the reactivity of the chlorine atoms. These deactivating groups are designed to be, in their turn, deactivated by an appropriate enzyme in the target tissue (Ross, 1962).

The carcinogenic action of simple alkylating agents is dealt with near the beginning of the next section. For further information on biological alkylating agents, see Ross (1962).

12.5 Lethal synthesis

The name 'lethal synthesis' was devised by Peters to describe the biochemical alteration of fluoroacetic acid, which is not toxic in itself but is changed by mammalian metabolism to a toxic substance, fluorocitric acid. This change, which occurs in the tricarboxylic acid cycle, depends on fluoroacetic acid being sterically so similar to acetic acid that it is accepted by a series of enzymes and undergoes similar enzymic changes until it ends as fluorocitric acid (12.39) (Peters, *et al.*, 1953; Liébecq and Peters, 1949). The toxic effect is due to this acid blocking the enzyme which dehydrates citric acid to *cis*-aconitic acid. Hence fluorocitric acid acts as a metabolite analogue of citric acid.

What distinguishes lethal synthesis from the cases of 'degradation before action' discussed in Section 3.5 is simply that synthesis is involved and not degradation: a substance having only two carbon atoms has been made into one having six carbons. Moreover, the raw material for this synthesis passes through at least three enzyme systems, and is changed a little by each, before it becomes toxic.

Fluoroacetic acid occurs in a South African plant *Dichapetalum*, and has killed many cattle in that country. The toxic action of fluoroacetic acid does not depend on any chemical reactivity on the part of fluorine, but on the small *size* of the fluorine atom (Table 9.1) (Bartlett and Barron, 1947).

Although fluoroacetic acid is being used to exterminate rabbits, its selectivity is not high, and hence it presents a hazard to human beings.

$$F—CH—CO_2H$$
$$|$$
$$HO—C—CO_2H$$
$$|$$
$$CH_2·CO_2H$$

Fluorocitric acid
(12.39)

Carcinogenesis.   This counter-selective phenomenon deserves a (small) place in this Chapter because of the opportunities it affords for comparison and contrast.

Many chemicals are known which can make cells grow in a less orderly, more random, pattern. This change, which is heritable, is called a 'transformation'. This has the nature of a mutation and, according to one school of thought, it is the initial step in a process that can result in the formation of cancer. However, relatively few chemicals are known which can convert normal human cells to cancerous ones. In most cases this takes many weeks during which time the *pro-carcinogen* molecule undergoes a covalent change to the *proximate carcinogen* which actually effects the carcinogenesis. The proximate carcinogen is usually of higher molecular weight, and positively charged (Miller, 1970). Such carcinogens are electrophilic reagents (like the anticancer nitrogen mustards described in the previous Section) and ready to attack the bases in DNA. However, unlike the mustards, they cannot form a (restraining) cross-link (Brookes, 1966).

Chemical carcinogenesis is usually recognized when a sufficient cluster of cases of a particular kind of cancer is reported for a particular trade, pastime, or other occupation. The first such correlation concerned the chimney sweeps of London, whose scrotal cancer was attributed by Potts in 1775 to contact with tar and soot. However, it was not until the 1930s that the causative chemicals were isolated from coal tar, namely benzo[a]pyrene (*12.41*) and 1,2,5,8-dibenzanthracene (Cook, Hewett, and Hieger, 1932, 1933).

Until that time, it had been assumed that cancers were the inevitable accompaniment of ageing. Today, because of the results of comparative studies of populations, the triggering of cancer is seen to be largely environmental. This follows from the great variation in the amount and types of cancer found in different communities in different parts of the world. The manifestations of cancer in migrants, too, changes in proportion as they adapt their life-style to the country of adoption. The International Agency for Research on Cancer, of WHO (1976), reported that 80% or more of all human cases are activated by exposure to sunlight, tobacco, alcohol, or polluted air (cf. Cairns, 1975). Genetic predisposition is important, too.

Because cancers are so easily produced in laboratory rats and mice, it is regrettable that no unambiguous criterion exists to extrapolate to man the results of experiments on rodents (International Agency for Research on Cancer, 1976). Thus, of the 272 reputedly carcinogenic substances that this Agency investigated in the first twenty years of its existence, only 20 proved carcinogenic in cultured human tissues, whereas 137 caused cancer in the experimental animals *only* (22 showed no carcinogenic effect in any test; 93 gave inconclusive results).

Much interest is now being shown, at governmental level, in two tests that can give more rapid results than those done on rodents. These are (i) the Ames test which looks for mutagenicity in a susceptible bacterium (Ames, Sims, and Grover, 1972), and (ii) the Styles cell transformation test (Purchase *et al.*, 1976). The former pronounces 2-naphthylamine positive but butter yellow negative, whereas the latter reports the exact opposite; however, both substances are known human carcinogens. At present, many fear that every mutagen is a potential carcinogen, but each gain in knowledge helps to define parameters beyond which this correlation does not exist.

Concerning *alkylating agents*, the medicinally useful ones (see previous Section) usually alkylate the 7-position of guanine. By way of contrast, the highly carcinogenic examples, using a S_N2 mechanism, alkylate on oxygen. Thus ethylnitrosourea and ethyl-N'-nitro-N-nitrosoguanidine attacks O-2 of cytosine and uracil in RNA, and O-2 of thymine and O-6 of guanine in double-stranded DNA (Singer, 1976).

Several *aromatic amines* are converted by the liver to N-hydroxy-derivatives (hydroxylamines), as Cramer, Miller, and Miller (1960) showed for 2-acetamidofluorene. The following aromatic amines also are converted in the mammalian body into carcinogenic aromatic hydroxyl-amines: 4-acetamidobiphenyl, benzidine, 2-acetamidophenol (Miller, Miller and Hartmann, 1961), 2-aminonaphthalene (Boyland, Dukes, and Grover, 1963), and 4-hydroxyaminoquinoline-1-oxide (from bioreduction of 4-nitroquinoline-1-oxide) (Endo, Ono and Sugimura, 1970). These hydroxylamines are then converted to the O-sulphuric esters ($RN \cdot O \cdot SO_2 \cdot O^-$), which hydrolyse to carbonium ions such as (12.40) and these seem to be the true carcinogens (Miller, 1970). Injections of inorganic sulphates into rats receiving N-hydroxy-2-acetamidofluorene greatly increase its toxicity (De Baun *et al.*, 1970).

(12.40)

Benzo [a] pyrene
(3,4-Benzpyrene)
(12.41)

The carcinogenic action of butter yellow (4-dimethylaminoazobenzene) is thought to depend on N-hydroxylation of the corresponding monomethyl analogue (which arises by bio-demethylation) (Poirier *et al.*, 1967).

The carcinogenicity of the *polycyclic hydrocarbons* depends on their becoming bound, after metabolism, to nucleic acid, as first shown by Brookes and Lawley (1964) (cf. Gelboin, 1969).

Benzo[a]pyrene (12.41), that universal contaminant of industrialized cities, is metabolized by mammalian cells to give the corresponding 7,8-dihydro-7,8-dihydroxy 9,10- epoxide, which binds strongly to DNA (Sims *et al.*, 1974), a result that has been widely confirmed (cf. Meehan, Straub, and Calvin, 1977). Moreover, it has been found that of the four enantiomers of this epoxide, the active one is the 7S, 8S, 9R, 10R isomer which forms a link between the 10-position of this molecule and the 2-amino-group of guanine in both DNA and RNA (Jeffrey *et al.*, 1977). Boyland (1950) was the first to suggest that metabolic conversion to epoxides may be the essential step in the carcinogenicity of the polycyclic hydrocarbons. At that time, a rival hypothesis held sway: that union with the target took place through a 'K region' whose contribution to the carcinogenicity rose as its electron-density rose (Robinson, 1946; Pullman and Pullman, 1955). This hypothesis was based on knowledge that several polycyclic hydrocarbons, such as 1,2-benzanthracene, were not carcinogenic, but became so when a methyl group was inserted in particular positions (Barry, *et al.*, 1935). Examples of the K-region are the 9,10 double-bond in phenanthrene, and the 4,5-bond in (*12.41*). Today the K-region hypothesis is out of favour, and the epoxidation approach is being found applicable to other carcinogenic polycyclic hydrocarbons.

Because some polycyclic hydrocarbons raise the T_m of double-stranded DNA, it has been suggested that intercalation (Section 10.3b) is a step in carcinogenesis. However, X-ray diffraction shows that even highly carcinogenic hydrocarbons are not flat [*see* e.g. Iball (1964)] an anomaly partly due to the overcrowding of substituents, partly to the presence of non-Kekulé rings, of which (*12.41*) has two.

The carcinogeneic properties of the various polycyclic hydrocarbons can be inhibited by the application of relatively harmless chemical analogues (Badger, *et al.*, 1941).

For further reading on chemical carcinogenesis, see Miller and Miller (1966): Freudenthal and Jones (1976).

Metabolite analogues. Azetidine-2-carboxylic acid (*12.42*) and 3,4-dehydro-DL-proline inhibit the growth of bacteria (and also of the seedlings of higher plants) by becoming incorporated into the protein in the place of proline (*12.43*) (Fowden, Neale, and Tristram, 1963).

Azetidine-2-
carboxylic acid
(*12.42*)

Proline
(*12.43*)

Several analogues of the purine and pyrimidine bases of nucleic acids have been dealt with in Section 4.0 (pp. 111–119) where their clinical uses are outlined. The most successful are those that undergo lethal synthesis in the cell, by being built up into analogues of deoxy-ribosides and ribotides which then compete with the normal nucleosides and nucleotides. In this category are to be found the anticancer drugs 5-fluorouracil (*3.3*) and 6-mercaptopurine (*3.12*), the antiviral drugs cytarabine (*4.10*), vidarabine (*4.11*), and Ald-Urd (*4.12*), the immunosuppressant azathioprine (*3.34*), and the oral fungicide flucytosine (*4.13*). Viewed with a mixture of gratitude and caution is 5-iododeoxyuridine (*4.9*), gratitude because it was the first successful antiviral drug, and caution because it is built into the body's DNA and hence is a potential mutagen never to be used internally. Also dealt with in Section 4.0 are analogues which affect RNA synthesis: 8-azaguanine (*4.23*) and 6-azauracil (*4.24*), the former a potent anticancer drug, the latter an agricultural fungicide.

Tubercidin (7-deaza-adenosine), an antibiotic extracted from *Streptomyces tubercidicus*, is incorporated into both RNA and DNA of mouse fibroblasts which it kills. Viruses infecting these cells are also killed (Acs, Reich, and Mori, 1964).

Some other examples. Aspirin (acetylsalicylic acid), the most heavily prescribed of all antirheumatic drugs, is thought to act by inhibiting prostaglandin synthetase (cyclo-oxygenase), a microsomal protein of mol. wt. 85 000. This irreversible effect is caused by the drug's acetylating the enzyme, which it does quite specifically within 15 minutes (Roth and Siok, 1978). Sodium salicylate, although equally active *in vivo*, has no action on the enzyme *in vitro*, which indicates that it may first be converted to a metabolite, possibly aspirin.

Carbon tetrachloride was introduced by M. C. Hall in 1921 for ridding man of the intestinal parasite, hookworm. Already by 1925, this drug's necrotic action on human liver and kidneys gave concern, and Hall endeavoured to have it replaced. Carbon tetrachloride is still used for worm infestations of cattle, sheep, and poultry, but more cautiously than before. Human beings are still being poisoned by this substance, which is widely used both as a solvent and a fire extinguisher.

It seems that mammalian toxicity is caused by homolytic splitting of carbon tetrachloride to the free radical $\cdot$ CCl_3 (Hove, 1948; Slater, 1966; Recknagel and Ghoshal, 1966). A flavoprotein, cytochrome-c reductase, appears to be the radical-forming centre. Free radical scavengers, such as propyl gallate, promethazine, or N,N'-diphenyl-p-phenylenediamine, were found to suppress this reaction strongly (Slater and Sawyer, 1971). Lipid peroxidation is known to require free radicals both for initiation and propagation. Even low concentrations of carbon tetrachloride can stimulate peroxidation in washed suspensions of liver 'microsomes' at $37°C$. The principal damage caused to liver by carbon tetrachloride is peroxidation of the double-bond of the β-aliphatic chains in the phospholipids of endoplasmic reticulum membrane, leading to the irreparable breakdown of this structure (May and McCay, 1968).

The (fortunately rare) sensitization of patients to penicillin occurs apparently through acylation of the ε-amino-group of lysine, in gammaglobulin, by the β-lactam ring of the drug (Hamilton-Miller and Abraham, 1971).

In Section 3.5 (p. 93) it was recounted how the herbicide 'MCP' injures only those weeds that, by β-oxidation within their tissues, degrade it to a highly toxic product.

For further examples of lethal synthesis, see Langen (1975).

12.6 Miscellaneous examples

The pharmacological effects, on the nervous system, of reserpine, and of the hydrazines that inhibit monoamineoxidase (Section 9.4), are irreversible. These facts suggest that covalency is involved.

The hormone that synthesizes thyroxine seems to be a protein bearing a sulphenyl iodide group (–CSI). It is thought that sulphur-bearing heterocycles such as 2-thiouracil (*12.44*) and its 6-propyl- and 6-methyl-derivatives, that are clinically used to control thyrotoxicosis, do so by covalently binding to this group, forming a S–S bond and liberating HI (Cunningham, 1964; Jirousek and Pritchard, 1971).

2-Thiouracil
(*12.44*)

Chlorine in aqueous solution can exist as an *element* only below pH 2. In less acid solutions it is converted to hypochlorous acid:

$$Cl_2 + H_2O = HOCl + H^+ + Cl^-$$

The pK of hypochlorous acid is 7.2, and the disinfectant activity is proportional to the concentration of neutral molecule. The marked efficiency of chlorine, which is active at 0.2 p.p.m. in water, indicates that its action is rather specific. It has been suggested that, after conversion to hypochlorous acid, which penetrates the cell as the neutral molecule, the sulphydryl (–SH)- groups of essential enzymes are attacked. The aldolase of *E. coli* is one of the essential enzymes of glycolysis sufficiently sensitive to hypochlorous acid to explain the bactericidal action of this substance (Knox *et al.*, 1948). Some organisms, presumed to have been killed by hypochlorous acid, have been revived by sodium thiosulphate (Mudge and Smith, 1935).

Hypochlorous acid reacts with ammonia to give the less active substance, chloramine (NH_2Cl), which is often used where a depot effect is required, e.g. in swimming pools. Similarly, hypochlorous acid forms substituted chloramines with aminoacids and proteins, both outside and inside the cell.

These can also act as depots, because they are in equilibrium with hypo-chlorous acid. Finally an artificial chloramine, p-toluenesulphonchloramide (Chloramine-T) is used by campers as a source of hypochlorous acid.

The bactericidal action of bromine above pH 6 is mainly due to non-ionized hypobromous acid (pK 9); below pH 3, the equilibrium is in favour of free bromine.

Iodine, in neutral aqueous solution, exists mainly as such and the sporicidal action is due to elementary iodine. At pH 8.5, the hypoiodous acid : iodine ratio rises to 1 : 1, with a consequent drop in sporicidal activity. Hypoiodous acid (pK 10) is a weak acid. Iodine does not form a depot substance with ammonia, but its complex (KI_3) with potassium iodide has depot properties. A great excess of potassium iodide is required to hold iodine as this tri-iodide in aqueous solution (Wyss and Strandskov, 1945).

Formaldehyde is believed to injure bacteria by combining with the amino-groups of proteins, which are thereby changed in nature and func-tion. Potassium permanganate and hydrogen peroxide can break down all kinds of organic matter by their violent oxidizing action. Hydrogen peroxide can initiate a self-propagating chain reaction in the presence of an oxidizable substrate (e.g. a thiol, or ascorbic acid) and a trace of a heavy-metal cation (e.g. iron).

13 Steric factors

13.0 Some fundamental considerations

The size and shape of a molecule can play a very important part in its biological action. For some types of action a flat molecule is required, whereas other types of action require a three-dimensionally bulky molecule. The benzene ring (*13.1*) is flat, and the six bonds leading from the ring to all attached atoms or groups also lie in the plane of the paper. All other conjugated systems (i.e. those where every second bond is a double-bond) are similarly flat.

On the other hand, aliphatic and alicyclic structures are non-planar. Thus *cyclo*hexane (*13.2*), which differs from benzene in having six more hydrogen atoms, is non-planar and the bonds leave the ring at different angles (only four of the six carbon atoms lie in the plane of the paper). Atropine (*7.14*) is an example of a drug which has a non-planar ring, whereas 9-aminoacridine (*10.7*) is typical of the drugs which have flat molecules. Both types of architecture are common in drugs, and sometimes both types occur in the one molecule, as in mepacrine (Fig. 10.8) and nicotine (*7.18*).

A biological requirement for a minimal area of flatness (in the molecule of a chemotherapeutic drug) was first observed in members of the amino-acridine series, which require about 38 Å^2 of planar surface in order to exhibit antibacterial properties (Section 10.3b) (Albert, Rubbo, and Burvill, 1949).

Benzene   *Cyclo*hexane
(*13.1*)   (*13.2*)

Each benzene or pyridine ring in a molecule permits 2–3 kcal/mol of adhesion, through van der Waals bonding, provided that it can rest on a flat area in the neighbourhood of the receptor. If it is desired to replace such a ring, in an agent, by a more hydrogenated ring, the following relationships become relevant. The *cyclo*pentyl ring, because of the crowding caused by substituents (even by hydrogen atoms) is nearly flat; this also applies to the five-membered ring of ribose. The *cyclo*pentenyl ring is flat, but the *cyclo*hexenyl and *cyclo*butyl rings are puckered, and the *cyclo*hexyl ring (*13.2*) is very much puckered. Even if the *cyclo*butyl ring were flat, it could have only two-thirds of the van der Waals attraction of a benzene ring. Another source of loss of van der Waals energy arises from the out-of-plane situation of the first atom of each substituent in a non-benzenoid ring.

Replacement of phenyl-groups has sometimes been carried out as a test for the necessity for a flat structure in a drug molecule. When the phenyl ring in amphetamine, and related phenylethylamine and phenylethanolamine drugs, was replaced by *cyclo*-butyl, -pentenyl, -hexenyl, and -hexyl rings, a decrease in the intensity of pharmacodynamic action was found in each case (Burger *et al.*, 1961, 1963).

Steric hindrance to effecting a simple chemical reaction is well known in preparative work. For example, it is much more difficult to esterify trimethylacetic acid (*13.3*) than acetic acid. Steric hindrance to the hydration of a double-bond was discussed in Section 2.3 (p. 43). Yet another type of steric hindrance, namely hindrance of a resonance, can profoundly change the reactivity of the group hindered, and penicillin (*12.6*) provides an example, as recounted in Section 12.1 (p. 450). The result is that penicillin is about a million times more reactive than an ordinary straight-chain amide.

Trimethylacetic acid   Bretylium   Stilboestrol
(*13.3*)   (*13.4*)   (*13.5*)

An example of a steric hindrance necessary to achieve the desired pharmacological response is afforded by bretylium (*13.4*), which has been used as a blood-pressure lowering drug. The bromine in this substance can be replaced by chlorine, iodine, a methyl- or a nitro-group without losing the biological effect, but the latter disappears when the bromine is replaced by hydrogen. This suggests that an *ortho*-substituent is necessary to force the basic side-chain out of the plane of the benzene ring (Boura, Copp, and Green, 1959).

Steric hindrance seems also to be responsible for the desirable biological action of stilboestrol (*13.5*). Evidence, from X-ray diffraction and u.v. spectroscopy, suggests that the angle of twist between the two benzene rings must exceed 60° for strong oestrogenic activity to become manifest (Jeffrey, Koch, and Nyburg, 1948). To secure this twist (and activity), four methyl-groups are as effective as two ethyl-groups (Laarhoven, Nivard, and Havinga, 1961).

The next three Sections will discuss some biological consequences of optical isomerism, geometrical isomerism, and conformational behaviour.

The solution of any problem with a stereochemical aspect requires access to molecular models. Of these, there are two major kinds. The first, the *skeletal* model (e.g. Dreiding, or Kendrew), indicates the centres of the atoms and the bonds that join them. The other type of model, *space-filling* (e.g. CPK, or Courtauld), shows both the shape of the molecule and the volume that if occupies. This kind is very useful for studying the conformations in which one molecule can interact with another. With practice, a chemist can learn to see a conformational drawing as a three dimensional skeletal shape, and eventually as space-filling molecule. Recently, other models (the CCS) have been made available which are fundamentally skeletal models that can be quickly converted to space-filling types and back again (Clarke, 1977).

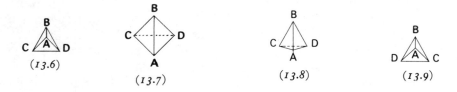

13.1 Optical isomerism

Carbon, far more than any other atom, is responsible for the principal forms of stereoisomerism dealt with in this and the following two Sections. Most of the examples of *optical* isomerism arise from the presence in the molecule of a carbon atom with four single-bonds, each of which is connected to a different kind of atom or group. Such a carbon atom, i.e. one with four different kinds of substituents, is called *asymmetric*.

The atom of carbon, although spherical, has its four bonds evenly (and rigidly) disposed, as if at the corners of a tetrahedron, namely a solid with four faces, all meeting at 109°. It may be tilted in all directions without changing the order of the four substituents. Thus in (*13.6*), BCD may be thought of as a triangular plane resting on a table, and A as an apex much nearer the eye. In other presentations of the same tetrahedron, B, C, or D in turn can be made the apex, leaving the other three groups in the plane. The presentation (*13.6*) can be tilted forward to (*13.7*) so that CD forms a line on the table, and AB is another line, parallel to the table, but above it. Presentation (*13.8*), an intermediate state between (*13.6*) and (*13.7*), has CD on the Table, B a little nearer the eye, and A much nearer the eye. These are all presentations of the *same* molecule, but if two substituents are interchanged, as in (*13.9*), a different substance is produced. The consequences of this can conveniently be examined with the help of lactic acid (*13.10*).

H
$H_3C \cdot \overset{|}{C} \cdot CO_2H$
OH

Lactic acid
(*13.10*)

B
|
C ---- | ---- D
|
A

(*13.11*)

B
|
D ---- | ---- C
|
A

(*13.12*)

When four different atoms, or groups, are attached to a central carbon atom, as in lactic acid (*13.10*), two different spatial arrangements, (*13.6*) and (*13.9*), are possible. One arrangement is the non-superposable mirror-image of the other, and hence they are related as one's right hand is to one's left. Between such isomers (enantiomers, also called enantiomorphs or optical 'antipodes'), no *chemical* differences exist, but each rotates the plane of polarized light in an opposite direction (to an equal degree). The enantiomers are absorbed selectively on optically active surfaces, such as protein, and hence although the two optical isomers of an agent often show the same biological effect, they usually show it to a very different degree.

For purposes of representation on paper, it is more convenient to think of the four bonds, which unite the four different substituents to the carbon atom, as proceeding from the centre of the atom but at the same angles as in (*13.6*) to (*13.9*). Then (*13.11*) becomes an acceptable representation of one of the enantiomers of lactic acid, and (*13.12*) of the other. The wedges imply that the atoms at their broad edges are nearer to the eye than those at the end of the lines of the dashes [(*13.11*) is presented in the same aspect as (*13.7*)]. In a crowded molecule, or for speed of handwriting, the wedges may be replaced by thick lines as in (*7.11*). In a crowded molecule, it is tempting to replace each dash by a dot; but the dashes cannot be replaced by three dots, the symbol for a hydrogen bond.

Often the use of heat, or of acid or alkali, converts one enantiomer into a mixture of equal parts of both enantiomers, which causes optical activity (as measured in a polarimeter) to disappear. The substance is then said to have been racemized. Both D- and L-lactic acid occur in nature, unracemized.

If a molecule has *two* asymmetric carbon atoms, provided that these are non-identical, there can be *four* possible stereoisomeric forms, and hence two completely different racemates. The relationship between an enantiomer from one racemate and one from the other cannot be a mirror-image, and members of such a pair are called diastereoisomers. The four ephedrines (*13.13*) to (*13.16*) present such a set of diastereoisomers (Witkop and Foltz, 1957). It will be seen that more than one change has to be made in passing from (*13.13*) to (*13.14*) to conserve the mirror-image relationship. A more quickly written notation (*13.30*) will be mentioned at the end of Section 13.3.

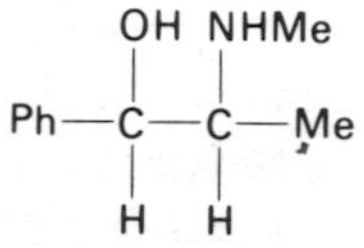

(−)-Ephedrine
(antiasthmatic drug)
3R 2S
(*13.13*)

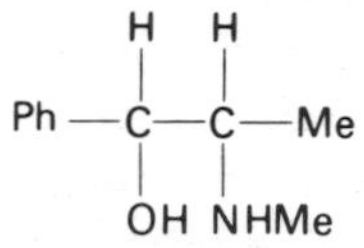

(+)-Ephedrine
(not used in medicine)
(*13.14*)

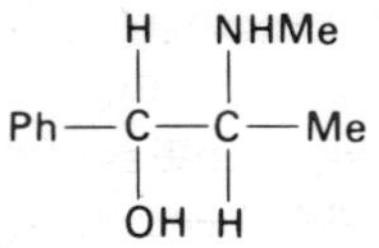

(+)-Pseudoephedrine
(local vasoconstrictor)
3S 2S
(*13.15*)

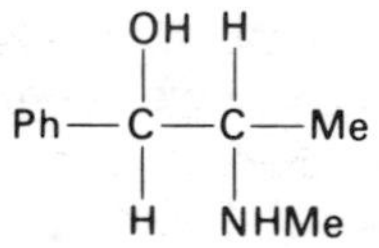

(−)-Pseudoephedrine
(not used in medicine)
(*13.16*)

Proteins are formed exclusively from aminoacids of the L-series, which means that they all have the configuration of L(−)-serine. However, (+)-glucose, (−)-deoxyribose, and (−)-fructose are derived (by synthesis or degradation) from the D-series, which means that they have the configuration of D(+)-glyceraldehyde. These configurations (D- and L-) of serine and glyceraldehyde are absolute, i.e. they have been determined by X-ray crystallography. The signs (− and +) give the direction of rotation of polarized light, and it will be noted that (−) is not necessarily equated with (L). The signs *d* and *l*, which often assumed that (−) was the same as (L), are no longer used.

Cushny (1926) was the first to realize that differences in the biological activity of enantiomers were caused by one antipode fitting the receptor surface much better than the other did. He also noted that something of the nature of the receptor could be learnt from this.

Optical isomers sometimes differ greatly in biological activity. Thus

D(−)-*iso*propylnoradrenaline (isoprenaline) has 800 times the broncho-dilator effect of its L(+)-isomer (Luduena *et al.*, 1957). Similarly, the natural D(−)-isomer of adrenaline has 12–20 times the activity of its enantiomer on various test-objects (Tainter, 1930; Blaschko, 1950). Again, the L(+)-form of acetyl-β-methylcholine is about 200 times more active on gut than the D(−)-form. Nicotine presents a very unusual feature: the difference in activity between the natural L(−)-form and the stereoisomeric D-form varies with the test-site, so that equipotent ratios for the two enantiomers vary from about 1 : 1 to 1 : 40. However, where, as is usual, one form is more active, that is always the L-form (Barlow and Hamilton, 1965).

Quite often, however, there is no difference in biological activity. This is understandable for structurally non-specific substances like hypnotics (see Chapter 15). Thus the (+)- and (−)-forms of barbiturates, made optically active by incorporating an asymmetric carbon atom in a 5-alkyl-group, act equally strongly (Kleiderer and Shonle, 1934). Both (+)- and (−)-cocaine (*7.11*) are equally powerful local anaesthetics (Gottlieb, 1923). Many such examples are known among synthetic drugs. Thus (+)- and (−)-chloroquine (*10.28*) have equal antimalarial action (Riegel and Sherwood, 1949). In such cases, it is assumed that the agent and the receptor make only a two-point contact at the asymmetric carbon atom, or else that this atom is not involved in the contact.

When one optical enantiomer is more biologically active than the other, antagonism between them is rarely found. This is because the space-relationship required for adsorption on the receptor is the very one altered by passing from D- to L-forms, or vice versa. For this reason, a mixture of two optical antipodes (or the racemized substance) usually has the averag-ed potency of both constituents, and there is no antagonism (see p. 296 for a rare exception).

Many adrenergic amines have been examined for the effect of optical isomerism on pressor activity. It is thought that D-adrenaline makes a three-point contact with its receptor through the following three groups: (a) the amino-group, (b) the benzene ring with its two phenolic hydroxyl-groups, and (c) the alcoholic hydroxyl-group in the side-chain. The biologically weak optical isomer, L-adrenaline, can make contact by only two groups (see Fig. 13.1, in which the shapes and sizes of the symbols have been chosen arbitrarily). Deoxyadrenaline (epinine) should therefore have much the same activity as L-adrenaline, as is indeed the case (Easson and Stedman, 1933). This hypothesis has been confirmed by further examples (Badger, 1947; Stedman, 1947).

Adrenaline is a convenient starting-point for a discussion on orientation in the D- and L-system. Natural (laevorotatory) adrenaline and noradrena-line have been shown by degradation to have the same configuration as D (−)-mandelic acid (Pratesi *et al.*, 1959), and L(+)-mandelic acid has

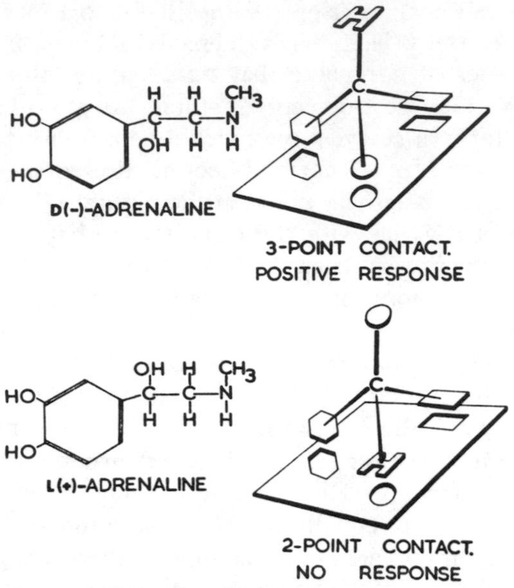

FIG. 13.1 Diagram illustrative of contact between optical isomerides and a surface complementary to one of them.

been related to the L-phenylalanine of proteins. One difficulty with such degradative approaches, especially for amphoteric substances, is that racemization followed by oppositely orientated resolution must be guarded against. Another objection is that the orientation of all known optically active substances by degradation would immobilize too many highly experienced chemists for too many decades. Fortunately, in series that are both simple and familiar, comparison of the substances' optical rotatory dispersions can yield the absolute configuration directly (the optical rotations of the compound are plotted against the various wavelengths of light at which they were determined, say, from 270 to 700 nm) (Klyne, 1962; Djerassi, 1960).

But a still more fundamental difficulty exists when, as in ephedrine, there are two centres of asymmetry. The fact that all the aminoacids of proteins are assigned to the L-series, whereas glucose and deoxyribose are assigned to the D-series (see above), does not imply that the living cell has made proteins and carbohydrates on spirals of opposite twist. On the contrary, it is known that both spirals have the same twist. The seeming divergence arose from the historical accident that glucose, with its many centres of asymmetry, was degraded first from one end of the molecule, and not from the other.

To surmount this difficulty, the Sequence Rule was invented, and is used as follows (Cahn, Ingold, and Prelog, 1956). The four substituents around each asymmetric centre in the molecule are named, a, b, c, d in order of decreasing weight. The group of lowest weight (d) is placed in the axis of an imaginary steering wheel. The three other groups thus lie on the rim of the wheel, which is rotated in the direction a → b → c. If such a rotation is to the right, the configuration is called R (*rectus*), but if rotation is to the left, the configuration is S (*sinister*). To apply this formula, the relative order of a, b, and c must be known from experimental work, preferably from diffraction analysis of a crystal using X-rays of a wavelength that will introduce a phase lag in the scattering of one of the atoms causing the asymmetry (Bijvoet, Peerdeman, and van Bommel, 1951). The greatest value of the Sequence Rule is to obtain consistency between systems (e.g. between aminoacids, carbohydrates, sympathicomimetics, and steroids). All are referred to dextrorotatory glyceraldehyde which is called R, and hence L(−)-serine is S. Within each system, degradative methods are still the most often used, because of the large amount of skill and time required to apply a Bijvoet X-ray analysis to each compound. However, some substances, especially monocyclic ketones because of their rigidity, have given good results with a theoretical treatment known as the Octant Rule based on the optical circular dichroism spectrum (Crabbé, 1967). Substances with as few as *two* fused rings are already too complex for reliable application of this rule.

Bearing the above minor qualifications in mind, it may be noted that natural (−)-adrenaline is R, and so are the synthetic analogues synephrine and phenylephrine (*7.46*) which merely lack one or other of the phenolic hydroxy-groups of adrenaline. The assignments for ephedrine (*13.13*) and pseudoephedrine (*13.15*) are given under their formulae. The preferred conformation for catecholamines, e.g. (*7.5*), is the fully extended staggered (*trans*) form in the solid state (Carlstrom and Bergin, 1967), and also in solution (Ison, Partington, and Roberts, 1973).

The *Atlas of Stereochemistry* lists the absolute configurations of about 3000 organic substances, with derivations. Apart from optical isomerism, it lists many examples whose chirality is owed to isotopic substitution, to chiral axes or planes, or to chiral centres other than carbon (Klyne and Buckingham, 1978).

The representation of carbohydrates.   Two systems are in use which antedate much of what has been described above. The older of these is the Fischer projection, e.g. (*13.17*) for D-glucose. In this representation of a monosaccharide, the carbon chain is written vertically with carbon atom number 1 at the top. The groups projecting to left and right of the carbon chain are considered as being in front of the plane of the paper. The optical antipode with the hydroxyl-group at the highest-numbered asymmetric carbon atom on the right is then regarded as belonging to the D-series. It is now known that this convention represents the absolute configuration.

Haworth later introduced the more realistic representations that bear his name, e.g. (*13.18*). In these, the monosaccharide ring is depicted perpendicular to the plane of the paper, the acetal-group being to the right, and the groups attached to the carbon atoms of that ring are above or below the ring. The carbon atoms of the ring are not shown.

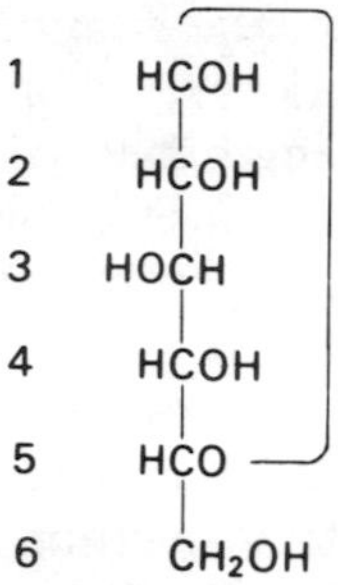

1   HCOH
2   HCOH
3   HOCH
4   HCOH
5   HCO
6   CH₂OH

D-Glucose
(*13.17*)

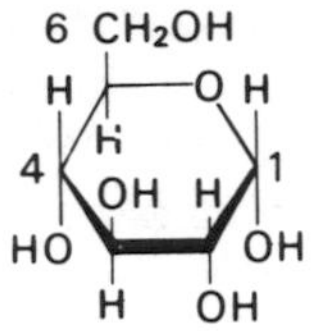

Haworth's representation
of D-glucose
(*13.18*)

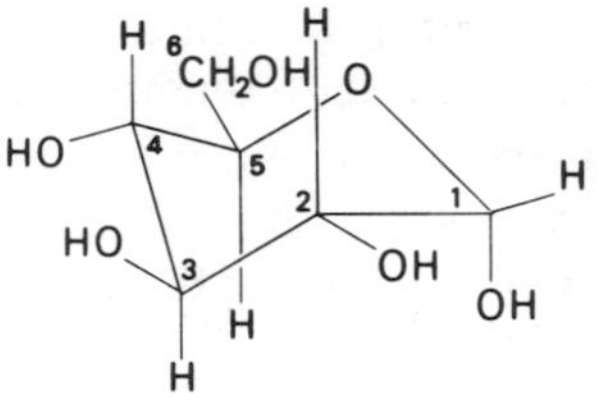

Conformational representation
of D-glucose
(*13.19*)

From contemporary X-ray diffraction work, it is known that the real structure of D-glucose is as shown in (*13.19*), which preserves the outlines of the saturated ring (*13.2*), and records the conformation (Section 13.3) which this particular example has been found to adopt. Although this conformational formula is much nearer to the truth than are the earlier representations, most people find that it takes longer to draw.

   Many agents, which ordinarily lack the molecular structure necessary for optical isomerism, display differences in activity between isomers once the possibility of isomerism is introduced. Thus the auxin types of plant-growth regulators usually lack an asymmetric carbon atom and hence are incapable of furnishing pairs of optical isomers. However, when an asymmetric carbon atom was deliberately introduced, as in α : 2,4,5-trichlorophenoxypropionic acid (*13.20*), it was found that the biological activity was confined mainly to the D(+)-form. This led to the formulation of the hypothesis that auxin-like action requires a three-point contact as depicted for adrenaline in Fig. 13.1. Substance (*13.20*), and related compounds, have a very unusual biological property: the action of the D-form is greatly decreased by the L-form (Smith, Wain, and Wightman, 1952). For a review of chemical structure in relation to auxin activity, see Wain and Fawcett (1969).

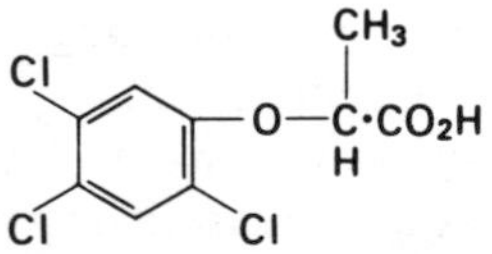

Trichlorophenoxypropionic acid
(*13.20*)

Optical isomerism can occur even in the absence of an asymmetric carbon atom when some other centre of asymmetry occurs in the molecule. The best-known examples are those biphenyls which are separable into (+) and (−) isomers when each of the two benzene rings has an *ortho*-substituent no smaller than a methyl-group. These *ortho*-groups sterically interfere with free rotation and hence introduce the necessary element of asymmetry.

For further reading on molecular asymmetry in biology, see Bentley (1969).

13.2 Geometrical isomerism

Geometrical isomers are found when rotation of atoms in a molecule is restricted by a double-bond, or by a fairly rigid non-planar ring-system. Such a pair of geometrical isomers is exemplified by maleic (*13.21*) and fumaric (*13.22*) acids (respectively *cis-* and *trans-*). Geometrical isomers, in spite of a similar fundamental structure, are not related to one another as an object is to its mirror-image. For this reason, geometrical isomers do not show optical activity, but it sometimes happens that one of them [e.g. the *trans*-1,2-dicarboxylic acid of *cyclo*hexane (*13.2*) has, in addition, an asymmetric structure and hence can be resolved into (+)- and (−)-isomers. *Cis-* and *trans-*forms, in general, have very different physical and chemical properties. Not surprisingly, they also have distinct biological properties (Butler, 1944).

The equilibrium between *cis-* and *trans-*isomers can often be disturbed by a beam of light. Indeed, human vision depends on the conversion by light of the 11-*cis*-isomer of retinal to the 11-*trans*-form. As soon as the excitatory beam is shut off, this carotenoid pigment reverts to the *cis*-form, thus terminating the impulses relayed to the brain (Gilardi *et al.*, 1971).

$$
\begin{array}{cc}
HC \cdot CO_2H & HC \cdot CO_2H \\
\parallel & \parallel \\
HC \cdot CO_2H & HO_2C \cdot CH \\
(cis) & (trans) \\
(13.21) & (13.22)
\end{array}
$$

Plant-growth substances provide some interesting examples of geometrical isomerism. Indoleacetic acid (*4.52*), and analogues like phenoxyacetic acids, e.g. (*6.46*), increase the size of cells, but not the rate of cell-division as the purine kinetins do. The structural requirements for a substance to have the indoleacetic acid type of action have been generalized as follows (Koepfli, Thimann, and Went, 1938): (i) a ring containing at least one double-bond, (ii) a side-chain possessing a $-CO_2H$-group, or a group easily converted to this, (iii) at least one carbon atom between the ring and the $-CO_2H$-group, (iv) a particular spatial relationship between the ring-system and the $-CO_2H$-group.

Requirement (iv), which is of special stereochemical interest, is exemplified by the large difference in activity between *cis*- and *trans*-pairs (geometrical isomerism). Thus *cis*-cinnamic acid is active, whereas the *trans*-isomer is inactive (Haagen-Smith and Went, 1935). Again, 2-phenyl-*cyclo*propane-1-carboxylic acid and 1,2,3,4-tetrahydro-naphthalidene-1-acetic acid are active only in the *cis*-form (Veldstra and van der Westeringh, 1951). In these examples, it is easily seen from molecular models that the ring and carboxylic acid groups are planar in the *trans*-isomer (inactive) but non-planar in the *cis*-isomer (active). Veldstra was the first to point out this connection between non-planarity and plant-growth activity. Hence requirement (iii) can be waived if enough steric hindrance to resonance can be supplied to produce an out-of-plane $-CO_2H$ group. Thus benzoic acid is kept flat by resonance, and is biologically inactive, whereas 2,6-dichlorobenzoic acid and 8-methyl-1-naphthoic acid are non-planar, and biologically active (Veldstra, 1953, 1963; Muir and Hansch, 1953).

Requirement (ii) applies only to substances of the highest activity, because $-CO_2H$ can be replaced by such negatively charged groups as $-NO_2$ and $-SO_3H$ without complete loss of biological action. These two groups are respectively totally non-ionized and totally ionized in the biological pH range, so that ionization can play only a secondary role. Moreover, the three groups $-CO_2H$, $-NO_2$, and $-SO_3^-$ have such entirely different chemical reactivities that there can be no question of covalent bond-formation with a receptor (Veldstra, 1956a). Although the receptor for auxins has not yet been identified, indoleacetic acid seems to unite with it by an induced conformational change (Kaethner, 1977).

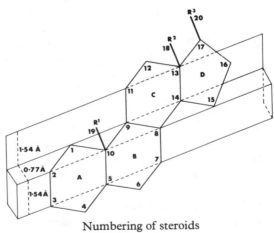

Numbering of steroids
(13.23)

Hydrocortisone
(as seen from front edge)
(*13.24*)

The geometrical isomerism of steroids has attracted much attention. This family of naturally occurring, and usually saturated, substances has the general structure (*13.23*). The formula shows the numbering of the carbon atoms and the lettering of the four rings. In all naturally occurring steroids, the junction between rings B and C is *trans* and they are both locked in a chair conformation. In the cardiac glycosides the junction between rings C and D is *cis*, but in the animal hormones, sterols and bile acids this is *trans*. Most biologically active steroids have a *trans* junction between rings A and B, and are therefore said to belong to the '5α' (formerly 'allo') series. This makes the four rings almost planar, at least to the extent shown in (*13.23*). That each ring is puckered can best be seen from a side-view, such as (*13.24*).

The meaning of '5α' is that the hydrogen atom in position 5 lies below the general plane of the rings. All substituents which lie below this plane in other positions are designated α, and those that lie above this plane are called β. The α-substituents are represented by dotted lines, and the β-substituents by thick lines.

In general, a high degree of any kind of mammalian biological activity, in the steroid series, is correlated with a lack of α-substituents along the edge of the molecule which runs from 1 to 17, and a lack of β-substituents from the bottom edge (from position 4 to 15). A side-view of the hydro-cortisone molecule (*13.24*) illustrates the above generalization (Sarett, Patchett, and Steelman, 1963). It is thought that interaction of steroid hormones with proteins takes place through the uncluttered underside (or α-surface) of the molecule. See Section 2.2 (p. 33) for specific protein transportation, as the first step in the biological action of steroid hormones.

The various steroids differ from one another mainly by variations in the nature of R^1, R^2, and R^3 (*13.23*), but extranuclear substituents are often present, and sometimes a degree of unsaturation is found. *Cyclo-hexenone* structure in ring A is usually necessary for progesterone, androsterone, and corticosteroid activity. Cortisone-type action requires, generally, oxygen atoms at positions 3, 11, and 17, as well as the characteristic $-CO.CH_2OH$ group in position 17. Androgenic and corticoid activity are highly dependent on these details of structure, but progestational activity persists when the 1-acetyl group is changed to the unnatural α-configuration, and replacement of the methyl-group in position 18 by an ethyl-group actually furnishes increased progestational activity, an example of which is norgestrel, the 'minipill' oral contraceptive. Of all steroid hormones, the oestrogens are the least dependent on structure. Provided that ring A is aromatic, and carries the acidic hydroxy-group in the 3-position, the rest of the steroid structure assumes only secondary importance. The simple and very effective (although not quite benign) benzene analogues, particularly diethylstilboestrol (*13.5*), do not share so much of the shape of the oestrogenic steroid molecule as was thought when the first member was introduced in 1938. X-ray diffraction studies reveal a *trans*-structure, distorted by steric hindrance from the methylene fragments of the two ethyl-groups. As a result, the two benzene rings make a dihedral angle of 63° with the central ethylene framework, and the total picture is not at all like a steroid. However, the distance between the two oxygen atoms is roughly similar, namely 12.1 Å in diethylstilboestrol, and 10.7 to 11.1 Å in the steroidal oestrogens: but all these molecules are too rigid to accommodate to a fixed distance on the receptor. As it is known that hydrogen bonding to the receptor by two oxygen atoms is essential for oestrogenic activity, the required flexibility must exist *in the receptor* (Weeks, Cooper, and Norton, 1970). That the action of diethylstilboestrol is also dependent on its molecular thickness was first suggested by Oki and Urushibara in 1952. It has since been measured as 4.5 Å, identical to that of steroidal oestrogens at C-18 (Weeks *et al.*, 1970).

For the cardioactive glycosides, see Section 14.1. For further reading on the mode of action of steroids, see Smellie, 1971; for steroid stereo-chemistry, see Shoppee (1964), and for steroid biochemistry and pharma-cology, see Briggs and Brotherton (1970).

Cis-4-aminocrotonic acid, an analogue of the central neurotransmitter GABA, has the folded conformation (*13.26*) and is biologically inactive, whereas the *trans* isomer (*13.25*) acts as efficiently as GABA in the mammalian central nervous system. This shows that the extended, rather than the folded, conformation of GABA is the important one in neurotransmission (Johnston *et al.*, 1975).

$H_3\overset{+}{N}$⌃⌄CO_2^-

Trans-4-Aminocrotonic acid
(*13.25*)

⌃CO_2^-
$\overset{+}{N}H_3$

Cis-4-Aminocrotonic acid
(*13.26*)

13.3 Conformational behaviour

Even when a bond is perfectly free to rotate, as every *single*-bond is, an infrared spectrum often reveals that the atoms of the molecule assume various preferred positions. The rules governing conformational analysis were established by D. Barton about 1950. Other methods which have greatly helped in conformational analysis include X-ray (and electron) diffraction, microwave spectra, dipole moments, chemical reactivity (see below), optical rotation (optical rotatory dispersion, circular dichroism), and n.m.r., often with application of the Karplus equation (see Appendix IV).

The commonest conformation is that where two non-hydrogen substituents take up positions as far from one another as possible. Thus 1-chloropropane in (*13.27*) contains much more of the *staggered* (sometimes confusingly, called *trans*, a term long associated with geometrical isomerism) form, than of either of the two *gauche* forms [e.g. (*13.28*)]. For the majority of molecules, the energy barriers between different conformations are too low to allow the separation of pure conformational isomers. However congestion, caused by the mutual interference of large groups or atoms in a molecule, has sometimes permitted the separation of pairs of conformers stable in the solid state, and many steroid examples are known (see also Section 13.7).

CH₃   H
　C—C—H
H   Cl
 H

Chloropropane
(staggered)
(*13.27*)

CH₃   Cl
　C—C—H
H   H
 H

Chloropropane
(gauche)
(*13.28*)

Conformational analysis has been vigorously developed in the chemistry of alicyclic rings, including the steroids, and already in Section 13.2 some conformational data were introduced to supplement the geometrical. Conformational analysis is concerned both with ring-shape and substituents. Concerning the former, *cyclo*hexane (*13.2*) can exist in three conformations: chair (*13.29*), boat (*13.30*), and twist (*13.31*). The chair from is less strained and hence highly preferred (in the chair form, each axial hydrogen atoms is 2.5 Å from the other two axial hydrogens on the same side of the ring). The twist form, intermediate between boat and chair, and even the highly strained boat form, can be stabilized with two or more fused rings if appropriately substituted.

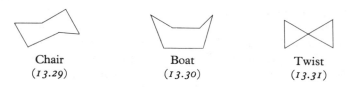

Chair   Boat   Twist
(*13.29*)   (*13.30*)   (*13.31*)

The two principal conformations into which substituents fall are classified as *equatorial* (i.e. in the general plane of the ring), and *axial* (i.e. perpendicular to this plane). In a mono-substituted *cyclo*hexane, the equatorial isomer predominates because this form has least interference from hydrogen atoms. In multi-substituted rings, some groups will necessarily be in the axial positions. Because axial groups are subject to greater steric hindrance, equatorial hydroxyl- and carboxyl-groups are the more readily esterified and the product the more readily hydrolysed. Often a conformational change is superimposed on geometrical isomerism, as in the pair: cocaine (*7.11*) and ψ-cocaine, the former having an axial, and the latter an equatorial methoxycarbonyl group.

Many other formulae embodying conformational information have been used in earlier chapters of this book, e.g. atropine (*7.14*), nicotine (*7.18*), morphine (*7.28a*), pyrethrin (*7.52*), and penicillin (*12.6b*), and other formulae of this kind will be used later in this chapter.

In thyroxine (*11.11*) and the more biologically active triiodothyronine, the iodine atoms in the 3- and 4- positions force the two rings into a conformation in which they are perpendicular to one another. Further work, with analogues, indicates that this arrangement is essential for thyroid function (Dietrich *et al.*, 1977).

Emetine and cycloheximide are two molecules that look quite dissimilar at first glance, but have conformationally similar areas which cause both of them to inhibit protein synthesis in the ribosomes of most living cells (Section 4.1, p. 127).

Acetylcholine has the same conformation in aqueous solution (as determined by n.m.r. in D_2O) as in the solid state (as determined by X-ray crystallography) (see Section 13.6). How widely does this correlation extend? Byrn, Graber, and Midland (1976) have reviewed the literature on this and, as X-ray diffraction analysis is exceedingly slow, they have devised a simple test: the infrared spectrum in the solid state is compared with that in chloroform. Although this test requires further examination, it is worth recording that they found very similar spectra for choline chloride, and also for the antihistaminic methapyriline; but very different spectra for histamine, and for the antihistaminic diphenhydramine. Strong distortion on binding to the enzyme lysozyme was shown by a tetrasaccharide fragment of murein (Section 5.1) when observed by Fourier-transform n.m.r. (Sykes, Patt, and Dolphin, 1971). On the other hand, no difference in conformation was found for *N*-acetyl-L-tryptophan when it combines with chymotrypsin, compared by both ^{13}C n.m.r. and X-ray crystal data (Rodgers and Roberts, 1973).

At this stage we would do well to pause and ask ourselves: Which conformation of a drug is of the most importance for its action? Is it the form assumed in aqueous solution, in lipid solution, or in the solid state, particularly that solvent-free and hence virtually solid state in which many drugs must exist when adsorbed on a macromolecule? Yet an even more fundamental question should take precedence. Can a receptor specifically attract a conformer that is only present to a very small extent in the total population of the drug molecules, a choice that must lead (through equilibration) to the generation of more of the selected conformer as fast as the receptor removes it, up to the point where a new equilibrium is reached? But there is a still more fundamental question: To what extent can the receptor create a preferred conformer when none of this is presented by the dissolved drug?

Burgen, Roberts, and Feeney (1975) carry the analysis still deeper. If a drug is flexible and hence can have many conformations, they ask: Does it have to wait until the molecule that collides with the receptor is in the right conformation for acceptance? Or does every colliding molecule become attached by *one* bond (whether a polar or a hydrogen bond) whereupon a series of conformational rearrangements of this partly-bound drug follow until each bondable segment of it conforms to the receptor and becomes totally bound? In the first mode, there is a large kinetic energy barrier and so binding must go slowly; but in the latter mode (called the 'zipper') there is a series of only small energy barriers and hence the binding goes faster. [The equilibrium constant must be the same for both modes.]

To all these questions, so difficult to answer at present, must be added the likelihood that some drugs induce a conformational change in their receptors. This aspect is discussed under the heading 'Allosteric hypothesis' in Section 7.5b. Certainly some substrates cause conformational changes in enzymes, clearly seen in X-ray diffraction studies (see, for example, the account of carboxypeptidase in Section 9.0). Another conformational change, studied by the same technique, is caused by the addition of oxygen to haemoglobin (to give oxyhaemoglobin). This reaction involves a movement of the proximal histidine residue towards the plane of the porphyrin ring by about 0.85 Å (Fig. *13.2*). This movement sets other tertiary-structural changes in motion because the iron atom is rigidly linked to a histidine residue. What happens is that Helix F of the globin is moved towards Helix H in the centre of the molecule and consequently expels the tyrosine moiety (140) from its pocket between helices F and H. The expelled tyrosine drags arginine (141) with it, thus breaking the latter's salt linkage. This conformational change facilitates the approach of a second oxygen atom by loosening the tight structure of the four haem units in the haemoglobin molecule.

An example nearer to drug action: the equilibrium conformation of bovine pancreatic RNAase is changed to different extents by the inhibitors cytidine 2'-, 3'-, and 5'-monophosphate, as seen in an n.m.r. study, and the change is proportional to the inhibition (Meadows, Roberts, and Jardetzky, 1969).

It is useful to keep in mind (many authors have overlooked this!) that

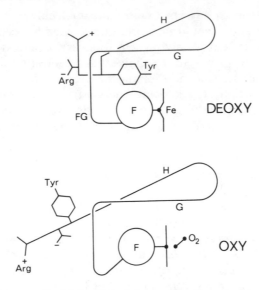

FIG. 13.2 Diagram of conformational change in tertiary structure of the haemoglobin sub-units on reaction with oxygen. (Perutz, 1970, modified in
correspondence.)

changes in conformation can change physical properties. Thus one conformer can be more lipophilic, or a stronger base, than the other [cf. (*13.70*)
and (*13.71*).] Hence biological activity can depend, in the last analysis, not
on the change in shape of the molecule but on the new physical properties
conferred by this change. If a drug-designer finds these new physical
properties advantageous, he should be able to provide them in other ways,
independent of conformation.

Conformational specificity has been demonstrated in the coenzyme
NADH (nicotinamide adenine dinucleotide) (*13.32*). Some apoenzymes
that use this coenzyme remove only the axial (and others the equatorial)
hydrogen atoms in the 4-position, as can readily be shown by replacing
each of these atoms, in turn, by a deuterium atom. The absolute conformation of the labile hydrogen atoms in NADH were determined by Cornforth
et al. (1962).

A shorthand notation that displays a good deal of information about both
optical isomerism and conformation is exemplified in (*13.33*). These
Newman projections are specially useful when both of two consecutive
carbon atoms are asymmetric, as in ephedrine (*13.13*). To use this notation,
these two carbon atoms are superimposed, so that six groups apparently
radiate from one point. For purposes of comparison it can also be used for
related substances that have only *one* asymmetric carbon atom, e.g. noradrenaline and its homologues (*13.34*).

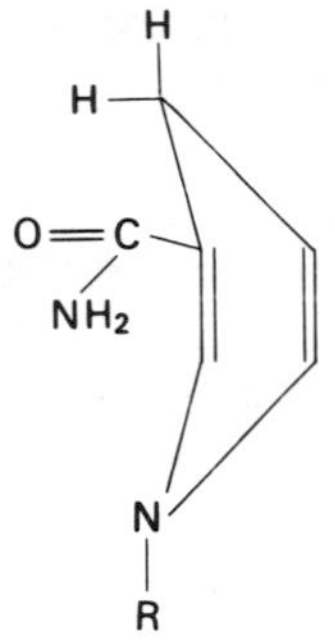

NADH (where R is ribosyl-
diphosphoadenosine)
(13.32)

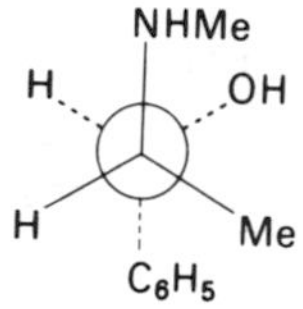

Ephedrine
(13.33)

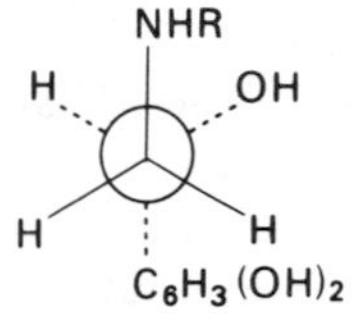

Noradrenaline (R = H), adrenaline (R = Me),
isoprenaline (R = CHMe$_2$)
(13.34)

Discussions of conformation often require knowledge of the torsion angle which, in a group XABY, is the angle that the plane XAB makes with the plane ABY. (See p. 506, for an example.)

For further reading on conformation, see Barton and Cookson (1956); Eliel *et al.*, 1965.

For further reading on general aspects of stereochemistry, see Eliel (1962), and especially Bentley (1969) where the biological consequences are discussed at length. The remainder of the present chapter summarizes what is known of the nature of several receptors important in pharmacodynamics, much of the information being derived from stereochemistry.

13.4 Catecholamine receptors

The pioneer work on the connection between constitution and activity in the phenylethylamine series of sympathomimetic drugs was carried out by Barger and Dale (1910). It has since become clear that *direct* action of the hormone and neurotransmitter type, is strongest in examples with hydroxy-groups in the 3- and 4-positions of the benzene ring, i.e. the 'catecholamines' such as noradrenaline, adrenaline, and dopamine. The *indirect* action of examples without these embellishments has been outlined in

Sections 9.4 (p. 320) and 7.6c (p. 266). As recounted in Section 13.1 the
D-catecholamines (Fig. 13.1) have much more biological activity than
their L-enantiomers.

The existence of two different adrenergic receptors was first suggested
by Ahlquist (1948). Those responses evoked most readily by noradrenaline
and least by isoprenaline (13.35) are credited to α-receptors. The activity of
adrenaline is intermediate between those of these two catecholamines.
Other responses, most readily evoked by both isoprenaline and adrenaline
but least by noradrenaline, were credited to β-receptors. Typical α-respon-
ses are: constriction of blood-vessels, stimulation of the uterus, relaxation
of the intestine. Typical β-responses are: dilatation of blood-vessels,
relaxation of the uterus, stimulation of muscle glycogenolysis, production of
tachycardia (Levy and Ahlquist, 1961).

Noradrenaline stimulates principally the α-receptors, N-tert-butyl-
noradrenaline (with its highly branched alkyl-group) stimulates principally
β-receptors, and adrenaline stimulates both. The increase in β-stimulating
effects with increased branching of the N-alkyl-group could be due to
increasing steric hindrance or, as Pratesi (1963) thinks, to increasing inductive effect of the alkyl-group and, contrariwise, to the increased ease of
hydrogen-bonding by the primary amino-group of noradrenaline. Both
α- and β-stimulating drugs are most effective if they are D-enantiomers.

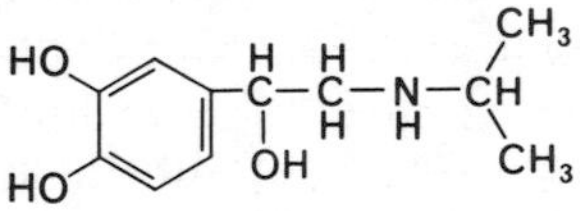

Isoprenaline
(13.35)

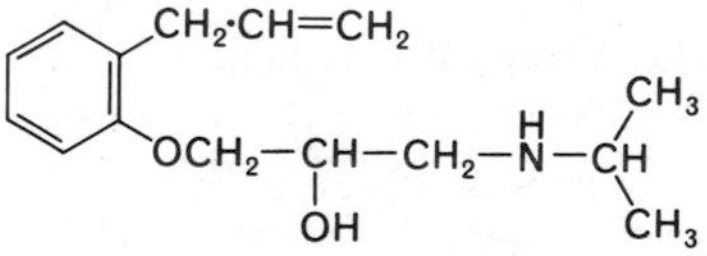

Alprenolol
(13.36)

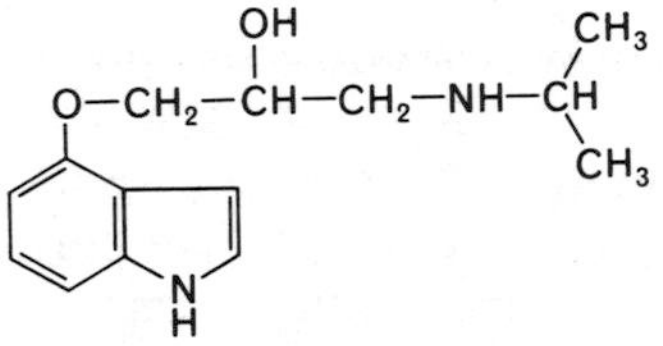

Pindolol
(13.37)

The ideal way to characterize catecholamine receptors would be to
isolate them. Although this has not yet been accomplished in more than
traces, considerable progress has been made with specific labelling.
[³H]dihydroergocryptine, an ergot alkaloid which is a potent α-adrenergic
antagonist, was used to label (reversibly) the receptors on uterine smooth
muscle. With its help, the relative specificity and potency of α-adrenergic
agonists and antagonists at the receptor sites were found to correspond

closely with evaluations made on the whole organ (Williams, Mullikin, and Lefkowitz, 1976).

A similar exploration of the β-receptor has been made with (−)[³H] dihydroalprenolol, a labelled derivative of the potent β-adrenergic antagonistic drug alprenolol (*13.36*). It selectively and reversibly bound β-adrenergic receptors in rat adipocytes. With this marker, it could be seen that β-adrenergic agonists and antagonists competed for the binding sites stereospecifically and in the same ratios as is found in therapy (Williams, Jarett, and Lefkowitz, 1976). Another potent β-adrenergic antagonistic drug, pindolol (*13.37*), has supplied a useful (reversible) marker, namely its C-[¹²⁵I]iodohydroxybenzyl-derivative. It was allowed to react with turkey erythrocyte membranes, and the labelled receptors were isolated, although only on a micro scale (E. Brown *et al.*, 1976). The same marker was applied to human fibroblasts and to rat glioma cells. Its displacement by β-adrenergic agonists and antagonists was found to be stereospecific and to occur in the same relative potencies as have been established in laboratory animals (Maguire *et al.*, 1976). The binding of these labelled antagonists was saturable, also it could be prevented by prior application of the same substance unlabelled. Measurement of dissociation constants showed that the number of β-adrenergic receptor sites on an avian erythrocytes is about 1000.

The β-adrenergic receptor is known to trigger adenylate cyclase so that the latter produces adenosine-3′,5′-cyclic monophosphate (cAMP) (*13.38*). The receptor and the enzyme are situated near together, the receptor in the outside layer of the membrane, near to the adenylate cyclase which is on the inner side. As soon as the receptor binds the neurotransmitter, the cyclase (with the help of guanosine triphosphate) produces cAMP (Perkins, 1973; Levitzki, 1977). When adenylate cyclase is blocked with guanyl-5′-yl imidodiphosphate, there is a conformational change that inhibits the β-receptor from taking up agonists, but its uptake of antagonists is unaffected (Lefkovitz, Mullikin, and Caron, 1976). It is noteworthy that these antagonists [including propranolol (*13.41*)] block the β-site without blocking adenyl cyclase; also the enzyme can be inactivated by heat without affecting uptake on the β-site (Schramm *et al.*, 1977). Injection of cAMP can bring about physiological responses similar to those evoked by the catecholamines.

Cyclic AMP
(*13.38*)

Until a workable laboratory preparation of adrenergic receptors (something corresponding to the acetylcholine micro-sacs of p. 502) is available, further efforts to understand receptor function must be concentrated on the structure-activity relationships of catecholamine agonists and their antagonists in a variety of biological systems. Studies of the loss or retention of activity by the omission of various groups point to the great importance of the basic group in the catecholamines. Thus a nitrogen-free isostere of noradrenaline, in which H_3N^+- is replaced by CH_3O-, is totally devoid of activity (Kaelin, 1947). Hence the principal mode of attachment of the catecholamines to all their receptors is thought to be by an ionic bond. The union between catecholamine and receptor brought about by this bond is likely to be reinforced further by a hydrogen bond from the β-hydroxy-group, the absence of which strongly diminishes the action, as was discovered by Barger and Dale (1910) (discussed also in Section 13.1 with the help of Fig. 13.1).

The α-receptors.   In smooth muscle, the α-receptors act by increasing the permeability of the cell membranes to inorganic ions (Jenkinson and Morton, 1967; Bülbring and Tomita, 1969). In intestinal muscle this increase favours K^+, so that hyperpolarization followed by muscular relaxation sets in. In most other kinds of smooth muscle, the permeability increase extends to Na^+ and Ca^{2+}, so that the membrane potential falls, and excitation is followed by contraction.

Dibenamine (*13.39*), which becomes physiologically active only after self-quaternization to the dibeniminium cation (*13.40*) (Nickerson, 1957; Henkel *et al.*, 1976), antagonizes the action of catecholamines at α-sites by alkylating them. Phenoxybenzamine [2-(*N*-benzyl-2-chloroethylamino)-1-phenoxypropane] acts similarly, and has the advantage of being active orally. Dibenamine blocks the receptors not only of catecholamines but also of acetylcholine and histamine. Hence it is not, as had been thought, a highly specific reagent, and it does not throw so much light on the mode of action of catecholamines at the α-site as had been hoped (van Rossum and Ariëns, 1962).

The use of α-site blockers in therapy is small compared to that of β-blockers. Imidazolines, like phentolamine (*7.41*) and tolazoline, are mainly α-blockers but have other actions too. The α-site blockers are used principally to restore peripheral circulation, as in frostbite, and to diagnose adrenaline-secreting tumours.

The topography of the α-site has been pictured by Belleau (1967). For a review of structure-action relationships in the dibenamine family of substances, see Graham (1962).

The β-receptor.   The most clinically useful inhibitors of the β-sympathetic receptors are the 1-*iso*propylamino-3-aryloxy-2-propanols such as propranolol (*13.41*) ('Inderal') which is one of the most used drugs in the treatment of moderately high blood-pressure. Although some of them

Dibenamine
(13.39)

Dibeniminimum cation
(13.40)

exert a small, helpful effect in reducing sympathetic nervous tone in the central nervous system, the main effect takes place in the heart, whose rate and contractility are decreased (Lewis and Haeusler, 1975). These drugs are much more clinically useful than those, such as guanethidine (7.45), which interfere with noradrenaline release into the synapse. The action develops only slowly, over 1 or 2 weeks, as though a suppression of an enzyme such as tyrosine hydroxylase were taking place (Raine and Chubb, 1977). Propranolol is also useful in the treatment of angina pectoris and cardiac arrhythmias.

Analogues of propranolol trying to establish a place by claiming heightened selectivity, include alprenolol (13.36), pindolol (13.37), metoprolol, acebutalol, oxprenolol ('Trasicor'), and timolol. Practolol, another analogue, which began to enjoy high favour because of its lack of bronchoconstricting properties, much appreciated by asthmatics, has been largely withdrawn because of serious side-effects.

Two kinds of β-receptors are now distinguished (Lands et al., 1967; Dunlop and Shanks, 1968). The β_1 receptors increase the force and rate of contraction of heart muscle, dilate coronary blood vessels, and relax smooth muscle in the gastro-intestinal tract, whereas β_2 receptors relax smooth muscle in the bronchi, uterus, and the arteries that supply skeletal muscle. The β_1 receptor exists in a less lipophilic environment than the β_2 receptor (Basil et al., 1976).

Specific blocking of β_1 receptors, desired for making more selective analogues of propranolol, can be achieved by replacing the isopropyl-group by a phenoxyethyl-group the benzene ring of which should carry either a methoxy- or an amido-substituent (Smith and Tucker, 1977).

Excellent agonists, for use as bronchodilators by asthmatics, became available by restricting the action to β_2 receptors in order to avoid the β_1-activated tachycardia which was a side-effect of the best of the hitherto used drugs, namely isoprenaline. To obtain a long-acting example, it is necessary to change the catechol hydroxyl-groups, which are not necessary for β_2 activity, but provide a site for degradation. Thus the excellent, purely β_2 and long-acting anti-asthmatic drug salbutamol (13.42) has a saligenin, instead of a catechol, structure, and another excellent example, terbutaline, has a resorcinol group. In general, activity increases with the size of the alkyl-group, at least up to the butyl-group [salbutamol is

1-(4-hydroxy-3-hydroxymethylphenyl)-2-*t*-butylaminoethanol]. For a discussion of the steric structure required for a β-adrenoreceptor antagonist, see Patel, Miller, and Trendelenberg (1974).

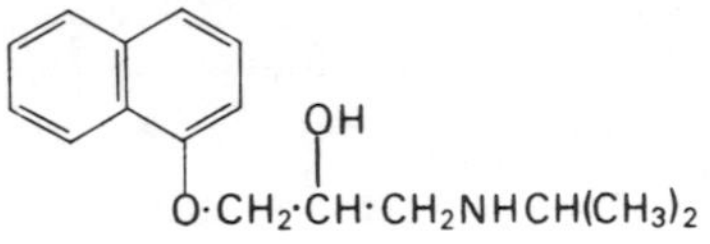

Propranolol
(*13.41*)

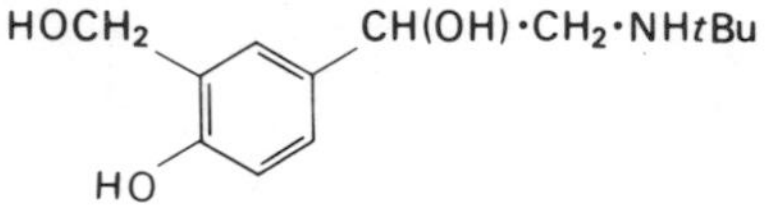

Salbutamol
(*13.42*)

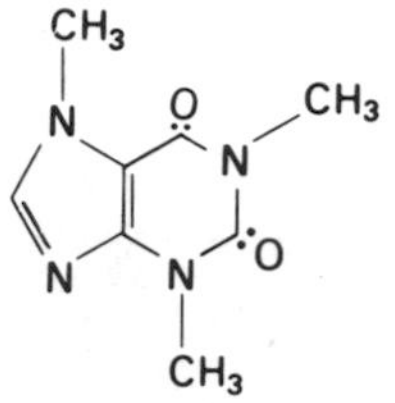

Caffeine
(*13.43*)

Dopamine. Like noradrenaline, this central neurotransmitter (3,4-dihydroxyphenylalanine) works by activating an adenylate cyclase. Human diseases are associated with both deficiency and excess. In Parkinson's disease, specific brain centres lack dopamine which is restored by treatment with levodopa. Major tranquillizers such as chloropromazine, work by blocking the dopamine receptor in the corpus striatum. Preliminary work has been done on isolation of the dopamine receptor. Meanwhile, receptor areas in the corpus striatum of the brain are monitored by their ability to bind ^{3}H-haloperidol, which correlates well with the pharmacological effect of other psycholeptics (see Section 13.8) (Schwarcz *et al.*, 1978).

The side-chain of dopamine is held in a rigid cyclic conformation in 2-amino-6,7-dihydroxyl-1,2,3,4-tetrahydronaphthalene. This substance, injected into the brain of a conscious rat, is taken up by brain synaptosomes where it mimics the actions of dopamine (Elkhawad and Woodruff, 1975).

Cyclic adenosine monophosphate. The physiological task of cAMP, when released indirectly by catecholamines either from an α- or a β-receptor site, is to energize the enzyme protein kinase which, it is thought, may phosphorylate a specific postsynapic membrane protein, thus creating a pore for the passage of inorganic cations, and this pore might be abolished by the rapid enzymatic hydrolysis of the phosphoester-group (Greengard, 1976). Clearly, much work remains to be done to establish the molecular basis of the postsynaptic potential. The methylated xanthines, such as caffeine (*13.43*) and theophylline, specifically hinder the destruction of cAMP by phosphodiesterase*. The anti-asthma prophylactic drug, sodium cromoglycate, is a strong inhibitor of phosphodiesterase, but also has powerful membrane-conserving properties which have placed it in Section 14.3.

Apart from mediating the action of catecholamines, cAMP and its congener cGMP are common secondary-transmitters of hormone action. For example, they play the main part in liberating insulin from the pancreas *in vivo*. Tolbutamide, and similar sulphonylureas, which are used to alleviate the diabetes of elderly people, somewhat selectively inhibit pancreatic phosphodiesterase and thus preserve cAMP from destruction (Goldfine *et al.*, 1971). Activity within a series of sulphonylureas is positively correlated with lipophilicity and also with binding by serum albumin (Seydel, Ahrens, and Losert, 1975). These cyclic phosphates also mediate the diuretic effect of vasopressin, and the action of ACTH and many other hormones (Sutherland, Øye, and Butcher, 1965).

For a review of the interaction of catecholamines with their receptors, see Triggle and Triggle (1977); Cooper, Bloom, and Roth (1974).

13.5 Acetylcholinesterase

The enzyme acetylcholinesterase, although available in a pure state, has so high a molecular weight (260 000) that X-ray diffraction has elucidated only a little of its structure. Aminoacid analysis of the C-terminal groups reveals that two different kinds of chain are present (each of the same molecular weight) and that each kind is present twice in the molecule (Leuzinger, 1971). This enzyme is obtainable, in a fairly pure state, by extracting the electric organ of the eel *Electrophorus electricus*. It is a general ester-hydrolysing enzyme, but differs from other esterases in the far greater efficiency of its action on those esters which have a cationic-group near the ethereal oxygen atom in the ester-group.

Acetylcholine (*13.44*) is a permanent cation, whose degree of ionization cannot be changed by variations in pH. Investigation of the molecular mechanism of its hydrolysis began with Wilson and Bergmann (1950) who found the dissociation constant of the acetylcholine-enzyme complex to be 2.6×10^{-4}. By observing changes in the efficacy of the enzyme with changing pH,[†] they concluded that the enzyme had a basic group of pK_a 7.2 (believed to be the imidazole ring of a histidine residue) and an acidic group of pK_a 9.3 (believed to be a tyrosine residue). The enzyme-substrate complex, they suggested, was formed by an ionic linkage between the

---

* It may be in this way that these methylxanthines perform their mentally-energizing and diuretic functions.

† This method of divining the pK_a values of enzyme sites is not without pitfalls (Kosower, 1962). A change in ionization of a group on the enzyme protein can precipitate a conformational change.

quaternary ammonium-group of acetylcholine and the anion of the pK_a 9.3 group on the enzyme protein, and by a simultaneous dipole-dipole bond between the doubly bound nitrogen of the imidazole ring (on the enzyme protein) and the fractional positive charge of the carbon atom in the C=O group of the ester (see review by Davies and Green, 1958). Thus the enzyme was said to have two binding sites, an *anionic site* which bound the cation of the substrate, and an *esteratic site* which first bound and then hydrolysed the ester-group ('esteratic' was coined as an adjective of the noun 'esterase', Wilson and Bergmann, 1950).

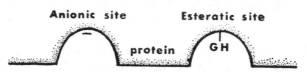

FIG. 13.3 The active patch on acetylcholinesterase (Wilson, 1962, after Wilson and Bergmann, 1950). (G stood for 'glyoxaline', a synonym for imidazole.)

A simplified representation* (Fig. 13.3) of the active patch on acetylcholinesterase came into use (Wilson, 1962). By applying various inhibitors, of rigid structure, the two main binding sites on the enzyme were located about 2.5 Å apart (Friess and Baldridge, 1956).

In a later modification of this hypothesis, it was postulated that the carbonyl oxygen atom of acetylcholine formed a covalent bond with the hydroxyl-group of a serine residue. This suggestion followed from the discovery that organic phosphates, such as di*iso*propyl fluorophosphonate phosphorylated a serine-group of the enzyme and that the sequence of aminoacids at this site is glu-ser-ala (Schaffer, May, and Summerson, 1954; see Section 9.0). It was concluded that the acetyl-group of acetylcholine is attracted to, and acetylates, the hydroxy-group of a serine residue in the enzyme. After that, the imidazole-group, located on another fold of the enzyme protein, was thought to assist hydrolysis of the acetylated serine-group (Wilson and Cabib, 1956). For a diagram suggesting distances in this more complex site, see Krupka and Laidler (1961).

The organic phosphates, which are strong inhibitors of cholinesterase, do not require any anionic site. See Section 12.3 for these and other in-activators and reactivators.

When it was found that 3,3-dimethylbutyl acetate (*13.45*) and acetylcholine are equally easily hydrolysed by acetylcholinesterase, it was realized that the van der Waals forces of the methyl-groups (surrounding the cation of acetylcholine) could be just as important as a positive charge in binding the natural transmitter to the enzyme (Whittaker, 1951).

---

* Such diagrams, symbolic of the disposition of the active groups in an enzyme, were introduced by Haldane (1930).

$$Me_3N^+ —CH_2—CH_2—O—\overset{O}{\overset{\cdot\cdot}{C}}CH_3$$

Acetylcholine cation
(13.44)

$$Me_3C—CH_2—CH_2—O—\overset{O}{\overset{\cdot\cdot}{C}}—CH_3$$

3,3-Dimethylbutyl acetate
(13.45)

In the absence of enzymes, acetylcholine, in cold aqueous solution, is stable to acid, but unstable to alkali above pH 10. The velocity constants for its hydrolysis show that the charge on the nitrogen atom attracts the attacking hydroxyl ions to the neighbourhood of the ester-group; hence acetylcholine is much more susceptible to alkaline hydrolysis than ordinary esters such as ethyl acetate (Butterworth, Eley, and Stone, 1953).

There is enough acetylcholinesterase in the end-plate of the muscle to split a thousand million molecules of acetylcholine in a millisecond, that is a thousand times as many molecules as are needed to depolarize the end-plate (Nachmansohn, 1940).

Apart from inhibition by organic phosphates and other acylating agents, acetylcholinesterase can also be reversibly blocked by simple quaternary ammonium compounds. As the size of the alkyl-groups in these was increased, the increased affinity (measured as $-\Delta F$) contributed by each methylene group (CH_2) was found to be about 300 cal/mol for *bis*quaternary compounds. For a given chain length, the *mono-* was bound more strongly than the *bis*-quaternary inhibitor (Bergmann and Segal, 1954). For a study of the hydrophobic areas on cholinesterases, see Kabachnik *et al.*, (1970).

A different method for terminating the action of acetylcholine occurs in the hearts of bivalent molluscs which have no cholinesterases. The release of ACh from the nerve ending causes the muscle to excrete an ATP-like substance which lowers the sensitivity of the ACh receptors, apparently by an allosteric change. This mechanism persists in the hearts of higher animals, but is overshadowed by the more efficient ACh-esterase (Turpaev and Sakharov, 1973).

13.6 Acetylcholine receptors

Acetylcholine is the natural transmitter at several different kinds of synaptic site, e.g. (a) the somatic nerve → voluntary muscle junctions, (b) the ganglionic synapses which are nerve → nerve junctions in the autonomic system, (c) such postganglionic nerve-endings as are parasympathetic. In addition it has some transmitting duties in the central nervous system, e.g. between spinal cord root fibres and Renshaw cells.

Nicotine mimics acetylcholine at sites (a) and (b), whereas muscarine does so at site (c) (see Table 7.1). Hence it is usual to divide acetylcholine receptors into 'nicotinic' and 'muscarinic' receptors, a useful classification first made by Dale (1914). The work of muscarinic and nicotinic receptors is carried out on very different time scales. A single nervous stimulus affects muscarinic receptors for at least 500 ms, a long duration that is preceded by a long latency (about 100 ms). In contrast to this, nicotinic receptors at voluntary neuromuscular junctions are stimulated for only 0.2 ms, and even the nicotinic synapses, which are slower, average only 60 ms. Cyclic GMP is thought to be a necessary mediator of muscarinic responses. One consequence of interest is that smooth muscle reacts far more slowly than voluntary muscle. Heart muscle is distinguished from both by the fact that acetylcholine increases its polarization, whereas it decreases polarization elsewhere.

Of all the synapses which have cholinergic transmission, that at the motor end-plate (at the voluntary neuromuscular junction) has been most studied. Its structure, visible even in the light microscope and sketched in Fig. 7.1, has revealed yet further complexities to the electron microscope, to electro-physiological measurements, to assays of acetylcholine vesicles and of acetylcholinesterase, and to autoradiography. The chemical nature of the receptors in the end-plate is imperfectly known, but a di-sulphide (S-S) group is essential for its functioning. This follows from the inhibition of the receptor by dithiothreitol (a disulphide reducer) and restoration of sensitivity by 5,5'-dithio-*bis*-2-nitrobenzoic acid (which restores a dithiol to the disulphide state) (Karlin and Bartels, 1966).

A practical detail, useful in recognizing the receptor, is that the Formosan snake toxin, α-bungarotoxin (*acetyl*-^{3}H), binds only to the acetylcholine (ACh) receptor site (in mouse diaphragm muscle), whereas di*iso*propyl-phosphorofluoridate (^{3}H) (*12.15*) binds specifically to the active site of acetylcholinesterase. An equal number (3×10^7 per end-plate) of the receptor and the enzyme sites is found, i.e. one active molecule per 5000 Å^2 of the membrane, which is consequently densely occupied by these two proteins. Blockade becomes marked only when 70 per cent of the ACh receptor sites are occupied, and hence there are not many spare receptors at this site (Barnard, Wieckowski, and Chiu, 1971).

The isolation and nature of the acetylcholine receptor was described in Section 2.1. Of the various products of this work, Changeux's micro-sacs are particularly welcome, as they enable much experimentation with drugs to be carried out under conditions more versatile than when the receptors are in the synapse. We shall learn much more about the chemical nature of the active site when the receptor is available, quite pure and in greater quantity, for determination of aminoacid sequence and then for X-ray diffraction study.

This revolutionary change of direction in studying the ACh receptor has stimulated work on other receptors of neurotransmitters and hormones, but the acetylcholine work remains the furthest advanced. However, until much more fundamental work has been done with the isolated ACh receptor, our knowledge of its active site must be supplemented by indirect methods. The best of these have been studies of structure-activity relationships in agonists that mimic the action of acetylcholine. Most information of this kind has been obtained at the postganglionic synapses, i.e. those mimicked by muscarine (*7.39*). Hence the following discussion will begin with the muscarinic receptors, and the nicotinic receptors will be taken up on p. 511. Some attention will also be given to information derived from antagonists, but these are from their very nature so much less dependent on structure that conclusions based on their behaviour is necessarily uncritical.

(a) *Muscarine and the muscarinic receptor for acetylcholine.*
The receptors for the synaptic transmitter substances show a high degree of specificity. Thus methacholine (L-acetyl-β-methyl-choline) (*13.46*), has the full muscarinic action of acetylcholine, but almost none of the latter's nicotinic action. Moreover, it is at least 200 times as active as its D-enantiomer (Ellenbroek and van Rossum, 1960).

L(+)-Acetyl-β-methylcholine
Methacholine
(*13.46*)

Because the ACh receptor does not hydrolyse acetylcholine, the esteratic site of acetylcholinesterase (see Fig. 13.3) must be absent. Other fundamental differences in the two sites are indicated by the following: (a) dimethylbutyl acetate (*13.45*), which is such a good substrate for the enzyme, barely activates the receptor which requires a basic group for marked activity, (b) muscarine is not a substrate for the enzyme and yet it is a powerful agonist for the receptor, (c) the specificity of antagonists mentioned above (p. 502).

The equilibrium distance of the quaternary nitrogen atom of acetylcholine from the negatively charged group of the receptor has been calculated as 3.29 Å from the difference in free energy of the receptor-interaction of (a) acetylcholine (*13.44*) and (b) dimethylbutyl acetate (*13.45*). The latter has a non-basic head-group isosteric with the basic head-group of acetylcholine. This distance is practically identical with the distance of closest approach found by molecular models (Burgen, 1965).

In recent years, the conformations of many of the more rigid ACh agonists have been determined by X-ray crystallography in order to predict (a) which of the many conformations, assumable by the loosely-jointed molecule of acetylcholine, is the one active at a given receptor, and hence

(b) the stereochemistry of the receptor itself. Because of the known de-
formability of receptors (see Section 13.3), this approach is of only limited
value but must be discussed.

A two-dimensional projection of the X-ray diffraction diagram of
acetylcholine (bromide) is shown in (*13.47*) (Canepa, Pauling, and Sörum,
1966). The interatomic distance from one *N*-methyl carbon atom to the
ethereal oxygen (i.e. the oxygen that links two carbons) is 3.02 Å in the
original, and from the nitrogen to the ethereal oxygen is 3.29 Å (both
these distances are shorter than usual). The two oxygen atoms are coplanar
with the three carbon atoms that are nearest the right-hand side of (*13.47*).
Thus the molecules of acetylcholine and muscarine (*13.49*) X-ray data
by Jellinek, 1957 have remarkably similar shapes in the solid state. However, the conformation of the acetylcholine molecule could be very different
in aqueous solution, where it would be unconstrained by neighbouring
molecules of the same substance. Hence its conformation was examined in
deuterium oxide solution by analysing the vicinal coupling constants deriv-
able from the proton magnetic resonance spectrum (Culvenor and Ham,
1966). The results (*13.48*) support the X-ray analysis except that the
ester group has a more normal ester conformation. The *gauche* arrangement of the $^{+}$NCCO sequence, which is the prominent feature of (*13.47*),
(*13.48*), and (*13.49*), is that preferred by very many 1,2-disubstituted
ethanes in solution. It must be concluded that the preferred conformation of acetylcholine is remarkably normal: yet contact with the receptor
could change the conformation completely.

Acetylcholine
(X-ray diffraction data; bond-lengths in Å)
(*13.47*)

Acetylcholine (p.m.r. data)
(*13.48*)

Muscarine (X-ray diffraction data)
(*13.49*)

The rigid nature of the ring-system in muscarine makes more definite
information available about the dimensions of the muscarinic receptor
of acetylcholine than can be obtained from the latter directly (Waser,

1961). There are seven stereoisomers of muscarine, but only natural L(+)-muscarine has strong acetylcholine-like activity. The nitrogen atom must be quaternary, and the ring-oxygen atom must not be replaced by sulphur, otherwise all activity is lost. These facts led Waser to postulate that muscarine is bound to the receptor by the nitrogen and the ring-oxygen atoms.* Although the conformational freedom of muscarine is much less than that of acetylcholine, the trimethylammonium side-chain is free to move over almost the whole area of the rest of the molecule (Waser, 1961).

Values for the equipotent ratios of L-muscarine (relative to acetylcholine), at various postganglionic cholinergic receptors, vary from about 0.1 to 5.4. Marked activity (among isomers and analogues of muscarine) is restricted to those substances in which the arrangement of the methyl, the hydroxyl, and the onium side-chain groups is the same as in muscarine.

It may now be asked what further structural modifications of the acetyl-choline and muscarine molecules are compatible with the possession of strong acetylcholine-like activity. The data is only semi-quantitative, pending laborious experimental work. This is because the 'activity' of each substance is made up of two factors, the *efficacy* and the *affinity* (see. p. 259). Thus the cation of dimethylaminoethyl acetate (*13.50*), which is the unquaternized analogue of acetylcholine (*13.44*), has been described as having almost no muscarinic activity. Actually it has a higher intrinsic activity than acetylcholine, and its poor performance is due to its feeble affinity, which is a thousand times less than that of acetylcholine (Gloge, Lüllmann, and Mutschler, 1966).

                                                    CH₂
                                    Me₃N⁺—CH |
                      O   C—O—C—Me
Me₂N·CH₂·CH₂·O·C·CH₃   H   O

Dimethylaminoethyl acetate   2-Acetoxy*cyclo*propyl trimethylammonium
         (*13.50*)   (cation)
                                              (*13.51*)

H₃C   O   CH₂—N⁺Me₃
         (*13.52*)

2-acetoxy*cyclo*propyl trimethylammonium iodide (*13.51*) is of special interest as a substance in which the N – C – C – O structure of acetylcholine is held rigid by covalent bonds. It was obtained as a mixture of four isomers,

---

*However, conformational studies (by X-ray diffraction) of several substances with strong muscarinic action persuaded Chothia that muscarine could bind the receptor only by the nitrogen atom and the *C*-methyl group of (*13.49*) (Chothia, 1970).

whose configurations were determined by X-ray diffraction (Chothia and Pauling, 1970a). The (+) *trans*-isomer had the full muscarinic activity of acetylcholine, but the other isomers had very little activity. (The active isomer had only one per cent of the activity of acetylcholine at nicotinic sites, and the other isomers were even less active.) It was concluded that, at least for muscarinic activity, acetylcholine must adopt the IS–2S conformation (see p. 483) possessed by the active isomer of (*13.51*). 5-methyl-2-trimethylammoniomethylfuran (*13.52*) (5-methylfurmethide, or 5-methylfurtrethonium) has about the same amount of muscarinic activity as acetylcholine and almost no nicotinic activity (Armitage and Ing, 1954). As with muscarine, the ring is flat and rigid, and (thanks to the double-bonds) the $-CH_2$ portion of the $-CH_2N^+Me_3$-group is held firmly in the plane of the paper and hence the shape of the molecule is largely defined. It should be noted that the hydroxy-group of muscarine is *not* represented in this molecule, and no stereoisomers are possible. The X-ray crystallography of this substance has been reported (Baker, *et al.*, 1971) and the details in part resemble those reported for muscarine and acetylcholine, and yet so strongly differ in other ways as not to advance knowledge of the muscarinic conformation. Loss of the 5-methyl-group from (*13.52*) greatly lessens the muscarinic activity. As this loss must cause depletion of electrons from the ethereal oxygen atom, but no change in conformation, one may suspect that the electron-distribution exerts more control on muscarinic activity than conformation does. Also furmethide and 5-methyl-furmethide exemplify the five-atom side-chain rule (see below).

Great difficulty has been encountered in trying to prepare completely rigid agonists (Martin-Smith, Smail, and Stenlake, 1967). A closer look at the great conformational latitude of the acetylcholine molecule (*13.53*) may be appropriate here, to help follow the literature. The conformations of acetylcholine depend on the four torsion angles: C5-C4-N-C3, O1-C5-C4-N, C6-O1-C5-C4, and O2-C6-O1-C5. The first of these (from analogy with all similar structures) is probably invariable, an antiplanar extended chain with torsion angle of 180°. This invariance is caused by the steric hindrance exerted by the *N*-methyl-groups, and the restraint on closer packing imposed by van der Waals radii (see Section 8.0, p. 283). The last of these parameters (O2-C6-O1-C5) is also fixed because all ester-groups are planar, due to the C6-O1 bond. X-ray diffraction studies have shown that the other two torsion angles can vary greatly in the crystals of various acetylcholine agonists. Such studies have suggested to one group of workers that muscarinic activity requires only that C1 and C7 of acetylcholine (*13.53*) must be on the same side of the molecule (Baker *et al.*, 1971). Others, from similar evidence (coupled with that obtained from antagonists, which is necessarily of less significance), have postulated that acetylcholine reacts with muscarinic receptors through the ester oxygen atom as well as the ammonium cation (Beers and Reich, 1970).

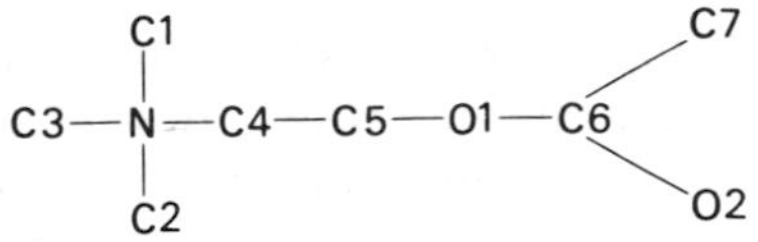

```
     C1                    C7
      |                   /
C3 — N — C4 — C5 — O1 — C6                 R — N⁺Me₃
      |                   \
     C2                    O2               (13.54)
        (13.53)
```

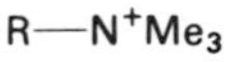

$R—N^{+}Me_{3}$

$$(13.54)$$

$$(13.53)$$

The cationic head of acetylcholine. It is useful to pause here and compare acetylcholine cations with inorganic cations likely to be present at the receptor surface. Whereas potassium has a stimulant action on all of the muscle, the action of acetylcholine is normally confined to the small end-plate region. The shielding effect of the alkyl-groups (on the nitrogen atom in a quaternary amine) ensures that the ion is virtually anhydrous in aqueous solution (Robinson and Stokes, 1959). Thus the effective ionic radius in solution may be taken as the same as the radius obtained from X-ray crystallography. It is seen from Table 13.1 that the tetramethylammonium ions has a radius of 2.41 Å, and this must also be the radius of the cationic head of acetylcholine.

Table 13.1

THE SIZE OF SOME CATIONS

Cation	Anhydrous radius (from crystal data)[a] Å	Supposed hydrated radius (from mobility in water at 25°C)[b] Å
Li^{+}	0.60	2.30
Na^{+}	0.95	1.79
K^{+}	1.33	1.22
NH_{4}^{+}	1.48	
NMe_{4}^{+}	2.41[c]	
Mg^{2+}	0.65	3.44
Ca^{2+}	0.99	3.05

[a]Pauling, 1960; [b]Hartley and Raikes, 1927; [c]Johnson, 1960.

Whereas the radius of every inorganic ion, in the anhydrous state, is well established, those of low mass are strongly hydrated in solution so that their effective radius is much greater. Just how much greater cannot be said because an exact method for measurement is lacking. However, the figures for Li^{+} and Na^{+} in the last column of Table 13.1 are indicative. There seems little doubt that the cation of acetylcholine is much broader than those of the monovalent inorganic cations which it might encounter near the receptor; the similarity to the presumed size of the hydrated calcium cation may indicate a significant competition. The head is the widest part of the ACh molecule: what happens if it is made wider?

Before discussing the effect of increasing the size of the cationic head of acetylcholine, we shall have to note the acetylcholine-like effect of simple aliphatic quaternary amines. These have only a feeble action on muscarinic sites, although their action on nicotinic sites is considerable (see below). Tetramethylammonium salts, for example, have only about one-thousandth of the activity of acetylcholine on the gut and heart (Clark and Raventós, 1937). Tetraethylammonium salts, and still higher homologues, are only antagonists. However, the series of alkyltrimethylammonium salts (*13.54*) is full of interest. Affinity for the receptor increases as the alkyl chain is lengthened, but efficacy falls from tetramethylammonium to ethyltrimethylammonium, and then climbs to a maximum at *n*-pentyltrimethylammonium [tested on mammalian gut: Stephenson (1956); van Rossum and Ariëns (1959); on frog's heart: Raventós (1937); on dog blood-pressure: Alles and Knoefel (1939)]. This, and related discoveries, led to the formulation of the 'five-atom rule' (see below). However, even the most potent members have no more than 1 per cent of the activity of acetylcholine.

Alterations to the cationic head of acetylcholine. Successive replacement of methyl-groups, in acetylcholine (*13.44*), by either hydrogen or ethyl causes a steep decline in parasympathomimetic activity of all kinds (Ing, 1949). It was pointed out above that replacement by hydrogen lowers affinity but increases efficacy. Ethyl, on the other hand, seems to increase affinity but lower efficacy (Barlow, Scott, and Stephenson, 1963). Tertiary amines, like (*13.50*), are at least 99 per cent ionized at pH 7.3. Hence the loss in affinity is not due to loss of basic strength. However, the acetylcholine receptors seem to require strong van der Waals linkages with the head-group of acetylcholine (Holton and Ing, 1949). All evidence suggests that a basin-like depression exists in the receptor and is shaped for the maximal van der Waals contacts from four carbon atoms tetrahedrally disposed on the quaternary nitrogen atoms (Belleau and Puranen, 1963).

The adverse effect of replacing three methyl- by three ethyl-groups has been observed in many other series of substances with acetylcholine-like properties (Barlow, 1964).

Although *simple* tertiary amines do not show marked muscarinic properties, this deficiency can be remedied if the remainder of the molecule binds powerfully to the receptor. Thus increased binding power can be given to the carbonyl-group if the lone pair of electrons on the oxygen atom is more strongly delocalized than it is in esters ($Y = OR$) in the resonance hybrid shown in (*13.55*). Amides ($Y = NH_2$ or NR_2) support this resonance much better, because nitrogen is better equipped than oxygen to carry a positive charge. The infrared absorption frequency of the carbonyl-group is considered to be a measure of this effect. As it decreases from the value typical of esters (1735 cm^{-1}) to that of amides (1690 for free, and 1650 for associated, amides), the muscarinic activity of tertiary bases, such as (*13.56*), rises steadily until it almost reaches that of quaternary

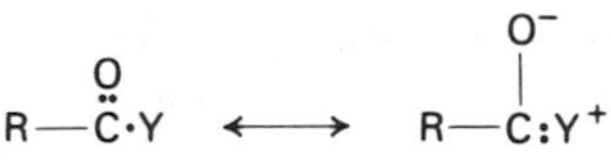

$$R—\overset{O}{\overset{\|}{C}}·Y \quad\longleftrightarrow\quad R—\overset{O^-}{\overset{|}{C}}:Y^+$$

(13.55)

$$\overset{O}{\overset{\|}{\big[}} N·CH_2·C\vdots C·CH_2·NMe_2$$

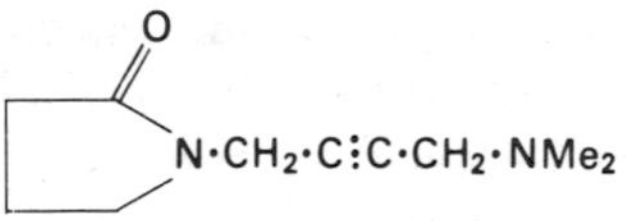

Tertiary base related to
oxotremorine
(13.56)

bases (the amide-group is contained in the pyrrolidone structure) (Bebbington, Brimblecombe, and Shakeshaft, 1966).

However, this is not the full story: arecoline (13.57), a most potent muscarinic drug, has a tertiary basic and an ordinary ester-group. Arecoline has a higher intrinsic activity than acetylcholine, but (like some other cyclic amines) is a more powerful drug than its quaternary (methyl) analogue, which has too high an affinity and is hence mainly inhibitory (Gloge et al., 1966). The structure-activity relationship of arecoline becomes clearer if studied in conjunction with 'Reversed acetylcholine' (13.62). Pilocarpine (13.58), another tertiary amine with an ester-group (actually it is a cyclic ester) has only moderately strong muscarinic activity tempered by some antagonistic effect (van Rossum et al., 1960).

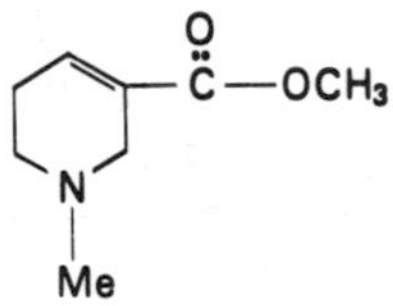

Arecoline
(13.57)

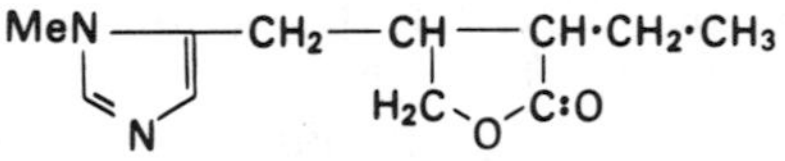

Pilocarpine
(13.58)

Analogues of acetylcholine in which the nitrogen atom is replaced by phosphorus or arsenic have only from 1 to 10 per cent of the activity of acetylcholine (at a variety of sites). This replacement of nitrogen does not alter the bond angles, but increases the mean distance between the methyl-groups by 27 to 35 per cent, because of the increased length of the $P-C$ and $As-C$ bonds (Holton and Ing, 1949).

The five-atom side-chain rule. The need for a chain of *five* atoms in order to achieve efficacy in acetylcholine-like substances was first conceived by Alles and Knoefel (1939), and consolidated by Ing (1949). In acetylcholine, and its analogues of the general type $R-^+NMe_3$, the most active member of any series of homologues is usually the one where R is a *five*-atom chain (excluding hydrogen atoms). This was discussed above for the case where R is an alkyl-group, but it is equally true if some of the carbon atoms are replaced, e.g. by oxygen. Thus acetylcholine (13.44) is much more active than formyl or propionyl-choline; and butyryl- and valeryl-choline have scarcely any muscarinic activity. Both the nitrous and the nitric esters of choline, which have such five-atom chains, have considerable muscarinic activity (Dale, 1914). The acetic esters of $HO \cdot CH_2 \cdot {}^+NMe_3$ and of $HO \cdot (CH_2)_3 \cdot {}^+ NMe_3$ are both less active than that of choline $(HO \cdot (CH_2)_2 \cdot {}^+ NMe_3)$ (Hunt and Taveau, 1911).

Similarly ethoxycholine [the ethyl ether of choline (*13.59*)] is more active than either the methyl or propyl ether (Dale, 1914); also, the *n*-propyl ether is the most active in the $HO \cdot CH_2 \cdot {}^+ NMe_3$ series. In the dioxolane (or 'acetal') series of substances with muscarinic action, e.g. (*13.60*), the compound in which R is Me is far more active than those in which R is H or Et (Fourneau *et al.*, 1944). The isomer illustrated [L(+)-*cis*] is six times as potent as acetylcholine (Belleau and Lacasse, 1964). For the factors underlying the five-atom rule, see under '*Antagonists of acetylcholine*', below.

$$H_3C—CH_2—O—CH_2—CH_2—N^+Me_3$$
$$\quad\quad\quad _4 \quad\quad _3 \quad _2 \quad\quad _1$$

Ethoxycholine (cation)
(*13.59*)

(*13.60*)

The optimal position for an oxygen atom in the side-chain.   The ether (*13.59*) has approximately 1 to 10 per cent of the activity of acetylcholine, and is more active at muscarinic than at nicotinic sites. This activity is diminished if the oxygen atom is moved from the 3- to the 2- or 4-position. The ketone (*13.61*) has little muscarinic (but from 0.2 to 100 per cent of the nicotinic) action of acetylcholine on various test preparations. If the carbonyl-group is moved from the 4- to the 3- or 2-position, the action is diminished (Ing, Kordik, and Williams, 1952). Thus both the ethereal and carbonyl oxygen atoms have maximal activity in the positions where they occur in acetylcholine (*13.44*).

The methyl ester of β-trimethylammoniopropionate (*13.62*) may be regarded as acetylcholine in which the order of the ethereal and carbonyl oxygen atoms has been reversed. It is a very poor substrate for acetylcholinesterase, and does not inhibit this enzyme. However, it has strong muscarinic and moderate nicotinic properties, as well as some small measure of individuality in the pharmacological properties (Bass *et al.*, 1950). The resemblance between this structure and that of arecoline (*13.57*) is noteworthy.

$$CH_3—\overset{\overset{\textstyle O}{\|}}{C}—CH_2—CH_2—CH_2N^+Me_3$$
$$\quad\quad\quad\quad _4 \quad\quad _3 \quad _2 \quad\quad _1$$

Ketone analogue of acetylcholine
(*13.61*)

$$CH_3—O—\overset{\overset{\textstyle O}{\|}}{C}—CH_2—CH_2—N^+Me_3$$

'Reversed acetylcholine'
(*13.62*)

Muscarone, obtained by oxidizing the secondary alcoholic-group in muscarine (13.49) to a carbonyl-group, not only has increased muscarinic properties, but considerable nicotinic properties also. It has both ethereal and carbonyl oxygen atoms, but more widely separated than in acetylcholine.

(b) *Nicotine and the nicotinic receptors for acetylcholine.*
It will be recalled that nicotine (7.18) mimics acetylcholine at two sites in vertebrates, (a) the neuromuscular junction of voluntary muscle (to be more exact, at the motor endplate of the muscle), and (b) at the ganglia of both sympathetic and parasympathetic nerves. Site (a) is the more accessible to it, as is evident when a mammal is poisoned by nicotine. However, in insects, which have no acetylcholine at the neuromuscular junction, nicotine exerts its principal effect on the ganglia of the central nervous system (Yaeger and Munson, 1945). Nicotine is now much less used as an insecticide. Nicotine-like insecticides have been synthesized (Kamiura et al., 1963): for high activity, an intact pyridine ring is required with a basic substituent (in the 3-position) which may be aliphatic, as in (7.19), but must not be quaternized because this prevents penetration. For an effect in mammals, quaternization of the pyrrolidine ring-nitrogen is permissible, but brings no advantage. The fact that nicotine, in excess, has an anti-acetylcholine (blocking) action on ganglia adds a difficulty to discovering the nature of the nicotinic receptor by using this alkaloid and its analogues (Barlow and Hamilton, 1962).

In general, it may be said that the requirements for nicotinic action are less rigid than those for muscarinic action. Simple quaternary salts are more effective at nicotinic, than at muscarinic, receptors. The ganglia are particularly susceptible. In the alkyltrimethylammonium series (13.54), maximal activity is reached at the *n*-pentyltrimethylammonium salts which are about eight times as active as acetylcholine (and about as active as nicotine) at nicotinic receptors (Willey, 1955). D-Lactoylcholine has strong nicotinic, but little muscarinic, potency (Sastry, Lasslo, and Pfeiffer, 1960). Phenolic ethers of choline, such as (13.63), have a strong nicotinic (but little muscarinic) activity (Hey, 1952); however, this ratio is reversed by inserting two methyl-groups into the two *ortho*-positions of the benzene ring, which gives xylocholine.

Tetramethylammonium salts and acetylcholine salts are equipotent at autonomic ganglia sites (Burn and Dale, 1915), but the former have only one-hundreth of this potency at the skeletal neuromuscular junction which is also a nicotinic site, and only one-thousandth at smooth muscle junctions (muscarinic). Only transient demands are made on the transmitter at autonomic ganglia, whereas a nerve-muscle junction requires a lingering action greatly facilitated by molecules that permit hydrogen-bonding as in acetylcholine. Apparently the tetramethylammonium cation is the only necessary effector-group in acetylcholine, and the rest of the molecule exists to supply extra bonding for those actions that do not take place quickly.

Using X-ray crystallography of acetylcholine and of the agonists that mimic it at nicotinic sites, a uniform conformation has been suggested for drugs with nicotinic action (Chothia and Pauling, 1970b; Chothia, 1970). A similar approach, leaning more on antagonists, which is always risky, has suggested a uniform conformation quite different from this (Beers and Reich, 1970, 1971).

The following evidence casts doubt on the assumption that the preferred conformations of nicotinic agonists are of overriding importance at the site of action. The great majority of these agonists have been found to carry a $-^+N \cdot C \cdot C \cdot O-$ group in the *gauche* (synclinal) conformation (Baker *et al.*, 1971; Culvenor and Ham, 1966; Canepa, *et al.*, 1966), whether studied in the solid state or in solution. One rare exception, carbachol (*2.11*) is *staggered* (antiplanar) in the crystal but *gauche* in solution (Barrnas and Clastre, 1970; Baker *et al.*, 1971). It has been assumed that the *gauche* conformation is fundamental to the action on the receptor of acetylcholine and related agonists.

This hypothesis is challenged by agonists containing the $-^+N \cdot C \cdot C \cdot S$ and $-^+N \cdot C \cdot C \cdot Se-$ groups which prefer the *staggered* (antiplanar) conformation, both in the crystal (Shefter and Mautner, 1969) and (on p.m.r. evidence) in solution (Cushley and Mautner, 1970). For example, cholinethiol and *S*-methylthiocholine (both *staggered*) are potent agonists whereas their oxygen analogues choline and *O*-methylcholine (both *gauche*) are not (Mautner, Bartels, and Webb, 1966). Moreover, replacement of the carbonyl oxygen of ACh by sulphur leaves the conformation *gauche* (Mautner, Dexter, and Low, 1972), and both acetylcholine and acetylthiocholine (*13.64*) are highly active in various biological tests (Scott and Mautner, 1967; Mautner *et al.*, 1966; Mautner, 1969). Thus it looks as if the resting conformation is not so important an ingredient of agonist activity as the electron distribution. It has been calculated that a receptor site need expend no more than one kilocalorie of energy to change the preferred *gauche* form of acetylcholine into the *staggered* form (Liquori, Damiani, and de Coen, 1968).

Choline phenyl ether
(*13.63*)

Acetylthiocholine
(*13.64*)

In an immunochemical approach to learning more about the receptor site, an antibody was prepared against choline phenyl ether (*13.63*) in the rabbit. Unfortunately, when this antibody was used as a model for nicotinic receptors, it was found unable to distinguish between muscarinic and nicotinic agents, nor between agonists and antagonists (Marlow, Metcalf, and Burgen, 1969).

Antagonists of acetylcholine. The connection between structure and activity of inhibitors is not so well defined as it is for agonists. The response of atropine (*7.14*) (the most studied antagonist of muscarinic action) to structural modifications was discussed in Section 7.3. The well-known principle that a stimulant may be turned into an antagonist by increasing the molecular weight is seen in the alkyltrimethylammonium homologues (*13.54*). Kinetic studies showed that all members of this series go on to the muscarinic receptor at the same rate, but the rate of dissociation from the receptor falls as the number of methylene-groups increases (see Section 10.3b, p. 356, for explanation). Hence, the lower members are pure muscarinic stimulants, but when $R = C_6H_{13}$ some residual atropine-like blocking is seen as well, and when $R = C_{12}H_{25}$ the action is purely atropinic (Paton, 1961). The intrusion of antagonistic action when R is > 5 may explain why a five-membered side-chain gives maximal muscarinic action in so many series (see above).

Ganglion-blocking activity in the polymethylene *bis*trimethyl-ammonium series is maximal when the two cationic heads are separated by five or six methylene-groups (Paton and Zaimis, 1949). Hexamethonium (*7.24*, $n = 6$), the most efficient ganglion-blocker in this series, competes with acetylcholine without causing any depolarization of the receptor (Paton and Perry, 1953).

The inter-nitrogen distance in hexamethonium was found by conductimetry to be 6.3 Å (Elworthy, 1963). If fully extended, hexamethonium would have an inter-nitrogen distance of about 9 Å.

Turning now to antagonists acting at the (voluntary) neuromuscular junction (a nicotinic site) two main types can be recognized. Members of the first class (e.g. tubocurarine) prevent acetylcholine from depolarizing the post-synaptic membrane but do not themselves possess any acetylcholine-like activity at this site. They are competitive with acetylcholine. The synthesis, liberation, and breakdown of acetylcholine are not interfered with, but this transmitter is excluded from its receptor, and hence profound muscular relaxation occurs. Because the cationic heads of tubocurarine (*2.6*) (which has only one quaternized amino-group) and gallamine (*7.23*) seem to be too sterically hindered to fit into an acetylcholine receptor, Waser (1960) assumed that these molecules merely cover a pore in which the acetylcholine receptor lies. The second class of antagonist at the neuromuscular junction, e.g. decamethonium (*7.20*) and suxamethonium (*7.21*), prevent acetylcholine from depolarizing the post-synaptic membrane but possess enough acetylcholine-like activity to cause depolarization before neuromuscular blockade sets in. These substances have unhindered trimethylammonium-groups; hence at least one end should be able to combine with the anionic site on the acetylcholine receptor, while the whole molecule is bulky enough to block the pore.

There is remarkable specificity in the affinities of these *bis*-onium salts towards the three main kinds of acetylcholine receptor. All of them are practically inactive at the postganglionic receptor; but activity at ganglia and at the neuromuscular junction is dramatic if, for each of these sites, the right homologue has been chosen. One hundred times that dose of decamethonium which completely blocks the neuromuscular junction does not affect the ganglia. Likewise, 100 times the dose of hexamethonium which blocks ganglia does not affect the neuromuscular junction (Paton and Zaimis, 1949, 1952). This specificity is illustrated in Table 13.2.

Table 13.2

THE SPECIFICITY OF *BIS* TRIMETHYLAMMONIUM CATIONS, OF DIFFERENT CHAIN-LENGTHS, FOR TWO IMPORTANT ACETYLCHOLINE RECEPTORS

(Potencies are relative; 1.0 is maximal for each site)

Type of cholinergic block	Number of methylene groups								
	4	5	6	7	8	9	10	11	12
Nerve-nerve junction	0.01	0.8	1.0	0.1	0.02				
Nerve-muscle junction	—	—	—	—	0.07	0.7	1.0	0.55	0.2

A drug which can combine with two sites at the one time should have a very high affinity because (a), when one end of the molecule dissociates and hence leaves the surface temporarily, the attached part must hold the liberated end within striking distance for recombination, and (b), van der Waals forces should cause the molecule to be strongly held on the biological surface that lies between the two binding sites. The introduction of ester groups into the molecules of *bis*-onium neuromuscular blockers strongly increases their ability to produce depolarizing inhibition. This effect becomes maximal in the compounds having 14–16 atoms in the inter-introgen chain (*13.65*). (Such compounds are simply esters of choline with dicarboxylic acids.) In this series, the second trimethylammonium group can be replaced by hydrogen without much reduction in potency (Danilov, *et al.*, 1974). One is led to expect that one trimethylammonium group in decamethonium could be replaced by another hydrophilic group (such as methoxy) without harm to the action, and that only one acidic group exists on the receptor for binding each molecule of this drug.

$$Me_3N^+-CH_2CH_2-O-\overset{O}{\overset{..}{C}}-(CH_2)_n-\overset{O}{\overset{..}{C}}-O-CH_2CH_2\cdot N^+Me_3$$

$$(13.65)$$

Pancuronium (dication)
$$(13.66)$$

$$Me_3^+N\cdot CH_2\cdot CH_2\cdot O\cdot \overset{O}{\overset{..}{C}}\cdot NH\cdot (CH_2)_6\cdot NH\cdot \overset{O}{\overset{..}{C}}\cdot O\cdot CH_2\cdot CH_2\cdot {}^+NMe_3$$

Carbolonium (dication)
$$(13.67)$$

The suxamethonium series (7.21) shows maximal activity when ten atoms separate the two quaternized nitrogens, and this provides vague information about the distance that separates the two binding groups (see below for clarification). More direct evidence is provided by pancuronium bromide (13.66) ('Pavulon'), a potent non-depolarizing neuromuscular blocking agent that has proved clinically useful (Baird and Reid, 1967). The evident rigidity of this molecule has been confirmed by n.m.r. in solution. X-ray crystallography reveals that the distance between the two nitrogen atoms is 11.08 Å, which should be compared with 10.7 Å, the $N^+ - N^+$ distance in the crystals of N, O, O'-trimethyl-d-tubocurarinium diiodide, and presumably this distance is the same in tubocurarine. It must be pointed out that pancuronium has much more of the acetylcholine structure than is found in the *bis*-onium series, in fact it has the sequence $Me\cdot CO(:O)\cdot CHR\cdot CHR\cdot N^+R_3$ twice over (Savage *et al.*, 1970).

In the crystal, where it lies fully extended, decamethonium (7.20) has an inter-nitrogen separation of 13.7 Å (Lonsdale, Milledge, and Pant, 1965), but it seems to be more puckered in solution [Elworthy (1963) found 9.5 Å by his conductimetric method]. Succinylcholine, flexible like all depolarizing agents, has given values from 7.8 to 11.9 Å for the inter-nitrogen distance in the crystal, depending on which anion forms the salt! The very flexibility of these agents permits the conformational change which seems to underlie the observed depolarization (Pauling and Petcher, 1973).

A cholinoreceptor sensitive to N-16-N compounds appeared earlier in the course of evolution, and is more widely spread in the animal kingdom. By 'N-16-N' is meant those *bis*-onium compounds where the two nitrogen atoms are separated by a chain of 16 atoms, not necessarily all carbon; examples: suberyldicholine and sebacinyldicholine; also carbolonium bromide ('Imbretil') which is used a little in human surgery. The neuro-muscular junctions of molluscs, echinoderms, and protochordates (Table 1.1) are inhibited by '16', but not by '10' compounds; some annelid worms respond to '10' inhibitors but all are inhibited by the '16' types. Amphibians respond more strongly to '16' than to '10' inhibitors; higher vertebrates are roughly equally sensitive to both types. The receptors for both '16' and '10' compounds, when both are present, must share some atoms, because it is not possible to block one type of receptor without blocking the other (Khromov-Borisov and Michaelson, 1966; Michelson and Zeimal, 1973). These results have led to a model in which each of four active sites on the muscle receptor contribute one anionic group to each corner of a square; in this hypothesis, the sides of the square anchor the '10' structures such as suxamethonium whereas the '16' structures sit on the diagonals (Khromov-Borisov and Michelson, 1966).

For further reading on the interaction of acetylcholine and its agonists and antagonists, with receptors, see Triggle and Triggle (1977); Cooper, Bloom, and Roth (1974).

13.7 Morphine, and the opioid receptors

The term opioid (synonym, *narcotic analgesic*) includes both natural and synthetic agents with morphine-type pain-relieving properties. Their action is exerted on the central nervous system and on smooth muscle.

Morphine, the principal analgesic alkaloid of opium, is the standard by which other opioids are measured. Simplification of the morphine molecule (*7.28a*) was briefly discussed in Section 7.3 (p. 246). Substances with mor-phine-like analgesic properties almost always have a quaternary carbon atom (i.e. one with no hydrogen directly attached to it). One of the groups attached to this saturated atom is usually a benzene ring, as such or occa-sionally as part of a larger ring-system, or else thiophen which is isosteric with benzene. Another of the groups is usually a tertiary nitrogen atom on a two-carbon chain (e.g. $-CH_2-CH_2-NMe_2$). An electron-attracting group (ketone, ester, double-bond) is also often present in analgesics. These features are clearly seen in the structure of methadone (*7.30*), pethidine (meperidine) (*7.29*), and also morphine, the molecule of which is in two planes, inclined to one another at about 70° (Mackay and Hodgkin, 1955).

Pethidine has no stereoisomers and, perhaps as a consequence, it has a rather weak analgesic action. The most potent of the synthetic analgesics, such as methadone (7.30), are optically active. Determinations of the stereochemistry of atom C-2 in the piperidine ring of morphine, by degradation (Corrodi and Hardegger, 1955) and by X-ray diffraction (Mackay and Hodgkin, 1955), have related this alkaloid to the D-series. Although it was originally thought that the aromatic ring in all synthetic analgesics must have an axial conformation (Beckett, 1959; Beckett and Casy, 1962), it is now clear that the steric relationship of the phenyl ring is often unimportant. It must be realized that earlier representations of the receptor site were made, in ignorance of this fact, before the ready availability of X-ray diffraction, nuclear magnetic resonance, and optical rotatory dispersion. Particularly when applied to the more rigid molecules, these new methods have thrown strong light on the problem.

The most convincing demonstration that analgesic action is independent of the conformation of the aromatic ring was furnished by the synthesis of 1-methyl-4-phenyl-*trans*-decahydro-4-propionoxyquinoline, where the two conformers [(13.68) equatorial and (13.69) axial] are separable and, because of close steric crowding, cannot be interconverted. Although possessing only one-tenth of the analgesic action of morphine (mouse), there was no difference in potency between the two conformers (Smissman and Steinman, 1966).

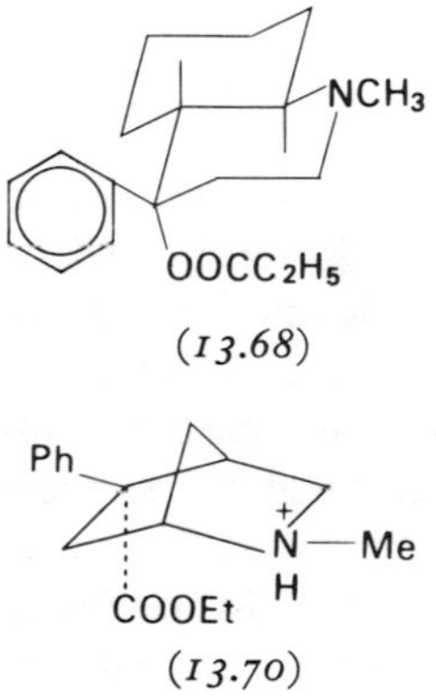

(13.68)

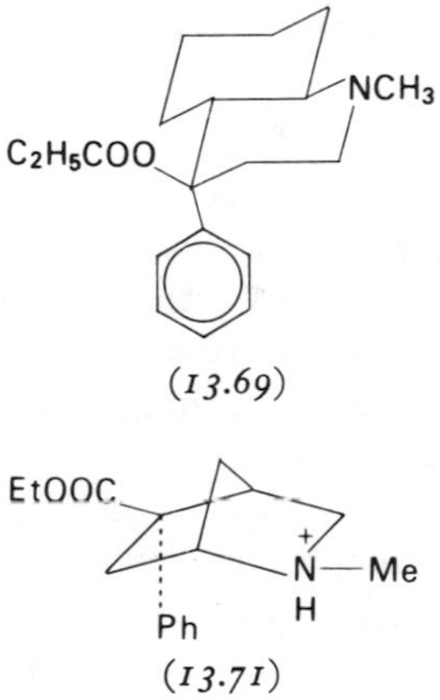

(13.69)

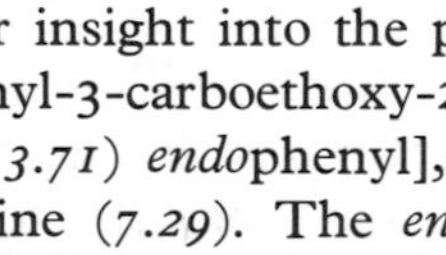

(13.70)

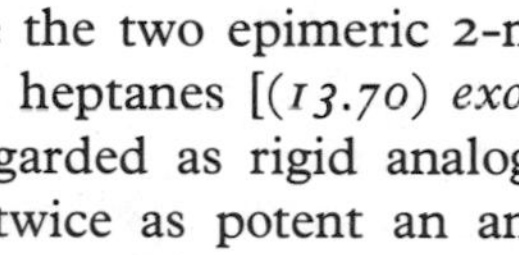

(13.71)

Another pair of rigid, non-interconvertible conformers have provided further insight into the problem. These are the two epimeric 2-methyl-5-phenyl-3-carboethoxy-2-azabicyclo [2.2.1] heptanes [(13.70) *exo*phenyl and (13.71) *endo*phenyl], which may be regarded as rigid analogues of pethidine (7.29). The *endo*phenyl-epimer, twice as potent an analgesic as pethidine, was four times as potent as the *exo*-epimer (13.70) (mouse). Analysis of the brain showed that it was penetrated twice as readily by the *endo*-epimer; in addition to this difference in partition coefficients between the two epimers, a difference of 0.16 unit was found in the pK_a values

(Portoghese, Mikhail, and Kupferberg, 1968). This work provides another example of a change in conformation of the aromatic ring having no drastic effect on analgesic activity. More importantly, it gives a timely reminder that physical properties change when conformations change, and that an altered physiological response may spring from these new properties rather than the mere change in shape of the molecule. On the evidence of this pair of substances, the conformational requirement for analgesia is low: the distance from the centre of the benzene ring to the nitrogen atom is about 6 Å for (*13.70*) but only 4 Å for (*13.71*), a truly enormous difference.

Because the molecule of morphine is rigid and undeformable, it should be capable of yielding information about the dimensions of groups in the morphine receptor. The first step is to nominate, in the morphine molecule, those features which observations on simpler analogues have indicated to be essential for analgesic action. There seem to be three such features: the benzene ring, the nitrogen atom, and possibly the α,β-unsaturated secondary alcohol. Using existing X-ray diffraction data, French workers have laboriously calculated many of the distances separating these centres in morphine and codeine, and corresponding ones in alphaprodine and methadone (Jung and Lami, 1970; Jung, Koffel, and Lami, 1971). Collectively, these measurements indicate a receptor of such elastic dimensions, that there must be more than one kind of analgesic receptor.

The opioid receptors.   Avram Goldstein first demonstrated the existence of an opioid receptor in the mouse brain by studying the stereospecific interactions of levorphanol (a morphine congener) and other morphine agonists, and the antagonist naloxone (*13.72*), on subcellular fractions (Goldstein, Lowney, and Pal, 1971). Partial purification furnished the receptor as a lipoprotein of estimated mass 60 000 daltons. It was suggested that combination of receptor with agonist (but not with antagonist) produces a conformational change that initiates the analgesic response. The existence of more than one kind of opioid receptor was suspected at this stage (Lowney, *et al.*, 1974). Pert and Snyder (1973) confirmed the presence of opiate receptors in nervous tissue and went on to demonstrate a differential effect exerted by sodium ions on the binding of opioid agonists and antagonists by the opioid receptor. Sodium ions, by increasing the number of sites available for antagonists, were thought to be reversing a conformational change favoured by agonists (Pert and Snyder, 1974).

Naloxone
(*13.72*)

What task has morphine to perform in its medicinal uses? Administration of a prostaglandin, either E_1 or E_2, to the rat brain elicited the main symptoms that morphine is used clinically to subdue, namely pain, diarrhoea, and cough. This was accompanied by liberation of cyclic adenosine monophosphate, a flux which was terminated by giving morphine in small doses (Collier and Roy, 1974).

The next question concerned the normal, physiological function of the opioid receptor, insofar as morphine is foreign to the animal organism. Hughes (1975) extracted from brain a pentapeptide (H-*tyr-gly-gly-phe-met*-OH), called *met*-enkephalin, which was accompanied by a small amount of a less active analogue in which the methionine was replaced by leucine. Both enkephalins mimic the ability of morphine to block muscular contractions (electrically evoked) of the ileum (guinea-pig) and vas deferens (mouse). They also inhibit the stereospecific receptor binding of an opiate antagonist, ^{3}H-naloxone (*13.72*), in brain homogenates. These substances were put into the brain of a living mouse with a cannula, because the enkephalins do not cross membranes, and are readily hydrolysed (in about 10 minutes) by brain enzymes. The more powerful of the two, *met*-enkephalin, was found only one twentieth as potent as morphine, but cross-tolerant with it (Hughes *et al.*, 1975). Swiss workers, by making stepwise changes to the molecule of *met*-enkephalin, have produced 'FK 33–824' which is 1000 times as potent as morphine by intra-cerebroventricular injection in laboratory animals (Roemer *et al.*, 1977), but has anaphylactoid side-effects in man.

Meanwhile interest had broadened to include natural polypeptides of higher molecular weight. C.H. Li had isolated lipotropin from brain tissue in 1964, and Guillemin of the Salk Institute (La Jolla, California) submitted this to partial hydrolysis (in 1966). Among the products was beta-endorphin, a polypeptide which contained the amino-acids of lipotropin from 61 through 91, and produced analgesia in rats, long-lasting and twice as intense as that produced by morphine. Naloxone (*13.72*) instantly abolished this analgesia. Laboratory hydrolysis of this endorphin gave *met*-enkephalin (residues 61–65).

Although no clear picture has yet emerged, there is a current tendency to think of enkephalins as neurotransmitters, and of beta-endorphin as a hormone that suppresses the output of many other neurotransmitters. It is not at all clear what might cause the body to liberate a pain-neutralizing substance under some conditions and not under so many others.

Up to the present, four different kinds of opioid receptors have been distinguished in mammals, each of them specific for particular kinds of opiates or of antagonists (Lord *et al.*, 1977). There are, for instance, sites activated by β-endorphin and enkephalin but not by morphine. In receptors that are activated by both enkephalin and morphine, the phenolic hydroxyl-group of each substance is probably bound to the same site.

Tolerance and dependence. The number and binding affinity of opioid receptors are the same in morphine-dependent rats as in controls. There is no increased breakdown of drug in tolerant animals (Klee and Streaty, 1974). Collier (1965) was the first to suggest that morphine inhibits a pathway, in the central nervous system, that depends on a serotoninergic synapse, leading to compensatory over-production of 5-HT. This causes (the hypothesis continues) unbearable irritability, requiring the dose of morphine to be raised to retrieve a former level of analgesia (Schulz, Cartwright, and Goldstein, 1974). This hypothesis is supported by the action of cyproheptadine, a specific blocker of 5-HT receptors, which abolishes most withdrawal phenomena (Opitz and Reimann, 1973). Long-term exposure to opiates evokes a compensatory adenylate cyclase activity which both Klee and Collier think can reinforce addiction.

The state of analgesia in mice, brought about by acupuncture and thought to be caused by release of endorphin, is lost when naloxone is injected (Mayer *et al.*, 1977; Pomeranz and Chiu, 1976). Patients receiving intra-cerebral electric stimulation, for relief of chronic pain, produce raised levels of circulating opioids (Terenius and Wahlstrom, 1978).

Although the induction of sleep is not an important action of the opioids, it is appropriate to mention the sleep-inducing nonapeptide '*dsip*' isolated from, and tested on, the rabbit brain. It is *trp-ala-gly-gly-asp-ala-ser-gly-glu* (Schoenenberger and Monnier, 1977).

*   *   *   *   *

For further reading on structure-activity relationships in morphine and its congeners, see Lewis, Bentley, and Cowan (1971); Robinson (1971); Casy (1970); for antagonists in this series, see Archer, Albertson, and Pierson (1973); and Kosterlitz, Collier, and Villarreal (1972).

13.8 Psychotherapeutic agents

Psycholeptic (mind-calming) drugs. The phenothiazine neuroleptic drugs, such as chlorpromazine (*13.73*), revolutionized the treatment of schizophrenia, formerely considered the most intractable form of insanity. Thanks to these agents, most schizophrenic patients now live at home instead of in an asylum, and very many are capable of earning a living. Before 1950, nearly two-thirds of schizophrenic patients admitted to hospital were still there two years later, whereas now less than 10 per cent remain in hospital. The benefit to society has exceeded even these economic gains by making it evident that the basis of mental illness is biochemical.

Drugs which act like the phenothiazines are variously called psycholeptics, ataractics, and neuroleptics. Although their action is strongly depressant, it is remarkably specific and consciousness is not clouded:

hence they are not related to the general biological depressants of Chapter 15. They are also called major tranquillizers, a vague name because anti-anxiety drugs (see below) are often called tranquillizers.

Chlorpromazine, introduced into medicine by the French surgeon Laborit (1952) for the management of surgical shock, was at once applied to the treatment of schizophrenia by Delay *et al.*, (1952). Eventually, long-acting forms of this type of therapy were devised for out-patients. Thus an injection of 25 mg of fluphenazine enanthate, dissolved in oil, provides maintenance therapy for 2–3 weeks. Fluphenazine is 10-{3-[4-(2-hydroxyethyl)piperazin-1-yl]propyl}-2-trifluoromethylphenothiazine.

The psycholeptic action, characteristic of these phenothiazines, was later found in other series, notably among the thioxanthenes [e.g. chlorprothixine (*13.74*), 'Taractan'], and the phenylbutyrophenones introduced by Janssen in Belgium about 1958 [e.g. haloperidol (*13.75*)]. To-day a distinction is made between the high-dose psycholeptics, such as chloropromazine and chlorprothixen, which have an additional sedative effect, and the low-dose psycholeptics, such as perphenazine, trifluoperazine, fluphenazine, haloperidol, and thiothixene, which have a strong, but purely psycholeptic, action.

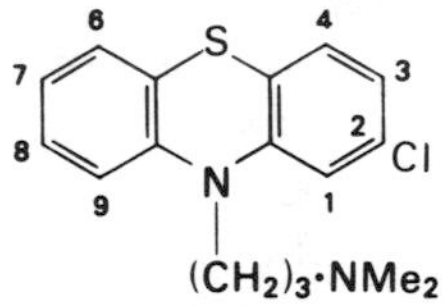

Chlorpromazine
(*13.73*)

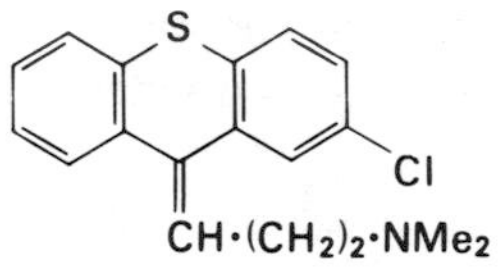

Chlorprothixene
(*13.74*)

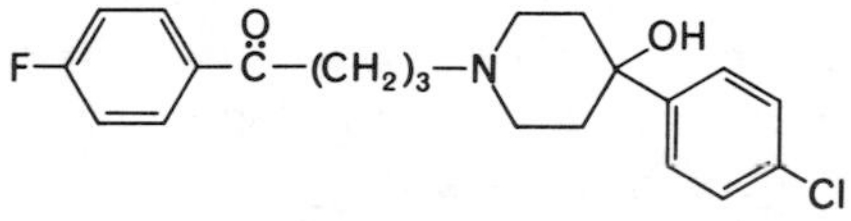

Haloperidol
(*13.75*)

It was found that psycholeptic drugs, such as haloperidol and chlorpromazine, block the dopamine receptor in mouse brain (Carlsson and Lundqvist, 1963; van Rossum, 1966), and this antagonism was found to take place also in the schizophrenic patient (Horn and Snyder, 1971). The clinically beneficial effects of flupethixol (a thioxanthene) are confined to the *cis*-isomer, the one that blocks the dopamine receptor *in vitro* (Crow and Johnstone, 1977). Patients overdosed with psycholeptics show parkinsonian symptoms. While there is little doubt that schizophrenia is accompanied by excessive and deleterious accumulation of dopamine in the striatum and possibly other parts of the brain, the biochemical cause of this disease may lie deeper. Many of the symptoms of schizophrenia seem to be derived from the cholinergic activity that dopamine provokes in the striatum.

The phenothiazines are readily oxidized to red free-radicals (Borg and Cotzias, 1962) but, at the present time, this is not thought to be correlated with their psycholeptic action. Unsubstituted phenazine, which was formerly much used as an oral anthelmintic in sheep, has been thought to owe its action to a stable free-radical formed in the worm (Craig *et al.*, 1960).

Anti-depressant drugs. Because a quite different class of psycho-therapeutic agent, the anti-depressant, shares the three-ring system with the psycholeptics, an exploration was made of the structure-action relations in the two systems (Wilhelm and Kuhn, 1970). The topology of the tricyclic skeleton determines the type of activity, but this is modified by the side-chain.

The shape of the skeleton (ring-system) is determined by four steric parameters: the bending angle α, the annellation angle β, the torsion angle γ, and the interatomic distance δ. Of these variables, the bending angle is most responsible for giving the drug its characteristic pharmacological action. A relatively flat molecule, such as a phenothiazine or thioxanthene ($\alpha = 25°$), has mainly neuroleptic (schizophrenia controlling) properties, whereas a decidedly bent skeleton, such as a dibenzo*cyclo*heptadiene (55°), imidodibenzyl (55°), or dibenzdiazepin (65°), produces thymoleptic (anti-depressant) drugs. The bending angle α is defined as the angle which the planes of the two lateral aromatic rings would make if projected towards one another. It is 0° for a totally planar molecule like anthracene, and would be 90° if the two lateral rings were inclined at a right angle to one another. The annelation angle β is defined as the rotation of the two lateral aromatic rings away from a straight line. It is 0° for dihydroanthracene, 60° for dihydrophenanthrene, and 40° for imidodibenzyl. The torsion angle γ measures any twisting of the planes of the two lateral aromatic rings relative to one another. Torsion is introduced by the presence of a seven-membered central ring; it varies only between 0° and 20° in the drugs under discussion.

X-ray diffraction analysis has shown that an unbranched side-chain, exactly three carbon atoms in length, conserves the psycholeptic or anti-depressant effect originated by the skeleton; departure from this rule introduces hypnotic properties. This chain needs to be free to take up a position where its terminal basic group can be near (for psycholeptic action) or actually overlap (for anti-depressant action) a benzene ring. These structures seem to indicate small, and yet smaller, receptor cavities for these two kinds of biological activity.

Typical tricyclic antidepressants are amitryptyline ('Laroxyl') (*13.76*) (a dibenzo*cyclo*hexadiene), and imipramine (*3.30*) (an imidobibenzyl). Consideration of the principles demonstrated by Wilhelm and Kuhn has led to more rigid molecules, such as the potent anti-depressant maprotoline ('Ludiomil') now entering clinical use. In general, tricyclic antidepressants tend to have a pK_a near to 10, and a partition coefficient of 4 in the system octanol/water. They inhibit the uptake of noradrenaline and 5-hydroxy-tryptamine into presynaptic membranes in the central nervous system, and their therapeutic action seems to depend on this (Iversen, 1971).

Amitryptyline
(13.76)

Diazepam
(13.77)

Anti-anxiety drugs.   The most used of the anxiolytics are the benzo-diazepines which not only relieve anxiety, and relax skeletal muscle, but can suppress convulsions, all accomplished apparently by augmenting the inhibitory transmission effected by gamma-aminobutyric acid in the spinal cord (Choi, Farb, and Fischbach, 1977). Discovered in 1933, the benzodiazepines gained clinical acceptance about 1965 (Zbinden and Randall, 1967). The first used member was chlordiazepoxide ('Librium'), followed by the simpler, but more potent, diazepam (13.77) ('Valium'). Some think that diazepam is a pro-drug for oxazepam ('Serax') which is a N-demethylated and 3-hydroxylated metabolic product, and is frequently prescribed as such. Related benzodiazepines such as nitrazepam ('Mogadon') and flurazepam are much used as hypnotics in the place of barbiturates.

Workers in Denmark claim to have found the receptor for benzodiaze-pines in the human brain (autopsy material); the cerebral and cerebellar cortical regions contain the highest density. Half-saturation by ^{3}H diazepam was obtained at the very low concentration of 2.6 nM. The potencies of 21 related substances ran parallel to their ease in displacing this labelled diazepam. The receptor had no feature in common with the opioid receptor, but its physiological functions are not yet known (Braestrup, Albrechtsen, and Squires, 1977). However Young *et al.*, (1974) found that the pharmaco-logical and behavioural action of a series of 21 benzodiazepines correlated with their ability to displace bound [3H] strychnine from synaptosomes, obtained from the rat brain stem, and thought to be rich in the glycine receptor. Others think hypoxanthine normally occupies the receptor.

For further reading on the benzodiazepines, see Garattini, Mussini, and Randall, 1973.

13.9 Conclusion

The study of steric factors has clearly contributed much to the understanding of structure-action relationships in biologically active agents,
and is also beginning to provide information about the nature of the various
receptors, some of which have been discussed in this chapter. Yet other
receptors have been investigated by similar competitive methods, among
them those for insulin and thyroxin. It may safely be said that the present
interest in this subject will continue to grow as its ability to throw light on
the action of agonists is appreciated. Meanwhile, as if in expectation of
early, definite knowledge of receptors (perhaps even of a ready supply
of purified receptors), the old, conjectural diagrams of receptor sites
(like Fig. 13.3) are vanishing from the literature (but for a collection of them,
see Ehrenpreis, Fleisch, and Mittag, 1969).

For further reading on steric factors, see Bentley (1969).

14 Surface chemistry.
The modification of membranes
by surface-active agents

The intense cytological studies of the last two decades have shown that cells, as well as most of the organelles within them, are covered with lipoprotein membranes (see Section 5.2). It is now widely thought that life is possible only because of the presence of these biphasic membranes (lipophilic within, and often hydrophilic on both outer surfaces), which provide for the separation of reactants. They also impose on the sequence of reactions an order that would otherwise be almost impossible to arrange. Often in, but sometimes apart from, these membranes, enzymes offer surfaces of the very greatest biological importance.

Macromolecules, including enzymes and other large protein molecules, whether particulate or 'dissolved' in the bulk phase, present interfaces for reactions. Human blood serum, which has 100 m² of protein surface in each cubic centimetre, exemplifies the large interfaces available in protein 'solutions'.

14.0 Surface phenomena *in vitro*

The short-range (van der Waals) forces, described in Section 8.0, exert an attraction between all molecules which are in contact with one another. The presence of these forces in liquids becomes particularly evident at surfaces. Molecules in the bulk of the liquid are subject to these forces equally and in all directions. However, the molecules located at an air-water interface experience almost no force from the gas phase, so that the attractive forces of the liquid phase are unopposed. Hence the molecules of the surface layer tend to be pulled into the bulk phase, and the surface is forced to assume the least area possible (this explains the spherical shape of gas bubbles and drops of liquid). The situation is shown in Fig. 14.1a. Constant exchange is taking place between those solvent molecules that are in the surface and those in the bulk phase.

A liquid-liquid interface (i.e. the surface between two immiscible liquids) behaves something like an air-water surface, but the contrast in pull exerted on the interfacial molecules is naturally much less. The surface tension at such an interface is often near to the difference of the individual tensions of the two liquids at the air-liquid interface.

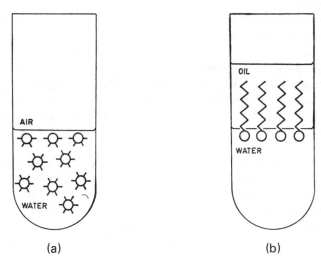

(a)   (b)

FIG. 14.1 (a) Diagram showing the unequal attractions experienced by molecules at the air-water interface.
(b) Orientation of an amphiphilic substance at an oil-water interface.

Amphiphilic substances tend to become concentrated at interfaces. The molecules of these substances often consist of a long hydrocarbon chain attached to a short head which is polar. In most cases this head owes its polarity to the presence of oxygen or nitrogen atoms, and the lone pairs of electrons on these atoms form hydrogen bonds with water molecules. The hydrocarbon tail, on the other hand, can only be accommodated in the aqueous phase by breaking hydrogen bonds between water molecules, which energetically oppose this fission. Hence amphiphilic molecules find their position of least energy at the oil-water interface where the hydrophilic head groups can remain in the water, and the lipophilic chains can enter the oil where they associate freely with the similar chains of the solvent (see Fig. 14.1,b). It will be evident that such a concentration of the amphiphile must stop as soon as a monomolecular layer of it is present at the interface. However, such a monolayer is always the site of turbulent exchange with other molecules of the amphiphile which are seeking places at the interface. Such an interface has a reduced surface tension and can easily become deformed. Both soluble and insoluble substances can be accumulated at interfaces.

It has long been recognized that factors operating at surfaces, especially orientation of molecules and increased concentration, can lead to chemical behaviour differing markedly from that observed in a bulk phase (Adam, 1941). For example, the molecules in a surface film of the *trans*-isomer of an unsaturated aliphatic acid can be pressed together so tightly that permanganate ion in the underlying aqueous phase does not reach the double-bonds. Hence only the *cis*-isomer is oxidizable under these conditions, whereas both isomers are oxidized at the same rate in a bulk phase (Rideal, 1945).

Micelles. Dilute aqueous solutions of surface-active substances have normal physical properties, but at a higher concentration (characteristic for each substance) there occurs an abrupt change in surface tension, osmotic pressure, and electrical conductivity. These changes are due to the formation of a new, dispersed phase which takes the form of aggregates named micelles. These are often roughly spherical: the hydrocarbon chains are in the interior of the sphere and the hydrophilic groups occupy the outside of the micelles in contact with the solvent water. The lowest concentration at which micelle formation occurs is called the *critical micelle concentration*.

For further reading on colloidal dispersion and micelles, see Mittal (1975).

14.1 Surface phenomena and drug action. Diuretics. Cardiac glycosides. Other ionophoric effects

Because most drugs are acting at surfaces, it is often said that the physical properties of these agents would have more biological significance if measured after adsorption on monomolecular films. Interesting results have been obtained in this way, but too few to form a coherent picture. This slow development is due not only to the scarcity of workers with both physical and biological backgrounds, but it also arises because some of the fundamental laws of surface chemistry remain incompletely known.

Micellar equilibria. A section of surface chemistry that offers few difficulties, and can greatly assist the study of selective toxicity, is the investigation of equilibria between monomers and micelles in aqueous solution. For example, the ions of agents with molecular weight over 150 usually polymerize reversibly to form micelles in concentrated solution. Examination of the effect of substituents on the *critical micelle concentrations (c.m.c)*, and relating this to biological activity, is a potentially rewarding field. Convenient methods for the investigation of c.m.s. include high-precision optical interferometry, deviations from Beer's Law (proportionality between concentration and optical density) in the ultraviolet, search for maxima in specific conductivity (a micelle is a better conductor than the ions of which it is composed), and detection of a sudden, relative decrease in gegen-ion (e.g. Cl^- or Na^+) concentration as the concentration of the drug is increased.

The use of soaps to solubilize phenols in water, for use as disinfectants, depends on the formation of *mixed micelles* of the soap and the phenol. It has been found that variation in the proportion of soap to phenol leads to several zones, as shown in Fig. 14.2 (Berry, Cook, and Wills, 1956). The first of these exists below 0.03 M potassium laurate and is poorly bactericidal; the maximal bactericidal effect is obtained when the soap reaches 0.03M, a figure which is identical with the critical micelle concentration for this soap. It was concluded that this bactericidal action is a combined attack of the phenol (mainly) and the soap on the protoplasmic membrane (see Section 14.2 for membrane damage). The next zone, up to 0.045 M soap, is one of greatly diminished bactericidal effect. The interpretation is that the phenol has entered the micelles, many more of which must have formed, and hence little of it is available for disinfection. When still more soap is introduced, a final zone (vigorous disinfection) appears, due to the toxicity of the soap itself. All the phenols commonly used as disinfectants, including *p*-chloro-*m*-xylenol, form zones like these.

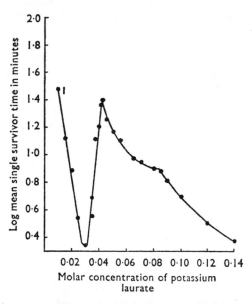

FIG. 14.2 Bactericidal action at 20°C of 4-benzylphenol (0.0016 M) in aqueous potassium laurate (concentration varied, as shown). Organism: *E. coli*, 2×10^9 organisms per ml. (Berry *et al.*, 1956).

The anthelmintic action of phenols is similarly potentiated by soaps and again it is important to avoid excess of the soap, because micelles can retain most of the phenol and deny it to the worms (Alexander and Trim, 1946). Below the critical micelle concentration of the soap, an adjuvant effect of the soap on the phenol is observable. No soap penetrates into the worms.

The formation of mixed micelles is well known in physical chemistry. An example: potassium myristate (C_{14}) develops micelles at one-quarter the concentration at which potassium laurate (C_{12}) does. Because of mixed micelle formation, as little as 15 per cent of potassium myristate halves the critical micelle concentration of potassium laurate (Klevens, 1948).

A related phenomenon is the accumulation by serum albumin of drugs of sufficiently high oil/water partition coefficients (Brodie and Hogben, 1957) as discussed in Section 3.3 (p. 76). The following recounts a further variant. Several species of bacteria require oleic acid for growth, but are inhibited by more than faint traces. However, in the presence of serum albumin, they will tolerate several hundred times the usual bacteriostatic concentration. This is because each molecule of albumin can bind nine molecules of fatty acid so tightly that the acid is no longer even haemolytic. Yet the mixed micelles remain in equilibrium with enough free oleic acid to nourish the bacteria (Davis and Dubos, 1947).

The destructive effect of phenol on the human skin was ameliorated by the introduction of lipophilic (alkyl- or chloro-) groups into the molecule, a change initiated by Bechhold and Ehrlich (1906). Because these are lipophilic groups, those phenols which are least harmful to the skin are the most strongly antagonized by serum, because, having higher oil/water partition coefficients, they enter the albumin core. Solutions of *p*-chloro-*m*-xylenol, a typical chlorinated phenol, are widely used for rapidly disinfecting intact skin and mucous membranes, but are harmful if used out of this context.

Micelle formation of phospholipids and bile salts plays an important part in the transport, by solubilization, of fatty material in the blood-stream and small bowel respectively.

For further reading on micelles and their biological importance, see Elworthy, Florence, and Macfarlane, 1968.

Plasma membranes. Lamellar, and partly micellar, mosaics of lipids and proteins form a thin, semi-permeable membrane around the exterior of every cell, and also around each organelle in the cell (see Section 5.2). The permeability of natural membranes was discussed in Section 3.1. The interaction of these membranes with diuretics, cardiac glycosides, and other ionophoric effects will now be considered.

Diuretics. Changing the permeability of the membrane that lines the kidney tubules is fundamental to the action of most diuretics. An activated process, which pumps sodium ions from the urine into the renal tubules, utilizes the mercapto-groups in the protein of the membrane. If these groups are blocked by the mercuric cation, a decreased resorption of salt and water occurs. The action of the mercurial diuretics, such as mersalyl ('Salyrgan'), is commonly attributed to the formation of Hg–S bonds in the kidneys (e.g. Baba, Smith, and Townshend, 1966). That organic mercurial diuretics act by liberation of the inorganic mercuric ion (Hg^{2+}) was shown by Clarkson, Rothstein, and Sutherland (1965), who injected rats with [203]Hg-labelled chloromerodin. The highest concentration of this drug was found in the kidney on the first day, but there was little diuresis. Maximal diuresis occurred on the third and fourth days after injection when no detectable amount of chloromerodin could be found in extirpated kidneys, but they were rich in Hg^{2+}. Mercurial diuretics are reviewed by Cafruny (1968).

Modern diuretics contain no mercury. Many of them, like amiloride (N-amidino-3,5-diamino-6-chloropyrazine-2-carboxamide) and the pteridine diuretic, triamterene ('Dytac') (14.1), act on the membrane lining the distal tubule, preventing resorption of sodium ions (and hence of water) (Crabbé, 1968; Wiebelhaus et al., 1965). The simpler molecule 2,4-diamino-6,7-dimethylpteridine is almost as active. Others, like frusemide and ethacrynic acid, seem to act somewhat similarly. It is less certain that the thiazides, such as (14.2), act in this way. For more information on the action of diuretics, see Suki, Eknoyan, and Martinez-Maldonado (1973).

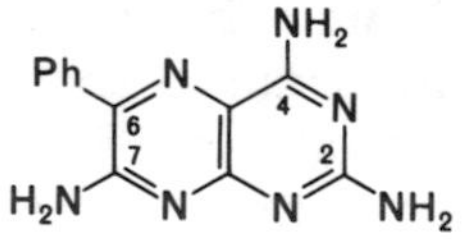

Triamterene
(14.1)

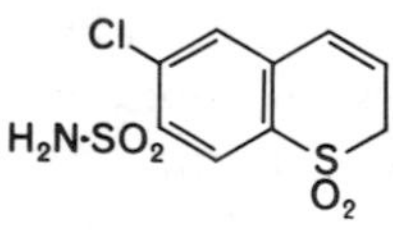

Chlorothiazide
(14.2)

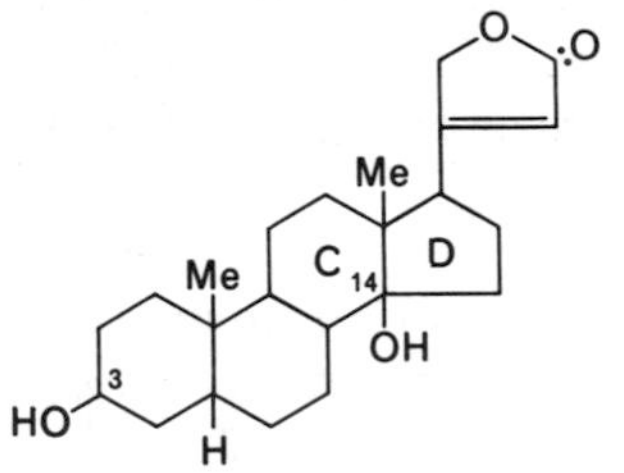

Digitoxigenin
(14.3)

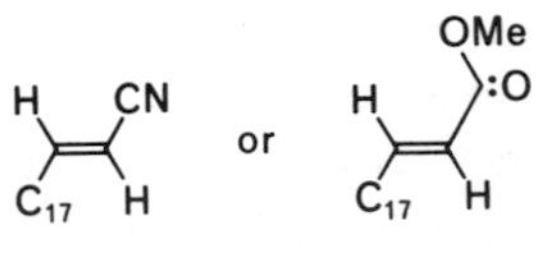

Non-lactone cardioactive
steroids
(14.4)

Cardiac glycosides.   The most used sources of these are two species of Digitalis (foxglove), and various species of Strophanthus (for ouabain). All these glycosides have a 19-carbon steroid nucleus (see Section 13.2

for chemistry). The β-hydroxy-group at C-14 ensures the unusual *cis* junction of rings C and D which some think is important for the positive inotropic (muscular-contracting) action which these drugs reinforce in patients with failing hearts. A much-used example, digitoxin, is the glycoside of a steroid aglycone called digitoxigenin (*14.3*), and has one molecule of glucose and three of digitoxose bound in the 3-position. The presence of sugar moieties greatly improves the uptake and distribution of the glycosides as contrasted with the aglycones (Wright, 1960).

After oral administration, some molecules of the glycoside reach the heart where they strongly inhibit the enzyme sodium-potassium adenosinetriphosphatase (Bonting, 1970). Either this enzyme is the glycoside receptor, or it undergoes a conformational change by being next to the receptor. When fractions containing this enzyme were extracted from the hearts of various mammals, dosed with tritiated glycosides, it was found that those species (such as man and dog) which are highly sensitive to cardiac glycosides, showed a high degree of association between the glycoside and the enzyme. Other species (such as rat) with only a low sensitivity to the glycosides, showed little affinity for the analogous enzyme (Schwartz, Matsui, and Laughter, 1968). The same authors showed that chemically related but inotropically inactive glycosides did not become bound to the human enzymes.

It is commonly supposed that when this enzyme becomes inhibited, the concentration of sodium ions builds up in the cell, causing calcium ions to be liberated during contraction (Klaus and Lee, 1969). (The nerve impulse which initiates each heart beat does so by releasing about 50 micromoles of calcium ions per kilogram of heart. This Ca^{2+} interacts with troponin, and then is removed from the scene by the sarcoplasmic reticulum.) Opposed to this view, that cardiac glycosides deliver extra calcium to the contractile apparatus, evidence has recently been presented that the inhibition of Na^+K^+-ATPase does not happen at therapeutic dose levels, and that these levels actually stimulate this enzyme, leading to increased ingress of potassium ions (Godfraind and Ghysel-Burton, 1977).

The prominence of the lactone ring in cardiac glycosides prompted the examination of simpler lactones for inotropic activity. Following preliminary work by Chen in 1942, Giarmann (1949) examined 28 simple, nonsteroidal lactones and found one with about 5% of the activity of the best cardiac glycosides. However, later work showed that the lactone ring in the glycosides can be substituted by unsaturated ester or nitrile groups without loss of biological activity (Thomas, Boutagy, and Gelbart, 1974). Both the stereochemical and the electronic requirements are stringent, leading to a postulated 2-point binding on the receptor. [See (*14.4*) for examples of activity-retaining substituents.]

An important question remains: why do cardiac glycosides selectively affect the heart although they are distributed from the bloodstream to the liver and kidneys also? The answer seems to be that, of these organs, the heart muscle is susceptible to far lower concentrations, because the analogous enzymes in other types of muscle do not take up the glycosides.

It is remarkable that *Erythrophleum* alkaloids, so completely different chemically, have a physiological action identical to that of the cardiac glycosides, although little is yet known of the molecular basis (Thorp and Cobbin, 1967). The margin of safety with all cardiac glycosides is very small, and it is most unlikely that, if they were newly discovered drugs, they would receive a government licence for clinical use. Nevertheless, patients, many of them elderly and frail, have had their lives extended for many years by the intelligent use of these agents, and fatalities are extremely rare. For all that, discovery of new, more-selective types, preferably with a non-steroid nucleus, would be warmly welcomed.

Other ionophoric effects. Although diuretics and cardiac glycosides are concerned with the transfer of ions, they are not themselves ionophores. Even Na^+K^+-ATPase is probably not an ionophore, although it must supply the energy for the ion-transfer. The fact is that the natural ionophores acting in mammals are not yet very well known. A K^+/Ca^{2+} ionophore, from mitochondria, was found to be a peptide of mol. wt. 1600 (Blondin *et al.*, 1977), and a calcium-specific ionophore, a peptide of mol. wt. 3000, was later isolated from this source (Jeng *et al.*, 1978). Gramicidin (see below) can transfer sodium and potassium ions into mitochondria, but is normally found only in bacteria. Prostaglandins and the oil-soluble vitamins are also suspected of playing ionophoric roles in mammals.

In contrast to the process of chelation (Chapter 11) in which a hydrogen ion on the ligand is replaced by an inorganic cation, transportation by ionophores requires only a stepwise replacement of the water molecules (attached to the co-ordination sphere of the cations) by the ionophore. The energy of desolvation must be compensated by the ionophore's binding energy. First the solvated cation must strike, through thermal agitation, the polar ligand groups of the ionophore, which then enfolds the cation, so that the complex presents a wholly lipophilic exterior to the plasma membrane which then accepts it. The conformational change of enfolding the cation is fast, but has been measured (for valinomycin) by relaxation techniques, such as sound-wave absorption, or fast temperature jumps (Grell, Eggers, and Funck, 1972).

Several fungal metabolites have been found which enhance the passive uptake of potassium. Some, like nonactin and monactin (*14.5*), are macro-tetrolides; others, like valinomycin, are depsipeptides. Valinomycin (from *Streptomyces fulvissimus*) is a macrocycle (mol. wt. 111) composed of three residues of each of L-valine, D-valine, L-lactic acid, and D-α-hydroxy-*iso*valeric acid, linked alternately by ester and amide bonds to form a 36-membered ring (Shemyakin *et al.*, 1963). It is soluble in lipids but insoluble in water. The perimeter of this flat molecule is lipophilic whereas the interior has a large hole surrounded by uncharged hydrophilic groups. The uptake of K^+ produces a conformational change which yields a bracelet-shaped molecule.

Valinomycin assists potassium ions to penetrate erythrocytes, mito-chondria (Moore and Pressman, 1964), and bacterial plasma membranes (Harold and Baarda, 1967) but has little effect on the permeability of sodium, lithium, or hydrogen ions. Nonactin acts similarly, but monactin also slightly assists the permeability of sodium (Henderson, McGivan, and Chappell, 1969).

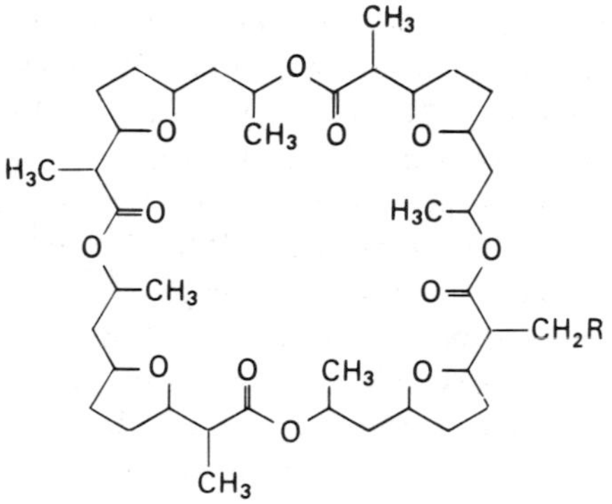

(a) Nonactin (R = H),
(b) Monactin (R = Me)
(14.5)

X-ray diffraction studies have shown that nonactin co-ordinates a potassium ion by four ether and four carbonyl oxygen atoms (Dobler, Dunitz, and Kilbourn, 1969), whereas valinomycin uses six carbonyl oxygens. The previously hydrated potassium ion is thus provided with a totally lipoid exterior which enables it to pass more easily into the cell membrane. In the collisions of this complex with the distal membrane-water boundary, a small percentage of the molecules pass through, and some of the potassium ions manage to exchange the nonactin molecule for water (this is the slow stage of the penetration). It will be realized that an anion (say, Cl^-) must accompany K^+ on these travels, but at a little distance, and constantly undergoing exchange. The preference of nonactin for K^+ (over Na^+) depends on the lower energy of dehydration of the former ion rather than on the dimensions of the central cavity (Prestegard and Chan, 1970).

Alamethacin, a cyclic polypeptide formed from 18 aminoacids, produces transient ion-channels in artificial lipid membranes. The time course of the rise and fall of electrical conductance in this system is studied as a model for potassium conductance in axons, and for one phase of the action of trans-mitters at synapses (Mauro, Nanavati, and Heyer, 1972).

Avatec (*14.6*) (X-537A, 'Lasalocid') is a poly-ether ionophore isolated from a *Streptomyces* found in New England soil (Berger, *et al.*, 1951). Chemically it is a substituted tetrahydropyranyl-tetrahydrofurylheptyl-derivative of salicylic acid, mol. wt. 591. X-ray diffraction of the barium salt showed that every oxygen (except the salicylic hydroxy-group) is bound to the cation. Many chemically-altered analogues have been made and their pKs and partition-coefficients recorded (Westley *et al.*, 1973). This substance readily transports calcium ions (and also catecholamines) through biological membranes (Pressman and Guzman, 1974). Its inotropic effect on the heart (Osborne, Wenger, and Zanko, 1977) is reminiscent of that evoked by digitalis, but the selectivity seems to be borderline. It is in regular use, however, as a remedy for the protozoal disease coccidiosis in fowls.

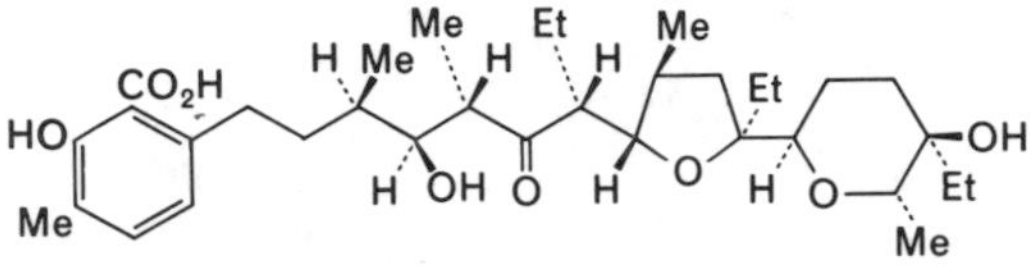

Avatec
(X-537 A)
(*14.6*)

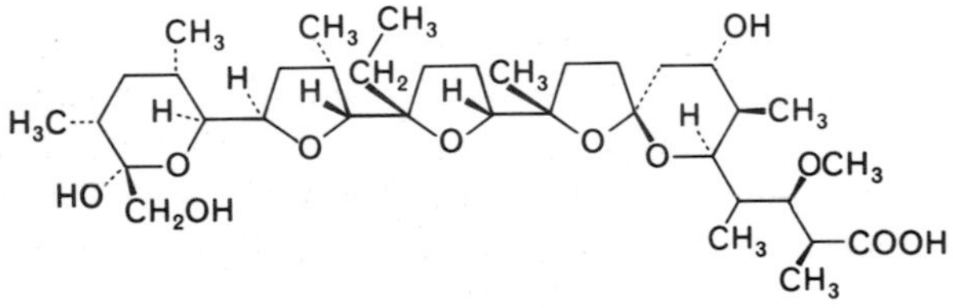

Monensin
(*14.7*)

Valinomycin and nonactin are electrically neutral, cause mitochondria to swell (apparently by forming channels), and generally accelerate the passage of cations *into* cells. A very different type of ionophore is represented by monensin and nigericin, which are acids, cause mitochondria to contract, and generally accelerate the passage of cations *out* of cells (Wipf and Simon, 1970). Monensin (*14.7*) ('Coban') was isolated from *Streptomyces cinna-monensis*. Chemically it is a fully hydrogenated pyranyl-furyl-furyl-dioxa-spirodecyl derivative of butyric acid, mol. wt. 670 (Lutz, Winkler, and Dunitz, 1971). The sodium salt is more soluble in hydrocarbons than in water. It is used to promote growth of cattle, acting by changing active transport in anaerobic rumen bacteria, which favours survival of strains which produce nutritive aliphatic acids. It is also used to treat coccidiosis in chicks.

Simple and inexpensive synthetic chemicals, known as 'Crowns', show great specificity in transporting alkali and alkaline earth metal cations from aqueous to lipophilic solvent layers. One of the most active is (*14.8*), which is, essentially, two molecules of 1,2-dihydroxy*cyclo*hexane fused with two molecules of diethyleneglycol. The complexing power of the Crowns is relatively low, that of (*14.8*) with K^+ being only 2, even though the cation is gripped by six oxygen atoms (Izatt *et al.*, 1971). Crowns can render lipophilic such unpromising substances as potassium hydroxide and permanganate. The Crown illustrated here prefers potassium to sodium, but one with a slightly smaller ring prefers sodium, and a still smaller one lithium. Conformational changes often accompany their uptake of salts (Pedersen, 1970).

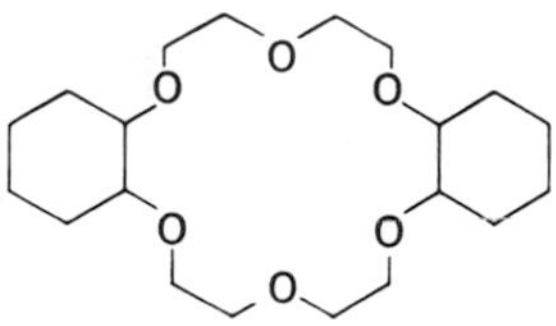

Di*cyclo*hexyl-18-crown-6
(*14.8*)

The Crowns were found in the U.S.A. The 'Cryptates', a more recent French discovery, are mixed ether-amine macrocycles that not merely encircle the salts of inorganic cations, as Crowns do, but actually surround them in all directions, leading to somewhat tighter binding (Lehn, Sauvage, and Dietrich, 1970), and to very strong binding of strontium *vis à vis* calcium. Of the alkali metals, potassium is often preferred to sodium and lithium.

The Crowns and Cryptates tend to be host-toxic. Example (*14.8*) is a skin and eye irritant and higher homologues affect the central nervous system (Pedersen, 1972). So far, they have not found much application in therapy.

14.2 The injury of membranes by biologically-active agents

Cholesterol, in various proportions, is a natural constituent of most biological membranes, but if the proportion is allowed to increase, membrane function is usually diminished. Thus, the membrane that surrounds the sarcoplasmic reticulum vesicles in muscle progressively loses the calcium-transporting function of its ATPase when cholesterol starts replacing the phospholipids. Similarly, ox-heart mitochondria, when exposed to cholesterol, progressively lose the activity of ATPase, succinate dehydrogenase, and β-hydroxybutyrate dehydrogenase (Warren *et al.*, 1975).

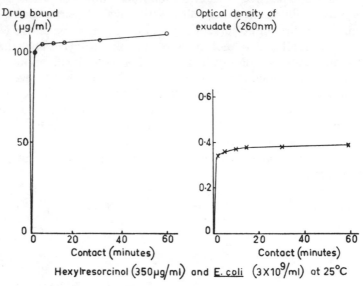

Hexylresorcinol (350μg/ml) and E. coli (3×10⁹/ml) at 25°C

FIG. 14.3 The quick rupturing effect of hexylresorcinol on *E. coli* (3 × 10⁹ organisms per ml). (Beckett, *et al.*, 1959.)

The alkyl-phenols [e.g. (*14.9*), the long-chain quaternary amines [e.g. (*14.10*)], and the polypeptide antibiotics all have the property of cracking bacterial cell walls (Gale and Taylor, 1947). Experiments conducted on protoplasts in hypertonic media indicate that all three classes of substances disintegrate cytoplasmic membranes and that the effect on cell walls is secondary to this. The disruptive effect of these substances has also been studied by measuring the time taken for the cell contents to be extruded. This is conveniently done by plotting optical density at 260 nm against time, as in Fig. 14.3, which shows the effect of hexylresorcinol (*14.9*) on *E. coli*. The action is almost complete in 2 minutes. Similar results have been recorded for quaternary amines such as CTAB (*14.10*) (Salton, 1951). The nature of these disintegrations of the membrane seems to be the creation of pores, which are large enough to permit cytochrome-c to diffuse out.

Hexylresorcinol
(*14.9*)

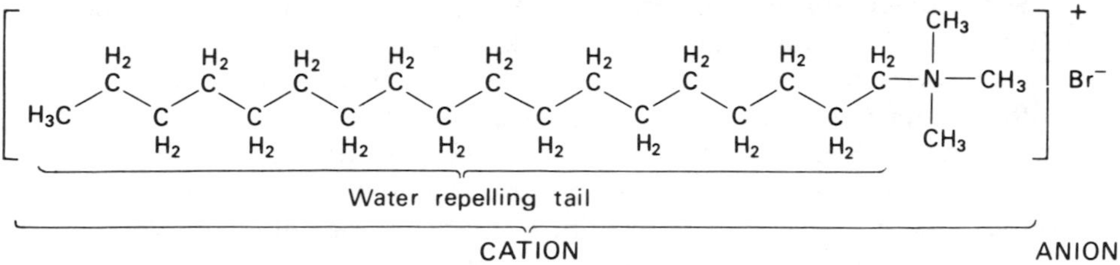

Water repelling tail

CATION   ANION

Cetyltrimethylammonium bromide (CTAB)
(14.10)

One of the mildest of these plasma membrane injuring drugs is polymyxin B (14.11), which is injected intramuscularly into patients with infections caused by Gram-negative bacteria, particularly *Pseudomonas*, a bacterium unaffected by most other antibacterial agents. It is a cyclic heptapeptide with a tripeptide side-chain N-acylated by a lipophilic acid (Suzuki *et al.*, 1964), and is obtained from a strain of *Bacillus polymyxa*. Other polymixins, with two D-aminoacids, are particularly kidney-damaging (Wilkinson and Lowe, 1966). Because of the presence of six residues of 2,4-diaminobutyric acid in each molecule, the polymixins are strong bases. This property, and the long hydrocarbon chain of the acylating group, give to these antibiotics a structure and amphiphilic properties akin to those of CTAB. The principal use of alkyl-phenols, quaternary amines, and polypeptide antibiotics is as topical antibacterials.

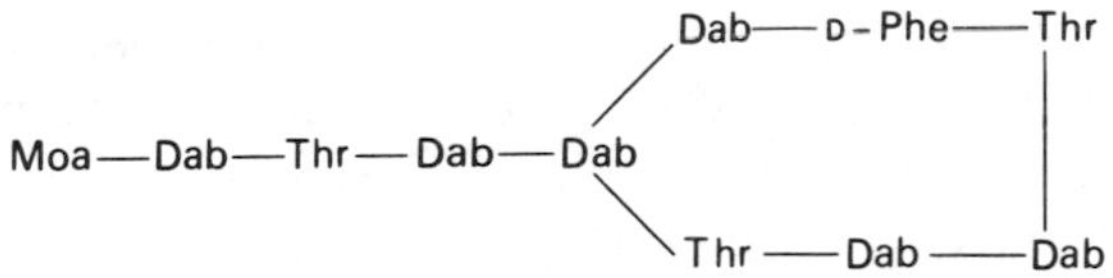

Polymixin B₁
(Moa = 6-methyloctanoic acid, Dab = diaminobutyric acid,
Thr = threonine, D-Phe = D-phenylalanine)
(14.11)

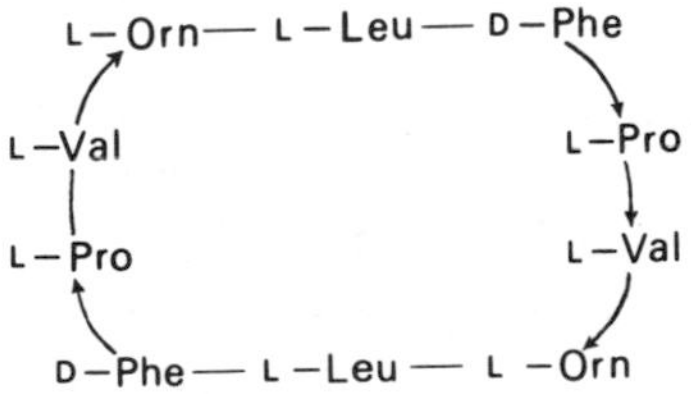

Gramicidin S
(14.12)

Some other antibiotics derived from bacillary bacteria will now be discussed. A cyclic decapeptide antibiotic, gramicidin S (*14.12*), has two residues of D-phenylalanine as its sole unusual aminoacid. X-ray diffraction, combined with n.m.r., has shown that the structure is a ladder of which four N–H . . . O bonds form the rungs (Conti, 1969). Gramicidin S is membrane-damaging but does not transport cations. Tyrocidine B has a rather similar structure. Gramicidin D, Dubos's original gramicidin, is an ion-channel-forming, linear polypeptide of 15 aminoacids, many of which are D. It injures bacteria by the removal of potassium (as valinomycin does, but more strongly), without injury to the plasma membrane. Gramicidin A, the principal constituent of commercial 'gramicidin' is similar (Haydon and Hladky, 1972). It is used in antibacterial ointments.

Although the alkylphenols, the quaternary amines, and the polypeptide antibiotics are surface-active, this property alone can not cause biological action, Luduena *et al.* (1955). Ordinary surface-active substances of the three charge-types (cationic, anionic, and neutral) are highly antibacterial, slightly antibacterial, and inert, respectively, when examples of equal surface-activity are compared. Thus high surface-activity does not of itself cause damage, but only helps a substance to become concentrated on the bacterial surface. Any damage to bacteria arises from structure-specific loosening of the components of the cell membrane.

The membrane-injury being discussed in this section is essentially the collapse of a mixed film, which has been much studied in model systems. If the adsorbed surface-active substance merely forms a new monolayer *over* the film, nothing more unusual may occur than that separate areas of the film sometimes adhere to one another (the phenomenon of agglutination). To collapse a film, the adsorbed agent must neutralize the film's characteristic charge (e.g. by an adsorbed cation if the film is anionic), or the agent must enter *into* the film, as happens when the agent is more surface-active than the components of the film, or can form stronger bonds with one of the components of a mixed film and hence displaces the other component. In the latter way, red blood cells are haemolysed by saponins or phospholipids (Schulman and Rideal, 1937). It is possible for a film to be made stronger by interpenetration, thus avoiding collapse, but normal biological function may no longer be maintained. Further examples of membrane-injuring agents will now be reviewed.

Two much-used agricultural fungicides are cationic surface-active agents: dodine (*n*-dodecylguanidine) and glyodin (2-heptadecyl-2-imidazol-ine). These rupture the cytoplasmic membranes of some fungi but kill others by merely increasing the permeability of this membrane, after which they enter the cell and destroy *intra*cellular membrane structure (Somers and Pring, 1966).

Chlorohexidine (*10.24*), a much-used local antiseptic, was found to release the cell contents of *E. coli* when these bacteria were placed in a

1 : 10000 aqueous solution for 5 minutes at 20°, and most of them died
(Rye and Wiseman, 1966). Both tetrachlorosalicylanilide and hexachlorophane (*11.37*) released 260 nm-absorbing material (a sign of damage to the
cytoplasmic membrane) from bacteria which then died. Both substances are
liposoluble skin disinfectants (Woodroffe and Wilkinson, 1966; Joswick,
1961).

Streptomycin (^{14}C) is initially accumulated by the bacterial cell wall.
This local concentration makes the cytoplasmic membrane swell and
become porous (Anand, Davis, and Armitage, 1960). Streptomycin then
enters the cell more easily (cf. the behaviour of dodine, above) and the final
site of action is on the ribosomes (see Section 4.1, p. 126).

A polymer, useful to experimental pharmacologists and known as
'48/80', selectively bursts the membrane of mast cells in living mammals,
and so causes the release of histamine in large amounts (Norton, 1954).
This substance is a trimer of N-methyl*homo*anisylamine and formaldehyde.

The 'Tritons' are non-ionic, polymeric emulsifying agents of the general
formula (*14.13*) (Cornforth, *et al.*, 1955). When administered to mice
infected with tuberculosis, these polyoxyethylene ethers accumulate in
lysosomes (including those of the macrophages) which then liberate an anti-
tuberculosis lipid (D'Arcy Hart, Gordon, and Jacques, 1969). The Tritons
unfortunately have too much mammalian toxicity for use in the clinic,
but this work embodies an excellent idea which may later become fruitful.

The discovery of the polyene antibiotics, isolated from species of
Streptomyces, found in soils about 1950, ushered in a treatment for systemic
fungal infections that was biochemically unique.

These polyene antifungal agents are macrolides containing a highly
hydroxylated portion in each molecule and from four to seven conjugated
double-bonds in a lactone ring. According to the number of these double-

where R is $-(CH_2 \cdot CH_2O)_{16-19}CH_2CH_2OH$
The Triton
(*14.13*)

Nystatin
(14.14)

bonds, they are called tetraenes, heptaenes, etc. The conjugated portion is unsubstituted and all-*trans* in configuration. It can be seen from the formula of nystatin (14.14) that the ring has a relatively planar lipophilic section and a less rigid hydrophilic section. Various substituents occur in different members of the family: e.g. amino-sugars, carboxyl-groups, epoxides, aliphatic and aromatic side-chains. Polyene antibiotics are lethal to the majority of fungi, protozoa, flat-worms, snails, and the higher algae. Bacteria are quite unaffected, and the higher plants and animals are intermediate in susceptibility.

These polyenes injure fungi by binding to the ergosterol of the plasma membranes (Hamilton-Miller, 1973). *Mycoplasma laidlawii*, for example, was unaffected by filipin when grown in the absence of the sterol, but lysed when grown in its presence (Weber and Kinsky, 1965). When polyene antibiotics were injected under mixed lipids, present as a monolayer in a surface-trough, it was found that the polyene interpenetrated the film and increased its area. Reorientation of the sterol component, caused by interaction with the polyene, seemed to make the film leaky (Demel, Van Deenen, and Kinsky, 1965). Mitochondrial and nuclear membranes are not affected by the polyenes, nor is the cell wall (Kinsky, 1962).

A whole spectrum of damage to the cytoplasmic membrane is shown by the various polyenes, from filipin, which produces severe damage and bursting, to *N*-acetylcandidin, which produces only a leakage of potassium ions and sorbose, and *N*-succinylperimycin, which released only potassium (Borowski and Cybulska, 1967). In general, members of lower molecular weight cause the most damage (Cirrillo, Harsch, and Lampen, 1964). Both nystatin and amphotericin B produce ion-permeable, water-filled pores of radius about 4 Å in fungal membranes (Dennis, Stead, and Andreoli, 1970).

Polyene antibiotics are used clinically as fungicides for internal infections. They are rather toxic to the patient, but are the best drugs available. The two most clinically useful members are (a) nystatin (14.14), whose complex composition was worked out by Birch *et al.* (1964), and Chong and Rickards

(1970), and (b) amphotericin (5.7). The latter's structure, determined by X-ray diffraction (Ganis *et al.*, 1971), is based on a 35-membered heptaene lactone ring, a long thin molecule, with hydrophilic and hydrophobic halves well separated, and ten hydroxy-groups capable of forming hydrogen bonds.

Nystatin is given orally (often as a suspension for it is only feebly water-soluble) for treating moniliasis of the throat, intestines, and rectum. It is not absorbed from the intestine. Amphotericin B is administered intravenously as a colloidal suspension to treat deep-lying, systemic fungal infections of the lung, bone-marrow, and meninges. Its selectivity is not high but, so far, there is no effective substitute.

Much of the pain and inflammation experienced by sufferers from gout are caused by the contents of lysosomes which rupture when crystals of sodium urate, phagocytosed from the blood-stream by polymorphonuclear leucocytes, rupture the plasma membrane of these cells.

14.3 The preservation of membranes by biologically-active agents

Biological membranes are under constant threat of rupture by noxious substances present in the same cell, or in neighbouring cells, once these materials (normally restrained by another membrane) become liberated as the result of a pathological process, such as an infection, allergy, or auto-immune phenomenon. Of these substances, histamine produces a violent but short-lived reaction, but there are many long-acting alternatives.

The principal spasmogenic substance released from sensitized human lungs in SRS-A (slow-reacting substance) which is prostaglandin-related (Bach *et al.*, 1977), and which is thought to play the dominant role in causing the bronchospasm of human asthma. A substance which is claimed to be the first specific antagonist of SRS-A has the composition 7-[3-(4-acetyl-3-hydroxy-2-propylphenoxy)-2-hydroxypropoxy]-4-oxo-8-propyl-1-benzopyran-2-carboxylic acid (Augstein *et al.*, 1973), but has had little use yet.

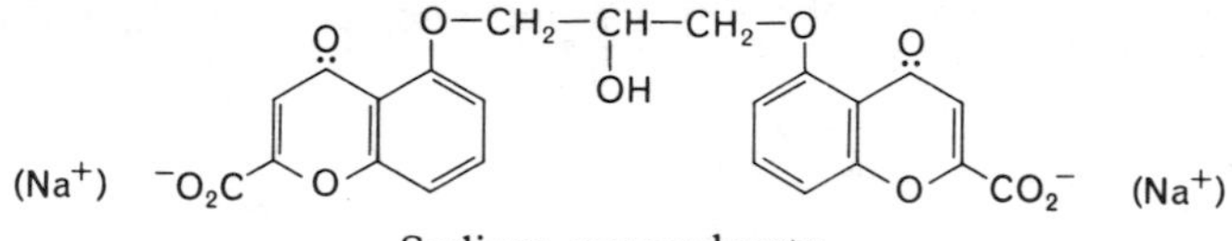

Sodium cromoglycate
(*14.15*)

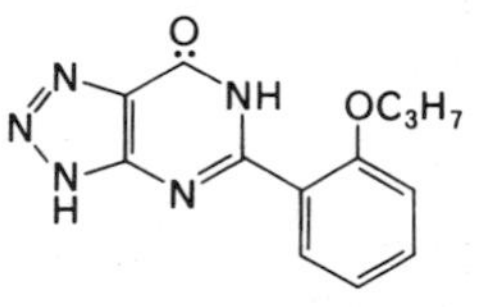

(*14.16*)

At present, the treatment of allergic asthma depends to a large degree on a prophylactic drug with a wider base of action. This is sodium cromoglycate (*14.15*) (cromolyn sodium, 'Intal') introduced in Britain in 1968. It is inhaled into the lungs daily, as a dust, and is thought to act by inhibiting the rupture of pulmonary mast cells, which are rich in both histamine and SRS-A (Cox *et al.*, 1970). Its use is now extended to the prevention of hay fever, under the name 'Rynacrom'.

Many more potent analogues of (*14.15*) have since been found, and many of them have molecules only half as large. They all seem to require an acidic group, a planar structure, and a ring-nitrogen or -oxygen placed diametrically opposite an oxo-group (C : O). Apart from stabilizing mast cells, some also keep the plasma membranes of lymphocytes intact, and others inhibit prostaglandin synthesis. In most cases, the results of clinical trials are awaited. Potent examples have been found in the 8-azapurine series, such as 2-*o*-propoxyphenyl-8-azapurin-6-one (*14.16*), which is 40 times as potent as sodium cromoglycate (Broughton *et al.*, 1975). In this molecule, the propoxy-group exerts sufficient steric hindrance to force the phenyl-group into the plane of the azapurine nucleus, thus extending the flat area.

Many other injurious agents are liberated in pathological conditions, including bradykinin (and other kinins), some of the prostaglandins (although others have a healing function), and even potassium ions in certain situations. Something is known about the role of calcium in maintaining the integrity of membranes: the use of zinc and aluminium preparations to accelerate healing in dermatology may be seen as the provisional use of more powerful calcium substitutes. The stabilization of membranes by corticoid drugs, both in dermatology and internal medicine, seems to form the principal basis of their use (Weissman and Dingle, 1961), but their total action is more broadly based.

Considerable developments in treating inflammatory diseases by the prophylactic conservation of membranes seem certain to play a much greater part in medical treatment than formerly.

For further reading on the physics and chemistry of interfacial phenomena, see Matijevic and Eirich, (1969).

15 Biological activity unrelated to structure. Ferguson's principle

As has been abundantly shown in the foregoing chapters, most biologically active substances are highly sensitive to small changes in structure (see, for example, the introduction to Chapter 2). However, no such strictures exist for one class of substance: the biological depressants. These are substances which depress many cellular functions in most forms of life. In man they are used as hypnotics and general anaesthetics. In higher concentrations, if volatile, they make useful insecticides, particularly for the fumigation of stored grain. Antimitotic effects (mentioned in Section 15.1) are also evident at low concentrations and seem to be independent of structure.

15.0 General biological depressants (hypnotics, general anaesthetics, and volatile insecticides)

General biological depressants are substantially non-ionized substances. They may be hydrocarbons (aliphatic or aromatic), chlorinated hydrocarbons, alcohols, ethers, ketones, sulphones, weak acids, weak bases, or aliphatic nitro-compounds. Aldehydes, esters, strong acids, and strong bases usually act differently. Many hypotheses have been put forward to explain the action of depressants, and these will be briefly reviewed here.

As mentioned in Section 2.0, the first coherent hypothesis was developed independently by E. Overton and H. Meyer (Meyer, 1899, Overton, 1901), and stated as three principles:

(a) all chemically indifferent substances which are soluble in lipids have depressant properties;
(b) the depressant effect is quickest and strongest in cells which are particularly rich in lipids;

(c) the depressant effect of a series of unrelated substances increases with
     rising partition coefficient between a lipid and water. That is, the
     examples with higher coefficients have greater depressant action.

This hypothesis still forms the basis of current thinking, but it is now
recognized that the correlation of paragraph (c) is not linear but parabolic
(Hansch *et al.*, 1968). This follows from the fact that any substance that is so
lipophilic that it has virtually no solubility in water cannot have depressant
properties, because it will accumulate in the first oily 'site of loss' which it
encounters and be unable to leave it.

The most important use of depressants is in human beings, as hypnotics
and general anaesthetics. In small doses they induce sleep, in larger doses
lack of sensation, in still larger doses muscular relaxation. The introduction
of specific muscle relaxants, like suxamethonium (*7.21*), which is short-
acting, and tubocurarine (*2.6*), which is long-acting, made it unnecessary
to push the dose of a general anaesthetic so high as was done before 1940.
In highly industrialized countries the most used anaesthetics have become:
nitrous oxide (usually after prior induction by intravenous thiopentone)
and the fluorinated hydrocarbons. The most used of these are *halothane*
(the first of them all, introduced in Britain about 1955), which is 2-bromo-
2-chloro-1,1,1,-trifluorethane; the more analgesic *methoxyflurane*, which
is 2,2-dichloro-1,1-difluoroethyl methyl ether; and the newly introduced
enflurane, which is 2-chloro-1,1,2-trifluoroethyl difluoromethyl ether.
Unsubstituted hydrocarbons, such as cyclopropane and ethylene are
avoided because of fire risk from the electrical apparatus so much used in
modern surgery. Thus, thanks to the muscle-relaxing drugs, anaesthetics
that would have been considered too light 25 years ago, now dominate the
field. Heavy (i.e. deep) anaesthetics such as ether are now used only in
developing countries where highly skilled anaesthetists are still rare.

Analyses of nerve membranes have brought to light the unusually high
ratio of cholesterol to phospholipid, namely about 1 to 3 (Chacko *et al.*,
1976). Because the spinal cord and brain are clad in lipid-rich membranes, a
lower dose of a depressant is effective for the central nervous system as
compared with the musculature. Thus the partition coefficient of halothane
is 6.80 for brain (grey matter), but only 2.92 for muscle (tissue/gas, $37°C$)
(Lowe, 1968). In detail, the site of action of a general anaesthetic is not yet
exactly known; some favour the polysynaptic sites in the central nervous
system, others the bulk of the cytoplasmic membrane. The molecular
nature of this site is discussed later in this chapter. (For general information
on partition coefficients, see Section 3.2 and Appendix II.)

Table 15.1 shows a small selection of the many results correlating partition
coefficients with depression of physiological activity. The results in the
last column, obtained by multiplying the values in the other two columns,
are an attempt to estimate the concentration of the depressant in the cell
lipids. With oleyl alcohol, a value ranging around 0.03 was usually obtained,

but older results, in which olive oil was the test-lipid, were more variable (see Table 2.1, which has historical value). Hansch (1971) worked out that the 17 examples of volatile anaesthetics in this Meyer and Hemmi (1935) series had an r (correlation coefficient) of 0.99 which is virtually complete agreement. Octyl alcohol is often favoured for the determination of partition coefficients because it less readily forms emulsions and is more easily removed by vacuum distillation should concentration be necessary (Hansch and Anderson, 1967). As was explained in Section 3.2, varying the non-aqueous solvent produces different absolute values for partition coefficients, but members of a series of substances still retain the same ranking order.

Meyer and Hemmi (1935) also measured the partition coefficients of anaesthetic *gases*, work that has been resumed by Hansch *et al.*, (1975) whose determinations were made easier by quantitative gas chromatography. Excellent agreement between general anaesthetic properties and the partition coefficients was found.

Table 15.1

CORRELATION OF MINIMAL HYPNOTIC DOSE WITH
PARTITION COEFFICIENT

Substance	Partition coefficient, oleyl alcohol/water	Concentration immobilizing tadpoles, mole/litre (water)	Calculated depressant concentration, mole/litre (cell lipoid)
Ethanol	0.10	0.33	0.033
n-Butanol	0.65	0.03	0.020
Valeramide	0.30	0.07	0.021
Benzamide	2.50	0.013	0.033
Salicylamide	5.90	0.0033	0.021
Phenobarbitone	5.90	0.008	0.048
o-Nitroaniline	14.0	0.0025	0.035
Thymol	950.0	4.7×10^{-5}	0.045

(Meyer and Hemmi, 1935.)

Meyer and Hemmi (1935) supplied the evidence that led to the rejection of two alternative attempts to explain depressant activity, (i) the Traube hypothesis of relative surface-tension, and (ii) the Warburg hypothesis of comparative adsorbability.

In 1939, the correlation between depressant action and lipophilicity was incorporated into a broader thermodynamic generalization by Ferguson, who saw the problem in terms of F, the free energy liberated in passing from an existing state to an equilibrium. The derivative of F which he chose for the correlation was $\bar{F}$, the partial molar free energy (PMFE), also known as the Chemical Potential. Lewis and Randall (1923) showed that:

$$\bar{F} = F_{\text{o}} + RT \ln A + k$$

where F_{o} is the PMFE in the standard state and A is the thermodynamic activity (as opposed to concentration). It follows from this that the change in PMFE is proportional to the thermodynamic activity. This led Ferguson (1939) to point out that the chemical potentials of isohypnotic solutions, of various hypnotic substances, must be the same.

Because few relevant thermodynamic activity values were known, and they are usually difficult to determine, Ferguson employed the following relationship (suitable for volatile compounds only):

Let the thermodynamic activity of a pure substance (i.e. one existing under its own vapour pressure) be taken as unity, then the thermodynamic activity of any concentration of its vapour *in air* is equal to the relative saturation of the vapour. Thus,

$$A = p_{\text{t}}/p_{\text{s}}$$

where p_{t} is the partial pressure of the vapour in air, and p_{s} is the saturated vapour pressure of the substance.

It is remarkable, when a general anaesthetic is being administered to a patient, how rapidly equilibration seems to occur. If the flow of anaesthetic gas is turned down, that patient at once achieves a measure of consciousness, and when the former flow-rate is resumed, the patient is very quickly back on the lower plane of anaesthesia. Actually, because of the complexity of the systems concerned, these are only 'steady states' but, to a first approximation, Ferguson felt justified in treating them as equilibria, in order to make use of simple thermodynamic principles.

Given this assumption of equilibrium, it follows that the thermodynamic potential of the depressant is the same in all phases. This means that one has only to measure the thermodynamic activity in the external phase to learn the thermodynamic activity in the biophase, for both activities must be the same. This is true even though the location and chemical nature of the biophase are unknown (by *biophase* is meant the nerve membrane, or other site, where the depressant exerts its characteristic physiological action). The nature of the biophase is discussed on p. 553.

Equation (i) gives A for volatile substances, applied as vapours. The thermodynamic activity *in aqueous solution* is roughly equal to the relative saturation of the solution, provided that the substance is not exceedingly soluble.

Hence the important figure for the correlation of depressants is the *relative saturation* of these substances in the vehicle (air or water) in which they are administered, and not the *concentration*. This principle has been confirmed on a variety of biological test-objects (Ferguson, 1939, 1951; Ferguson and Pirie, 1948; Burtt, 1945).

It has been found that many structurally non-specific agents produce equal biological effects at roughly the same relative saturation. Thus, a substance soluble in water to the extent of 1 per cent will exhibit, in a 0.2 per cent solution, the same degree of depressant activity as a substance soluble to the extent of only 0.1 per cent does in a 0.02 per cent solution. It is evident that all changes in structure that lower water solubility will tend to intensify depressant action in the sense that the new substance will act at a lower concentration than its parent. In ascending a series of homologues, aqueous solubilities decrease from member to member, and the concentrations of these required to produce a specified biological effect rapidly decrease. However, in such a series, the thermodynamic activities necessary to produce a given degree of depressant action are found to increase gradually until a member is reached that is effective only in saturated solution (i.e. a solution that is in equilibrium with undissolved material and hence is at a thermodynamic activity of 1). The next higher homologue inevitably has little or no biological action (Ferguson, 1939, 1951).

Structurally non-specific agents seem to act by becoming accumulated in some vitally important part of a cell, thus disorganizing a chain of metabolic processes. In short, they act *simply as foreign bodies*. Obviously they owe the property of being accumulated by cells to a favourable physical property conferred upon them by their chemical constitution. The required physical property depends only on the balance between two common variables in molecular structure, namely hydrophilic atoms and lipophilic atoms. Suitable proportions of these atoms can always be reached by ascending innumerable homologous series of many different chemical types.

Exemplifying Ferguson's principle, Table 15.2 shows the effect of various hydrocarbons, halogenated paraffins, nitro-hydrocarbons, and weak bases on the wireworm (larva of *Agriotes*). These substances were applied as vapours diluted with air. It is seen from this Table that when equimolar concentrations are compared in column two, a 4000-fold variation in activity appears. However, a much more uniform result is obtained when *proportional saturations* are compared by calculating the least fraction of the saturated vapour pressure required to kill the test-animal. Here (within the much narrower limits of a ninefold variation) a reasonably constant figure (around 0.5) is obtained. This means that the air becomes lethal when it is about half saturated. On the other hand, non-Fergusonian substances such as hydrocyanic acid, carbon bisulphide, ammonia, and strong organic bases give low and non-concordant figures (e.g. ammonia, 0.00008).

Were the figure 0.5 a constant for the action of structurally non-specific substances on every kind of cell, it would be idle to expect them to show any *selectivity* in their toxicity. However, this 'relative saturation' varies, for different cells, between 0.01 and 1. For example, it is approximately 0.03 for the production of narcosis in mice and tadpoles and for the inhibition of the development of sea-urchin eggs. A higher value, 0.5, has been found for the minimal concentrations of aniline, phenols, aliphatic alcohols, and ketones required to kill *B. typhosus* in aqueous solution, i.e. approximately half-saturated solutions are required (Ferguson, 1939).

The great value of this principle to those who are working with toxic agents is that it becomes easy to find out if a new biological action is structurally non-specific or not. To get this information, the Ferguson value for the biological effect under study must first be determined, using about a dozen examples of the chemical types suggested by Table 15.2. If the new drug, when tested, gives a similar figure, the likelihood of its being structurally non-specific is high. Hence one would not expect it to show particularly novel biological properties and would not map out a programme in which the molecule was to be altered in minute particulars, e.g. by inserting a methyl-group in various positions.

Another utilitarian conclusion that can be derived from Ferguson's principle is that, when investigating a new agent, it is economical to alter the molecule so that it becomes less soluble in water, up to the limit discussed above.

Table 15.2

AGREEMENT BETWEEN THE RELATIVE SATURATIONS OF
THE TOXIC CONCENTRATIONS OF VARIOUS SUBSTANCES,
TESTED ON WIREWORMS

Substance	Toxic concentration, millionths moles/litre lethal in 1000 min. at 15°C	p_s (vapour pressure at 15°C, mm)	p_t/p_s (relative saturation of toxic concentration)
Monomethylaniline	3.7	0.22	0.3
Dimethylaniline	6.6	0.28	0.4
Pyridine	76	10.4	0.1
Bromoform	94	3.2	0.5
Tetrachloroethane	141	4.2	0.6
Chlorobenzene	200	6.8	0.5
Toluene	420	17.0	0.4
Nitromethane	710	23	0.6
Benzene	775	58	0.2
Heptane	800	27	0.5
Chloroform	1040	128	0.2
Trichlorethylene	1200	52	0.4
Carbon tetrachloride	1600	73	0.4
Hexane	3000	96	0.6
Dichlorethylene	3100	230	0.2
Pentane	16000	320	0.9

(Ferguson, 1939.)

Although discussed here, so far, only in connection with insecticides, Ferguson's principle applies equally for hypnotics in warm-blooded (Table 15.3) or cold-blooded (Table 15.4) mammals. Table 15.4 demonstrates how six depressants can vary in potency over a 400-fold range, if calculated on a molar basis, but be contained within a twofold range when calculated on the basis of thermodynamic activities.

One of the most exciting and challenging aspects of the study of anaesthetics was the early realization that chemically-inert gases can be as profound biological depressants as any substance in the preceding Tables (provided the comparison is made in thermodynamic activities). This is well illustrated by the anaesthetic properties of nitrogen. Deep-sea divers, more than a hundred years ago, experienced dizziness and inco-ordination, symptoms which were eventually traced to breathing, under pressure, the nitrogen component of their compressed air (Unsworth, 1861). When several experienced divers were subjected, in a laboratory, to mixtures of oxygen (20%) with either nitrogen, or argon, or both, these mixtures had no effect at atmospheric pressure, but a pronounced hypnotic effect at pressures corresponding to depths of 90–300 feet (Behnke and Yarbrough, 1939). They recognized that these two chemically inert gases are lipophiles, and that the oil/water partition coefficient of argon is even higher than that of ether.

Table 15.3

CORRELATION OF MINIMAL HYPNOTIC DOSE (MOUSE) WITH THERMODYNAMIC ACTIVITY

(Vapour phase work)

Substance	Saturation pressure at 37°C (p_s) mm	Narcotic conc. % by volume	Thermodynamic activity p_t/p_s
Nitrous oxide	59 300	100	0.01
Acetylene	51 700	65	0.01
Methyl ether	6 100	12	0.02
Methyl chloride	5 900	14	0.01
Ethylene oxide	1 900	5.8	0.02
Ethyl chloride	1 780	5.0	0.02
Diethyl ether	830	3.4	0.03
Methylal	630	2.8	0.03
Ethyl bromide	725	1.9	0.02
Dimethylacetal	288	1.9	0.05
Diethyformal	110	1.0	0.07
Dichlorethylene	450	0.95	0.02
Carbon disulphide	560	1.1	0.02
Chloroform	324	0.5	0.01

(Ferguson, 1939.)

Table 15.4

SUPPRESSION OF MOTILITY OF TADPOLES

(Liquid phase work)

Substance	Minimal depressant concentration, moles/litre	Minimal depressant thermodynamic activity, $\times 10^2$
Ethanol	0.41	2.8
Butanol	0.02	2.1
Octanol	0.0001	2.8
Acetone	0.28	3.0
Chloroform	0.001	1.9
Ether	0.03	4.0
	400- fold	2- fold

(Brink and Posternak, 1948.)

Helium, the lightest of the inert gases, is free from narcotizing properties which increase with molecular weight. Argon (mol. wt. 40) is more narcotizing than nitrogen (mol. wt. 28). When a diver is 200 feet below the surface of the sea, he is working under seven times the pressure to which he is accustomed in ordinary life. If air is used for breathing, the extra nitrogen, more lipophilic than oxygen, decreases the ability to think clearly and to take sensible decisions. To prevent this 'nitrogen nacrosis', a helium-oxygen (4 : 1) mixture is now used and this has been found compatible with clear decision-taking, even at a depth of 1000 feet.

It was found that xenon (mol. wt. 131), at atmospheric pressure, caused temporary loss of reflexes in mice (Lawerence *et al.*, 1946). In this experiment, the gas was effective at a thermodynamic activity of only 0.01 and thus was highly potent. But would it produce anesthesia in man? To find out, xenon was administered to patients undergoing operations in the University of Iowa's Hospital (Cullen and Gross, 1951). It was diluted with 20 per cent of oxygen, and administered without prior medication with barbiturates or muscle relaxants. Loss of consciousness was prompt, relaxation of muscle good, and recovery rapid. The degree of anaesthesia was as deep as with ethylene but not quite so deep as with ether. Surgeons performed orchidectomy, and ligation of the Fallopian tubes, and considered xenon a satisfactory anaesthetic. This result leads to the important generalization that anaesthesia by inert molecules, of which xenon is outstanding for its high potency and low chemical reactivity, takes places *as soon as a constant fraction of some phase of the nerve cell is occupied by foreign molecules.*

What is the nature of this biophase, so sensitive to anaesthetics? The amoeba, a monocellular protozoon, is often taken as the simplest possible model for a nerve cell. Hiller (1927) showed that amoebae were anaesthetized when placed in a dilute solution of a depressant, but not when the depressant was injected into the animal. When the depressant was allowed to diffuse away from the amoebae, their sensitivity was restored to normal.

In mammals, the most sensitive phase is certainly a similar lipoprotein membrane, one that is localized in the central nervous system and which may be a mitochondrial, synaptosomal, or plasma membrane. Accumulation of a depressant in such a membrane may cause swelling. The simple physics of swelling is that lipophilic substances become intercalated between the hydrocarbon side-chains of proteins and possibly lipids in a membrane (see Section 5.2 and Fig. 5.5). Moreover, inert gases, in bioactive concentrations, have been found to expand lipoprotein membranes (Clements and Wilson, 1962), and such common general anaesthetics as halothane, methoxyflurane, and ether were shown to expand human erythrocyte membrane (Seeman and Roth, 1972). Swelling is likely to bring about the mechanical separation of enzymes responsible for an orderly sequence of reactions (Quastel, 1965), particularly if the membrane in question is mitochondrial. More likely, swelling closes the pores which exist for the cations, so important in the propagation of impulses in nerves (see Section 7.5a).

Although pressure can introduce anaesthesia, *excess* pressure can abolish it. Thus, newts, anaesthetized with nitrogen under 34 atmospheres, were restored to consciousness by increasing the pressure to 140 atmospheres. Similarly newts anaesthetized (without pressure) by ether, halothane, or sodium pentobarbitone, were deanaesthetized by applying hydrostatic pressure outside their bodies (Lever *et al.*, 1971). This effect of excess pressure is interpreted as a reversal of the membrane expansion (about 0.4% suffices) required for anaesthesia (Miller, *et al.*, 1973).

Contrary to what had earlier been supposed, there is no parallel between the anaesthetic doses of a series of depressants and their inhibition of the various enzymes isolated from the respiratory chain (see review by Butler, 1950). The concentrations of depressants required to inhibit respiration in tissues, *in vitro*, has always proved to be much higher than those used to produce surgical anaesthesia in humans. Thus the observed drop in cellular respiration caused by depressants is more likely to be a result of reduced nervous activity rather than a cause of it (McIlwain, 1962).

In 1961 a quite new hypothesis of anaesthetic action was put forward. Linus Pauling and Stanley Miller independently proposed that each molecule of an anaesthetic acts as a stabilizing centre around which water molecules join to form a more compact state of water which produces anaesthesia. It was thought that these denser water molecules may form a cover over nerve cell-membranes, thus hindering the passage of ions which could, in turn, impede depolarization. In support of these hypotheses, the authors claimed that a close correlation existed between the partial pressures required for anaesthesia by various gases and the partial pressures of their *hydrates*, in fact that the former divided by the latter pressure equalled a constant (Pauling, 1961; Miller, 1961). (An exposition of the structure of water was given at the end of Section 3.0.)

Concerning hydrates, although hydrocarbons and the rare gases form true hydrates, these are stable only under several atmospheres of pressure (cf. v. Stackelberg, 1954). In the Pauling hypothesis, it is assumed that anaesthetics form ice clathrates like propane does. Because they could not be stable at 37°C and atmospheric pressure, a further assumption had to be made: that the clathrates were stabilized by the charged side-chains of protein molecules, leading to a decrease in neural conduction. It will be noted that these hypotheses resemble the others described above in one important way: they connect depressant action with a process of reversible disorganization. However, the water-organization hypotheses have certain weaknesses, which will now be discussed.

A sensitive test as to whether a special structure is induced in water by non-polar groups was provided by the rate constant for breaking the hydrogen bond that unites a tertiary amine to water, as in $R_3N \cdot HOH$. Here, R is a hydrocarbon group whose size was systematically increased in a series of measurements. The results showed no evidence of the induction of ice-like water by hydrophobic groups (Grunwald and Ralph, 1967). Another difficulty preventing acceptance of the hydrate hypotheses is that the cavity within ice clusters can accommodate only *spherical* molecules and hence, when a hydrocarbon series is ascended, the ability to form hydrates is lost whereas anaesthetic activity increases. Diethyl ether, most typical of the anaesthetics, is a rather flat, butterfly-shaped molecule that forms no crystalline hydrate.

The fluorocarbons provide another test of the hydrate hypothesis because they are noted for the weakness of their intermolecular associations. The tendency of the various anaesthetics to form hydrates was appropriately compared by plotting the reciprocal of the dissociation pressure at 0° against anaesthetic potency. It was then seen that fluorinated compounds were much less hydrated than other anaesthetics when compared in equi-anaesthetic concentrations (K. Miller, Paton, and Smith, 1965).

In another investigation of the comparative value of lipid and hydration hypotheses (Eger *et al.*, 1969), the minimal anaesthetic concentrations of the following agents were plotted against the relevant physical properties: carbon tetrafluoride, sulphur hexafluoride, nitrous oxide, xenon, cyclopropane, fluorexene (trifluoroethyl vinyl ether), diethyl ether, enflurane (see above), halothane, chloroform, and methoxyflurane (see above). (These anaesthetics have been arranged here in order of increasing lipid/water solubility.) The results of this study showed an excellent correlation between anaesthetic potency and lipophilicity, and little correlation with hydrate formation. Thus, although the m.a.c. (minimal anaesthetic concentration) varied from 0.0023 to 26 atmospheres (a range of 11 000-fold) the lowest product of m.a.c. and the partition coefficient was 1.44 and the highest 2.86, a difference of only two-fold. On the other hand, the ratio of m.a.c. to hydrate dissociation pressures varied from 0.12 to 6.4 (a range of 53-fold), apart from the fact that the following anaesthetics apparently formed *no* hydrate: halothane, ether, methoxyflurane, fluorexene, and enflurane ('Ethrane').

However, the site of action was shown not to be purely lipoidal by the following work. Nitrous oxide, halothane, and cyclopropane (in the concentrations found during surgery) were led over a film of cholesterol (40%) in dimyristoyl lecithin, a composition designed to represent nerve membranes. Neither X-ray nor neutron diffraction analysis showed any change, even when concentrations of the anaesthetics were increased tenfold. The authors suggest that these drugs act at a lipid-protein interface, presumably in ion pores (Franks and Lieb, 1978).

Barbiturates. The barbiturates, e.g. pentobarbitone (15.1a), were introduced in 1903 as hypnotics to replace simple aliphatic amides and sulphones. In the course of time, the therapeutic index of barbiturates has been much improved by making one side-chain of such a nature that it would be degraded in a few hours by the body's detoxifying mechanisms (see Section 3.4). Whereas barbitone ('Veronal') is excreted entirely unchanged, pentobarbitone ('Nembutal') is readily oxidized in the body. A double-bond or a small branch in the side-chain assists degradation. With this degradation assured, it became safe to administer higher doses, and secure deeper hypnosis, even to the extent of light surgical anaesthesia.

To secure rapidity of onset, the partition coefficient of barbiturates has been raised by one of the three following devices: (a) increasing the number of saturated carbon atoms in the side-chain, (b) substituting a sulphur atom for an oxygen atom, or (c) repressing ionization by *N*-alkylation. Convulsant properties arise if lipophilicity is pushed too high, e.g. if a side-chain is lengthened beyond six carbon atoms or if *both* nitrogen atoms are methylated. Molecules which are more lipophilic still, such as dibenzylbarbituric acid, are simply inactive.

(a) Pentobarbital (X = O)
(b) Thiopental   (X = S)
(*15.1*)

Phenobarbital
(*15.2*)

Thiobarbiturates such as thiopental (*15.1b*) are administered intravenously to begin surgical anaesthesia, and a few very short-acting
oxobarbiturates, notably methohexital, have the same use. Employment of
barbiturates as sedatives has been discontinued in recent years, and their
place taken by the many benzodiazepines such as diazepam (Section 13.8).
Barbiturates given orally to induce sleep include the highly effective
pentobarbital ('Nembutal'), secobarbital (quinalbarbitone, 'Seconal'),
and amobarbital ('Amytal'), but these have been replaced to some extent
by the more hypnotic of the benzodiazapines, such as nitrazepam. The
decline is prescribing barbiturates as hypnotics stems from tardy recognition
that they are insidiously habituating, and that even 12 hours after a single
dose, error in judgment, loss of attention, and lapses in driving performance
are common.

From time to time, attempts have been made to find some individuality
in the hypnotic action of barbiturates, such as would exclude them from the
class of general depressants. However, no acceptable evidence has been
presented that would separate them from the general class. The small
amount of ionization of which they are capable actually hinders their action
a little (Mautner and Clemson, 1970; Hansch and Anderson, 1967).

When the free prescribing of barbiturates began to be frowned upon,
manufacturers were quick to market similarly substituted piperidines
(i.e. rings with one nitrogen atom instead of two) such as methyprylone
('Noludar') and glutethimide ('Doriden'), without any notable gain in
selectivity (Mautner and Clemson, 1970; Hansch et al., 1968).

For a comparison of physical and biological properties of the oxo-,
thio-, and seleno-barbiturates, see Krackov, Lee, and Mautner, 1965.

Bemegride ('Megimide'; β,β-methylethylglutarimide) (*15.3*), a strong
antagonist of barbiturates, has proved useful in cases of poisoning. The
structure is somewhat reminiscent of that of the barbiturates, but its
analeptic action is not specifically directed against barbiturates. In Section
7.5b, it was pointed out that increasing the size of the alkyl-group converts
these stimulants into hypnotics (Laycock and Shulman, 1963; Schulman,
Laycock, and Henry, 1965), whereas the contrary is true for barbiturates.

Bemegride
(*15.3*)

Phenytoin
(*15.4*)

Anti-epileptic drugs.　Phenobarbitone (*15.2*), in addition to its hypnotic
properties, is a powerful antiepileptic drug. The phenyl-group is essential
for this action, which is available without the hypnotic effect in phenytoin

(*15.4*) (5,5-diphenylhydantoin), and methoin (*3.27*). Antiepileptic drugs act by specifically curbing the high-voltage, high-frequency brain distribution of grand mal (Greengard and McIlwain, 1955). How they begin to do so is indicated by the specific inhibitory action of phenytoin on the resting sodium permeability in the central nervous system (Perry *et al.*, 1978). Sodium valproate (dipropylacetate) acts differently, apparently inhibiting an enzyme that degrades GABA (p. 254).

Δ¹-Tetrahydrocannabinol
(*15.5*)

Cannabis indica. Δ¹-tetrahydrocannabinol (*15.5*), the principal active constituent of marihuana, has both likenesses and disparities when compared to general biological depressants. Its high partition-coefficient (about 8000 in the octanol/water system) seems responsible for the slowness of its kinetics and its persistence in the body. It keeps subjects in a mildly narcotized state for hours without being able to effect a higher degree of anaesthesia. This result is reminiscent of the cut-off effect found when the molecular weight of aliphatic alcohols is steadily increased (Section 2.3 and Fig. 2.2) (Paton, 1975). Moreover there are indications that an acyl-transferase, in the synaptosomes of brain membranes, is specifically inhibited (Greenberg, *et al.*, 1978).

For a discussion of physical mechanisms in biological depressants and convulsants, see Shulman and Laycock (1967); Mautner and Clemson (1970).

15.1 Mitotic disorganizers

Many simple biological depressants have an adverse effect on mitosis. They allow the chromosomes to divide, but the daughter chromosomes remain side by side instead of moving to two opposite spindle-poles. Thus the spindle is disorganized and the chromosomes do not proceed beyond metaphase. Among the large number of inert substances that act in this way are: hexane and other aliphatic hydrocarbons, alcohols, ether, chloroform, acetone, paraldehyde, acetamide, urethane, acetophenone, benzophenone, acetanilide, benzene, chlorobenzene, and sulphonal (Östergren, 1951); also nitrogen and argon under pressure (Ferguson, Hawkins, and Doxey, 1950).

This effect appears to be a straightforward case of biological depression. The effect is readily reversed when the concentration of the agent falls. Colchicine is a mitotic disorganizer of another kind, because it gives results at a very low thermodynamic activity and is sensitive to small changes in molecular structure. Again, substances which cause drastic and irreversible changes such as chromosome breakage (e.g. phenols, coumarins, and mustard gas) have physical properties quite different from those of the structurally indifferent depressants.

16 The perfection of a discovery

Let us suppose that a substance has been discovered with a rare and much desired biological property. It may have been found by application of the principles of selectivity, or from a chance laboratory observation, or by a tedious mechanical screening programme. Usually it is neither potent nor selective enough to be thought of as a candidate drug, heading towards clinical trial, but it can be nevertheless a very promising lead.* What steps can be taken to improve it, by finding the most selective example among its many chemical relatives? Moreover, how can this goal be reached by making the fewest possible examples?

Some useful preliminaries can be extracted from earlier Chapters. For example, tests can determine whether the ion or the molecule is the biologically-active species (Section 10.7). Whether it can chelate with a metal cation may be suggested by a glance at the structure (Section 11.2) followed by a quick pH test (Section 11.3). Whether the molecule is structurally non-specific can be found by comparing the minimal hypnotic activity with that of an established example such as chloroform, or by similar comparison of partition coefficients (Section 15.0).

From this point onwards, the paths diverge. One pathway is to pursue the scientific study of the cytological, biochemical, and distributive clues that provided the lead in the first place. The other pathway is the statistical correlation of several physical properties of the lead molecule with its biological actions. It must be emphasized that statistics lies remote from experimental science and can, at best, indicate only a probability. However, these statistical methods are much used, particularly in industry, and it is proposed to give a brief account of them.

Quite the most popular of these approaches is *multiple regression analysis*, introduced by Hansch in 1968. In this method, the most favoured variables are (i) partition coefficients (P), from the system octanol/water (Section 3.2); (ii) the sigma (σ) and rho (ρ) values from Hammett's Linear Free Energy Equation (Appendix III); and (iii) Taft's steric factors† (E_s) which are

---

* In this use, 'lead' rhymes with 'seed' and not with 'said' (unlike Pb).

† Taft (1953) obtained these values from a study of reaction-equilibria of molecules that bore bulky groups adjacent to a (non-biological) reactive centre. Not many Taft values are yet known. Molar refraction has been tried as a not very satisfactory substitute (Hansch, *et al.*, 1973).

used to determine what space for substituents exists between a nominated small region of the lead molecule and its receptor. These variables are correlated in the following equation:

$$\log 1/C = -k(\log P)^2 + k_2(\log P) + \sigma\rho + k_3 E_s + k_4$$

where C is the least concentration eliciting the biological effect on the uneconomic cells, or (in another set) on the economic cells. Other terms are sometimes added, e.g. hydrogen-bonding (Fujita et al., 1977). When the molecule has only a low partition coefficient, the $(\log P)^2$ term is dropped.

It is evident that multifactorial equations cannot fail to give good correlations with experimental data, because the values of the various constants (k) are systematically altered by the computer until they do so, a result which does not necessarily contribute to a solution of the main problem (Topliss and Costello, 1972; Unger and Hansch, 1973).

To operate the above equation so as to obtain values for all the different kinds of k, one takes a set* of compounds whose biological effects have been evaluated, and which are related to the lead in as many different ways as possible. After supplying the equation with their values of C, P, $\sigma\rho$, and E_s, the computer multiple regression programme (operating by the method of least squares) will provide the values of the coefficients. These values are then evaluated for appropriateness for (i) correlating all the data, and (ii) extrapolating to a new set of compounds which will yield values of C in advance of any syntheses.† Evaluation makes use of n (the number of data points used), s (the standard deviation for the regression), and r (the correlation coefficient, which should be 1.00, ideally). From these results is calculated an assessment of the probability (p) that the derived relationship is only a chance one. It is usual to regard a probability of 1 in 20 ($p = 0.05$) as sufficient to establish significance, and if p is as low as 0.01, the results are called 'highly significant'. [For further reading on pharmacologists' statistics, see Lewis (1970)]. If all has gone well, so far, the results should indicate that the biological activity correlates highly with one or more of the variables, such as P.

In choosing the first compounds to submit to multiple regression analysis, tremendous help can be derived from Craig's sigma-versus-pi scatter diagram (Fig. 16.1). Representative compounds must be drawn from each of the four quadrants to discover the σ/π region of maximal activity.

---

* It is recommended to take five compounds for each variable being investigated. Thus, if one is looking only into lipophilicity and Hammett values, ten compounds should suffice, provided they are equipped with substituents that cover a wide range of values for these variables (Topliss and Costello, 1972; Hansch, Unger, and Forsythe, 1973).

† In such cases, P must be calculated from the old π values, or better from the **f** values of Appendix II, but, in any case, this method is subject to serious errors only some of which can be guarded against (Section 3.2).

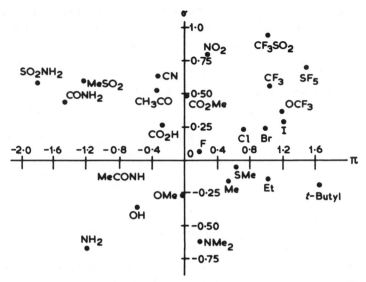

FIG. 16.1 Relationship between the Hammett σ and Hansch π values of some commonly used para-substituents.
(Craig, 1971; redrawn by Redl, Cramer, and Berkoff, 1974.)

Those who prefer to work without computers or statistics may derive great help from the 'Decision Tree' of Topliss (1972). He begins by assuming that the lead-molecule is dominated by a benzene ring. In this case, one should first make the p-chloro-derivative and find if it is less or more active than the parent lead. If the potency is increased, the gain can be attributed to $+\pi$, $+\sigma$, or both together (for signs of substituents, see Appendices II and III). If the chloro-derivative is equipotent with the parent, this should be interpreted as a small favourable π-effect (almost all drugs show a small biologically-favourable π-effect) counterbalanced by an unfavourable σ-relationship. To test this interim conclusion, the 4-methyl-derivative should be made. This ought to show increased potency because it is $+\pi$ and $-\sigma$. If the 4-Me-derivative is less potent than the 4-chloro analogue, an unfavourable steric effect may be assumed for *para*-substitution. Hence analogues should be made with chlorine, and methyl, in the 3-position. Finally if the 4-chloro-derivative is significantly less potent than the parent, the most likely cause is control by $-\sigma$, because $-\pi$ is rare. This should be tested by making the 4-dimethylamino-derivative, where the effects of $-\sigma$ would become more evident. Topliss goes on to suggest how a side-chain could be similarly manipulated, starting with steady increases in π, while keeping steric effects low by preferring, e.g. a cyclobutyl substituent to open-chain groups. For a further development along these lines, see Topliss (1977).

Historically the most valuable achievement of multiple regression analysis was exposure of areas of neglect. For example, let us suppose that a good lead had turned up, and that it was a quinoline substituted in the heterocyclic ring. Chemists were asked to submit, say, 20 examples with alternative substituents, and when they had done this they felt satisfied that they had submitted a representative cross-section. In this, they were self-deceived. Inspection of the σ values, long before any regression analysis was begun, would show that one end of the Hammett σ-scale was unrepresented. This happened because any standard synthetic reaction, that seemingly can make an endless variety of products, is always partial to producing examples up one horn of the Hammett scale, and (for good Hammett-related reasons) neglecting the other. The chemists therefore had to find a quite different reaction to complete their project, and as a favourable reaction did not exist, they were obliged to discover one. Appreciation of this concept has caused no small revolution in the thinking of the chemical staff of drug-seeking teams.

The greatest weakness in multiple regression analysis seems to be the stereochemical term. Although the exact fit of an agonist on its receptor is easily visualized with molecular models, and is instantly comprehensible in terms of stereochemistry, so much touching and folding and fitting, involving so many atoms and each to a different degree, and with conformational changes likely in both drug and receptor: all of this is simply not reducible to a single term in a regression equation. The best that one can do is to test for space around each position in the agent by inserting a bulky substituent into each place, in turn. However, this is a tedious procedure.

Sometimes it is claimed that the biological activity of a series depends on the group dipole moment (μ) rather than on σ. Actually it is not possible to make this differentiation for mono-substituted derivatives because the two constants are mathematically related. They can be distinguished, however, in di-substitution, when σ will prove simply additive, but μ vectorially additive, and hence often self-cancelling. For values of μ, see Sutton (1955).

A healthy aspect of this work is that multiple regression analysts view one another's work with a highly critical eye (e.g. Cammarata, et al., 1970; Martin, 1970). The following quotations from the Pomona School are worth keeping in mind. 'Space limitation has not allowed a discussion of many instances where no combination of constants has yielded even moderate correlations' (Hansch, 1971). After cautioning against over-reliance on statistical criteria to the neglect of common sense, Unger and Hansch (1973) add: 'Without such a qualitative perspective, one is apt to generate statistical unicorns, beasts that exist on paper, but not in reality. For example, it has recently become all too clear that one can correlate a set of dependent variables using random numbers as independent variables'. In this connexion, see also Topliss and Costello (1972).

The Free and Wilson additive method.   This is a contemporary refinement of an old hypothesis that biological activity is an additive property to which every substituent in the molecule makes a mathematically predetermined contribution (Free and Wilson, 1964). As Hansch (1971) remarked, this approach is completely unencumbered by any attempt to apply thermodynamics or physical chemistry. Instead, a computer is used to determine substituent constsnts for structure-activity relationships. This is accomplished by employing the method of least-squares as a data-fitting device to find 'best numbers' for each substituent in a drug when furnished with biological data from a standard laboratory test. From these constants, estimates are made of the degree of biological activity of *combinations* of substituents. The claimed advantage of the Free-Wilson method is that it can be used when no physical data are available. However, in like circumstances, the terms in a multiple regression analysis equation can be taken from tables. Under these circumstances, the more reliable results will be obtained when both methods are combined. A real disadvantage of the Free-Wilson method is that it is a *linear* combination, whereas physical properties (especially P) can be *parabolic*. For further reading on this method, see James (1974), also Purcell, Bass, and Clayton (1973) which requires little mathematical background.

Molecular orbital calculations.   Since the introduction of electron-density calculations, by Pullman in 1945, to explain the carcinogenicity of the polycyclic hydrocarbons by the fractional charge on K-regions (see Section 12.5), attempts have been used to apply molecular orbital calculation to the prediction of optimal drug activity. Up to now, different calculations on the same molecules have yielded different conformational energy-profiles depending on the values of the bond-lengths and bond-angles selected, and the particular MO method chosen for the calculations. Whether this method, which seems to have possibilities, could be more successful if agreement were reached on these fundamentals is not yet clear, but its practitioners are enthusiastic. For reading in the topic, see Kier (1971); Richards (1977).

Molecular connectivity.   This recently developed method attempts to determine quantitative structure-action relationships by a simple and rapid calculation following inspection of the structural formula. This method has been used for predicting thermodynamic (non-biological) properties for 100 years, mainly in Croatia, but its application (by graphical topology) has had to be limited to hydrocarbons. In the application of this method to drugs, Kier and Hall (1976) have had to depart radically from this earlier work, because of the necessity for including oxygen, nitrogen, or suphur atoms for which existing theory can make no provision. In its absence these authors proceed, sometimes empirically and sometimes with the help of a regression programme, to select values for all atoms commonly found in drugs, values which vary according to the number of non-hydrogen substituents which they carry. In spite of the uncertain theoretical basis of this method, it has shown itself, on occasion, to be capable of correlating structure with both physical properties and biological activity no less accurately than what has been obtained by application of Hansch's multiple regression analysis. Molecular connectivity, although it has so far achieved few predictions, is certainly a method to watch as it develops. In its present state, it cannot deal with several heteroatoms in one heteroaromatic molecule, nor can it account for any three dimensional physicochemical behaviour.

For a useful discussion of the various statistical methods for the prefection of a discovery, see Redl, Cramer, and Berkoff (1974). For suggestions on the strategy and tactics of chemotherapeutic drug development, see Hahn (1975).

Appendices

Appendix I

CALCULATIONS OF PERCENTAGE IONIZED, GIVEN pK_a AND pH

pK_a − pH	If anion	If cation
− 6.0	99.99990	0.0000999
− 5.0	99.99900	0.0009999
− 4.0	99.9900	0.0009990
− 3.5	99.968	0.0316
− 3.4	99.960	0.0398
− 3.3	99.950	0.0501
− 3.2	99.937	0.0630
− 3.1	99.921	0.0794
− 3.0	99.90	0.09991
− 2.9	99.87	0.1257
− 2.8	99.84	0.1582
− 2.7	99.80	0.1991
− 2.6	99.75	0.2505
− 2.5	99.68	0.3152
− 2.4	99.60	0.3966
− 2.3	99.50	0.4987
− 2.2	99.37	0.6270
− 2.1	99.21	0.7879
− 2.0	99.01	0.990
− 1.9	98.76	1.243
− 1.8	98.44	1.560
− 1.7	98.04	1.956
− 1.6	97.55	2.450
− 1.5	96.93	3.07
− 1.4	96.17	3.83
− 1.3	95.23	4.77
− 1.2	94.07	5.93
− 1.1	92.64	7.36
− 1.0	90.91	9.09
− 0.9	88.81	11.19
− 0.8	86.30	13.70
− 0.7	83.37	16.63
− 0.6	79.93	20.07
− 0.5	75.97	24.03
− 0.4	71.53	28.47
− 0.3	66.61	33.39
− 0.2	61.32	38.68
− 0.1	55.73	44.27

Appendix I (*contd.*)

pK_a – pH	If anion	If cation
0	50.00	50.00
+ 0.1	44.27	55.73
+ 0.2	38.68	61.32
+ 0.3	33.39	66.61
+ 0.4	28.47	71.53
+ 0.5	24.03	75.97
+ 0.6	20.07	79.93
+ 0.7	16.63	83.37
+ 0.8	13.70	86.30
+ 0.9	11.19	88.81
+ 1.0	9.09	90.91
+ 1.1	7.36	92.64
+ 1.2	5.93	94.07
+ 1.3	4.77	95.23
+ 1.4	3.83	96.17
+ 1.5	3.07	96.93
+ 1.6	2.450	97.55
+ 1.7	1.956	98.04
+ 1.8	1.560	98.44
+ 1.9	1.243	98.76
+ 2.0	0.990	99.01
+ 2.1.	0.7879	99.21
+ 2.2	0.6270	99.37
+ 2.3	0.4987	99.50
+ 2.4	0.3966	99.60
+ 2.5	0.3152	99.68
+ 2.6	0.2505	99.75
+ 2.7	0.1991	99.80
+ 2.8	0.1582	99.84
+ 2.9	0.1257	99.87
+ 3.0	0.09991	99.90
+ 3.1	0.0794	99.921
+ 3.2	0.0630	99.937
+ 3.3	0.0501	99.950
+ 3.4	0.0398	99.960
+ 3.5	0.0316	99.968
+ 4.0	0.0099990	99.9900
+ 5.0	0.0009999	99.99900
+ 6.0	0.0000999	99.99990

Appendix II

TABLE AND DISCUSSION: FRAGMENTAL CONSTANTS AND
PARTITION COEFFICIENTS OF ORGANIC MOLECULES

This appendix supplements the discussion on partition coefficients in Section 3.2.

Partition coefficients of solids and liquids are conveniently measured in a 250 ml glass-stoppered centrifuge tube. This is charged with the weighed solute and such proportions of the two solvents as are suggested by previous runs or analogous solutes. The tube is inverted 100 times in 5 minutes, although equilibrium will probably occur within the first 2 minutes. The mixture is then centrifuged, allowed to settle, and inspected for traces of emulsification (if this has occurred, a fresh start must be made). Either phase can now be analysed for its content of solute (Leo, Hansch, and Elkins, 1971).

Partition coefficients of gases are measured by bubbling the gas through a mixture of the two solvents, then withdrawing a sample of the organic layer and analysing it by gas-liquid partition chromatography (Leo, *et al.*, 1975; Hansch *et al.*, 1975).

For a table of 5806 partition coefficients, see Leo, Hansch, and Elkins (1971).

A machine known as the 'Akufve', equipped with devices for mixing, centrifuging, and u.v. sensing, is available for routine determinations of partition coefficients. Its principal disadvantage is the large quantity of organic solvent required: about 500 ml (Davis *et al.*, 1976).

The accompanying Table presents a useful selection of fragmental constants (f) derived from octanol/water partition coefficients (P). Other values, such as -NMe$_2$, can be constructed from the Table. These f values, which replace the former π values, tend to be about 0.2 higher but not consistently so.

The lipophilic effect of hydrocarbon fragments is evident from the Table. When a carbon-carbon double bond is present, it makes a definite (-0.55) contribution to hydrophilicity whereas a C—C triple bond makes a much larger one (-1.42). The aliphatic equivalent to phenyl, as a lipophilic substituent, lies between ethyl and propyl, whereas naphthyl approximates to pentyl. The hydrophilic properties of lone pairs of electrons are clearly reflected in the f values of nitrogen- and oxygen-containing groups.

Table II.1

SOME COMMON FRAGMENTAL CONSTANTS

A. No carbon (hydrogen absent)	Aliphatic	Aromatic		C. With carbon (hydrogen absent)	Aliphatic	Aromatic
-I	0.59	1.35		-C̩-	0.20	0.20
-Br	0.20	1.09		-CN	− 1.27	− 0.34
-Cl	0.06	0.94		-CON <	− 3.04	− 2.80
-F	− 0.38	0.37		-CO-	− 1.90	− 1.09
-N <	− 2.18	− 0.93		-CO$_2$-	− 1.49	− 0.56
-NO		0.11		-CO$_2$-	− 5.19	− 4.13
-NO$_2$	− 1.16	− 0.03		-SCN	− 0.48	0.64
-O-	− 1.82	− 0.61				
-SO$_2$N <		− 2.09				
-SO-	− 3.01	− 2.12				
-SO$_2$-	− 2.67	− 2.17				
-SO$_2$F		0.30				
-S-	− 0.79	0.03				

B. No carbon (hydrogen present)	Aliphatic	Aromatic		D. With carbon (hydrogen present)	Aliphatic	Aromatic
-H	0.23	0.23		-CH$_3$	0.89	(*)
-NH-	− 2.15	− 1.03		-CH$_2$-	0.66	
-NH.N <	− 3.06	− 0.62		-CH <	0.43	
-OH	− 1.64	− 0.44		C$_6$H$_5$	1.90	
-NH$_2$	− 1.54	− 1.00		C$_6$H$_4$	1.67	
-SH	− 0.23	0.62		-CO.NH-	− 2.71	− 1.81
-SO$_2$NH$_2$		− 1.59		> C.NOH	− 1.25	− 0.38
				-O.CONH-		− 1.51

H. In heteroaromatic rings					Aliphatic	Aromatic
-N =	− 1.12			-CO$_2$H	− 1.11	− 0.03
-NH-	− 0.67			-CONH$_2$	− 2.18	− 1.26
-O-	− 0.08			-NHCONH-		− 1.57
-S-	0.36			-NCHONH$_2$	− 2.18	− 1.07
-CO.NH-	− 2.00					
-N = N-	− 2.14					

(*) Hydrocarbon fragments are allotted the aliphatic values when attached to aromatic nuclei.

(Source: Leo *et al.*, 1975; Dr. A. J. Leo, personal communication, 1977).

Appendix III

TABLES AND DISCUSSION: ELECTRONIC EFFECTS IN MOLECULES
(HAMMETT AND TAFT SIGMA VALUES)

A knowledge of the effects of various substituents on any ionizable group allows each substituent to be classed as electron-attracting or electron-releasing, and placed in ranking order. This operation was quantified, about 1940, by the introduction of Hammett's *Linear Free Energy Equation*:

$$\log K - \log K_0 = \rho\sigma$$

where K_0 is the ionization constant of benzoic acid, which is the standard, K is the ionization constant of a benzoic acid bearing the substituent under investigation, ρ (rho) is a constant pertaining to the nucleus under investigation, and σ (sigma) is the constant pertaining to the substituent (ρ was given the value of 1.00 for the ionization of benzoic acid). The subject has been lucidly explained by Hammett (1970). Extensive lists of ρ values are available (Jaffé, 1953; Wells, 1963), and even longer ones of σ values (Jaffé, 1953; Wells, 1963; Ritchie and Sager, 1964; also Barlin and Perrin, 1966 for heterocycles), and recently a selection of 191 Hammett sigma values have been assembled specially for multiple regression analysts (Hansch *et al.*, 1973).

The list of σ values in Table III.1 should suffice here for the quantified ranking of substituents according to their electronic effects. For the aromatic series, values obtained from *meta*-substituted benzoic acids have the greatest reproducibility. Some values from *para* substituents are subject to a through-resonance interaction as in *p*-nitrophenol; when this occurs they are greatly changed. Through-resonance, discussed further by Clark and Perrin (1964), is illustrated in (III.1). *Ortho* substituents are complicated by steric effects and hydrogen bonding.

Through-resonance in *p*-nitrophenol
(III.1)

The principal groups evoking through-resonance are $-NO_2$ and $-CN$ in conjunction with one of the following: $-OH, -OMe, -NH_2$, and $-NMe_2$. Because of this resonance, the σ_p value of $-OMe$ may lie anywhere from -0.80 to 0.00, and that of $-NO_2$ anywhere between 0.60 to 1.4 (van Bekkum, Verkade, and Wepster, 1959; Bordwell and Andersen, 1953). Although several attempts have been made to introduce special values for use when cross-resonance is likely, the extent of the latter varies so greatly in different molecules that only a semi-quantitative estimate can be made.

Returning to Table III.1, the values marked with a minus sign are electron-releasing; all others are electron-attracting. It will be seen at once that the whole span of values is only about one unit; hence quite small changes in σ values may indicate fairly large electronic effects. Much attention should not be given to the second place of decimals, because σ values are the difference between two pK_a values each of which may have a small uncertainty in the second place. Again, if σ values are recalculated from other sources than the ionization of benzoic acid, even after applying the ρ correction, they show considerable differences from those of Table III.1, although the ranking order remains unchanged. When zwitterion formation is possible (as in m-aminobenzoic acid where there is much, although p-aminobenzoic acid has only a little), the change in σ values may be quite substantial.

Taft and Lewis (1959) took the first step to separate field from resonance effects, in sigma constants, by comparison with the (necessarily resonance-free) values which Taft had obtained for aliphatic acids (see below). This dual substituent parameter (DSP) approach can be applied to new results as a multiple correlation, using statistical methods, e.g. Snedecor (1946). This separation was further refined by Swain and Lupton (1968) (who were the first to show that the field effects of m- and p-positioned groups were quite different) into $\mathfrak{F}$ (field) and $\mathfrak{R}$ (resonance) effects. A systematic arithmetical error in the latter work has been ironed out by Hansch et al., (1973) who present a list of nearly 200 such values. From a theoretical point of view, it is an achievement to know from this work that the ranking order of resonance (mesomeric) effects is: (most negative) $-NH_2$, $-OMe$, F, $-NHAc$, Cl, Me, tBu, Ph, H, (neutral), $-NMe_3^+$ (neutral), $-CO_2^-$, $-CO_2H$, $-NO_2$ (most positive). Swain and Lupton also gave the following ranking order of field (inductive) effects in aromatic substituents (necessarily the same as in aliphatic substituents) : (most negative) $-CO_2^-$, tBu, Me, H (neutral), $-NH_2$, Ph, $-OMe$, $-NHAc$, $-CO_2H$, Cl, F, $-NO_2$, $-NMe_3^+$ (most positive). For a fresh look at the separation of field and resonance contributions, see Taft and Grob (1974).

For *aliphatic compounds*, completely saturated, Taft (1953) proposed a series of σ_I values, similarly derived from acetic acid:

$$\sigma_r = 0.262 \log K/K_o$$

Table III.1

SIGMA VALUES

	From benzoic acid[a]		From acetic acid[b]
	Meta substituents σ_m	Para substituents σ_p	σ_1
CH_2SiMe_3	− 0.19	− 0.22	− 0.19
CO_2^-	− 0.10	0.00	
t-Bu	− 0.10	− 0.20	− 0.07
Me	− 0.07	− 0.17	− 0.05
NH_2	− 0.04[c, d]	0.17[c]	0.11[h]
NMe_2	− 0.05[c]	0.17[c]	0.11[h]
OMe	0.12	− 0.27	0.27
OH	0.12	− 0.37	0.25
SMe	0.15	0.00	0.19
SH	0.25	0.15	0.25
$NH.COMe$	0.21	0.00	0.28
$CO.NH_2$	0.28[e]	0.36[f]	
CO.OMe	0.39	0.31	0.33
CO.OH	(0.37)	(0.45)	0.30
CHO	0.35[e]	0.42[g]	
COMe	0.38	0.50	0.31
F	0.34	0.06	0.57
Cl	0.37	0.23	0.51
Br	0.39	0.23	0.49
I	0.35	0.18	0.43
OCF_3	0.40	0.35	
SCF_3	0.40	0.50	
CN	0.56	0.66	0.63
SO_2NH_2	0.55	0.62	
SO_2Me	0.56	0.68	0.59
NO_2	0.71	0.78	0.69
SO_2CF_3	0.79	0.93	0.80
Me_3N^+	0.88	0.82	0.92

[a] Taken from Hammett (1970), supplemented by McDaniel and Brown (1958) except where otherwise indicated.

[b] Taken from Hammett (1970), supplemented by Taft and Lewis (1958), and Taft et al., (1963).

[c] These are σ^n values, thought to be freed from all zwitterionic contamination and cross-resonance (van Bekkum et al., 1959), and represent Hammett's own choice (1970); McDaniel and Brown (1958) gave, suprisingly, − 0.16 and − 0.66 for NH_2 (σ_m and σ_p respectively) and − 0.15 and − 0.83 for NMe_2 (respectively) (Hansch et al., 1973, list these values).

[d] The raw σ for NH_2 is 1.1, but m-aminobenzoic acid is largely zwitterionic so that this is really a $^+NH_3$ value.

[e] Jaffé (1953).

where K_0 is the ionization constant of acetic acid, K is the ionization constant of a substituted acetic acid, and 0.262 is a reciprocal ρ value to assist comparison between the two series. The effect of a substituent in acetic acid is far greater than in the m-position of benzoic acid because the distance is much less; hence the large size of ρ (about 4). A selection of Taft's σ_I values is given in the last column of Table III.1, from which it can be seen that they are very similar to σ_m values.

The usually electron-attracting vinyl- and phenyl-groups become mildly electron-releasing when a conjugated aliphatic chain intervenes between these substituents and the ionizing group. The doubly bound nitrogen in heterocycles (e.g. pyridine) is strongly electron-attracting, whereas the singly bound nitrogen atom (as in pyrrole) is strongly electron-releasing.

---

[f] Charton (1963).
[g] Charton (1965).
[h] Corrected for abundant zwitterionic species (glycine).

Appendix IV

TABLE AND DISCUSSION: NUCLEAR MAGNETIC RESONANCE

Introduction. The magnetic moments possessed by atomic nuclei with odd values of either mass or atomic number cause them to *precess* when placed in a powerful magnetic field. The frequency of this precession, which is directly proportional to the field strength, is characteristic of the type of nucleus and falls within the radio-frequency range. Of the elements most commonly encountered in organic chemistry, ^1H, ^{13}C, ^{14}N, ^{19}F, and ^{31}P give this effect, whereas ^{12}C and ^{16}O do not. Because the most readily accessible apparatus is specialized for the detection and measurement of ^1H, the nuclear magnetic resonance (n.m.r.) discussion will begin with that of the hydrogen nucleus (i.e. 'proton magnetic resonance').

A solution of the compound to be studied is irradiated, commonly in a slightly variable magnetic field of about 15 000 gauss, with an electromagnetic (radio) beam of frequency 60 megacycles (or more) per second. The transitions to a higher energy level which this irradiation causes in each hydrogen nucleus are detected by measuring the adsorption of energy from the transmitting circuit. This absorption unbalances a radio-frequency bridge, and the out-of-balance signal is then amplified, detected, and recorded.

The field experienced in each hydrogen nucleus is less than that applied by the instrument because of the diamagnetic shielding effect of the extra-nuclear electron cloud. Hence different magnetic fields must be applied so that nuclei in different electronic environments can be brought into resonance. This variation in magnetic field is usually arranged by sweeping some auxiliary magnetic coils into the environment of the specimen. The difference between the resonance frequencies of various hydrogen nuclei is called the 'chemical shift' and is usually measured in parts per million (p.p.m.). The value 0.00 p.p.m. has been arbitrarily assigned to the resonance of the hydrogen atoms in tetramethyl-silane, enabling a table of delta (δ) values to be drawn up, e.g. Table IV.1. A high δ value indicates a decrease in the applied field necessitated by much shielding in the molecule. (In another used scale, tetramethyl-silane is given the value of 10, and the results are recorded as tau values ($\tau = 10 - \delta$).

The commonest use of n.m.r. in chemistry is to decide whether certain groups are present or absent. Hence it is much used in finding the constitution of newly synthesized or isolated substances. It is also valuable in investigating potentially tautomeric molecules. When the tautomeric equilibrium is reached slowly (as usually occurs when the mobile proton is attached to a *carbon* atom in one tautomeric form), signals from both tautomeric forms are recorded independently, and a kinetic study may be made. The equilibrium is reached almost instantaneously when the mobile proton is attached to a *nitrogen* or *oxygen* atom.

Table IV.1

APPROXIMATE δ VALUES FOR HYDROGEN NUCLEI IN DIFFERENT MOLECULAR ENVIRONMENTS

Environment	δ(p.p.m.)	Environment	δ(p.p.m.)
CH_3—C	0.9	NH_2—Ar	3.5[a]
C—CH_2—C } C—CH(R)—C }	1.2–1.5	CH_3—O—CO	3.8
		CH_3—O—Ar	3.8
H_2N—CR_2	1.6[a]	CH_2 : C	4.7
CH_3C : C	1.8	HR(R) : C	5.3
CH_3—C : O	2.0	HO—C	5.3[a]
CH_3—S	2.0	H_2N—CO	7.0[a]
CH_3—N	2.2	H—Ar	7–8
CH_3—Ar	2.4	HO—Ar	7.7[a]
CH_3—N(R)—CO	2.8	R.CHO	9.8
CH_3—O	3.3	R.COOH	10.8

[a]Positions variable because of hydrogen bonding (see text). (Jones and Katritzky, 1962.)

Most n.m.r. spectra have separate peaks for each kind of hydrogen atom that is present in a different environment, and the peak area is always proportional to the number of hydrogen nuclei which contribute to the peak. An electronic device, in the spectrometer, *integrates* the area of each peak to give the number of hydrogen atoms (per molecule) contributing to that peak.

Because *hydrogen-bonding* alters the environment of a hydrogen nucleus, it can have a large effect on the δ value. For example, concentrated solutions of alcohols in carbon tetrachloride usually give δ 5.3 for the $-OH$ proton, but when they are diluted (or heated) sufficiently, the signal moves upfield in the direction of 0.5 as intermolecular bonding is lost. However, substances with intramolecular hydrogen bonds retain their high δ values on dilution, and this is diagnostic.

Apart from the shielding effects mentioned above, the external field of the instrument can induce electron currents which strongly shield acetylenic hydrogen atoms (δ 2.3) whereas aromatic protons are strongly deshielded (δ 7–7).

The peaks of a n.m.r. spectrum are often split, e.g. into doublets, triplets, quartets. This fine structure arises from *spin-spin interaction* between hydrogen nuclei of different δ values. This is caused by the magnetic nucleus in an atom producing small magnetic fields at other positions in the molecule. This splitting, which is independent of the strength of the applied magnetic field, is usually recorded, in Hertz (cycles per second) as $\mathfrak{J}$, the spin-spin coupling constant. Coupling of hydrogen nuclei by σ-bonds is strong but rapidly attenuated by distance, whereas couplings transmitted through π-electron systems in aromatic molecules are relatively small although not greatly diminished by increased distance. Hence spin-spin multiplets are useful, either to assign the peaks in substances of known structure, or to determine the structure of a molecule from its spectrum. Most modern instruments have a spin-spin decoupling device which can be made to irradiate the specimen with a second radio frequency, so chosen as to make the multiplet structure collapse, even to a single peak, but this operation is usually lengthy.

The most useful *solvents* in nuclear magnetic resonance studies are those that are free from hydrogen atoms (e.g. carbon tetrachloride), or are completely deuterated, or else have only hydrogen atoms of low δ (e.g. dimethyl sulphoxide or acetone). In work of biological interest, however, the demand is always for water as the solvent and this injects a swamping hydrogen signal in mid-field. A compromise may be reached with deuterium oxide as the solvent, which contributes no signals but removes signals caused by the rapidly exchangeable hydrogen atoms attached to nitrogen, oxygen, and sulphur. In some compounds, the chemical shift of a hydrogen atom in a particular position is unusually solvent-dependent. Thus, in indole the 2-hydrogen atom shows marked differences in chemical shift between a polar and a non-polar solvent, whereas the 3-hydrogen atom does not.

The high concentrations that are required in most n.m.r. measurements sometimes lead to conclusions incompatible, or only partly compatible, with those derived from other physical techniques, and often traceable to association. One way of overcoming this is to work in a more dilute solution which is scanned several hundreds of times and the cumulated readings plotted after passage through a 'cat' (computer of average transients) to improve the ratio of signal to noise.

It is often helpful to examine a specimen that has been deuterated in chosen positions, e.g. by replacing a mobile chlorine atom by deuterium, or by D^+-catalysed electrophilic attack on a relatively electron-rich position in the molecule. The signal formerly given by the hydrogen atom (that has been replaced by deuterium) completely disappears without altering the chemical shifts (but with considerable change in the spin-spin coupling constants) of the remaining ^1H nuclei.

For a collection of analysed spectra, see Simons and Zanger (1972).

For reading on nuclear magnetic resonance spectra, see Jackman and Sternhell (1968); Batterham (1973).

Applications of n.m.r. in biological and medicinal chemistry. Many conformational and configurational problems have been solved by use of the Karplus equation which correlates the coupling constant between vicinal protons with the torsional angles (defined in Section 13.3) between different carbon-hydrogen planes (Karplus, 1959; Roberts, 1968). In this way, each of the four isomers of cocaine (*7.11*) was assigned a conformation (Sinnema et al., 1968).

N.m.r. is esteemed as one of the most powerful physical techniques to investigate the reaction between a small molecule and a polymer. Because many of the resonances in the spectrum of the biopolymer will overlap, special techniques are used, such as perturbation of the resonances by introducing paramagnetic ions. Also ^{13}C and ^{19}F make useful labels in such cases (Dwek et al., 1977).

Part of the n.m.r. spectrum of an agent undergoes broadening after adsorption has occurred on to a macromolecule. Briefly, the technique is based on the fact that the relaxation rate $(1/T_1)$–and hence the width of the n.m.r. spectral line–depends on the motion of the molecule which gives rise to the line. If the motion of the molecule is restricted, the relaxation time of the nuclei is shortened and the width of its n.m.r. spectral lines is increased. Thus when a small molecule is bound to a macromolecule the lines of its n.m.r. spectrum broaden by a factor of 100–1000, very roughly in proportion to the increase in effective molecular weight. If only a part of the small molecule becomes attached, its spectral line is broadened selectively while the lines of the unattached parts of the molecule remain narrow by comparison. The part of the molecule firmly held on the macromolecule is therefore readily identifiable. Thus when atropine (*7.14*) was bound by acetylcholinesterase, the signals for both phenyl- and *N*-methyl-groups were broadened, and equally so, showing that both ends of the molecule were firmly bound. Physostigmine (*7.25*) was similarly shown to be firmly bound by both of its *N*-methyl-groups (Kato, Yung, and Ihnat, 1970).

For some years, Jardetzky and his colleagues have been using this technique to obtain information about factors concerned in attaching small molecule to their receptors (Jardetzky and Jardetzky, 1962; Jardetzky and Wade-Jardetzky, 1966). Two general types of complexes were distinguished, (a) van der Waals complexes where the binding (also the n.m.r. relaxation rate for the bound molecule) increases with increasing polarity of the solvent, and (b) electrostatic complexes where the reverse is true. Examples of the former are the binding of penicillin side-chains and the sulphanilamide moiety to serum albumin (Fischer and Jardetzky, 1965); examples of the latter are the binding of choline derivatives to an anti-choline antibody. Such an antibody was prepared against phenoxycholine to provide an immunochemical model for cholinergic receptors. Unhappily the specificity of this antibody turned out to be too low to permit differentiation between agonists and antagonists, or between muscarinic and nicotinic cholinomimetics (Marlow, Metcalf, and Burgen, 1969). This antibody showed, by line-broadening, that interaction with the tetramethylammonium ion imposed a barrier to the rotation of the methyl-groups (Burgen, 1967).

Particularly convenient for study by this technique is the common type of complex for which the binding constants K_s falls in the range 10^3–10^5. Such complexes exist in rapid equilibrium with the uncomplexed species, the rate of complex formation k_R in these systems being of the order of 10^8–10^{10} litres mol^{-1} s^{-1}, and the rate of dissociation k_D, by virtue of the relationship $K_s = k_R/k_D$, of the order 10^3–10^5 s^{-1}.

High-resolution n.m.r. combined with information from X-ray diffraction, is revealing much about the active sites and mechanisms of action of various enzymes, such as chymotrypsin (Gerig, 1968) and lysozyme (Cohen and Jardetzky, 1968), and the same benefits are expected for drugs and their receptors. Selective deuteration of the enzyme is a great help in these studies (Putter et al., 1969).

For further reading on proton molecular spectroscopy in medical and biological chemistry, see Casy (1971).

Non-proton n.m.r. spectra.   Recent years have witnessed an intensification of interest in the spectra of nuclei other than protons. Commercially available instruments can produce spectra of such nuclei as ^{13}C and ^{15}N in their natural abundance, and the introduction of Fourier transform devices immensely reduces the time and effort spent in this work.

Usually a (proton-decoupled) natural-abundance ^{13}C n.m.r. spectrum is more finely resolved than the corresponding protonic spectrum because nearly every non-equivalent carbon atom yields a well-resolved single-carbon resonance. This high resolution permits measurement of individual ^{13}C spin-lattice relaxation times (T_1) using a partially relaxed Fourier transform (PRFT) spectrum. The ^{13}C spin-lattice relaxation times of protonated carbon atoms in the larger drug molecules can easily be related to dynamic properties in solution, such as rotational motion of a molecular backbone or the internal rotations in a side-chain. Gramicidin S, for instance, has been investigated in this way (Allerhand and Komorowski, 1973).

In nitrogen-heterocyclic drugs, the ring-nitrogen atoms, whose natural ^{15}N label can now be routinely observed, are usually the sites where tautomerism, and association with the receptor, have their greatest effects.

For further reading on the applications of n.m.r. to interactions between small molecules and biopolymers, see James (1975); Dwek et al., (1977).

References

Ågren, A. (1954), *Acta Chem. Scand.*, **8**, 1059.

Ågren, A., and Bäck, T. (1973), *Arch. Pharm. Suecica* (Sweden), **10**, 223.

Abelson, H. and Penman, S. (1972), *Nature New Biol.*, **237**, 144.

Abraham, E. (1957), *Biochemistry of Some Peptide and Steroid Antibiotics*, New York: Wiley.

Abraham, E. (1962), *Pharmacol. Rev.*, **14**, 473.

Abraham, E. (1967), *Quart. Rev. Chem. Soc. Lond.*, **21**, 231.

Acs, G., Reich, E., and Mori, M. (1964), *Proc. Nat. Acad. Sci., U.S.*, **52**, 493.

Adam, N. K. (1941), *The Physics and Chemistry of Surfaces*, 3rd Edn, Oxford: Oxford University Press.

Adams, J. (1958), *J. Pharm. Pharmacol.*, **10**, 507, 516.

Adams, M., McPherson, A., Rossmann, M., Schevitz, R. and Wonscott, A. (1970), *J. Mol. Biol.*, **51**, 31.

Adamson, R., Bridges, J., and Williams, R. (1966), *Biochem. J.*, **101**, 71P.

Adcock, E. (1940), *J. exp. Biol.*, **17**, 449.

Addanki, S., Cahill, F. and Sotos, J. (1967), *Nature, Lond.*, **214**, 400.

Adler, R., and Snoke, J. (1962), *J. Bact.*, **83**, 1315.

Adler, S. and Tchernomoretz, I. (1942), *Ann. Trop. Med. Parasit.* **36**, 11.

Adler, T. (1963), *J. Pharmacol.*, **140**, 155.

Aeschlimann, J. and Reinert, M. (1931), *J. Pharmacol.*, **43**, 413.

Africk, J. and Fulton, J. (1971), *Brit. J. Dermatol.*, **84**, 151.

Agrawal, K., Booth, B., Moore, E. and Sartorelli, A. (1972), *J. Med. Chem.*, **15**, 1184.

Agrawal, K. and Sartorelli, A. (1975), Antineoplastic and Immunosuppressive Agents, (ed. Sartorelli, A. and Johns, C.), Berlin: Springer.

Ahlquist, R. (1948), *Amer. J. Physiol.*, **153**, 586.

Aigami, K., Inamoto, Y., Takaishi, N. and Fujikura, Y. (1976), *J. Med. Chem.*, **19**, 536.

Aigami, K., Inamoto, Y., Takaishi, N., Hattori, K., Takatsuki, A., and Tamura, G. (1975), *J. Medicin. Chem.*, **18**, 713.

Albert, A. (1944), *Med. J. Australia, i*, 245.

Albert, A. (1950), *Biochem. J.*, **47**, 531.

Albert, A. (1952), *Biochem. J.*, **50**, 690.

Albert, A. (1953), *Biochem. J.*, **54**, 646.

Albert, A. (1956), *Nature, Lond.*, **177**, 525.

Albert, A. (1957), *Biochem. J.*, **65**, 124.

Albert, A. (1966), *The Acridines, Their Preparation, Properties, and Uses*, 2nd Edn, London: Edward Arnold.

Albert, A. (1967), *Angew. Chem. Internat. Edn.*, **6**, 919.

Albert, A. (1968), *Heterocyclic Chemistry, an Introduction*, 2nd Edn, London: Athlone Press.

Albert, A. (1975), *The Selectivity of Drugs*, London: Chapman and Hall; New York: Wiley-Halsted.

Albert, A. (1976), *Adv. Heterocyclic Chem.*, **20**, 117 (Review).

Albert, A., Armarego, W. and Spinner, E. (1961), *J. Chem. Soc.*, 2689, 5267.

Albert, A. and Brown, D. (1954), *J. Chem. Soc.*, 2060.

Albert, A., Brown, D. and Cheeseman, G. (1952a), *J. Chem. Soc.*, 1620.

Albert, A., Brown, D. and Cheeseman, G. (1952b), *J. Chem. Soc.*, 4219.

Albert, A., Falk, J. and Rubbo, S. (1944), *Nature, Lond.*, **153**, 712.

Albert, A., Gibson, M. and Rubbo, S. (1953), *Brit. J. Exper. Path.*, **34**, 119.

Albert, A. and Goldacre, R. (1946), *J. Chem. Soc.*, 706.

Albert, A. and Goldacre, R. (1948), *Nature, Lond.*, **161**, 95.

Albert, A., Goldacre, R. and Phillips, J. (1948), *J. Chem. Soc.*, 2240.

Albert, A. and Hampton, A. (1952), *J. Chem. Soc.*, 4985.

Albert, A. and Hampton, A. (1954), *J. Chem. Soc.*, 505.

Albert, A., Hampton, A., Selbie, F. and Simon, R. (1954), *Brit. J. Exper. Path.*, **35**, 75.

Albert, A. and Howell, C. (1962). *J. Chem. Soc.*, 1591.

Albert, A., Howell, C. and Spinner, E. (1962), *J. Chem. Soc.*, 2595.

Albert, A. and Rees, C. (1956), *Nature, Lond.*, **177**, 433.

Albert, A., Rees, C. and Tomlinson, A. (1956), *Brit. J. Exper. Path.*, **37**, 500.

Albert, A. and Reich, F. (1961), *J. Chem. Soc.*, 127.

Albert, A., Rubbo, S. and Burvill, M. (1949), *Brit. J. Exper. Path.*, **30**, 159.

Albert, A., Rubbo, S. and Goldacre, R. (1941), *Nature, Lond.*, **147**, 332.

Albert, A., Rubbo, S., Goldacre, R. and Balfour, B. (1947), *Brit. J. Exper. Path.*, **28**, 69.

Albert, A., Rubbo, S., Goldacre, R., Davey, M. and Stone, J. (1945), *Brit. J. Exper. Path.*, **26**, 160.

Albert, A. and Serjeant, E. (1960), *Biochem. J.*, **76**, 621.

Albert, A. and Serjeant, E. (1971), *Ionization Constants, a Laboratory Manual*, 2nd Edn, London: Chapman and Hall; New York: Wiley-Halsted.

Albiston, H., Bull, L., Dick, A. and Keast, J. (1940), *Austral. Vet. J.*, **16**, 233.

Aldridge, W., (1958), *Biochem. J.*, **69**, 367.

Aldridge, W. and Barnes, J. (1952), *Nature, Lond.*, **169**, 345.

Aldridge, W. and Davison, A. (1952), *Biochem. J.*, **52**, 663.

Alexander, A. and Trim, T. (1946), *Proc. Roy. Soc. B*, **113**, 220.

Allen, P. and Gottlieb, D. (1970), *Appl. Microbiol.*, **20**, 919.

Allerhand, A. and Komorowski, R. (1973), *J. Amer. Chem. Soc.*, **95**, 8228.

Alles, G. and Knoefel, P. (1939), *Univ. Calif. Publ. Pharmacol.*, **1**, 187.

Allison, J., O'Brien, R. and Hahn, F. (1965), *Science*, **149**, 1111; *Antimicrob. Agents and Chemother.*, 310.

Allman, D., Wakabayashi, T., Korner, E. and Green, D. (1970), *Bioenergetics*, **1**, 73.

Alt, F., Kellems, R., Bertino, J. and Schimke, R. (1978), *J. Biol. Chem.*, **253**, 1357.

Alving, C., Steck, E., Chapman, W., Waits, V., Hendricks, L., Swartz, G. and Hanson, W. (1978), *Proc. Nat. Acad. Sci., U.S.A.*, **75**, 2959.

Ames, A., Tsukada, T. and Nesbett, F. (1967), *J. Neurochem.*, **14**, 145.

Ames, B. and Dubin, D. (1960), *J. Biol. Chem.*, **235**, 769.

Ames, B., Sims, P. and Grover, P. (1972), *Science*, **176**, 47.

Anand, N., Davis, B. and Armitage, A. (1960), *Nature, Lond.*, **185**, 23.

Anderson, B., Buckingham, D., Robertson, G., Webb, J., Murray, K. and Clark, P. (1976), *Nature, Lond.*, **262**, 722.

Anderson, B. and Swaby, R. (1951), *Austral. J. Sci. Res., B.*, **4**, 275.

Anderson, J., Matsubashi, M., Hoskin, M. and Strominger, J. (1965), *Proc. Nat. Acad. Sci., U.S.A.*, **53**, 881.

Anderson, K. and Liao, S. (1968), *Nature, Lond.*, **219**, 277.

Anker, R. and Cook, A. (1946), *J. Chem. Soc.*, 58.

Anon. (1974), *WHO Chronicle*, No. 8, p. 386.

Anon. (1975), *Chem. Eng. News*, Oct. 6th, p. 6.

Anton, A. (1960), *J. Pharmacol.*, **129**, 282.

Anzai, K. and Suzuki, S. (1961), *J. Antibiot. (Japan) A*, **14**, 253, 340. (*Chem. Abs.*, 1962, **56**, 8849, 10677.)

Arcamone, F., Cassinelli, G., Fantini, G., Grein, A., Orezzi, P., Poli, C. and Spalla, C. (1969), *Biotechnol. Bioeng.*, **11**, 1101.

Archer, S., Albertson, N. and Pierson, A. (1973), in *Agonist and Antagonist Actions of Narcotic Analgesic Drugs* (ed. Kosterlitz, H., Collier, H. and Villarreal, J.), Baltimore: University Park Press.

Ariëns, E. (1954), *Arch. internat. Pharmacodyn. Thér.*, **99**, 32.

Ariëns, E. (1960), in *Adrenergic Mechanisms* (ed. Vane, J., Wolstenholme, G. and O'Connor, M.), London: Churchill.

Ariëns, E., van Rossum, J. and Simonis, A. (1957), *Pharmacol. Rev.*, **9**, 218.

Armitage, A. and Ing, H. (1954), *Brit. J. Pharmacol.*, **9**, 376.

Armstrong, G., Bradbury, F. and Standen, H. (1951), *Ann. Appl. Biol.*, **38**, 555.

Armstrong, R. and Panzer, N. (1972), *J. Amer. Chem. Soc.*, **94**, 7650.

Arunlakshana, O. and Schild, H. (1959), *Brit. J. Pharmacol.*, **14**, 48.

Ashton, F. and Crafts, A. (1973), *Mode of Action of Herbicides*, New York: Wiley.

Ashe, H. (1964), *Arch. Environ. Health*, **9**, 545.

Atkinson, M., Jackson, J. and Morton, R. (1961), *Nature, Lond.*, **192**, 946.

Atkinson, M. and Murray, A. (1965), *Biochem. J.*, **94**, 64.

Audus, L. (ed.) (1976), *Herbicides* (2 vols), New York: Academic Press.

Augstein, J., Farmer, J., Lee, T. Sheard, P. and Tattersall, M. (1973), *Nature New Biol.*, **245**, 215.

Austin, W., Courtney, W., Danilewicz, J. and 7 others, (1966), *Nature, Lond.*, **212**, 1273.

Avery, O., MacLeod, C. and McCarty, M., (1944), *J. Exper. Med.*, **79**, 137.

Aviado, D., Brugler, B. and Bellet, J. (1968), *Exper. Path.*, **23**, 294.

Axelrod, J., Weil-Malherbe, H. and Tomchick, R. (1959), *J. Pharmacol.*, **127**, 251.

Baba, W., Smith, A. and Townshend, M. (1966), *Brit. J. Pharmacol.*, **28**, 238.

Babin, D., Forrest, T., Valenta, Z. and Wiesner, K. (1962), *Experientia*, **18**, 549.

Bach, M., Brashler, J. and Gorman, R. (1977), *Prostaglandins*, **14**, 21 (*per Chem. Abs.* 1977, **87**, 132152.)

Bacon, J., Milne, B., Taylor, I. and Webley, D. (1965), *Biochem. J.*, **95**, 28C.

Baddiley, J. (1962), *J. Roy. Inst. Chem.*, **86**, 366.

Baddiley, J., Hancock, I. and Sherwood, P. (1973), *Nature, Lond.*, **243**, 43.

Badger, G. (1946), *Nature, Lond.*, **158**, 585.

Badger, G. (1947), *Nature, Lond.*, **159**, 194.

Badger, G. Elson, L., Haddow, A., Hewett, C. and Robinson, A. (1941), *Proc. Roy. Soc. B*, **130**, 255.

Baird, W. and Reid, A. (1967), *Brit. J. Anaesth.*, **39**, 755.

Baker, B. (1967), *Design of Active Site-Directed Irreversible Inhibitors*, New York: Wiley.

Baker, B., Lee, W., Martinez, A., Ross, L. and Goodman, L. (1962a), *J. Org. Chem.*, **27**, 3283.

Baker, B., Lee, W., Tong, E., Ross, L. and Martinez, A. (1962b), *J. Theoret. Biol.*, **3**, 446.

580 References

Baker, B. and Patel, R. (1964), *J. Pharm. Sci.*, **53**, 717.
Baker, B. and Shapiro, H. (1966), *J. Pharm. Sci.*, **55**, 308.
Baker, P. (1968), *Brit. Med. Bulletin*, **24**, 179.
Baker, R., Chothia, C., Pauling, P. and Petcher, T. (1971), *Nature, Lond.*, **230**, 439.
Baldwin, B., Clarke, C. and Wilson, I. (1968), *Biochim. Biophys. Acta*, **162**, 614.
Baldwin, E. (1948a), *An Introduction to Comparative Biochemistry*, 3rd Edn, Cambridge: Cambridge University Press.
Baldwin, E. (1948,b), *Brit. J. Pharmacol. Chemother.*, **3**, 91.
Ball, W. and French, O. (1935), *Bull. Univ. Calif. Agric. Exper. Station*, **596**, 5.
Ballard, B. and Nelson, E. (1962), *J. Pharm. Sci.*, **51**, 915.
Bangham, A., Standish, M. and Weissman, G. (1975), *J. Mol. Biol.*, **13**, 253.
Bard, R. and Gunsalus, L. (1950), *J. Bact.*, **59**, 387.
Barger, G. and Dale, H. (1910), *J. Physiol.*, **41**, 19.
Barker, H., Smyth, R., Weissbach, H., Toohey, J., Ladd, J. and Volcani, B. (1960), *J. Biol. Chem.* **235**, 480.
Barlin, G. and Perrin, D. (1966), *Quart. Rev. Chem., Soc., London*, **20**, 75.
Barlow, R. (1964), *Chemical Pharmacology*, 2nd Edn, London: Methuen (revised printing, 1968).
Barlow, R. and Hamilton, J. (1962), *Brit. J. Pharmacol.*, **18**, 510, 543.
Barlow, R. and Hamilton, J (1965), *Brit. J. Pharmacol.*, **25**, 206.
Barlow, R. and Ing, H. (1948), *Brit. J. Pharmacol.*, **3**, 298.
Barlow, R., Scott, K. and Stephenson, R. (1963), *Brit. J. Pharmacol.*, **21**, 509.
Barnard, E., Wieckowski, J. and Chiu, T. (1971), *Nature, Lond.*, **234**, 207.
Barnes, J. and eight others (1957), *Nature, Lond.*, **180**, 62.
Barnes, J. and Stoner, H. (1958), *Brit. J. Industr. Med.*, **15**, 15.
Barnett, J., Ralph, A. and Munday, K. (1970), *Biochem. J.*, **116**, 537.
Barrett, P. (1974), *Proc. Brit. Weed Control Conf.*, **12**, 229.
Barrett, W., Rutledge, R., Plummer, A. and Yonkman, F. (1953), *J. Pharmacol.*, **108**, 305.
Barrnas, Y. and Clastre, J. (1970), *Compt. rend. Acad. Sci. Paris*, **270**, C, 306.
Barry, G., Cook, J., Haslewood, G., Hewett, C. and Kennaway, E. (1935), *Proc. Roy. Soc. B*, **117**, 318.
Barry, V. (1954), *J. Proc. Roy. Inst. Chem.*, **78**, 313.
Barlett, G. and Barron, E. (1947), *J. Biol. Chem.*, **170**, 67.
Barton, D. and Cookson, R. (1956), *Quart. Rev. Chem. Soc. London*, **10**, 44.
Bartz, Q. (1948), *J. Biol. Chem.*, **172**, 445.
Basil, B., Clark, J., Coffee, E., Jordan, R., Loveless, A., Pain, D. and Wooldridge, K. (1976), *J. Med. Chem.*, **19**, 399.
Basolo, F. and Pearson, R. (1967), *Mechanisms of Inorganic Reactions*, 2nd Edn, New York: Wiley.
Bass, W., Schueler, F., Featherstone, R. and Gross, E. (1950), *J. Pharmacol.*, **100**, 465.
Batchelor, F., Chain, E., Richards, M. and Robinson, G. (1961), *Proc. Roy. Soc. B*, **154**, 522.
Bateman, J. (1958), *Ann. N.Y. Acad. Sci.*, **68**, 1057.
Bate-Smith, E. and Westhall, R. (1950), *Biochim. Biophys. Acta*, **4**, 427.
Batterham, T. (1973), *NMR Spectra of Simple Heterocycles*, New York: Wiley.
Bauer, D. and Sadler, P. (1961), *Nature, Lond.*, **190**, 1167.
Bauer, D., St. Vincent, C., Kempe, C. and Downie, A. (1963), *Lancet*, ii, 494.
Bauer, W. and Vinograd, J. (1970), *J. Mol. Biol.*, **47**, 419.
Baum, F. (1899), *Arch. exper. Path. Pharmakol.*, **42**, 119.
Baur, E. and Preis, H. (1936), *Z. phys. Chem.*, **32**, B, 65.

References 581

Beaudet, A. and Caskey, C. (1971), *Proc. Nat. Acad. Sci. U.S.A.*, **68**, 619.
Bebbington, A., Brimblecombe, R. and Rowsell, D. (1966), *Brit. J. Pharmacol. Chemother.*, **26**, 68.
Bebbington, A., Brimblecombe, R. and Shakeshaft, D. (1966), *Brit. J. Pharmacol.*, **26**, 56.
Bebbington, R., Brooks, D., Geoghegan, M. and Snell, B. (1969), *Chem. and Indust.*, 1512.
Beccari, E. (1938), *Boll. Soc. ital. Biol. sper.*, **13**, 6.
Baccari, E. (1941), *Boll. Soc. ital. Biol. sper.*, **16**, 214; *Arch. Sci. biol.*, Bologna, **27**, 204.
Bechhold, H. and Ehrlich, P. (1906), *Z. physiol. Chem.*, **47**, 173.
Beckett, A. (1959), *Arzneimittelforschung* (Basel), **1**, 455.
Beckett, A., Boyes, R. and Triggs, E. (1968), *J. Pharm. Pharmacol.*, **20**, 92.
Beckett, A. and Casy, A. (1962), *Progress Medicinal Chem.*, **2**, 43.
Beckett, A., Harper, N. and Clitherow, J. (1963), *J. Pharm. Pharmacol.*, **15**, 362.
Beckett, A., Patki, S. and Robinson, A. (1959), *J. Pharm. Pharmacol.*, **11**, 360.
Beckett, A., Vahora, A. and Robinson, A. (1958), *J. Pharm. Pharmacol.*, **10**, 160T.
van Beek, W., Smets, L. and Emmelot, P. (1975), *Nature, Lond.*, **253**, 457.
Beers, W. and Reich, E. (1970), *Nature, Lond.*, **228**, 917.
Beers, W. and Reich, E. (1971), *Nature, Lond.*, **232**, 422.
Behnke, A. and Yarbrough, O. (1939), *Amer. J. Physiol.*, **126**, 409.
van Bekkum, H., Verkade, P., and Wepster, B. (1959), *Rec. Trav. chim. Pays-Bas*, **78**, 815.
Belisario, J. (1970) in *Current Dematologic Management*, (ed. Maddin, S., and Brown, T.), St. Louis (U.S.A.): Mosby.
Bell, C. (1976), *Principles and Applications of Metal Chelation*, Oxford: Oxford University Press.
Bell, P. and Roblin, R. (1942), *J. Amer. Chem. Soc.*, **64**, 2905.
Bell, R. (1973), *The Proton in Chemistry*, 2nd edn, London: Chapman and Hall; New York: Wiley-Halsted.
Bell, R. and Matschiner, J. (1972), *Nature, Lond.*, **237**, 32.
Belleau, B. (1967), *Ann. N.Y. Acad. Sci.*, **139** (art. 3), 580.
Belleau, B. and Lacasse, G. (1964), *J. Med. Chem.*, **7**, 768.
Belleau, B. and Puranen, J. (1963), *J. Med. Chem.*, **6**, 325.
Belleau, B., Tani, H. and Lie, F. (1965), *J. Amer. Chem. Soc.*, **37**, 2283.
Bellville, J. and Forrest, W. (1968), *Clin. Pharmacol. Ther.*, **9**, 142.
Belozersky, A. and Spirin, A. (1958), *Nature, Lond.*, **182**, 111.
Benda, L. (1912), *Ber. deutsch. chem. Ges.*, **45**, 1787 (with appendix by Ehrlich, P.).
Bender, M. (1971). *Mechanisms of homogeneous catalysis from protons to proteins*, New York: Wiley-Interscience.
Bender, M., van Etten, R., Clowes, G. and Sebastian, J. (1966), *J. Amer. Chem. Soc.*, **88**, 2318.
Benesi, H. and Hildebrand, J. (1948), *J. Amer. Chem. Soc.*, **70**, 3978.
Bennett, J. (1977), *Ann. Intern. Med.*, **86**, 319 (review).
Bennett, J. and Bueding, L. (1973), *J. Molec. Pharmacol.*, **9**, 311.
Bennett, L., Simpson, L., Golden, J. and Barker, T. (1963), *Cancer Res.*, **23**, 1574.
Bent, K. (1970), *Ann. Appl. Biol.*, **66**, 103.
Bentley, R. (1969), *Molecular Asymmetry in Biology*, Vol. *1*, London: Academic Press.
van den Bercken, J. and Narahashi, T. (1974), *Europ. J. Pharmacol.*, **27**, 255.
Berends, F., Posthumus, C., van der Sluys, I. and Deierkauf, F. (1959), *Biochim. et Biophys. Acta*, **34**, 576.
van der Berg, G., Bultsma, T., Rekker, R. and Nauta, W. (1975), *Eur. J. Med. Chem.*, **10**, 242.

582   References

Bergel, F. (1958), *Ann. N.Y. Acad. Sci.*, **68**, 1238.
Bergel, F. and Morrison, A. (1948), *Quart. Rev. Chem. Soc. London* **2**, 349.
Bergel, F. and Stock, J. (1954), *J. Chem. Soc.*, 2409.
Bergel, F., and Todd, A. (1937), *J. Chem. Soc.*, 1504.
Berger, J., Rachlin, A., Scott, W., Sternbach, L. and Goldberg, M. (1951), *J. Amer. Chem. Soc.*, **73**, 5295.
Berger, M. (1957), *J. Neurochem.*, **2**, 30.
Bergmann, F., Kwietny, H., Levin, G. and Brown, D. (1960), *J. Amer. Chem. Soc.*, **82**, 598.
Bergmann, F. and Segal, R. (1954), *Biochem. J.*, **58**, 692.
Bernard, C. (1856), *Compt. rend. Acad. Sci. Paris*, **43**, 825.
Bernheim, F. and Bernheim, M. (1939), *Cold Spring Harbor Symp. Quant. Biol.*, **7**, 174.
Berry, H., Cook, A. and Wills, B. (1956), *J. Pharm. Pharmacol.*, **8**, 425.
Bertino, J., Cashmore, A., Fink, N., Calabresi, P. and Lefkowitz, E. (1965), *Clin. Pharmac. Ther.*, **6**, 763.
Bertino, J. and Johns, D. (1967), *Ann. Rev. Med.*, **18**, 27.
Bessman, S., Rubin, M. and Leikin, S. (1954), *Pediatrics*, **14**, 201.
Beutler, E. (1959), *Blood*, **14**, 103.
Biagi, G., Barbaro, A., Guerra, M., Forti, G. and Fracasso, M. (1974), *J. Med. Chem.*, **17**, 28.
Bickel, H., Hall, G., Schierlein, W., Prelog, V., Vischer, E. and Wettstein, A. (1960), *Helv. Chim. Acta*, **43**, 2129.
Bicker, V. (1974), *Nature, Lond.*, **252**, 726.
Bijvoet, J., Peerdeman, A. and van Bommel, A. (1951), *Nature, Lond.*, **168**, 271.
Birch, A., Holzapfel, C., Rickards, R., Djerassi, C., Seidel, P., Suzuki, M., Westley, J. and Dutcher, J. (1964), *Tetrahed. Lett.*, 1491.
Bird, A. and Marshall, A. (1967), *Biochem. Pharmacol*, **16**, 2275.
Bittar, E. (1964), *Cell pH*, Washington, D.C.: Butterworths.
Bittar, E. (Ed.) (1970–1), *Membranes and Ion Transport*, (3 vols), New York: Wiley.
Bjerrum, J. (1941), *Metal Amine Formation in Aqueous Solution*, Copenhagen: Haase.
Black, J., Durant, G., Emmett, J. and Ganellin, C. (1974), *Nature, Lond.*, **248**, 65.
Blackman, G. (1946), *Agriculture*, **53**, 16.
Blackman, G. (1948), *J. Roy. Horticult. Soc.*, **73**, 134.
Blackman, G. (1951), *Ann. Rev. Plant Physiol.* **2**, 199.
Blackman, G. (1954), *Nature, Lond.*, **174**, 1179.
Blackwood, R. (1970), *Advances Appl. Microbiol.*, **13**, 237.
Blair, D., Clarke, V., Fontanilles, F., Yokogawa, M., Sano, M., Tsuji, M., Kojima, S., Iijima, T. and Ito, Y. (1969), *Ann. N.Y. Acad. Sci.*, **160**, 811, 915, and 933.
Blake, C., Johnson, L., Main, G., North, T., Phillips, D. and Sarma, V. (1967), *Proc. Roy. Soc. B*, **167**, 378.
Blake, J. (1848), *Amer. J. Med. Sci.*, **15**, 63.
Blakley, R. (1969), *The Biochemistry of Folic Acid and Related Pteridines*, Amsterdam: North-Holland.
Blanz, E. and French, F. (1968), *Cancer Res.*, **28**, 2419.
Blaschko, H. (1950), *Proc. Roy. Soc. B*, **137**, 307.
Blaschko, H. (1952), *Pharmacol. Rev.* **4**, 415.
Blaschko, H. (1959), *Pharmacol. Rev.*, **11**, 307.
Block, S. (1956), *J. Agr. Food Chem.*, **4**, 1042.
Blokhina, N., Vozny, E. and Garin, A. (1972), *Cancer*, **30**, 390.
Blokhuis, G. and Veldstra, H. (1970), *F.E.B.S. Letters (Amsterdam)*, **11**, 197.
Blomäck, B. and Yamashina, I. (1958), *Arkiv. Kemi*, **12**, 299.

Blondin, G., Kessler, R. and Green, D. (1977), *Proc. Nat. Acad. Sci.*, *U.S.A.*, **74**, 3667.

Blubaugh, L., Botts, C. and Gerwe, E. (1940), *J. Bact.*, **39**, 51.

Blum, R. and Carter, S. (1974), *Ann. Intern. Med.*, **80**, 249.

Boakes, R., Bradley, P., Brookes, N., Candy, J. and Wolstencroft, J. (1971), *Brit. J. Pharmacol.*, **41**, 462.

Bock, L., Miller, G., Schaper, K. and Seydel, J. (1974), *J. Med. Chem.*, **17**, 23.

Boehme, E., Applegate, H., Toeplitz, B., Dolfini, J. and Gougoutas, J. (1971), *J. Amer. Chem. Soc.*, **93**, 4324.

Bollag, W. (1972), *Eur. J. Cancer*, **8**, 689.

Bolliger, A. (1939), *Analyst*, **64**, 416.

Bonadonna, G., Brusamolino, E., Valagussa, P., and many others, (1976), *New England J. Med.*, **294**, 405.

Bondi, A. (1964), *J. Phys. Chem.*, **68**, 441.

Bonner, J., and Varner, J. (1976), *Plant Biochemistry*, 3rd Edn, New York: Academic Press.

Bonting, S. (1970), in *Membranes and Ion Transport* (ed. Bittar, E.), vol. 1, Chap. 8, New York: Wiley-Interscience.

Bordwell, F. and Andersen, H. (1953), *J. Amer. Chem. Soc.*, **75**, 6019.

Borg, D. and Cotzias, G. (1962), *Proc. Nat. Acad. Sci. U.S.A.*, **48**, 623, 643.

Borisy, G. and Taylor, E. (1967), *J. Cell. Biol.*, **34**, 525, 535.

Borkovec, A. (1966), *Insect Chemosterilisants*, New York: Wiley.

Borowski, E. and Cybulska, B. (1967), *Nature, Lond.*, **213**, 1034.

van den Bossche, H. (Ed.), (1972), *Comparative Biochemistry of Parasites*, London: Academic Press.

van den Bossche, H. and Janssen, P. (1969), *Biochem. Pharmacol.*, **18**, 35.

Bosund, I. (1960), *Physiol. Plantarum*, **13**, 793.

Bouanchaud, D., Scavizzi, M. and Chabbert, Y. (1968), *J. Gen. Microbiol.*, **54**, 417.

Boura, A., Copp, F. and Green, A. (1959), *Nature, Lond.*, **184**, 70.

Boura, A. and Green, A. (1965), *Ann. Rev. Pharmacol.*, **5**, 183.

Bourne, G. (1970), *Division of Labor in Cells*, 2nd Edn, New York: Academic Press.

Bourne, G. (Ed.) (1973), *The Structure and Function of Muscle*, New York: Academic Press (in 4 volumes).

Bovet, D. (1947), *Rendiconti Istituto superiore di Sanità*, Rome, **10**, 1161.

Bovet, D. and Bovet-Nitti, F. (1949), *Rendiconti Istituto superiore di Sanità*, Rome, **12**, 7.

Bovet, D., Lepierre, F. and Lestrange, Y. (1947), *Compt. rend.*, **225**, 74.

Bovet, D., Horclois, R. and Walthert, F. (1944), *Comt. rend. Séanc. Soc. Biol.*, **138**, 99.

Bowers, W., Ohta, T., Cleere, J. and Marsella, P. (1976), *Science*, **193**, 542.

Boyce, C., Jones, T. and van Tongeren, W. (1967), *Bull. World Health Org.*, **37**, 1.

Boyd, G. and Smellie, R. (1972), *Biological Hydroxylation Mechanisms*, London: Academic Press.

Boyd, I. and Pathak, C. (1965), *J. Physiol.*, **176**, 191.

Boyer, P. (Ed.) (1970–   ), *The Enzymes*, 3rd Edn, New York: Academic Press (in 13 + volumes).

Boyland, E. (1947), *The Biochemical Reactions of Chemical Warfare Agents*, Symp. Biochem. Soc., 2, Cambridge: Cambridge University Press.

Boyland, E. (1950), *Biochem. Soc. Symp.*, **5**, 40.

Boyland, E., Dukes, C. and Grover, P. (1963), *Brit. J. Cancer*, **17**, 79.

Boyland, E., Wallace, D. and Williams, D. (1955), *Brit. J. Cancer*, **9**, 62.

Bradbury, F. and Standen, H. (1959), *Nature, Lond.*, **183**, 983.

584 References

Braestrup, C., Albrechtsen, R. and Squires, R. (1977), *Nature, Lond.*, **269**, 702.
von Brand, T. (1974), *Z. Parasitenkund.*, **45**, 109 (in English).
Brandes, D., Anton, E., Schofield, B. and Barnard, S. (1966), *Cancer Chemotherapy Report*, **50**, 47. (C.A. 1966, **64**, 20 452.)
Branton, D. (1966), *Proc. Nat. Acad. Sci., U.S.A.*, **55**, 1048.
Bratkowska-Seniów, B., Kaniak, T., Stumpf, A., Wahl-Mugeńska, M. and Wojnarska, J. (1976), *Materia Medica Polona, Warsaw*, **8**, 316.
Bresnick, E. and Hitchings, G. (1961), *Cancer Research*, **21**, 105.
Breyer, B., Buchanan, G. and Duewell, H. (1944), *J. Chem. Soc.*, 360.
Brian, R. (1965), *Chem. and Indust.*, 1955.
Briggs, G. and Haldane, J. (1925), *Biochem. J.*, **19**, 338.
Briggs, M. and Brotherton, J. (1970), *Steroid Biochemistry and Pharmacology*, London: Academic Press.
Brink, F. and Posternak, J. (1948), *J. Cell. Comp. Physiol.*, **32**, 211.
Brock, T. and Brock, M. (1959), *Arch. Biochem. Biophys.*, **85**, 176.
Brockman, R. (1963), *Cancer Res.*, **23**, 1191.
Brockman, R., Kelley, G., Stutts, P. and Copeland, V. (1961), *Nature, Lond.*, **191**, 469.
Brockman, R., Shaddix, S., Laster, W. and Schabel, F. (1970), *Cancer Res.*, **30**, 2358.
Brockman, W., Carter, W., Li, L.-H., Reusser, F. and Nichol, F. (1971), *Nature, Lond.*, **230**, 249.
Brockmann, H. (1960), *Forts. Chem. Org. Naturstoffe*, **18**, 1.
Brodie, B. (1956), *J. Pharm. Pharmacol.*, **8**, 1.
Brodie, B. (1962), *Enzymes and Drug Action*, (ed. Mongar, J., and de Reuck, A.) London: Churchill.
Brodie, B. (1964), *The Pharmacologist, Washington*, 6, 12.
Brodie, B. (1971), *Chem. Biol. Interactions, Amsterdam*, 3, 247.
Brodie, B., Aronow, L., and Axelrod, J. (1952), *J. Pharmacol.*, 106, 200.
Brodie, B., and Axelrod, J. (1948), *J. Pharmacol.*, **94**, 29.
Brodie, B., and Axelrod, J. (1949), *J. Pharmacol.*, **97**, 58.
Brodie, B., Gillette, J. and Ackerman, H. (1971), *Concepts in Biochemical Pharmacology*, Parts 1 and 2, Berlin: Springer. (For Part 3, see Gillette and Mitchell, 1975.)
Brodie, B. and Hogben, C. (1957), *J. Pharm. Pharmacol.*, **9**, 345.
Brodie, B., Kurz, H. and Schanker, L. (1960), *J. Pharmacol.*, **130**, 20.
Brodie, B., Udenfriend, S., Baer, J., Chenkin, T. and Dill, W. (1945), *J. Biol. Chem.*, **158**, 705.
Brookes, G. and Harrison, A. (1963), *Biochem. J.*, **87**, 5P.
Brookes, P., (1966), *Cancer Research*, **26**, 1994.
Brookes, P. and Lawley, P. (1964), *Nature, Lond.*, **202**, 781.
Brotzu, G. (1948), *Lav. Ist. Igiene Cagliari, Sardinia*.
Broughton, B., Chaplen, P., Knowles, P., Lunt, E., Marshall, S., Pain, D. and Woodridge, K. (1975), *J. Med. Chem.*, **18**, 1117.
Brown, A. Crum, see Crum Brown, A.
Brown, D. J. (1962), *The Pyrimidines*, New York: Wiley-Interscience.
Brown, D. J. and Mason, S. (1956), *J. Chem. Soc.*, 3443.
Brown, E., Aurbach, G., Hauser, D. and Troxler, F., (1976), *J. Biol. Chem.*, **251**, 1232.
Brown, G. M. (1962), *J. Biol. Chem.*, **237**, 536.
Brown, H., Matzuk, A., Ilves, I., Peterson, L., Harris, S., Sarett, L., Egerton, J., Yakstis, J., Campbell, W. and Cuckler, A. (1961), *J. Amer. Chem. Soc.* **83**, 1764.
Brown, H. and Rogers, E. (1950), *J. Amer. Chem. Soc.*, **72**, 1864.
Brown, M. and Richards, R. (1965), *Nature, Lond.*, **207**, 1391.
Brown, N., Hollinshead, D., Kingsbury, P. and Malone, J. (1962), *Nature, Lond.*, **194**, 379.

Brown, P. (1967), *Nature, Lond.*, **213**, 363.

Brown, W. and Pearce, L. (1919), *J. Exper. Med.*, **30**, 483.

Browning, C. (1929), in *A System of Bacteriology in Relation to Medicine*, London: H. M. Stationery Office for The Medical Research Council.

Browning, C. (1955), *Nature, Lond.*, **175**, 570, 616.

Browning, C., Cohen, J., Gaunt, R. and Gulbransen, R. (1922), *Proc. Roy. Soc. B*, **93**, 329.

Browning, C. and Gilmour, W. (1913), *J. Path. Bact.*, **18**, 144.

Browning, C. and Gulbransen, R. (1922), *J. Path. Bact.*, **25**, 395.

Browning, C., Gulbransen, R. and Kennaway, E. (1919), *J. Path. Bact.*, **23**, 106.

Browning, C., Gulbransen, R., Kennaway, E. and Thornton, L. (1917), *Brit. Med. J.*, **i**, 73.

Browning, C., Morgan, G., Robb, J. and Walls, L. (1938), *J. Path. Bact.*, **46**, 203.

Brugmans, J., Thienpont, D., van Wijngaarden, I. *et al.*, (1971), *J. Amer. Med. Assoc.*, **217**, 313.

Bruice, T. and Benkovic, S. (1966), *Bioorganic Mechanisms*, New York: Benjamin.

Brulé, G., Eckhardt, S., Hall, T. and Winkler, A. (1973), *Drug Therapy of Cancer*, Geneva: WHO.

Bryan, S. and Frieden, E. (1967), *Biochemistry*, **6**, 2728.

Buchanan, J. (1957), in *Chemistry and Biology of Purines, (Ciba Symposium)*, (ed. Wolstenholme, G., and O'Connor, C.), London: Churchill, p. 233.

Buchheim, R. (1872), *Über die 'scharfen' Stoffe, Arch. Heilk.*, 1.

Büchel, K. (ed.) (1977), *Pflanzenschutz und Schädlings Bekämpfung*, Stuttgart: Thieme.

Büchel, K. and Draber, W. (1969), *Prog. in Photosyn. Res.*, **3**, 1777.

Büchel, K. and Schäfer, G. (1970), *Zeits. Naturforsch.*, **25b**, 1465.

Bueding, E. (1962), *Drugs, Parasites and Hosts* (eds. Goodwin, L., and Nimmo-Smith, R.), London: Churchill, p. 15.

Bueding, E. and Fisher, J. (1966), *Biochem. Pharmacol.*, **15**, 1197.

Bueding, E. and Fisher, J. (1970), *Molecular Pharmacol.*, **6**, 532.

Bülbring, E. and Tomita, T. (1969), *Proc. Roy. Soc., B*, **172**, 103.

Bukatsch, F. and Haitinger, M. (1940), *Protoplasma*, **34**, 515.

Bull, G. and Hemsworth, B. (1965), *Brit. J. Pharmacol. Chemother.*, **25**, 228.

Bullen, J. and Rogers, H. (1969), *Nature, Lond.*, **224**, 380.

Bunting, J. and Meathrel, W. (1972), *Canad. J. Chem.*, **50**, 917.

Bunting, J. and Perrin, D. (1967), *J. Chem. Soc., (B)*, 950.

Burchall, J. and Hitchings, G. (1965), *Mol. Pharmacol.*, **1**, 126.

Burchenal, J., Lester, R., Riley, J. and Rhoads, C. (1948), *Cancer*, **1**, 399.

Burchenal, J., Murphy, M., Ellison, R., Karnofsky, D., Sykes, M., Tan, T., Leone, L., Craver, L., Dargeon, H. and Rhodes, C. (1953), *Blood*, **8**, 965.

Burgen, A. (1965), *Brit. J. Pharmacol. Chemother.*, **25**, 4.

Burgen, A. (1967), *Proc. Nat. Acad. Sci. U.S.A.*, **58**, 447.

Burgen, A. and Iversen, L. (1965), *Brit. J. Pharmacol. Chemother.*, **25**, 34.

Burgen, A., Roberts, G. and Feeney, J. (1975), *Nature, Lond.*, **253**, 753.

Burger, A. (1970), *Medicinal Chemistry*, 3rd Edn., New York: Wiley-Interscience.

Burger, A., Standridge, R. and Ariëns, E. (1963), *J. Med. Chem.*, **6**, 221.

Burger, A., Standridge, R., Stjernström, N. and Marchini, P. (1961), *J. Med. Pharm. Chem.*, **4**, 517.

Burger, M., and Noonan, K. (1970), *Nature, Lond.*, **228**, 512.

Burgoyne, L. (1974), *Biochem. Pharmacol.*, **23**, 1619.

Burkitt, D., Hutt, M. and Wright, D. (1965), *Cancer, Philadelphia*, **18**, 399.

Burn, J. (1950), *Brit. Med. J.*, **ii**, 691.

Burn, J. and Dale, H. (1915), *J. Pharmacol.*, **6**, 417.

586   References

Burn, J. and Rand, M. (1958), *J. Physiol.*, **144**, 314.

Burns, B. and Paton, W. (1951), *J. Physiol.*, **115**, 41.

Burns, J., Yü, T., Dayton, P., Gutman, A. and Brodie, B. (1960), *Ann. New York Acad. Sci.*, **86**, 253.

Burnstock, G., Campbell, G., Satchell, D. and Smythe, A. (1970), *Brit. J. Pharmacol.*, **40**, 668.

Burnstock, G. and Costa, M. (1975), *Adrenergic Neurones*, London: Chapman and Hall; New York: Wiley-Halsted.

Burton, A. and Carter, A. (1964), *Biochemistry*, **3**, 411.

Burton, D., Clarke, K. and Gray, G. (1964), *J. Chem. Soc.*, 1314.

Burton, D., Lambie, A., Ludgate, J., Newbold, G., Percival, A. and Saggers, D. (1965), *Nature, Lond.*, **208**, 1166.

Burtt, E. (1945), *Ann. Appl. Biol.*, **32**, 247.

Buss, E. (1875), *Zentrabl. f.d. med. Wiss.*, 276.

Busvine, J. (1957), *Trans. Roy. Soc. Trop. Med.*, **51**, 11.

Butler, A., Freeman, K. and Wright, D. (1977), *J. Chem. Soc.*, Perkin I, 765.

Butler, H., Hurse, A., Thursky, E. and Shulman, A. (1969), *Aust. J. Exper. Biol. Med. Sci.*, **47**, 541.

Butler, T. (1944), *J. Pharmacol.*, **81**, 72.

Butler, T. (1948), *J. Pharmacol.*, **92**, 49.

Butler, T. (1950), *Pharmacol. Rev.*, **2**, 121.

Butler, T. (1955), *J. Amer. Pharm. Assoc.*, **44**, 367.

Butterworth, J., Eley, D. and Stone, G. (1953), *Biochem. J.*, **53**, 30.

Byrde, R. and Woodcock, D. (1957), *Nature, Lond.*, **179**, 539.

Byrn, S., Graber, C. and Midland, S. (1976), *J. Org. Chem.*, **41**, 2283.

Cade, J. (1949), *Med. J. Austral.*, **36**, 349.

Cafruny, E. (1968), *Pharmacol. Rev.*, **20**, 89.

Cahn, A. and Hepp, P. (1887), *Berl. klin. Woch.*, **24**, 4, 26.

Cahn, R., Ingold, C. and Prelog, V. (1956), *Experientia*, **12**, 81.

Cain, B., Atwell, G. and Denny, W. (1976), *J. Med. Chem.*, **19**, 772.

Cairns, J. (1962), *Cold Spring Harbor Symp. Quant. Biol.*, **27**, 311.

Cairns, J. (1963), *J. Mol. Biol.*, **6**, 208.

Cairns, J. (1975), *Sci. Amer.*, **233**, 64.

Calabresi, P., McCollum, R. and Welch, A. (1963), *Nature, Lond.*, **197**, 767.

Calabresi, P. and Turner, R. (1966), *Ann. Intern. Med.*, **64**, 352.

Calvin, M. and Wilson, K. (1945), *J. Amer. Chem. Soc.*, **67**, 2003.

Cama, L. and Christensen, B. (1974), *J. Amer. Chem. Soc.*, **96**, 7582.

Cammarata, A. (1967), *Pharm. Chem.*, **10**, 525.

Cammarata, A., Yau, S., Collett, J. and Martin, A. (1970), *Molec. Pharmacol.*, **6**, 61.

Camp, H., Fukuto, T., and Metcalf, R. (1969), *J. Agr. Food. Chem.*, **17**, 243.

Campbell, H. and Link, K. (1941), *J. Biol. Chem.*, **138**, 21.

Campbell, P. and Kilby, B. (1975), *Basic Biochemistry for Medical Students*, London: Academic Press.

Canellakis, E., Shaw, Y., Hanners, W. and Schwartz, R. (1976), *Biochim. Biophys. Acta*, **418**, 277.

Canepa, F., Pauling, P. and Sörum, H. (1966), *Nature, Lond.*, **210**, 907.

Canfield, C. and Rozman, R. (1974), *Bull. World Health Org.*, **50**, 203.

Cantley, L., Resh, M. and Guidotti, G. (1978), *Nature, Lond.*, **272**, 552.

Carlsson, A. and Lundqvist, M. (1963), *Acta Pharmacol. Toxicol.*, **20**, 140.

Carlstrom, D. and Bergin, R. (1967), *Acta Cryst.*, **23**, 313.

Carmichael, J. and Bell, F. (1944), *J. Comp. Path. Therap.*, **54**, 49.

Carpenter, K. and Heywood, B. (1963), *Nature, Lond.*, **200**, 28.

Carrasco, L. (1978), *Nature, Lond.*, **272**, 694.
Carson, S., Godwin, S., Massoulie, J. and Kato, G. (1977), *Nature, Lond.*, **266**, 176.
Carter, G., Huppatz, J. and Wain, R. (1976), *Ann. Appl. Biol.*, **84**, 333.
Carter, S. (1967), *Nature, Lond.*, **213**, 261.
Carter, S. and Blum, R. (1976), *Prog. Biochem. Pharmacol.*, **11**, 158.
Carter, S. and Friedman, M. (1972), *European J. Cancer*, **8**, 85.
Casemore, D. (1970), *J. Clin. Path.*, **23**, 649.
Casida, J. (1970), *J. Agric. Food. Chem.*, **18**, 753.
Casida, J. (1973), *Ann. Rev. Biochem.*, **42**, 259.
Casida, J., McBryde, L., and Niedermeir, R. (1962), *J. Agric. Food Chem.*, **10**, 370.
Casselton, P. (1964), *Nature, Lond.*, **204**, 93.
del Castillo, J. and Katz, B. (1957), *Proc. Roy. Soc. B*, **146**, 339.
del Castillo, J., Mello, W. and Morales, T. (1964), *Brit. J. Pharmacol.*, **22**, 463.
Caswell, A. and Hutchison, J. (1971), *Biochem. Biophys. Res. Commun.*, **43**, 625.
Casy, A. (1970), in *Progress in Medical Chemistry*, 7 (ed Ellis, G., and West, G.), Part 2, London: Butterworth.
Casy, A. (1971), *PMR Spectroscopy in Medicinal and Biological Chemistry*, New York: Academic Press.
Casy, A. and Ison, R. (1970), *J. Pharm. Pharmacol.*, **22**, 270.
Cathey, H. (1964), *Ann. Rev. Plant Physiol.*, **15**, 271.
Cattell, W., Chamberlain, D., Fry, I., McSherry, M., Broughton, C. and O'Grady, F. (1971), *Brit. Med. J.*, **1**, 377.
Cavalli-Sforza, L. and Lederberg, J. (1956), *Genetics*, **41**, 367.
Cervello, V. (1882), *Arch. per le Sci. med.*, **6**, 177.
Chacko, G., Villegas, G., Barnola, F., Villegas, R. and Goldman, D. (1976), *Biochim. Biophys. Acta.*, **443**, 19.
Chain, E. (1948), *Ann. Rev. Biochem.*, **17**, 657.
Chambers, R. and Chambers, E. (1961), *Explorations into the Nature of the Living Cell*, Princeton: Harvard University Press.
Chambron, J., Daune, M. and Sadron, C. (1966), *Biochim. Biophys. Acta*, **123**, 306, 319.
Chance, B. (1960), in *Free Radicals in Biological Systems*, (ed. M. Blois *et al.*), New York: Academic Press.
Chance, B., Lee, C.-P., Blasie, J., Yonetani, T., and Mildvan, A. (1971), *Probes of Structure and Function, of Macromolecules and Membranes*, New York: Academic Press.
Chance, B. and Sacktor, B. (1958), *Arch. Biochem. Biophys.*, **76**, 509.
Changeux, J.-P. (1969), in *Proceedings of the Nobel Symposium on Symmetry Functions in Biological Systems* (eds. Engstrom, A., and Almqvist, W.), **11**, 235, New York: Wiley.
Changeux, J.-P., Meunier, J.-C., and Huchet, M. (1971), *Molec. Pharmacol.*, **7**, 538.
Chao, L. (1978), *Nature, Lond.*, **271**, 385.
Chapman, D. and Wallach, D. (1973), *Biological Membranes*, vol. 2, London: Academic Press.
Chapman, D. and Wallach, D. (1976), *Biological Membranes*, vol. 3, London: Academic Press.
Chappell, J. (1966), *Biochem. J.*, **100**, 43P.
Chappell, J., and Crofts, A. (1965), *Biochem. J.*, **95**, 707.
Charton, M. (1963), *J. Org. Chem.*, **28**, 3121.
Charton, M. (1965), *J. Org. Chem.*, **30**, 552.
Chatterjee, A. and Park, J. (1964), *Proc. Nat. Acad. Sci. U.S.A.*, **51**, 9.
Chen, M., Ward, D. and Prusoff, W. (1976), *J. Biol. Chem.*, **251**, 4833.

588　References

Cheng, C., Fugimura, S., Grunberger, D. and Weinstein, I. (1972), *Cancer Res.*, **32**, 22.

Chick, H. (1908), *J. Hygiene*, **8**, 92.

Chignell, C. (1970), *Molec. Pharmacol.*, **6**, 1.

Childs, A., Davies, D., Green, A. and Rutland, J. (1955), *Brit. J. Pharmacol.*, **10**, 462.

Childs, C. (1970), *Inorg, Chem.*, **9**, 2465.

Choi, D., Farb, D. and Fischbach, G. (1977), *Nature, Lond.*, **269**, 342.

Choi, Y. and Carr, C. (1968), *Nature, Lond.*, **217**, 556.

Chong, C. and Rickards, R. (1970), *Tetrahedron Letters*, 5145.

Choo-Kang, Y., Simpson, W. and Grant, I. (1969), *Brit. Med. J.*, **2**, 287.

Chothia, C. (1970), *Nature, Lond.*, **225**, 36.

Chothia, C. and Pauling, P. (1970a), *Nature, Lond.*, **226**, 541.

Chothia, C. and Pauling, P. (1970b), *Proc. Nat. Acad. Sci. U.S.A.*, **65**, 477.

Chow, A., Foerster, J. and Hryniuk, W. (1970), *Antimicrob. Agents and Chemother.*, 214.

Christophers, S. (1947), *J. Hygiene, Camb.*, **45**, 176.

Christopherson, J. (1918), *Lancet*, **ii**, 325.

Chu, M. and Fischer, G. (1965), *Biochem. Pharmacol.*, **4**, 333.

Cigén, R. (1958), *Acta Chem. Scand.*, **12**, 1456.

Cirillo, V., Harsch, M. and Lampen, J. (1964), *J. Gen. Microbiol.*, **35**, 249.

Clark, A. (1933), *The Mode of Action of Drugs on Cells*, London: Edward Arnold.

Clark, A. (1937), in *Handbuch der experimentellen Pharmakologie* (eds. Heffter, A., and Heubner, W.), Berlin: Springer; Erganz., **4**, p. 63 (in English).

Clark, A. and Raventós, J. (1937), *Quart. J. Expl. Physiol.*, **26**, 375.

Clark, E. and O'Donnell, S. (1965), *J. Chem. Soc.*, 6509.

Clark, J. and Perrin, D. (1964), *Quart. Rev. Chem. Soc. London*, **18**, 295.

Clark, N., Croshaw, B., Leggetter, B. and Spooner, D. (1974), *J. Med. Chem.*, **17**, 977.

Clark, R. and Panchen, A. (1971), *Synopsis of Animal Classification*, London: Chapman and Hall.

Clarke, F. (1977), *J. Chem. Educ.*, **54**, 230.

Clarkson, A. and Brohn, F. (1976), *Science*, **194**, 204.

Clarkson, B. (1972), *Cancer*, **30**, 1572.

Clarkson, T., Rothstein, A. and Sutherland, R. (1965), *Brit. J. Pharmacol. Chemother.*, **24**, 1.

Cleland, W. (1970), in *The Enzymes* (ed. Boyer, P.), 3rd Edn., New York: Academic Press, **2**, 1.

Clements, A. and May, T. (1974), *J. Expl. Biol.*, **60**, 783.

Clements, J. and Wilson, K. (1962), *Proc. Nat. Acad. Sci. U.S.A.*, **48**, 1008.

Clemons, G. and Sisler, H. (1969), *Phytopathology*, **59**, 705.

Clowes, G. and Keltch, A. (1931), *Proc. Soc. Expl. Biol. Med.*, **29**, 312.

Clowes, G., Keltch, A. and Krahl, M. (1940), *J. Pharmacol.*, **68**, 312.

Cohen, J. and Changeux, J. (1975), *Ann. Rev. Pharmacol.*, **15**, 83.

Cohen, J., and Jardetzky, O. (1968), *Proc. Nat. Acad. Sci., U.S.A.*, **60**, 92.

Cohen, N. (1966), *Biological Rev.*, **41**, 503.

Cohen, S. (1963), *Ann. Rev. Biochem.*, **32**, 83.

Cohen, S. (1971), *Polyamines*, New Jersey: Prentice-Hall.

Cohen, S. (1976), *Nature, Lond.*, **263**, 731.

Cohen, S., Flaks, J., Barner, H., Loeb, M. and Lichtenstein, J. (1958), *Proc. Nat. Acad. Sci., U.S.A.*, **44**, 1004.

Cohen, S. and Yielding, K. (1965), *Proc. Nat. Acad. Sci., U.S.A.*, **54**, 521.

Cohn, E., McMeekin, T., Edsall, J. and Weare, J. (1934), *J. Amer. Chem. Soc.*, **56**, 2270.

Cohn, M. and Leigh, J. (1962), *Nature, Lond.*, **193**, 1037.

Colburn, R. and Maas, J. (1965), *Nature, Lond.*, **208**, 37.

Colebrook L. and Kenny, M. (1936), *Lancet*, **i**, 1279.

Coleman, R. (1973), *Biochem. Biophys. Acta*, **300**, 1 (review).

Collander, R. (1933), *Act. Bot. Fenn., Finland*, **11**, 1.

Collander, R. (1937), *Trans. Farad. Soc.*, **33**, 985.

Collander, R. (1947), *Acta Physiol. Scand.*, 1947, **13**, 363.

Collander, R. (1954), *Acta Chem. Scand.*, **5**, 774.

Collier, H. (1965), *Nature, Lond*, **205**, 181.

Collier, H. (1971), *Proc. Roy. Soc. Med.*, **64**, 1.

Collier, H. and Roy, A. (1974), *Nature, Lond.*, **248**, 24.

Collier, H. and Waterhouse, P. (1950), *Ann. Trop. Med. Parasit.*, **44**, 156.

Collins, G., Sandler, M., Williams, E. and Youdim, M. (1970), *Nature, Lond.*, **225**, 817.

Colquhoun, D., Dionne, V., Steinbach, J. and Stevens, C. (1975), *Nature, Lond.*, **253**, 204.

Commission on Enzymes (1972), *Enzyme nomenclature*, Amsterdam: Elsevier.

Connemacher, R. and Mandel, H. (1965), *Biochem. Biophys. Res. Commun.*, **20**, 98.

Conney, A. (1967), *Pharmacol. Rev.*, **19**, 317.

Conney, A. and Burns, J. (1962), *Advances Pharmacol.*, **1**, 31.

Conney, A., Levin, W., Ikeda, M., Kuntzman, R., Cooper, D. and Rosenthal, O. (1968), *J. Biol. Chem.*, **243**, 3912.

Connors, T., Cox, P., Farmer, P., Foster, A. and Jarman, M. (1974), *Biochem. Pharmacol.*, **23**, 115.

Connors, T. and Hare, J. (1974), *Brit. J. Cancer*, **30**, 477.

Connors, T., Jones, M., Ross, W., Braddock, P., Khokhar, A. and Tobe, M. (1972), *Chem. Biol. Interactions, Amsterdam*, **5**, 415.

Conti, F. (1969), *Nature, Lond.*, **221**, 777.

Cook, D. (1967), *J. Mol. Biol.*, **29**, 167.

Cook, J., Hewett, C. and Hieger, I. (1932), *Nature, Lond.*, **130**, 926.

Cook, J., Hewett, C. and Hieger, I. (1933), *J. Chem. Soc.*, 396.

Cooper, J., Bloom, F. and Roth, R. (1974), *The Biochemical Basis of Neuropharmacology*, 2nd edn, Oxford: Oxford University Press.

Cooper, P. (1956), *Bacteriol. Rev.*, **20**, 28.

Corbett, J. (1974), *The Biochemical Mode of Action of Pesticides*, New York: Academic Press.

Corbett, J. and Goose, J. (1971), *Biochem. J.*, **121**, 41P.

Cordes, E. (1973), *Reaction Kinetics in Micelles*, New York: Plenum Press.

Cornforth, J., D'Arcy-Hart, P., Nicholls, G., Rees, R. and Stock, J. (1955), *Brit. J. Pharmacol.*, **10**, 73.

Cornforth, J., Milborrow, B. and Ryback, G. (1965), *Nature, Lond.*, **206**, 715.

Cornforth, J., Ryback, G., Popják, G., Donninger, C. and Schroepfer, G. (1962), *Biochem. Biophys. Res. Commun.*, **9**, 371.

Corrodi, H. and Hardegger, E. (1955), *Helv. Chim. Acta*, **38**, 2038.

Cortés, H., Vicente, J., Baena, L., Otero, J. and Gosálvez, M. (1978), *Europ. J. Cancer.*, **14**, 1359.

Cotzias, G., Van Woert, M. and Schiffer, L. (1967), *New Engl. J. Med.*, **276**, 374.

Council on Pharmacy and Chemistry, U.S.A. (1936), *J. Amer. Med. Ass.*, **107**, 1132.

Cowles, P. (1942), *Yale J. Biol. Med.*, **14**, 599.

Cox, J., Beach, J., Blair, A. and 8 others (1970), *Adv. Drug Res.*, **5**, 115.

Crabbé, J. (1968), *Arch. internat. Pharmacodyn. Thér.*, **173**, 474.

Crabbé, P. (1967), *Topics in Stereochemistry*, **1**, 93.

590 References

Craddock, V. (1970), *Nature, Lond.*, **228**, 1264.

Crafts, A. (1964), in *Physiology and Biochemistry of Herbicides*, (ed. L. Audus), New York: Academic Press.

Craig, J., Tate, M., Warwick, G. and Rogers, W. (1960), *J. Med. Pharm. Chem.*, **2**, 659, 669.

Craig, P. (1971), *J. Med. Chem.*, 14, 680.

Cramer, F. and Martin, F. (1958), *Chem. Ber.*, **91**, 308.

Cramer, H. (1967), *Pflanzenschutz Nachr. Bayer*, **20**, 1.

Cramer, J., Miller, J. and Miller, E. (1960), *J. Biol. Chem.*, **235**, 885.

Crane, R. and Wilson, T. (1958), *J. Appl. Physiol.*, **12**, 145.

Crathorn, A. and Hunter, G. (1958), *Biochem. J.*, **69**, 47 P.

Cremer-Bartels, G. (1975), in *Chemistry and Biology of Pteridines*, (ed. Pfleiderer, W.), Berlin: de Gruyter.

Criss, W. (1973), *Cancer Res.*, **33**, 51, 57.

Crow, T. and Johnstone, E. (1977), *Brit. J. Pharmacol.*, **59**, 466 P.

Crowther, A. and Levi, A. (1953), *Brit. J. Pharmacol.*, **8**, 93.

Cruess, W. and Richert, P. (1929), *J. Bact.*, **17**, 363.

Cruickshank, I. (1963), *Ann. Rev. Phytopath.*, **1**, 351.

Crum Brown, A. and Fraser, T. (1869), *Trans. Roy. Soc. Edinburgh*, **25**, 151, 693.

Cuatrecasas, P., Wilcheck, M. and Anfinsen, C. (1968), *Proc. Nat. Acad. Sci., U.S.A.*, **61**, 636.

Cucinell, S., Conney, A., Sansur. M. and Burns, J. (1965), *Clin. Pharmacol. Therap.*, **6**, 420.

Cullen, S. and Gross, E. (1951), *Science*, **113**, 580.

Cullum, V., Farner, J., Jack, D. and Levy, G. (1969), *Brit. J. Pharmacol.*, **35**, 141.

Culp, L. and Black, P. (1972), *J. Virol.*, **9**, 611.

Culvenor, C. and Ham, N. (1966), *Chem. Comm.* (Chem. Soc., London), 537.

Cunningham, L. (1964), *Biochemistry*, **3**, 1629.

Curd, F. and Davey, D. (1949), *Nature, Lond.*, **163**, 89.

Curd, F., Davey, D. and Rose, F. (1945), *Ann. Trop. Med. Parasit.*, **39**, 208.

Curtis, D., Duggan, A., Felix, D. and Johnston, G. (1971), *Brain Research*, **32**, 69.

Curtis, D. and Johnston, G. (1970), *Handbook of Neurochemistry*, **4**, 115, New York: Plenum Press.

Curtis, D., Ryall, R. and Watkins, J. (1964), *Proc. 2nd Internat. Pharmacol. Meeting (Prague)*, Oxford: Pergamon Press.

Cushley, R. and Mautner, H., (1970), *Tetrahedron*, **26**, 2151.

Cushny, A. (1926), *Biological Relations of Optically Isomeric Substances*, Baltimore: Williams & Wilkins.

Cymerman-Craig, J., Rubbo, S., Willis, D. and Edgar, J. (1955), *Nature, Lond.*, **176**, 35.

Cymerman-Craig, J. and Willis, D. (1955), *J. Chem. Soc.*, 4315.

Dainton, F. (1966), *Chain Reactions*, London: Methuen.

Dale, H. (1914), *J. Pharmacol.*, **6**, 147.

Dale, H. (1933), *J. Physiol.*, **80**, 10 P.

Dale, H., Feldberg, W. and Vogt, M. (1936), *J. Physiol.*, **86**, 353.

Danielli, J. (1937), *Proc. Roy. Soc.*, B, **122**, 155,

Danielli, J. and Davson, H. (1934), *J. Cell. Compar. Physiol.*, **5**, 495.

Daniels, M. (1971), *Biochem. J.*, **122**, 197.

Danilov, A., Guli-Kevkhyan, R., Lavrentieva, V., Michelson, M., Mndjoyan, O., Shelkovnikow, A. and Starshinova, L. (1974), *Arch. Internat. Pharmacodyn. Thér.*, **208**, 35.

Danson, M. and Perham, R. (1976), *Biochem. J.*, **159**, 677.

D'Arcy Hart, P., Gordon, A. and Jacques, P. (1969), *Nature, Lond.*, **222**, 673.
Das, H., Goldstein, A. and Kanner, L. (1966), *Mol. Pharmacol.*, **2**, 158.
Datta, S. and Rabin, B. (1956), *Biochim. Biophys. Acta*, **19**, 572.
Dauwalder, M., Whaley, W. and Kephart, J., (1972), *Sub-cellular Biochem.*, **1**, 225.
Davenport, H. (1963), *Proc. Roy. Soc. B*, **157**, 332.
Davey, K. (1964), *Adv. Insect Physiol.*, **2**, 219.
Davidson, J. (1977), *The Biochemistry of the Nucleic Acids*, New York: Academic Press.
Davidson, M., Griggs, B., Boykin, D. and Wilson, W. (1977), *J. Med. Chem.*, **20**, 1117.
Davies, D. and Green, A. (1958), *Adv. in Enzymology*, **20**, 283.
Davies, F., Musa, M. and Dormandy, T. (1968), *J. Clin. Path.*, **21**, 363.
Davies, G. and Lowe, J. (1966), *Brit. J. Pharmacol. Chemother.*, **27**, 107.
Davies, J., Campbell, W. and Kearns, C. (1970), *Biochem. J.*, **117**, 221.
Davis, B. and Dubos, R. (1947), *J. Exper. Med.*, **86**, 215.
Davis, S. (1973), *J. Pharm. Pharmacol.*, **25**, 1, 293.
Davis, S., Elson, G., Tomlinson, E., Harrison, G. and Dearden, J. (1976) *Chem. and Indust.*, 677.
Davson, H. and Danielli, J. (1952), *The Permeability of Natural Membranes*, 2nd. Edn, Cambridge: Cambridge University Press.
Dawes, G. (1946), *Brit. J. Pharmacol.*, **1**, 90.
Day, M., Roach, A. and Whiting, R. (1973), *Europ. J. Pharmacol.*, **21**, 271.
Dean, R., and Barrett, A. (1976), *Essays Biochem.*, **12**, 1.
DeBaun, J., Smith, J., Miller, E. and Miller, J. (1970), *Science*, **167**, 184.
DeBruyn, P., Robertson, R. and Farr, F. (1950), *Anat. Record*, **108**, 279.
Dekker, J. (1968), *Neth. J. Plant Path.*, **74** (Suppl. 1), 127.
Delay, J., Deniker, P. and Harl, J. (1952), *Ann. méd.-psychol.*, **110**, 112.
DeLey, J. and Docky, R. (1960), *Biochim. Biophys. Acta*, **40**, 277.
Delp, C. and Klopping, H. (1968), *Plant Disease Reporter*, **52**, 95.
Demel, R., Van Deenen, L. and Kinsky, S. (1965), *J. Biol. Chem.*, **240**, 2749.
Dennis, V., Stead, N. and Andreoli, T. (1970), *J. Gen. Physiol.*, **55**, 375.
Deskin, W. (1958), *J. Amer. Chem. Soc.*, **80**, 5680.
Desowitz, R., Bell, T., Williams, J., Cardines, R. and Tamarua, M. (1970), *Amer. J. Trop. Med. Hyg.*, **19**, 775.
Dewhurst, W. (1968), *Nature, Lond.*, **218**, 1130.
De Wys, W. and Pories, W. (1972), *J. Nat. Cancer Inst.*, **48**, 375.
Diamond, J. and Wright, E. (1969), *Ann. Rev. Physiol.*, **31**, 581.
Dickerson, R. and Geis, I. (1969), *Structure and Action of Proteins* (with Stereo Supplement), New York: Harper and Row.
Dietrich B., Lehn, J. and Sauvage, J. (1969), *Tetrahedron Letters*, **34**, 2885, 2889.
Dietrich, S., Bolger, M., Kollman, P. and Jorgensen, E. (1977), *J. Med. Chem.*, **20**, 863.
Dill, W., Fisken, R., Reutner, T., Weston, J. and Glazko, A. (1957), *Antibiot. and Chemother.*, **7**, 99.
Dimond, A. and Horsfall, J. (1959), *Ann. Rev. Plant Physiol.*, **10**, 257.
Dittmer, K. (1949), *J. Amer. Chem. Soc.*, **71**, 1205.
Dittmer, K. and du Vigneaud, V. (1944), *Science*, **100**, 129.
Dixon, M. (1966), *Biochem. J.*, **100**, 41 P.
Dixon, M. and Webb, E. (1964), *Enzymes*, 2nd Edn. (1st Edn., 1958), London: Longmans.
Djerassi, C. (1960), *Optical Rotatory Dispersion*, New York: McGraw-Hill.
Dobbie, H. and Kermack, W. (1955), *Biochem. J.*, **59**, 246.

Dobkin, A. (1975), *Clin. Pharmac. Ther.*, **18**, 547.

Dobler, M., Dunitz, J. and Kilbourn, B. (1969), *Helv. Chim. Acta*, **52**, 2573.

Dockter, M. and Magnuson, J. (1973), *Biochem. Biophys. Res. Commun.*, **54**, 790.

Dodd, M. (1946), *J. Pharmacol.*, **86**, 311.

Doherty, D., Shapira, R. and Burnett, W. (1957), *J. Amer. Chem. Soc.*, **79**, 5667.

Doi, O., Miyamoto, N., Tanaka, N. and Umezawa, H. (1968), *Appl. Microbiol.*, 16, 1282.

Dolin, M. (1961) in *The Bacteria*, (eds. Gunsalus, I., and Stanier, R.), New York: Academic Press, **2**, p. 425.

Doluizio, J. and Martin, A. (1963), *J. Med. Chem.*, **6**, 16, 20.

Domagk, G. (1935), *Deutsch. med. Woch.*, **61**, 250.

Domagk, G. (1936), *Klin. Woch.*, **15**, 1585.

Dominguez, R. (1933), *Proc. Soc. Expl Biol. Med.*, **31**, 1146–1150.

Donald, C., Passey, B. and Swaby, R. (1952), *J. Gen. Microbiol.*, **7**, 211.

Donohue, J. (1968), *Arch. Biochem. Biophys.*, **128**, 591.

Douch, P. (1976), *Xenobiotica*, **6**, 531.

Douglas, C., Haldane, J.S. and Haldane, J.B.S. (1912), *J. Physiol.*, **44**, 275.

Douglas, W. (1968), *Brit. J. Pharmacol.*, **34**, 451.

Dreser, H. (1899), *Pflügers Arch. ges. Physiol.*, **76**, 306.

Drew, R. (1957), *Nature, Lond.*, **179**, 1251.

Dring, L., Smith R. and Williams, R. (1970), *Biochem. J.*, **116**, 425.

Druckrey, H. (1955), *Klin. Woch.*, 784.

Dubos, R. (1939), *J. Exper. Med.*, **70**. 1.

Duggar, B. (1948), *Ann. N. Y. Acad. Sci.*, **51**, 177.

Dunitz, J. (1952), *J. Amer. Chem. Soc.*, **74**, 995.

Dunlop, D. and Shanks, R. (1968), *Brit. J. Pharmacol.*, **32**, 201.

Dwek, R., Campbell, I., Richards, R. and Williams, R. (eds.) (1977), *NMR in Biology*, London: Academic Press.

Dwyer, F., Gyarfas, E., Koch, J. and Rogers, W. (1952), *Nature, Lond.*, **170**, 190.

Dwyer, F., Gyarfas, E. and O'Dwyer, M. (1951), *Nature, Lond.*, **167**, 1036.

Dyckes, D., Nestor, J., Ferger, M. and du Vigneaud, V. (1974), *J. Med. Chem.*, **17**, 969.

Dyson, G. (1928), *The Chemistry of Chemotherapy*, London: Benn.

Eagle, H. (1939), *J. Pharmacol.*, **66**, 10, 423, 436.

Eagle, H. (1945), *J. Pharmacol.*, **85**, 265.

Eagle, H. (1951), *Pharmacol. Rev.*, **3**, 107.

Easson, L. and Stedman, E. (1933), *Biochem. J.*, **27**, 1257.

Ebashi, S. and Endo, M. (1968), *Prog. Biophys. Mol. Biol.*, **18**, 123.

Ebeling, W. and Wagner, R. (1959), *J. Econ. Entomol.*, **52**, 190.

Eccles, J. (1957), *The Physiology of Nerve Cells*, Baltimore: Johns Hopkins Press, pp. 193–5.

Eccles, J. (1964), *Nobel Lecture*. Amsterdam: Elsevier.

Eccles, J. (1965), *Scient. Am*, **212** (no. 1), 56.

Edelman, I., Bogoroch, R., and Porter, G. (1963), *Proc. Nat. Acad. Sci. U.S.A.*, **50**, 1169.

Edgerton, L. and Blanpied, G. (1968), *Nature, Lond.*, **219**, 1064.

Edgington, L., Walton, G. and Miller, P. (1966), *Science*, **153**, 307.

Edlbacher, S., Baur, H. and Becker, M. (1940), *Z. physiol. Chem.*, **265**, 61.

Edsall, J., Martin, R. and Hollingworth, B. (1958), *Proc. Nat. Acad. Sci. U.S.A.*, **44**, 505.

Edson, E., Sanderson, D. and Noakes, D. (1964), *World Rev. Pest Control*, **4**, 36; (1966), *ibid*, **5**, 143.

Edwards, D., Dye, M. and Carne, H. (1973), *J. Gen. Microbiol.*, **76**, 135.

Edwards, D. and Mathison, G. (1970), *J. Gen. Microbiol.*, **63**, 297.
Eger, E., Lundgren, C., Miller, S. and Stevens, W. (1969), *Anaesthesiology*, **30**, 129.
Ehrenpreis, S., Fleisch, J. and Mittag, T. (1969), *Pharmacol. Rev.*, **21**, 131.
Ehringer, H. and Hornykiewicz, O. (1960), *Klin. Woch.*, **38**, 1236.
Ehrlich, P. (1900), *Proc. Roy. Soc. Lond.*, **66**, B, 424.
Ehrlich, P. (1908), *Nobel Prize Lecture, Münch. med. Woch.*, 1909, No. 5.
Ehrlich, P. (1909), *Ber. deutsch. chem. Ges.*, **42**, 17.
Ehrlich, P. (1911), *Theorie und Praxis der Chemotherapie*, Leipzig: Klinkhardt.
Ehrlich, P. (1912), in *Benda, L.* (1912) (*q.v.*).
Ehrlich, P. and Bertheim, A. (1907), *Ber. deutsch. chem. Ges.*, **40**, 3292.
Ehrlich, P. and Bertheim, A. (1912), *Ber. deutsch. chem. Ges.*, **45**, 756.
Ehrlich, P. and Hata, S. (1910), *Die experimentelle Chemotherapie der Spirillosen*, Berlin: Springer.
Ehrlich, P. and Morgenroth, J. (1910), in *Studies in Immunity* (ed. Ehrlich, P.), 2nd Edn., pp. 23, 24, 47. New York: Wiley (translation of a paper by Ehrlich and Morgenroth, *Berl. klin. Woch.*, 1900, No. 2).
Ehrlich, P. and Shiga, K. (1904), *Berl. klin. Woch.*, **41**, 329.
Einhorn, A. (1905), *Deutsch. med. Woch.*, **31**, 1668.
Eisenberg, D. and Kauzmann, W. (1969), *The structure and properties of water*, Oxford: Clarendon Press.
Eisleb, O. and Schaumann, O. (1938), *Deut med. Woch.*, **65**, 967.
Elderfield, R. (1946), *Chem. and Eng. News*, **24**, 2598.
Eliel, E. (1962), *Stereochemistry of Carbon Compounds*, New York: McGraw-Hill.
Eliel, E., Allinger, N., Angyal, S. and Morrison, G. (1965), *Conformational Analysis*, New York: Wiley-Interscience.
Elion, G. (1967), *Fed. Proc.*, **26**, 898.
Elion, G., Burgi E. and Hitchings, G. (1952), *J. Amer. Chem. Soc.*, **74**, 411.
Elion, G., Callahan, S., Rundles, R. and Hitchings, G. (1963), *Cancer Res.*, **23**, 1207.
Elion, G., Furman, P., Fyfe, J., de Miranda, P., Beauchamp, E. and Schaeffer, H. (1977), *Proc. Nat. Acad. Sci. U.S.A.*, **74**, 5716.
Elion, G., Kovensky, A., Hitchings, G., Metz, E. and Rundles, R. (1966), *Biochem. Pharmacol.*, **15**, 863.
Elkhawad, A. and Woodruff, G. (1975), *Brit. J. Pharmacol.*, **54**, 107.
Ellenbroek, B. and van Rossum, J. (1960), *Arch. Internat. Pharmacodyn. Thér*, **125**, 216.
Elliott, M. (ed.) (1977), *Synthetic Pyrethroids*, Washington, D.C.: American Chemical Society.
Elliot, M., Farnham, A., Janes, N., Needham, P. and Pulman, D. (1974), *Nature, Lond.*, **248**, 710.
Elliott, T, (1905), *J. Physiol.*, **32**, 401.
Elliott, W. (1963), *Biochem. J.*, **86**, 562.
Ellis, R. (1971), *Biochem. J.*, **124**, 52 P.
Elslager, E. and Worth, D. (1965), *Nature, Lond.*, **206**, 630.
Elworthy, P. (1963), *J. Pharm. Pharmacol.*, **15** (suppl), 137 T.
Elworthy, P., Florence, A. and Macfarlane, C. (1968), *Solubilization by Surface-active Agents*, London: Chapman and Hall.
Endo, H., Ono, T. and Sugimura, T. (1970), *Chemistry and Biological Actions of 4-nitroquinoline-1-oxide*, Berlin: Springer.
Ennor, A., Rosenberg, H., Rossiter, R., Beatty, I. and Gaffney, T. (1960), *Biochem. J.*, **75**, 179.
Enoch, H. and Lester, R. (1975), *J. Biol. Chem.*, **250**, 6693.

594 References

Ephrussi, B. and Hottinguer, H. (1950), *Nature, Lond.*, **166**, 956.

Ernster, L., Dallner, G. and Azzone, G. (1963), *J. Biol. Chem.*, **238**, 1124.

Estensen, R., Krey, A. and Hahn, F. (1969), *Molecular Pharmacol.*, **5**, 532.

Eto, M. (1974), *Organophosphorus Pesticides: Organic and Biological Chemistry*, Cleveland: CRC Press.

v. Euler, U. (1934), *Arch. exp. Path. Pharmakol.*, **175**, 78.

Evans, D., Fuller, A. and Walker, J. (1944), *Lancet*, **ii**, 523.

Everett, A., Lowe, L. and Wilkinson, S. (1970), *Chem. Comm., Chem. Soc. Lond.*, 1020.

Everett, J., Roberts, J. and Ross, W. (1953), *J. Chem. Soc.*, 2386.

Ewins, A., Ashley, J., Barber, H., Newbery, G., and Self, A. (1942), *J. Chem. Soc.*, 103.

Ewins, A. and Phillips, M. (1939), *Brit. Pat.* 512 145

Exer, B. (1958), *Experientia*, **14**, 135.

Fahmy, M., Fukuto, T., Metcalf, R. and Homstead, R. (1973), *J. Agr. Food Chem.*, **21**, 585.

Faigle, J., Keberle, H., Riess, W. and Schmid, K. (1962), *Experientia*, **18**, 1.

Fairlamb, A. and Bowman, I. (1975), *Trans Roy. Soc. Trop. Med. Hyg.*, **69**, 268.

Fairley, G. and Simister, J. (eds.) (1965), *Cyclophosphamide*, Baltimore: Williams & Wilkins.

Fairley, N. (1946), *Trans. Roy. Soc. Trop. Med. Hyg.*, **40**, 105.

Falco, E., Goodwin, L., Hitchings, G., Rollo, I. and Russell, P. (1951), *Brit. J. Pharmacol.*, **6**, 185.

Falkenmark, M. and Lindh, G. (1977), *Water for a Starving World*, Boulder, Colorado: Westview Press.

Falkow, S. (1975), *Infectious Multiple Drug Resistance*, New York: Academic Press.

Farber, S. (1952), *Blood*, **7**, 107.

Farber, S. and Mitus, A. (1968), in *Actinomycin*, (ed. Waksman, S.), New York: Wiley.

Farley, T., Strong, F. and Bydalek, T. (1965), *J. Amer. Chem. Soc.*, **87**, 3501.

Fastier, F. (1949), *Brit. J. Pharmacol.*, **4**, 315,

Fastier, F. (1964), *Ann. Rev. Pharmacol.*, **4**, 351.

Fastier, F. and Reid, C. (1952), *Brit. J. Pharmacol.*, **7**, 417.

Faust, R. and Shearin, S. (1974), *Nature, Lond.*, **248**, 60.

Fayard, C. (1949), *Thesis*, Paris (through *Sem. Hôp. Paris*, 1949, **35**, 1778).

Felber, T., Smith, E., Knox, J. *et al.*, (1973), *J. Amer. Med. Assoc.*, **223**, 289.

Fendler, J. and Fendler, E. (1975), *Catalysis in Micellar and Macromolecular Systems*, New York: Academic Press.

Fenner, F., McAuslan, B., Mims, C., Sambrook, J. and White, D. (1974), New York: Academic Press.

Fenner, F. and White, D. (1976), *Medical Virology*, 2nd Edn, New York: Academic Press.

Ferguson, J. (1939), *Proc. Roy. Soc. B*, **127**, 387.

Ferguson, J. (1951), *Colloques internationaux du Centre nationale de la Recherche scientifique (Paris)*, No. 26: *Mécanisme de la Narcose*, p. 25.

Ferguson, J., Hawkins, S. and Doxey, D. (1950), *Nature, Lond.*, **165**, 1021.

Ferguson, J. and Pirie, H. (1948), *Ann. App. Biol.*, **35**, 532.

Ferone, R., Burchall, J. and Hitchings, G. (1969), *J. Molec. Pharmacol.*, **5**, 49.

Ferreira, S. and Vane, V. (1974), *Ann. Rev. Pharmacol.* **14**, 57.

Festy, B., Sturm, J. and Daune, M. (1975), *Biochim. Biophys. Acta*, **407**, 24.

Fierlafijn, E. (1971), *J. Amer. Med. Assoc.*, **218**, 1051.

Fieser, L. and Fieser, M. (1935), *J. Amer. Chem. Soc.*, **57**, 491.

Fildes, P. (1940a), *Lancet*, **i**, 955.

Fildes, P. (1940b), *Brit. J. Exper. Path.*, **21**, 67.

Finch, J., Lutter, L., Rhodes, D., Brown, R., Rushton, B., Levitt, M. and Klug, A. (1977), *Nature, Lond.*, **269**, 29.

Finch, L. and Haeusler, G. (1973), *Brit. J. Pharmacol.*, **47**, 217.

Finean, J., Coleman, R. and Michell, R. (1974), *Membranes and their Cellular Function*, Oxford: Blackwell; New York: Wiley-Halsted.

Fischer, E. and v. Mering, J. (1903), *Therapie der Gegenwart*, **44**, 97.

Fischer, J. and Jardetzky, O. (1965), *J. Amer. Chem. Soc.*, **87**, 3237.

Fishman, W. (ed.) (1970–3), *Metabolic Conjugation and Metabolic Hydrolysis* (in three parts). New York: Academic Press.

Fleming, A. (1929), *Brit. J. Exper. Path.*, **10**, 226.

Flockhart, I., Large, P., Troup, D., Malcolm, S. and Marten, T. (1978), *Xenobiotica*, **8**, 97.

Florey, H., Abraham, E., Chain, E., Fletcher, C., Gardner, A., Heatley, N., Jennings, M., Orr-Ewing, J. and Sanders, A. (1940), *Lancet*, **ii**, 226; (1941), *ibid*, **ii**, 177.

Florey, H., Chain, E., Heatley, N., Jennings, M., Sanders, A., Abraham, E., and Florey, M. (1949), *Antibiotics*, Oxford: Oxford University Press.

Florkin, M. and Mason, H. (1960–4), *Comparative Biochemistry*, (7 vols.), New York: Academic Press.

Flower, R. (1974), *Pharmacol. Rev.*, **26**, 33.

Flower, R., Cheung, H. and Cushman, D. (1973), *Prostaglandins*, **4**, 425.

Flower, R. and Kingston, W. (1975), *Brit. J. Pharmacol.*, **55**, 239 P.

Fodor, G. (1960), in *The Alkaloids*, (eds. Manske, R., and Holmes, H.), **6**, 145, New York: Academic Press.

Fondy, T., Ghangas, G. and Reza, M. (1970), *Biochemistry*, **9**, 3272.

Foster, M., Jones, K. and Woods, D. (1961), *Biochem. J.*, **80**, 519.

Fourneau, E., Bovet, D., Bovet, F., and Montezin, G. (1944), *Bull. Soc. Chim. biol.*, **26**, 134, 516.

Fourneau, E., Tréfouël, J., Tréfouël, Mme J., and Vallée, J. (1924), *Ann. Institut Pasteur*, **38**, 81.

Fouts, J. (1962), *Fed. Proc.*, **21**, 1107.

Fowden, L., Neale, S. and Tristram, H. (1963), *Nature, Lond.*, **199**, 35.

Fox, H. (1953), *Trans. New York Acad. Sci.*, **15**, 234.

Franke, E., and Roehl, W. (1905), first recorded by Franke, E. (1905) in *Therapuetische Versuche bei Trypanosomenkrankung*, Jena; later by Browning, C. (1907), *Brit. Med. J.*, **ii**, 1405, and Ehrlich, P. (1907), *Berl. klin. Woch.*, **44**, 233, 341.

Franklin, M. (1972), *Xenobiotica*, **2**, 517.

Franklin, T. (1963a), *Biochem. J.*, **87**, 449.

Franklin, T. (1963b), *Biochim. Biophys. Acta*, **76**, 138.

Franklin, T. (1966), *Symp. Soc. General Microbiol.*, **16**, 192.

Franklin, T. (1971), *Biochem. J.*, **123**, 267.

Franklin, T., and Snow, G. (1975), *Biochemistry of Antimicrobial Action*, 2nd Edn., London: Chapman and Hall.

Franks, F. (1972), *Water, a Comprehensive Treatise*, London: Plenum Press.

Franks, N. and Lieb, W. (1978), *Nature, Lond.*, **274**, 339.

Frear, D. (1975), *Pesticide Handbook Entoma*, College Park, Maryland: Entomological Society of America.

Free, S. and Wilson, J. (1964), *J. Med. Chem.*, **7**, 395.

Freeman, K. (1970), *Canad. J. Biochem.*, **48**, 479.

Freese, E., Sheu, C. and Galliers, E. (1973), *Nature, Lond.*, **241**, 321.

Frenkel, J. and Hitchings, G. (1957), *Antibiotics Chemother.*, **7**, 630.

Freudenthal, R. and Jones, P. (eds.) (1976), *Carcinogenesis*, vol. 1, New York: Raven Press.

Friberg, L. Piscator, M. and Nordberg, G. (1971), *Cadmium in the Environment*, CRC Press: Cleveland, Ohio.

Fridborg, K., Kannan, K., Liljas, A., Lundin, J., Strandberg, B., Strandberg, R., Tilander, B. and Wirén, G. (1967), *J. Mol. Biol.*, **25**, 505.

Fridovich, I. (1975), *Ann. Rev. Biochem.*, **44**, 147.

Friedheim, E. (1951), *Amer. J. Trop. Med.*, **31**, 218.

Friess, S. and Baldridge, H. (1956), *J. Amer. Chem. Soc.*, **78**, 2482.

Fujita, T., Iwasa, J. and Hansch, C. (1964), *J. Amer. Chem. Soc.*, **86**, 5175.

Fujita, T., Nishioka, T. and Nakajima, M. (1977), *J. Med. Chem.*, **20**, 1071.

Fukuto, T. (1972), *Drug. Metab. Rev.*, **1**, 117.

Fuller, A. (1942), *Biochem. J.*, **36**, 548.

Fuller, R., Kidder, G., Nugent, N., Dewey, V. and Rigopoulos, N. (1971), *Photochem. Photobiol.*, **14**, 359.

Fuller, W. and Waring, M. (1964), *Ber. Bunsen. physik. Chem.*, **68**, 805.

Fulton, J. and Grant, P. (1956), *Ann. Trop. Med. Parasit.*, **50**, 381.

Gabbay, E. (1968), *J. Amer. Chem. Soc.*, **90**, 5257.

Gaddum, J. (1926), *J. Physiol.*, **61**, 141.

Gaddum, J. (1936), *Proc. Roy. Soc. Med.*, 29, 1373.

Gaddum, J. (1963), *Nature, Lond.*, **197**, 741.

Gage, J. (1953), *Biochem. J.*, **54**, 426.

Gage, P. (1971), in *Neuropoisons*, (ed. Simpson, L.), **1**, p. 187, New York: Plenum Press.

Gale, E. (1946), *Adv. Enzymol.*, **6**, 1.

Gale, E. (1947), *J. Gen. Microbiol.*, **1**, 53.

Gale, E., Cundliffe, E., Reynolds, P., Richmond, M. and Waring, M. (1972), *The Molecular Basis of Antibiotic Action*, London: Wiley.

Gale, E. and Folkes, J. (1953), *Biochem. J.*, **55**, 493, 730.

Gale, E., and Rodwell, A. (1949), *J. Gen. Microbiol.*, **3**, 127.

Gale, E., Shepherd, C. and Folkes, J. (1958), *Nature, Lond.*, **182**, 592.

Gale, E. and Taylor, E. (1947), *J. Gen. Microbiol.*, **1**, 77.

Galton, D. (1956), *Adv. Cancer Res.*, **4**, 73.

Ganis, P., Avitable, G., Mechlinski, W. and Schaffner, C. (1971), *J. Amer. Chem. Soc.*, **93**, 4560.

Garattini, S., Mussini, E. and Randall, L., (eds.) (1973), *The Benzodiazepines*, New York: Raven Press.

Gaskin, F. and Shelanski, M. (1976), *Essays, in Biochem.*, **12**, 115.

Gelboin, H. (1969), *Cancer Res.*, **29**, 1272.

Gelboin, H., Wortham, J., and Wilson, R. (1967), *Nature, Lond.*, **214**, 281.

Gelmo, P. (1908), *J. prakt. Chem.*, **77**, 369.

Gemmell, M. and Shearer, G. (1968), *Vet. Record*, **82**, 252.

Gent, M., and Prestegard, J. (1974), *Biochemistry*, **13**, 4027.

Gerhartz, H. (1960), *Der Internist* **1**, 278.

Gerig, J. (1968), *J. Amer. Chem. Soc.*, **90**, 2681.

Germar, B. (1936), *Z. angew. Ent.*, **22**, 603.

Gershenfeld, L. and Milanick, C. (1941), *Amer. J. Pharm.*, **113**, 306.

Ghiretti, F. (1962), in *Oxygenases*, (ed. Hayaishi, O.), New York: Academic Press.

Ghuysen, J., Leyh-Bouille, M., Frère, J., Dusart, J., Marquet, A., Perkins, H. and Nieto, M. (1974), *Ann. N.Y. Acad. Sci.*, **235**, 236.

Giarmann, N. (1949), *J. Pharmacol.*, **96**, 119.

Gibaldi, M. and Perrier, D. (1975), *Pharmacokinetics*, New York: Marcel Dekker.

Gibson, F. (1964), *Biochem. J.*, **90**, 256.
Gilardi, R., Karle, I., Karle, J. and Sperling, W. (1971), *Nature, Lond.*, **232**, 187.
Gilbert, B., Leme, L., Ferreira, A., Bulhoes, M. and Castleton, C. (1973), *Bull. World Health Org.*, **49**, 633.
Gilbert, L. (ed.) (1976), *The Juvenile Hormones*, New York: Plenum Press.
Giles, C., MacEwan, T., Nakhwa, S. and Smith, D. (1960), *J. Chem. Soc.*, 3973.
Gillespie, L., Oates, J., Crout, J. and Sjoerdsma, A. (1962), *Circulation*, **25**, 281.
Gillette, J. (1965), *Ann. N.Y. Acad. Sci.*, Art. 1,1.
Gillette, J. (1966), *Adv. Pharmacol.*, **4**, 219.
Gillette, J., Conney, A., Cosmides, G., Estabrook, R., Fouts, J. and Mannering, G. (eds) (1969), *Microsomes and Drug Oxidations*, New York: Academic Press.
Gillette, J. and Mitchell, J. (1975), *Concepts in Biochemical Pharmacology*, Part 3, Berlin: Springer.
Gilligan, D. and Plummer, N. (1943), *Proc. Soc. Exper. Biol. Med.*, **53**, 142.
Gilman, A. and Philips, F. (1946), *Science*, **103**, 409.
Gingell, R. and Bridges, J. (1973), *Xenobiotica*, **3**, 599.
Ginnings, P. and Baum, R. (1937), *J. Amer. Chem. Soc.*, **59**, 1111.
Globe, H., Lüllmann, H. and Mutschler, E. (1966), *Brit. J. Pharmacol. Chemother.*, **27**, 185.
Godfraind, T. and Ghysel-Burton, J. (1977), *Nature, Lond.*, **265**, 165.
Goggins, J., Johnson, G. and Pastan, I. (1972), *J. Biol. Chem.*, **247**, 5759.
Goksøyr, J. (1955), *Nature, Lond.*, **175**, 820; *Physiol. Plantarum*, **8**, 719.
Goldacre, R. (1977), *Brit. J. Cancer*, **35**, 247.
Goldacre, R., Loveless, A. and Ross, W. (1949), *Nature, Lond.*, **163**, 667.
Goldacre, R. and Phillips, J. (1949), *J. Chem. Soc.*, 1724.
Goldberg, I. and Friedman, P. (1971), *Ann. Rev. Biochem.*, **40**, 775.
Goldfine, I., Perlman, R. and Roth, J. (1971), *Nature, Lond.*, **234**, 295.
Goldshtein, B. and Gerasimova, V. (1966), *Ukr. khim. Zh.*, **32**, 1031.
Goldstein, A. (1954), *J. Pharmacol.*, **112**, 326.
Goldstein, A., Aronow, L. and Kalman, S. (1974), *Principles of Drug Action*, 2nd edn., New York: Wiley.
Goldstein, A., Lowney, L. and Pal, B. (1971), *Proc. Nat. Acad. Sci. U.S.A.*, 68, 1742.
Gomperts, B. (1977), *The Plasma Membrane*, London: Academic Press.
Gönnert, R. and Schraufstätter, E. (1960), *Arzneimittel-Forsch.*, **10**, 881.
Good, N. (1961), *Plant. Physiol.*, **36**, 788.
Good, N., Winget, G., Winter, W., Connolly, T., Izawa, S. and Singh, R. (1966), *Biochemistry*, **5**, 467.
Goodman, L. and Gilman, A. (1975), *The Pharmacological Basis of Therapeutics*, 5th Edn, New York: Macmillan.
Goodman, L., Wintrobe, M., Dameshek, W., Goodman, M., Gilman, A. and McLennan, M. (1946), *J. Amer. Med. Ass.*, **132**, 126.
Goodson, J., Henry, T. and Macfie, J. (1930), *Biochem. J.*, **24**, 874.
Goodwin, B. (1976), *Handbook of Intermediary Metabolism of Aromatic Compounds*, London: Chapman and Hall; New York: Wiley-Halsted.
Goodwin, L., Jayewardene, L. and Standen, O. (1958), *Brit. Med. J.*, **2**, 1572.
Goodwin, T. (ed.) (1965), *Aspects of Insect Biochemistry, Biochem. Soc. Symp.*, **25**.
Goodwin, T. (1966), *Biochemistry of Chloroplasts*, London: Academic Press.
Gosálvez, M. (1976), *Proc. X Internat. Congr. Biochem.*, Hamburg.
Gosálvez, M., Blanco, M., Vivero, C. and Vallés, F. (1978), *Europ. J. Cancer* 14, 1185.
Goss, W., Deitz, W. and Cook, T. (1965), *J. Bact.*, **89**, 1068.
Goto, T., Kishi, Y., Takahashi, S. and Hirata, Y. (1964), *Tetrahedron Letters*, 779.
Goto, T., Kishi, Y., Takahashi, S. and Hirata, Y. (1965), *Tetrahedron*, **21**, 2059.

Gottlieb, D. and Shaw, P. (eds.) (1967), *Antibiotics*, New York: Springer.

Gottlieb, J. and Hill, C. (1974), *New Engl. J. Med.*, **290**, 193.

Gottlieb, R. (1923), *Arch. exper. Path. Pharmakol.*, **97**, 113.

Gould, G. and Hitchins, A. (1963), *Nature, Lond.*, **197**, 622.

Gould, J. (1957), *Nature, Lond.*, **180**, 282.

Gourevitch, A., Pursiano, T. and Lein, J. (1962), *Nature, Lond.*, **195**, 496.

Graham, J. (1962), *Prog. Med. Chem.*, **2**, 132.

Graham-Smith, G. (1919), *J. Hyg., Cambridge*, **18**, 1.

Granick, S. and Gilder, H. (1945), *Science*, **101**, 540.

Grant, P. and Fulton, J. (1957), *Biochem. J.*, **66**, 242.

Grant, P. and Sargent, J. (1960), *Biochem. J.*, **76**, 229.

Grant, P., Sargent, J. and Ryley, J. (1961), *Biochem. J.*, **81**, 200.

Gray, G., Smith, I., McKenzie, I., Crean, G. and Gillespie, G. (1977), *Lancet, Lond.*, **i**, 4.

Greathouse, G., Block, S., Kovack, E., Barnes, D., Byron, C., Long, G., Gerber, D. and McLenny, J. (1954), *Research on Chemical Compounds for Inhibition of Fungi*, U.S. Corps of Engineers, Fort Belvoir, Virginia.

Green, A. (1937), in *Thorpe's Dictionary of Applied Chemistry*, 4th Edn, Ch. 1, p. 39.

Green, A., Heale, D. and Grahame-Smith, D. (1977), *Psychopharmacology*, **52**, 195.

Greenberg, J., Mellors, A. and McGowan, J. (1978), *J. Med. Chem.*, **21**, 1208.

Greengard, O. and McIlwain, H. (1955), *Biochem. J.*, **61**, 61.

Greengard, P. (1976), *Nature, Lond.*, **260**, 101.

Greenham, C. (1966), *Planta*, **69**, 150.

Greenstein, J. (1954), *Biochemistry of Cancer*, 2nd Edn, New York: Academic Press.

Gregoriadis, G. (1977), *Nature, Lond.*, **265**, 407.

Grell, E., Eggers, F. and Funck, T. (1972), *Chimia*, **26**, 632.

Griffin, M. and Brown, G. (1964), *J. Biol. Chem.*, **239**, 310.

Griffiths, J., Intarakosit, P., Taylor, H. and Wain, R. (1966), *Ann. App. Biol.*, **58**, 183.

Grigg, G. (1970), *Molec. General Genetics*, **106**, 228.

Grigg, G., Edwards, M. and Brown, D. (1971), *J. Bact.*, **107**, 599.

Grollman, A. (1966), *Proc. Nat. Acad. Sci. U.S.A.* **56**, 1867.

Grollman, A. (1968), *J. Biol. Chem.*, **243**, 4089.

Grollman, A. (1971), in *Drug Design*, (ed. Ariens, E.), **2**, 231 (review).

Grollman, A., and Horwitz, S. (1971), in *Drug Design*, (ed. Ariens, E.), **2**, 261 (review).

Gros, F., Beljanski, M., and Macheboeuf, M. (1950), *Compt. rend.*, **231**, 184.

Gross, F. and Turrian, H. (1957), *Experentia*, **13**, 401.

Grossmann, F. (1962), *Naturwissenschaft*, **49**, 138.

Grunberg, E. and Schnitzer, R. (1953), *Proc. Soc. Expl Biol. Med.*, **84**, 220.

Grunwald, E. and Ralph, E. (1967), *J. Amer. Chem. Soc.*, **89**, 4405.

Gull, K. and Trinci, A. (1973), *Nature, Lond.*, **244**, 292.

Gundorova, R., Lenkevich, M. and Tartakovskaya, A. (1967), *Vestn. Offalmol.* **80**, 42.

Gurson, C. and Saner, G. (1971), *Amer. J. Clin. Nutr.*, **24**, 1313.

Guth, P., Amaro, J., Sellinger, O. and Elmer, L. (1965), *Biochem. Pharmacol.*, **14**, 769.

Gutman, M., Coles, C., Singer, T. and Casida, J. (1971), *Biochemistry*, **10**, 2036.

Gutte, B. and Merrifield, R. (1969), *J. Amer. Chem. Soc.*, **91**, 501.

Guttmann, P. and Ehrlich, P. (1891), *Berl. klin. Woch.*, **28**, 953.

Guze, L. (1967), *Microbial Protoplasts, Spheroplasts, and L-forms*, Baltimore: Williams and Wilkins.

Gysin, H. (1962), *Chem. and Indust.*, 1393.

Haagen-Smit, A. and Went, F. (1935), *Proc. k. ned. Akad. Wetenschap.*, **38**, 852.

Habermann, E. (1974), *Ann. Rev. Pharmacol.*, **14**, 1.

Hackenbrock, C. (1968), *J. Cell Biol.*, **37**, 345.

Haddow, A. (1959), *Proc. Roy. Inst.*, **37**, 223.
Haddow, A., Harris, R., Kon, G. and Roe, E. (1948), *Proc. Roy. Soc. B*, **241**, 147.
Haddow, A., Kon, G. and Ross, W. (1948), *Nature, Lond.*, **162**, 824.
Haddow, A. and Timmis, G. (1953), *Lancet*, **i**, 207.
Haddow, A., Timmis, G. and Brown, S. (1958), *Nature, Lond.*, **182**, 1164.
Haefeley, W., Hürlimann, A. and Thoenen, H. (1966), *Brit. J. Pharmacol.*, **26**, 172.
Haest, C., de Gier, J., op den Kamp, J., Bartels, P. and van Deenen, L. (1972), *Biochem. Biophys. Acta*, **255**, 720.
Hahn, F. (1975), *Naturwissenschaften*, **62**, 449.
Hahn, F., Wisseman, C. and Hopps, H. (1954), *J. Bact.*, **67**, 674.
Hahn, P., Bale, W., Ross, J., Hettig, R. and Whipple, G. (1940), *Science*, **92**, 131.
Haldane, J. (1930), *Enzymes*, London: Longmans.
Haldar, D., Freeman, K. and Work, T. (1966), *Nature, Lond.*, **211**, 9.
Hall, D. and Evans, M. (1969), *Nature, Lond.*, **223**, 1342.
Hallman, P., Perrin, D. and Watt, A. (1971), *Biochem. J.*, **121**, 549.
Halpern, B. (1942), *Arch. Internat. Pharmacodyn. Thér.*, **68**, 339.
Halpern, R., Halpern, B., Stea, B. and eight others (1977), *Proc. Nat. Acad. Sci. U.S.A.*, **74**, 587.
Hamilton-Miller, J. (1973), *Bact. Rev.*, **37**, 166.
Hamilton-Miller, J. and Abraham, E. (1971), *Biochem. J.*, **123**, 183.
Hammett, L. (1970), *Physical Organic Chemistry*, 2nd Edn, New York: McGraw-Hill, pp. 355, 384.
Hampton, A. (1976), *J. Med. Chem.*, **19**, 1279.
Hansch, C. (1968), *J. Med. Chem.*, **11**, 920.
Hansch, C. (1971), *Drug Design*, (ed. Ariens, E.), **1**, 271 (review).
Hansch, C. and Anderson, S. (1967), *J. Med. Chem.*, **10**, 745.
Hansch, C. and Fujita, T. (1964), *J. Amer. Chem. Soc.*, **86**, 1610.
Hansch, C., Kim, K. and Sarma, R. (1973), *J. Amer. Chem. Soc.*, **95**, 6447.
Hansch, C., Leo, A., Unger, S., Kim, K., Nikaitani, D. and Lien, E. (1973), *J. Med. Chem.*, **16**, 1207.
Hansch, C., Quinlan, J. and Lawrence, G. (1968), *J. Org. Chem.*, **33**, 347.
Hansch, C., Steward, A., Anderson, S., and Bentley, D. (1968), *J. Med. Chem.*, **11**, 1.
Hansch, C., Unger, S. and Forsythe, A. (1973), *J. Med. Chem.*, **16**, 1217.
Hansch, C., Vittoria, A., Silipo, C. and Jow, P. (1975), *J. Med. Chem.*, **18**, 546.
Hardman, H. (1962), *Circulation Res.*, **10**, 598.
Harley, E., Rees, K. and Cohen, A. (1969), *Biochem. J.*, **114**, 289.
Harold, F. and Baarda, J. (1967), *J. Bact.*, **94**, 53.
Harris, J., Sanger, F. and Naughton, M. (1956), *Arch. Biochem. Biophys.*, **65**, 427.
Harrison, S., Hixon, E., Burdeshaw, J. and Denine, E. (1977), *Nature, Lond.*, **269**, 511.
Hartley, B. and Kilby, B. (1952), *Biochem. J.*, **50**, 672.
Hartley, H. and Raikes, H. (1927), *Trans. Farad. Soc.*, **23**, 393.
Hashimoto, Y., Makita, T., Miyata, H., Noguchi, T. and Okta, G. (1968), *Toxicology and Appl. Pharmacol.*, **12**, 536.
Hassell, C. (1950), *Experientia*, **6**, 462.
Hassell, C. (1958), *Progress in Organic Chemistry* (ed. Cook, J.), **4**, 115.
Hata, A. (1932), *Kitasato Arch. Exper. Med.*, **9**, 1.
Hatanaka, H. and Sano, K. (1973), *Zeits. Neurol.*, **204**, 309.
Haussler, M. and Norman, A. (1969), *Proc. Nat. Acad. Sci., U.S.A.*, **62**, 155.
Hawking, F. (1944), *J. Pharmacol.*, **82**, 31.
Hawkins, C. (1971), *Absolute Configuration of Metal Complexes*, London: Wiley.
Hawkins, C. and Perrin, D. (1962), *J. Chem. Soc.*, 1351.
Hawkins, C. and Perrin, D. (1963), *Inorg. Chem.*, **2**, 843.

Haydon, D. and Hladky, S. (1972), *Quart. Rev. Biophys.*, **5**, 187.

Hayes, W. (1967), *Proc. Roy. Soc. B*, **167**, 101.

Hayes, W., Durham, W. and Cueto, C. (1956), *J. Amer. Med. Assoc.*, **162**, 890.

Hazelbauer, G. and Changeux, J. (1974), *Proc. Nat. Acad. Sci.*, *U.S.A.*, 71, 1479.

Heath, D. (1956), *J. Chem. Soc.*, 3796.

Hecht, G. (1936), *Arch. exper. Path. Pharmakol.*, **183**, 87.

Hedberg, K., Hughes, E. and Waser, J. (1961), *Acta Cryst.*, **14**, 369.

Heidelberger, C., Griesbach, L., Cruz, O., Schnitzer, R. and Grunberg, E. (1958), *Proc. Soc. Expl Biol. Med.*, **97**, 470.

Helin, P. and Bergh, M. (1975), *New Engl. J. Med.*, **291**, 1311.

Hellberg, H. (1959), *Acta Chem. Scand.*, **13**, 1106.

Heller, E., Argaman, M., Levy, H. and Goldblum, N. (1969), *Nature, Lond.*, **222**, 273.

Hemker, H. (1962), *Biochim. Biophys. Acta*, **63**, 46.

Hemmerich, P., Veeger, C. and Wood, H. (1965), *Angew. Chem.*, **77**, 1.

Henderson, P., McGivan, J. and Chappell, J. (1969), *Biochem. J.*, **111**, 521.

Henkel, J., Portoghese, P., Miller, J. and Lewis, P. (1976), *J. Med. Chem.*, **19**, 6.

Hershenson, F., Prodan, K., Kochman, R., Bloss, J. and Mackerer, C. (1977), *J. Med. Chem.*, **20**, 1448.

Hewitt, R., Kushner, S., Stewart, H., White, E., Wallace, W. and Subbarow, Y. (1947), *J. Lab. Clin. Med.*, **32**, 1314.

Hey, P. (1952), *Brit. J. Pharmacol.*, **7**, 117.

Heymann, B. (1924), *Z. angew. Chem.*, **37**, 585.

Heymann, B. (1928), *Klin. Woch.*, **7**, 1305.

Heymann, B., Kothe, R., Dressel, O. and Ossenbeck, A. (1917), U.S. Pat. 1 218 654–5 (cf. 1 308 071).

Higashi, Y., Strominger, J. and Sweeley, C. (1967), *Proc. Nat. Acad. Sci. U.S.A.*, **57**, 1878.

Higuchi, T. and Stella, V. (eds.) (1975), *Pro-drugs as Novel Drug Delivery Systems*, Washington, D.C.: American Chemical Society.

Hildebrand, J. (1960), *J. Phys. Chem.*, **72**, 1841.

Hill, J., Loeb, E., MacLellan *et al.* (1975), *Cancer Chemother. Reports*, **59**, 647.

Hill, L. (1966), *J. Gen. Microbiol.*, **44**, 419.

Hill-Cottingham, D. and Lloyd-Jones, C. (1961), *Nature, Lond.*, **189**, 312.

Hille, B. (1966), *Nature, Lond.*, **210**, 1220.

Hiller, S. (1927), *Proc. Soc. Expl. Biol. Med.*, **24**, 427.

Hilton, J., Ard, J., Jansen, L. and Gentner, W. (1959), *Weeds*, **7**, 381.

Himmelweit, F. (ed.) (1956–   ), *The collected papers of Paul Ehrlich, with biography*, Oxford: Pergamon Press.

Hirai, T., Hirashima, A., Itoh, T., Takahishi, T., Shimoura, T. and Hayashi, Y. (1966), *Phytopathology*, **56**, 1236.

Hirom, P., Millburn, P. and Smith, R. (1976), *Xenobiotica*, **6**, 55.

Hirsch, J. (1942), *Science*, **96**, 1942.

Hirschmann, R., Nutt, R., Veher, D., Vitali, R., Varga, S., Jacob, T., Holly, F. and Denkewalter, R. (1969), *J. Amer. Chem. Soc.*, **91**, 507.

Hitchings, G. (1952), *Trans. Roy. Soc. Trop. Med. Hyg.*, **46**, 467.

Hitchings, G. and Burchall, J. (1965), *Advances Enzymol.*, **27**, 417.

Hitchings, G., Elion, G., Falco, E., Russell, P., Sherwood, M. and VanderWerff, H. (1950), *J. Biol. Chem.*, **183**, 1.

Hlubucek, J., Hora, J., Toube, T. and Weedon, B. (1970), *Tetrahedron Letters*, 5163.

Hobbiger, F. (1954), *Chem. and Indust.*, 415.

Hobbiger, F. (1955), *Brit. J. Pharmacol.*, **10**, 356.

Hochster, R. and Quastel, J. (1963), (eds.), *Metabolic Inhibitors*, Vols. 1 and 2, New York: Academic Press.

Hodgkin, A. (1964), *The Conduction of the Nervous Impulse*, Liverpool: Liverpool University Press.

Hodgkin, A. and Huxley, A. (1952), *J. Physiol., Lond.*, **117**, 500.

Hodgkin, A. and Katz, B. (1949), *J. Physiol.*, **108**, 37.

Hodgson, E. and Casida, J. (1962), *J. Agric. Food Chem.*, **10**, 208.

Höber, R. (1945), *Physical Chemistry of Cells and Tissues*, Philadelphia: Blakiston Co.

Hoffman, C., Schweitzer, T. and Dalby, G. (1940), *J. Amer. Chem. Soc.*, **62**, 988.

Hoffman, C., Schweitzer, T. and Dalby, G. (1941), *Indust. Eng. Chem.*, **33**, 749.

Hofschneider, P. and Martin, H. (1968), *J. Gen. Microbiol.*, **51**, 23.

Hogben, C., Schanker, L., Tocco, D. and Brodie, B. (1957), *J. Pharmacol.*, **120**, 540.

Hogben, C., Tocco, D., Brodie, B. and Schanker, L. (1959), *J. Pharmacol.*, **125**, 275.

Hokin, L. and Hokin, M. (1963), *Ann. Rev. Biochem.*, **32**, 553.

Holan, G. (1965), *Nature, Lond.*, **206**, 311.

Holan, G. (1969), *Nature, Lond.*, **221**, 1025.

Holan, G. (1971), *Nature, Lond.*, **232**, 644.

Hollenberg, C., Borst, P. and van Bruggen, E. (1970), *Biochim. Biophys. Acta*, **209**, 1.

Holley, R. (1953), *Science*, **117**, 23.

Hollingworth, R. (1975), in *Pesticide Selectivity*, (ed. Street, J.), New York: Dekker.

Hollingworth, R., Fukuto, T. and Metcalf, R. (1967), *J. Agr. Food. Chem.*, **15**, 235.

Holman, B. (1941), in *Thorpe's Dictionary of Applied Chemistry*, 4th Edn, **5**, p. 263.

Holmes, R. and Robins, E. (1955), *Brit. J. Pharmacol.*, **10**, 490.

Holton, P. and Ing, H. (1949), *Brit. J. Pharmacol.*, **4**, 190.

Homer, R., Mees, G. and Tomlinson, T. (1960), *J. Sci. Food. Agric.*, 309.

Horn, A. and Snyder, S. (1971), *Proc. Nat. Acad. Sci., U.S.A.*, **68**, 2325.

Horowitz, M. and Brayton, C. (1970), *Virology*, **48**, 690.

Horsfall, J. (1972), in *Pest Control: Strategies for the Future*, Washington, D.C.: Nat. Acad. Sciences, p. 216.

Horwitz, S. and Grollman, A. (1968), *Antimicrob. Agents Chemother.*, **21**.

Hotchkiss, R. (1951), *Cold Spring Harbor Symp. Quant. Biol.*, **16**, 457.

Hotchkiss, R. (1955), *J. Cell. Comp. Physiol.*, **45** (Supp. 2), 1.

Hou, J. and Poole, J. (1971), *J. Pharmaceut. Sci.*, **60**, 503.

Hove, E. (1948), *Arch. Biochem.* **17**, 467.

Howard, F. (1941), *Science*, **94**, 345.

Howells, R., Peters, W., Homewood, C. and Warhurst, D. (1970), *Nature, Lond.*, **228**, 625.

Huang, C. (1969), *Biochemistry*, **8**, 344.

Huang, M., Biggs, D., Clark-Walker, D. and Linnane, A. (1966), *Biochim. Biophys. Acta*, **114**, 434.

Huang, T. and Grollman, A. (1970), *Fed. Proc.* **29**, 609.

Hudson, C. and Neuberger, A. (1950), *J. Org. Chem.*, **15**, 24.

Hughes, D. (1962), *J. Gen. Microbiol.*, **29**, 39.

Hughes, J. (1975), *Brain. Res.*, **88**, 1.

Hughes, J., Smith, T., Kosterlitz, H., Fothergill, L., Morgan, B. and Morris, H. (1975), *Nature, Lond.*, **258**, 577.

Hughes, M. (1972), *The Inorganic Chemistry of Biological Processes*, London: Wiley.

Hunt, R. and Taveau, R. (1911), *Bull. Hyg. Lab.*, U.S. Treasury, No. 73.

Hunter, F. and Lowry, O. (1956), *Pharmacol. Rev.*, **8**, 89.

Hurly, M. (1959), *Trans. Roy. Soc. Trop. Med. Hyg.*, **53**, 410, 412.

Hurwitz, C., Doppel, H., and Rosano, C. (1964), *J. Gen. Microbiol.*, **35**, 159.

Hurwitz, J., Furth, J., Malamy, M. and Alexander, M. (1962), *Proc. Nat. Acad. Sci. U.S.A.*, **48**, 1222.

Hutner, S. (1949), *Science*, **110**, 548.

Hyman, J. (1949), *Brit. Pat.* 652 300

Iball. J. (1964), *Nature, Lond.*, **201**, 916.

I. G. Farbenindustrie, Pharmaceutical Dept. (1933–8), *Medicine in its Chemical Aspects, Reports from the Medico-Chemical Research Laboratories*, Leverkusen (Germany): Bayer, Vols. 1–3.

Ikeda, M., Suzyki, M. and Djerassi, C. (1967), *Tetrahedron Letters*, 3745.

Inbar, M., Ben-Bassat, H. and Sachs, L. (1972), *Nature, New. Biol.*, **236**, 3.

Ing, H. (1936), *Physiol. Rev.*, **16**, 527.

Ing, H. (1949), *Science*, **109**, 264.

Ing, H., Kordik, P. and Williams, T. (1952), *Brit. J. Pharmacol.*, **7**, 103.

Inoue, F. and Frank, G. (1962), *J. Pharmacol.*, **136**, 190.

Inoue, Y. and Perrin, D. (1962), *J. Chem. Soc.*, 2600.

International Agency for Research on Cancer, (1976), *Annual Report*, **1**, Lyon, France.

Iqbal, K. and Ottaway, J. (1970), *Biochem. J.*, **119**, 145.

Irving, H. and Mellor, D. (1962), *J. Chem. Soc.*, 5222, 5237.

Irving, H. and Rossotti, H. (1956), *Acta Chem. Scand.*, **10**, 72.

Irving, H. and Williams, R. (1953), *J. Chem. Soc.*, 3192.

Irving, S., Osborne, M. and Wilson, R. (1976), *Nature, Lond.*, **263**, 431.

Isaka, S. (1957), *Nature, Lond.*, **179**, 578.

Ison, R., Partington, P. and Roberts, G. (1973), *Molec. Pharmacol.*, **9**, 756.

Ito, K., Nakahara, I. and Sakamoto, Y. (1964), *Gann*, **55**, 379.

Iversen, L. (1967), *The Uptake and Storage of Noradrenaline in Sympathetic Nerves*, Cambridge: University Press.

Iversen, L. (1971), *Brit. J. Pharmacol.*, **41**, 571.

Iversen, L. (1974), *Nature, Lond.*, **252**, 630.

Ives, D. and Lemon, T. (1968), *Roy. Inst. of Chemistry Reviews*, **1**, 62.

Iwai, K., Akino, M., Goto, M. and Iwanami, Y. (eds.) (1970), *Chemistry and Biology of Pteridines*, Tokyo: International Academic Printing Co. (in English).

Iwasa, J., Fujita, T. and Hansch, C. (1965), *J. Med. Chem.*, **8**, 150.

Iyer, V. and Szybalski, W. (1964), *Science*, **145**, 55.

Izaki, K., Matsuhashi, M. and Strominger, J. (1966), *Proc. Nat. Acad. Sci. U.S.A.*, **55**, 656.

Izaki, K., Matsuhashi, M. and Strominger, J. (1968), *J. Biol. Chem.*, **243**, 3180.

Izatt, R., Nelson, D., Rylting, J., Haymore, B. and Christensen, J. (1971), *J. Amer. Chem. Soc.*, **93**, 1619.

Jackman, L. and Sternhell, S. (1968), *Applications of NMR Spectroscopy in Organic Chemistry*, 2nd Edn, Oxford: Pergamon Press.

Jackson, G., Muldoon, R. and Akers, L. (1963), *Antimicrob. Agents and Chemother.*, 703.

Jackson, K. and Mason, S. (1971), *Trans. Farad. Soc.*, **67**, 966.

Jacobs, M., Glassman, H. and Parpart, A. (1935), *J. Cell. Comp. Physiol.*, **7**, 197.

Jacobs, W. and Heidelberger, M. (1919), *J. Amer. Chem. Soc.*, **41**, 1587.

Jacobson, M. (1972), *Insect Sex Pheromones*, 2nd Edn, New York: Academic Press.

Jacoby, G., and Gorini, L. (1967), in *Antibiotics*, (eds. Gottlieb, D. and Shaw, P.), **1**, 726, New York: Springer.

Jaenicke, L. and Chan, P. (1960), *Angew. Chem.*, **72**, 753.

Jaffé, H. (1953), *Chem. Rev.*, **53**, 191.

Jaffe, J. and McCormack, J. (1967), *Molec. Pharmacol.* **3**, 359.

James, K. (1974), *Progress in Medicinal Chemistry*, (eds. Ellis, G. and West, G.), **10**, 205.

James, T. (1975), *Nuclear Magnetic Resonance in Biochemistry*, New York: Academic Press.

v. Jansco, N. (1931), *Zbl. Bakt., Abt. I. Orig.*, **122**, 393.
v. Janscó, N. (1932), *Klin. Woch.*, **11**, 1305.
Janssen, M. (1958), *J. Inorg. Nuclear Chem.*, **8**, 340.
Jardetzky, O. (1963), *J. Biol. Chem.*, **238**, 2498.
Jardetzky, O. and Jardetzky, C. (1962), *Methods of Biochem. Anal.*, **9**, 235.
Jardetzky, O. and Wade-Jardetzky, N. (1966), *Molec. Pharmacol.*, **1**, 214.
Jawetz, E. (1952), *Arch. Intern. Med.*, **90**, 301.
Jeffrey, A., Weinstein, I., Jennette, K. and 5 others (1977), *Nature, Lond.*, **269**, 348.
Jeffrey, G., Koch, H. and Nyburg, S. (1948), *J. Chem. Soc.*, 1118.
Jellinek, F. (1957), *Acta Cryst.*, **10**, 277.
Jencks, W. (1969), *Catalysis in Chemistry and Enzymology*, New York: McGraw-Hill.
Jenkinson, D. and Morton, I. (1967), *J. Physiol.*, **188**, 373.
Jeng, A., Ryan, T. and Shamoo, A. (1978), *Proc. Nat. Acad. Sci., U.S.A.*, **75**, 2125.
Jenner, P. and Testa, B. (1978), *Xenobiotica*, **8**, 1.
Jensen, E. and Jacobson, H. (1962), *Recent Prog. Hormone Res.*, **18**, 387.
Jensen, K. and Schmith, K. (1942), *Z. Immunitäts*, **102**, 261.
Jepson, J. and Smith, W. (1974), *Essentials of Organic Nomenclature*, Oxford: University Press.
Jirousek, L. and Pritchard, E. (1971), *Biochim. Biophys. Acta*, **243**, 230.
Johnson, Q. (1960), *U.S. Atom Energy Commiss.*, UCRL 9350.
Johnston, G., Curtis, D., Beart, P., Game, C., McCulloch, R. and Twitchin, B. (1975), *J. Neurochem.*, **24**, 433.
Jonas, A. and Weber, G. (1971), *Biochemistry*, **10**, 1335.
Jones, M. M. (1960), *Nature, Lond.*, **185**, 96.
Jones, O. and Watson, W. (1965), *Nature, Lond.*, **208**, 1169.
Jones, R. and Katritzky, A. (1962), *Chem. and Indust.*, 522.
Jordan, A. and Trevern, M. (1978), *Nature, Lond.*, **272**, 719.
Jordan, D. (1968), *Molecular Associations in Biology* (ed. Pullman, B.), New York: Academic Press, p. 221.
Jordan, D., and Sansom, L. (1971), *Biopolymers*, **10**, 399.
Josephson, E., Taylor, D., Greenberg, J. and Coatney, G. (1953), *J. Infect. Diseases*, **93**, 257.
Josephy, P., Palcic, B. and Skarsgard, L., (1978), *Nature, Lond.*, **271**, 370.
Joswick, H. (1961), *Mode of Action of Hexachlorophene*, Ph.D. thesis, University of Michigan.
Juan, S., Segura, E. and Cazzulo, J. (1978), *Internat. J. Biochem.*, **9**, 395.
Juel-Jensen, B. (1970), *Brit. Med. J.*, **2**, 154.
Jung, L. and Lami, H. (1970), *Bull. Chimie therap.*, **5**, 391.
Jung, L. Koffel, J.-C. and Lami, H. (1971), *Bull. Chimie therap.*, **6**, 341.
Kabachnik, M., Brestkin, A., Godovikov, N., Michelson, M., Rozengart, E. and Rozengart, V. (1970), *Pharmacol. Rev.*, **22**, 355.
Kadota, I. and Abe, T. (1954), *J. Lab. Clin. Med.*, **43**, 375.
Kadota, I. and Midorikawa, O. (1951), *J. Lab. Clin. Med.*, **38**, 671.
Kaelin, A. (1947), *Helv. Chim. Acta*, **30**, 2132.
Kaethner, T. (1977), *Nature, Lond.*, **267**, 19.
Kalnins, K. and Belenski, B. (1964), *Dokl. Akad. Nauk SSR*, **157**, 619.
Kalow, W. (1962), *Pharmacogenetics, Heredity, and Response to Drugs*, Philadelphia: Saunders.
Kamiura, H., Matsumoto, A., Miyazake, Y. and Yamamoto, I. (1963), *Agr. Biol. Chem., Tokyo*, **27**, 684.
Kaplan, A. and Ben-Proat, T. (1966), *J. Mol. Biol.*, **19**, 320.
Karle, I. and Brockway, L. (1944), *J. Amer. Chem. Soc.*, **66**, 1974.

Karlin, A. (1967), *J. Theoret. Biol.*, **16**, 306.

Karlin, A. (1974), *Life Sci.*, **14**, 1385.

Karlin, A., and Bartels, E. (1966), *Biochim. Biophys. Acta*, **126**, 525.

Karlson, P. and Sekeris, C. (1962), *Biochim. Biophys. Acta*, **63**, 489.

Karplus, M. (1959), *J. Chem. Phys.*, **30**, 11.

Kartha, G., Bello, J. and Harker, D. (1967), *Nature, Lond.*, **213**, 862.

Kasai, M. and Changeux, J.-P. (1971), *J. Membrane Biol.*, **6**, pp. 1, 24, 58.

Katic, F., Lavery, H., and Lowe, R. (1972), *Brit. J. Pharmacol.*, **44**, 779.

Kato, G., Yung, J. and Ihnat, M. (1970), *Molec. Pharmacol.*, **6**, 588.

Kato, N. and Eggers, H. (1969), *Virology*, **37**, 632.

Katz, B. (1962), *Proc. Roy. Soc. B*, **155**, 455.

Katz, B. (1966), *Nerve, Muscle, and Synapse*, New York: McGraw-Hill.

Katz, B. and Miledi, R. (1972), *J. Physiol. Lond.*, **224**, 665.

Katz, B. and Thesleff, S. (1957), *J. Physiol. Lond.*, **138**, 63.

Kaufman, H. (1962), *Proc. Soc. Expl Biol. Med.*, **109**, 251.

Kaufman, S. (1964), in *Pteridine Chemistry*, (eds. Pfleiderer, W. and Taylor, E.), Oxford: Pergamon Press.

Kauzmann, W. (1954), in *Mechanism of Enzyme Action*, (eds. McElory, W. and Glass, B.), Baltimore: Johns Hopkins Press.

Kaye, R. (1950), *J. Pharm. Pharmacol.*, **2**, 902.

Kaye, R. and Stonehill, H. (1951), *J. Chem. Soc.*, 2638.

Kearney, P. and Kaufman, D. (1969), *Degradation of Herbicides*, New York: Dekker.

Keberle, H. (1964), *Ann. N.Y. Acad. Sci.*, **119** (Art. 2), 758.

Kefford, N. (1966), *Botanical Gazette*, **127**, 159.

Keighley, E. (1962), *Brit. Med. J.*, **ii**, 93.

Keilin, D. (1933), *Ergebnis. Enzymforsch.*, **2**, 239.

Kelly, D. (1974), *J. Gen. Virol.*, **25**, 427.

Kennedy, B. and Yabro, J. (1966), *J. Amer. Med. Assoc.*, **195**, 1038.

Kerkut, G., Shapira, A. and Walker, R. (1965), *Comparative Biochem. Physiol.*, **16**, 37.

Kerr, M. and Wain, R. (1964), *Ann. Appl. Biol.*, **54**, 441.

Kessel, D. (1971), *Cancer Res.*, **31**, 1883.

Kessel, D., Hall, T. and Reyes, P. (1969), *Molec. Pharmacol.*, **5**, 481.

Kessel, D., Hall, T., Roberts, D. and Wodinsky, I. (1965), *Science*, **150**, 752.

Khorana, H., Buechi, H., Ghosh, H., Gupta, N., Jacob, T., Koessel, H., Morgan, R., Narang, S., Ohtsuka, E. and Wells, R. (1966), *Cold Spring Harb. Symp. Quant. Biol.*, **31**, 39.

Khromov-Borisov, N., Gmiro, V. and Magazanik, L. (1969), *Dokl. Akad. Nauk*, **186**, 236 (per *Chem. Abs.*, 1969, 71, 28959.)

Khromov-Borisov, N. and Michelson, M. (1966), *Pharmacol. Rev.*, **18**, 1051.

Kier, L. (1971), *Molecular Orbital Theory in Drug Research*, New York: Academic Press.

Kier, L. and Hall, L. (1976), *Molecular Connectivity in Chemistry and Drug Research*, New York: Academic Press.

Kikuth, W. (1932), *Deutsch. med. Woch.*, **58**, 530.

Kikuth, W. (1935), *Zbl. Bakt.*, *Abt. I, Orig.*, **135**, 135.

Kim, J. and Eidinoff, M. (1965), *Cancer Res.*, **25**, 698.

King, A. and Nicholson, B. (1969), *Biochem. J.*, **114**, 679.

King, H., Lourie, E. and Yorke, W. (1938), *Ann. Trop. Med. Parasit.*, **32**, 177.

King, H. and Strangeways, W. (1942), *Ann. Trop. Med. Parasit.*, **36**, 47.

Kini, M. and Cooper, J. (1962), *Biochem. J.*, **82**, 164.

Kinsky, S. (1962), *Proc. Nat. Acad. Sci. U.S.A.*, **48**, 1049; *J. Bact.*, **83**, 351.

Kisliuk, R. and Brown, G. (1979), *Chemistry and Biology of Pteridines*, New York: Elsevier.

Kittleson, A. (1952), *Science*, **115**, 84.
Klaus, W. and Lee, K. (1969), *J. Pharmacol.*, **166**, 68.
Klee, W. and Streaty, R. (1974), *Nature, Lond.*, **248**, 63.
Kleiderer, E. and Shonle, H. (1934), *J. Amer. Chem. Soc.*, **56**, 1772.
Kleinwächter, V. Bakarova, Z. and Bohacek, J. (1969), *Biochem. Biophys. Acta*, **174**, 188.
Klevens, H. (1948), *J. Physical Colloid Chem.*, **52**, 130.
Klyne, W. (1962), *Stereochemical Correlations*, (Roy. Inst. Chem. Lecture Series, No. 4).
Klyne, W. and Buckingham, J. (1978), *Atlas of Stereochemistry*, 2nd Edn, London: Chapman and Hall.
Kmetec, E. and Bueding, E. (1961), *J. Biol. Chem.*, **236**, 584.
Knorr, L. (1887), *Liebigs Annalen*, **238**, 137.
Knox, R. (1962), in *The Scientific Basis of Medicine, Annual Reviews*, London: Athlone Press.
Knox, W., Stampf, P., Green, D. and Auerbach, V. (1948), *J. Bact.*, **55**, 451.
Kober, T. and Cooper, G. (1976), *Nature, Lond.*, **262**, 704.
Koepfli, J., Thimann, K., and Went, F. (1938), *J. Biol. Chem.*, **122**, 763.
Kohn, K. and Spears, C. (1970), *J. Mol. Biol.*, **51**, 551.
Kohn, K., Waring, M., Glaubiger, D. and Friedman, C. (1975), *Cancer Res.*, **35**, 71.
Koller, K. (1884), *Wien. med. Wochschr.*, **34**, 1276, 1309.
Kollman, P. and Allen, L. (1972), *Chem. Rev.*, **72**, 283.
Kollonitsch, J., Barash, L., Kahan, F. and Kropp, H. (1973), *Nature, Lond.*, **243**, 347.
Konaka, K. and Matsuoka, T. (1967), *Kumamoto Med. J.*, **20**, 196.
Kopin, I. (1968), *Annual Rev. Pharmacol.*, **8**, 377.
Korman, E., Harris, R., Williams, G., Wakabayashi, T. and Green, D. (1970), *Bioenergetics*, **1**, 387.
Kortüm, G., Vogel, W. and Andrussow, K. (1961), *Dissoziationskonstanten organischer Säuren in wässeriger Lösung*, compiled for I.U.P.A.C., London: Butterworths.
Kosolapoff, G. and Maier, L. (1972), *Organic Phosphorus Compounds* (3 vols.), New York: Wiley-Interscience.
Koshland, D. (1964), *Fed. Proc.*, **23**, 719.
Koshland, D. and Neet, K. (1968), *Ann. Rev. Biochem.*, **37**, 359.
Kosower, E. (1962), *Molecular Biochemistry*, New York: McGraw-Hill.
Kosterlitz, H., Collier, H. and Villarreal, J. (eds.) (1972), *Agonist and Antagonist Actions of Narcotic Analgesic Drugs*, London: Macmillan; Baltimore: University Park Press.
Kowala, C., Murray, K., Swan, J. and West, B. (1971), *Austral. J. Chem.*, **24**, 1369.
Kozloff, M. and Lute, M. (1965), *J. Mol. Biol.*, **12**, 780.
Kozloff, L., Lute, M., Crosby, L., Rao, N., Chapman, V. and Delong, S. (1970), *J. Virol.*, **5**, 726.
Kozloff, L., Lute, M. and Henderson, K. (1957), *J. Biol. Chem.*, **228**, 511.
Krackov, M., Lee, C. and Mautner, H. (1965), *J. Amer. Chem. Soc.*, **87**, 892.
Krakoff, I., Brown, N. and Reichard, P. (1968), *Cancer Res.*, **28**, 1559.
Krebs, E. and Najjar, V. (1948), *J. Exper. Med.*, **88**, 569.
Krebs, H. (1957), *Endeavour*, **16**, 125.
Kritschewsky, J. (1927), *Zent. Bakt.*, **104**, 214.
Kritschewsky, J. (1928), *Z. Immunitäts*, **59**, 1.
Krnjević, K. (1966), *Endeavour*, **25**, 8.
Krueger, H. and O'Brien, R. (1959), *J. Econ. Entomol.*, **52**, 1063.
Krueger, H., O'Brien, R. and Dauterman, W. (1960), *J. Econ. Entomol.*, **53**, 25.
Krueger, R. and Mayer, G. (1970), *Science*, **169**, 1213.

Krüger-Thiemer, E. (1957), *Berichte Borstel, Germany*, **4**, 299.

Krüger-Thiemer, E. (1960), *Klin. Woch.*, **38**, 514.

Krüger-Thiemer, E. (1962), *Klin. Woch.*, **40**, 153.

Krüger-Thiemer, E. (1966), *J. Theoret. Biol.*, **13**, 212.

Krüger-Thiemer, E. and Bünger, P. (1961), *Arzneimittel Forsch.*, **11**, 867.

Krüger-Thiemer, E. and Bünger, P. (1965), *Chemotherapia*, **10**, 61, 129.

Kruger, P. (1955), *Radiation Research*, **3**, 1.

Kruger, R., and Mayer, G. (1970), *Science*, **169**, 1213.

Krupka, R. and Laidler, K. (1961). *J. Amer. Chem. Soc.*, **83**, 1458.

Kuchino, Y. and Borek, E. (1978), *Nature, Lond.*, **271**, 126.

Küntzel, H. and Noll, H. (1967), *Nature, Lond.*, **215**, 1340.

Kuhn, R. (1940), *Angew. Chem.*, **53**, 1.

Kuhn, R., Weygand, F. and Möller, E. (1943), *Ber. deut, chem. Ges.*, **76**, 1044.

Kumler, W. and Halverstadt, I. (1941), *J. Amer. Chem. Soc.*, **63**, 2182.

Kuntzman, R., Mark, L., Brand, L., Jacobson, M., Levin, W. and Conney, A. (1966), *J. Pharmacol.*, **152**, 151.

Kupchan, S., Komoda, Y., Branfman, A., Dailey, R. and Zimmerly, V. (1974), *J. Amer. Chem. Soc.*, **96**, 3706.

Kwan, S.-W. and Webb, T. (1967), *J. Biol. Chem.*, **242**, 5542.

Laarhoven, W., Nivard, R. and Havinga, E. (1961), *Experientia*, **17**, 214.

Laborit, H. (1952), *Réaction organique à l'agression et choc, Paris : Masson*

Ladd, M. (1968), *Theoret. Chim. Acta (Berlin)*, **12**, 333.

La Du, B., Mandel, H. and Way, E. (1971), *Fundamentals of Drug Metabolism and Drug Disposition*, Baltimore: Williams and Wilkins.

Läuger, P., Martin, H. and Müller, P. (1944), *Helv. Chim. Acta*, **27**, 892.

Lai, C. and Weisblum, B. (1971), *Proc. Nat. Acad. Sci. U.S.A.*, **68**, 856.

Laidlaw, P., Dobell, C. and Bishop, A. (1928), *Parasitology*, **20**, 207.

Laidler, K. and Shuler, K. (1949), *J. Chem. Phys.*, **17**, 851, 856.

Lambert, C. and Ferreira, F. (1965), *Bull. Org. mond. Santé*, **32**, 73.

Lambert, J., Simpson, R., Mohr, H. and Hopkins, L. (1970), *J. Assoc. Offic. Anal. Chem.*, **53**, 1145.

Lambley, D. and Ware, J. (1967), *Brit. J. Urol.*, **39**, 147.

Lampen, J. and Jones, M. (1946), *J. Biol. Chem.*, **166**, 435.

Lands, A., Arnold, A., McAuliff, J., Luduena, F., and Brown, T. (1967), *Nature, Lond.*, **214**, 597.

Landy, M. and Gerstung, R. (1944), *J. Bact.*, **47**, 448.

Lang, A. (1970), *Ann. Rev. Plant Physiol.*, **21**, 537.

Langen, P. (1975), *Antimetabolites of Nucleic Acid Metabolism* (trans., Scott, T.), London: Gordon and Breach.

Langley, J. (1878), *J. Physiol.*, **1**, 339.

Langmuir, I. (1916), *J. Amer. Chem. Soc.*, **38**, 2221.

Langmuir, I. (1917), *J. Amer. Chem. Soc.*, **39**, 1848.

Langmuir, I. (1918), *J. Amer. Chem. Soc.*, **40**, 1361.

Lapworth, M. (1940), in *Thorpe's Dictionary of Applied Chemistry*, 4th Edn, **4**, pp. 224, 235.

Large, E. (1940), *The Advance of Fungi*, London: Cape.

Lasser, N. (1966), *J. Lipoid Research*, **7**, 403, 413.

Latorre, R. and Hall, J. (1976), *Nature, Lond.*, **264**, 363.

Laveran, A. and Mesnil, F. (1902), *Ann. Inst. Pasteur*, **16**, 785.

Law, J., Yuan, C., and Williams, C. (1966), *Proc. Nat. Acad. Sci. U.S.A.*, 55, 577.

Lawley, P. and Brookes, P. (1959), *Ann. Rep. Brit. Emp. Cancer Camp.* **37**, 68.

Lawley, P. and Brookes, P. (1967), *J. Molec. Biol.*, **25**, 143.

Lawrence, J., Loomis, W., Tobias, C. and Turpin, F. (1946), *J. Physiol.*, 105, 197.

Lawrence, P. and Strominger, J. (1970), *J. Biol. Chem.*, **245**, 3653.
Laws, E., Curley, A. and Biros, F. (1967), *Arch. Environ. Health*, **15**, 766.
Laycock, G. and Shulman, A. (1963), *Nature, Lond.*, **200**, 849.
Laycock, G. and Shulman, A. (1967), *Nature, Lond.*, **213**, 995.
Lazarus, M. and Rogers, W. (1951), *Aust. J. Sci. Res.*, **4** B, 163.
Leake, C., Koch, D. and Anderson, H. (1930), *Proc. Soc. Expl Biol. Med.*, **27**, 717.
Lederberg, J. (1957), *J. Bact.*, **73**, 144.
Lederberg, J. and Lederberg, E. (1952), *J. Bact.*, **63**, 399.
Ledóchowski, A. (1976), *Materia Medica Polona, Warsaw*, **8**, 237.
Lee, R. and Hodsden, M. (1963), *Biochem. Pharmacol.*, **12**, 1241.
Lees, H. and Simpson, J. (1957), *Biochem. J.*, **65**, 297.
Leeson, L., Krueger, J. and Nash, A. (1963), *Tetrahedron Letters*, 1155.
Le Fevre, P. (1961), *Pharmacol. Rev.*, **13**, 39.
Le Fevre, P. (1975), *Current Topics in Membranes and Transport*, **7**, 109.
Lefkowitz, R., Mullikin, D. and Caron, M. (1976), *J. Biol. Chem.*, **251**, 4686.
Lehn, J., Sauvage, J. and Dietrich, B. (1970), *J. Amer. Chem. Soc.*, **92**, 2916.
Lehninger, A. (1970), *Biochem. J.*, **119**, 129.
Lehninger, A. (1971), *The Mitochondrion*, 2nd Edn, New York: Worth Publishers; Amsterdam: Addison-Wesley.
Lehninger, A. (ed.) (1975), Biochemistry: *The Molecular Basis of Cell Structure and Function*, 2nd Edn, New York: Worth.
Leitz, W., Winkler, F. and Dunitz, J. (1971), *Helv. Chim. Acta*, **54**, 1103.
Lemberg, R., Callaghan, J., Tandy, D. and Goldsworthy, N. (1948), *Aust. J. Expl Biol. Med. Sci.*, **26**, 9.
Leo, A. and Hansch, C. (1971), *J. Org. Chem.*, **36**, 1539.
Leo, A., Hansch, C. and Elkins, D. (1971), *Chem. Rev.*, **71**, 525.
Leo, A., Jow, P., Silipo, C. and Hansch, C. (1975), *J. Med. Chem.*, **18**, 865.
Lerman, L. (1961), *J. Mol. Biol.*, **3**, 18.
Lerman, L. (1963), *Proc. Nat. Acad. Sci., U.S.A.*, **49**, 94.
Lerman, L. (1964a), *J. Mol. Biol.*, **10**, 367.
Lerman, L. (1964b), *J. Cell. Comp. Physiol.*, **64** (Suppl. 1), 1.
Letham, D., Shannon, J. and McDonald, I. (1964), *Proc. Chem. Soc.*, 230.
Leuzinger, W. (1971), *Biochem. J.*, **123**, 139.
Levaditi, C. (1908), *Compt. rend. Soc. Biol.*, **64**, 911.
Lever, M., Miller, K., Paton, W. and Smith, E. (1971), *Nature, Lond.*, 231, 368.
Levey, G. (ed.) (1976), *Hormone-Receptor Interaction: Molecular Aspects*, New York: Dekker.
Levine, L. and Ohuchi, K. (1978), *Nature, Lond.*, **276**, 274.
Levine, R. and Goldstein, M. (1955), *Recent Prog. Hormone Research*, 11, 343.
Levine, R., Hall, T. and Harris, C. (1963), *Cancer*, **16**, 269.
Levine, R., Streeten, D. and Doisy, R. (1968), *Metabolism*, **17**, 114.
Levine, W. (Ed.) (1978), *The Chelation of Heavy Metals*, Oxford: Pergamon Press.
Levinson, W., Woodson, B. and Jackson, J. (1971), *Nature New Biology*, **232**, 116.
Levitzki, A. (1973), in *A Guide to Molecular Pharmacology-Toxicology*, (ed. Featherstone, R.), New York: Marcel Dekker, p. 305.
Levitzki, A. (1977), *Biochem. Biophys. Res. Commun.*, **74**, 1154.
Levy, B. and Ahlquist, R. (1961), *J. Pharmacol.*, **133**, 202.
Lewin, S. (1974), *Displacement of Water and its Control of Biochemical Reactions*, London: Academic Press.
Lewis, D. and Lowe, G. (1973), *Chem. Commun., Chem. Soc.*, 713.
Lewis, G. and Randall, M. (1923), *Thermodynamics and the Free Energy of Chemical Substances*, New York: McGraw-Hill.
Lewis, J. (1970), *Pharmacology* (revised by Crossland, J.), Edinburgh: Livingstone.

Lewis, J., Bentley, K. and Cowan, A. (1971), *Ann. Rev. Pharmacol.*, **11**, 241.

Lewis, P. and Haeusler, G. (1975), *Nature, Lond.*, **256**, 440.

Lewis, S., Waller, J. and Fowler, K. (1960), *J. Insect Physiol.*, **4**, 128.

Li, M. and Ross, S. (1976), *J. Amer. Med. Assoc.*, **235**, 2825.

Liébecq, C. and Peters, R. (1949), *Biochim. Biophys. Acta*, **3**, 215.

Liebermeister, K. (1950), *Z. Naturforsch.*, **5b**, 79.

Liebreich, O. (1869), *Wiener med. Wochenschr.*, 1087.

Lindberg, B. (1970), *Ark. Kemi*, **32**, 317.

Lineweaver, H. and Burk, D. (1934), *J. Amer. Chem. Soc.*, **56**, 658.

Linnane, A., Vitols, E. and Nowland, P. (1962), *J. Cell. Biol.*, **13**, 345.

Lipscomb, W. (1970), *Accounts of Chemical Research, Amer. Chem. Soc.*, **3**, 81.

Lipscomb, W., Hartsuck, J., Quiocho, F. and Reeke. G. (1969), *Proc. Nat. Acad. Sci. U.S.A.*, **64**, 28.

Liquori, A., Damiani, A. and deCoen, J. (1968), *J. Mol. Biol.*, **33**, 445.

Litchfield, J. (1961), *J. Amer. Med. Assoc.*, **177**, 34.

Lloyd, D. (1974), *The Mitochondria of Microorganisms*, London: Academic Press.

Loewenstein, W. and Kanno, Y. (1967), *J. Cell. Biol.*, **33**, 235.

Loewi, O. (1921), *Arch. ges. Physiol.*, **189**, 239.

Loewi, O. and Navratil, E. (1926), *Arch. ges. Physiol.*, **214**, 678.

London, F. (1937), *Trans. Farad. Soc.*, **33**, 8.

Long, J. and Siegel, M. (1975), *Chem.–Biol. Interactions Amsterdam*, **10**, 383.

Lonsdale, K., Milledge, H. and Pant, L. (1965), *Acta Cryst.*, **19**, 827.

Loo, J. and Riegelman, S. (1968), *J. Pharmaceut. Sci.*, **57**, 918.

Lord, J., Waterfield, A., Hughes, J. and Kosterlitz, H. (1977), *Nature, Lond.*, **267**, 495.

Lotspeich, W. and Peters, R. (1951), *Biochem. J.*, **49**, 704.

Lowe, H., (1968), in *Theory and Application of Gas Chromatography* (eds. Kroman, H. and Bender, S.), New York: Grune and Stratton.

Lowe, M. and Phillips, J. (1961), *Nature, Lond.*, **190**, 262.

Lowney, L., Schulz, K., Lowrey, P. and Goldstein, A. (1974), *Science*, **183**, 749.

Luduena, F., von Euler, L., Tullar, B. and Lands, A. (1957), *Arch. internat. Pharmacodyn. Thér.*, **111**, 392.

Luduena, F., Hoppe, J., Nachod, F., Martini, C. and Silvern, G. (1955), *Arch. internat. Pharmacodyn. Thér.*, **101**, 17.

Lueck, L., Wurster, D., Higuchi, T., Lemberger, A. and Busse, L. (1957), *J. Amer. Pharm. Assoc. Sci. Ed.*, **46**, 694, 698.

Lüttringhaus, A. and Gralheer, H. (1942), *Annalen*, **550**, 67.

Lukens, R. (1971), *Chemistry of Fungal Action*, London: Chapman and Hall.

Lumsden, J. and Hall, D. (1975), *Nature, Lond.*, **257**, 670.

Lundegardh, H. (1937), *Biochem. Z.*, **290**, 104.

Luongo, M. and Bjornson, S. (1954), *New Engl. J. Med.*, **251**, 995.

Lutz, W., Winkler, F. and Dunitz, J. (1971), *Helv. Chim. Acta*, **54**, 1103.

Luzzatto, L., Apirion, D. and Schlessinger, D. (1968), *Proc. Nat. Acad. Sci. U.S.A.*, **60**, 873.

Luzzi, L. (1970), *J. Pharm. Sci.*, **59**, 1367.

Lwoff, A. (1961), *Proc. Roy. Soc. B*, **154**, 1.

Maass, E. and Johnson, M. (1949), *J. Bacteriol.*, **57**, 415.

Macadam, R. and Williamson, J. (1972), *Trans. Roy. Soc. Trop. Med. Hyg.*, **66**, 897.

Macadam, R. and Williamson, J. (1974), *Ann. Trop. Med. Parasit.*, **68**, 291, 301.

McBryde, W. (1967), *Canad. J. Chem.*, **45**, 2093.

McBryde, W. and Atkinson, G. (1961), *Canad. J. Chem.*, **39**, 510.

McCalla, T. (1941), *Proc. Soil Sci. Soc. Amer.*, **6**, 165.

McCollister, R., Gilbert, W., Ashton, D. and Wyngaarden, J. (1964), *J. Biol. Chem.*, **239**, 1560.

McCormick, J., Jensen, E., Miller, P. and Doerschuck, A. (1960), *J. Amer. Chem. Soc.*, **82**, 3381.

McDaniel, D. and Brown, H. (1958), *J. Org. Chem.*, **23**, 420.

Macfarlane, M. (1961), *Biochem. J.*, **80**, 45 P.

Macfarlane, M. (1962), *Nature, Lond.*, **196**, 136.

Macheboeuf, M. (1948), *Bull. Soc. Chim. biol.*, **30**, 161.

McIlwain, H. (1941), *Biochem. J.*, **35**, 1311.

McIlwain, H. (1957), *Chemotherapy and the Central Nervous System*, London: Churchill.

McIlwain, H. (1962), in *Enzymes and Drug Action* (eds. Mongar, J. and de Reuck, A.), London: Churchill.

Macintosh, F., Birks, R. and Sastry, R. (1956), *Nature, Lond.*, **178**, 1181.

Mackay, M. and Hodgkin, D. (1955), *J. Chem. Soc.*, 3261.

Maclean, N. (1977), *The Differentiation of Cells*, London: Edward Arnold.

McMorris, T., Seshadri, R., Weihe, G., Arsenault, G. and Barksdale, A. (1975), *J. Amer. Chem. Soc.*, **97**, 2544.

Macomber, P., O'Brien, R. and Hahn, F. (1966), *Science*, **152**, 1374.

McQueen, E. (1968), *Brit. J. Pharmacol. Chemother.*, **33**, 312.

Macris, B. and Georgopoulos, S. (1969), *Phytopathology*, **59**, 879.

Maeda, T., Abe, H., Kakiki, K. and Misato, T. (1970), *Agric. Biol. Chem.*, (Japan), **34**, 700.

Magee, P. (1964), in Ciba Symp., *Cellular Injury* (eds. DeReuck, A. and Knight, J.), p. 1, London: Churchill.

Maggi, N., Furesz, S. and Sensi, P. (1968), *J. Med. Chem.*, **11**, 368.

Maggi, N., Pasqualucci, C., Ballotta, R. and Sensi, P. (1966), *Chemotherapia*, **11**, 285.

Maghidson, O. and Grigorovski, A. (1933), *Khim. Farm. Prom.*, *URSS*, 187.

Magrath, D. and Phillips, J. (1949), *J. Chem. Soc.*, 1940.

Maguire, M., Wiklund, R., Anderson, H. and Gilman, A. (1976), *J. Biol. Chem.*, **251**, 1221.

Mahler, H., Mehrotra, B. and Sharp, C. (1961), *Biochem. Biophys. Res. Commun.*, **4**, 79.

Mandelstam, J. (1962), *Biochem. J.*, **84**, 294.

Manifold, M. (1941), *Brit. J. Expl Path.*, **22**, 111.

Mann, T. and Keilin, D. (1940), *Nature, Lond.*, **146**, 164.

Manson, P. (1908), *Ann. Trop. Med.*, **2**, 49.

Mansour, T. and Bueding, E. (1953), *Brit. J. Pharmacol. Chemother.*, **8**, 431.

Mansour, T. and Bueding, E. (1954), *Brit. J. Pharmacol. Chemother.*, **9**, 459.

Mao, J., Putterman, M. and Wiegand, R. (1970), *Biochem. Pharmacol.*, **19**, 391.

Marantz, R. and Shelanski, M. (1970), *J. Cell. Biol.*, **44**, 234.

di Marco, A. and Arcamone, F. (1975), *Arzneimittel Forsch.*, **25**, 368.

Marcovich, H. (1953), *Ann. Inst. Pasteur*, **85**, 199, 443.

Maren, T., Wadsworth, B., Yale, E. and Lonso, L. (1954), *Johns Hopkins Hosp. Bull.*, **95**, 277.

Margoliash, E., Barlow, G. and Byers, V. (1970), *Nature, Lond.*, **228**, 723.

Margoshes, M. and Vallett, B. (1957), *J. Amer. Chem. Soc.*, **79**, 4813.

Margulis, L. (1970), *Origin of Eukaryote Cells*, New Haven: Yale University Press.

Mark, L., Burns, J., Brand, L., Campomanes, C., Trousof, N., Papper, E. and Brodie, B. (1958), *J. Pharmacol.*, **123**, 70.

Marlow, H., Metcalf, J. and Burgen, A. (1969), *Molec. Pharmacol.*, **5**, 156, 166.

Marquardt, R. and Brosemer, R. (1966), *Biochim. Biophys. Acta*, **128**, 454.

Marsh, R. (1972), *Systemic Fungicides*, Essex: Longman.

Marshall, E. (1937), *J. Biol. Chem.*, **122**, 263.

Marston, H., Allen, S. and Smith, R. (1961), *Nature, Lond.*, **190**, 1085.

Martin, A. (1973), *Biochem. Soc. Transactions*, **1**, 1206.

Martin, B. (1967), *Brit. J. Pharmacol. Chemother.*, **31**, 420.

Martin, H. (1964), *J. Gen. Microbiol.*, **36**, 441.

Martin, H. (1973), *The Scientific Principles of Crop Protection*, 6th Edn, New York: Crane, Russak Co.

Martin, H. and Worthing, C. (eds.) (1977), *Insecticide and Fungicide Handbook for Crop Protection*, 5th Edn, pub. for British Crop Protection Council, Oxford: Blackwell Scientific.

Martin, K. (1969), *Brit. J. Pharmacol.*, **36**, 458.

Martin, Y. (1970), *J. Medicin. Chem.*, **13**, 145.

Martinez-Carrion, M., Sator, V. and Raferty, M. (1975), *Biochem. Biophys. Res. Commun.*, **65**, 129.

Martin-Smith, M., Smail, G., and Stenlake, J. (1967), *J. Pharm, Pharmacol.*, **19**, 561.

Massey, V., Hofmann, T. and Palmer, G. (1962), *J. Biol. Chem.*, **237**, 3820.

Matijevic, E. and Eirich, F. (1969), *Surface and Colloid Science*, New York: Wiley.

Matsubara, T., Nakamura, Y. and Tochino, Y. (1975), *Xenobiotica*, **5**, 205.

Matthews, B., Sigler, P., Henderson, R. and Blow, D. (1967), *Nature, Lond.*, **214**, 652.

Matthews, D., Alden, R., Bolin, J. and 7 others, (1977), *Science*, **197**, 452.

Matthyse, A. and Abrams, M. (1970), *Biochim. Biophys. Acta*, **199**, 511.

Mauro, A., Nanavati, R. and Heyer, E. (1972), *Proc. Nat. Acad. Sci. U.S.A.*, **69**, 3742.

Mauss, H. and Mietzsch, F. (1933), *Klin. Woch.*, **12**, 1276.

Mautner, H. (1969), *J. Gen. Physiol.*, **54**, 271 S.

Mautner, H., Bartels, E. and Webb, G. (1966), *Biochem. Pharmacol.*, **15**, 187.

Mautner, H. and Clemson, H. (1970), in *Medicinal Chemistry*, 3rd. Edn, Part II (ed. Burger, A.), New York: Wiley.

Mautner, H., Dexter, D. and Low, B. (1972), *Nature, New Biol.*, **238**, 87.

May, H. and McCay, P. (1968), *J. Biol. Chem.*, **243**, 2288.

Mayer, D., Price, D. and Rafii, A. (1977), *Brain Res.*, **121**, 368.

Mayer, S., Maickel, R. and Brodie, B. (1959), *J. Pharmacol.*, **127**, 205.

Meade, T. (1975), *Brit. J. Prevent. and Social Med.*, **29**, 157.

Meadows, D., Roberts, G. and Jardetzky, O. (1969), *J. Mol. Biol.*, **45**, 491.

Meehan, T., Straub, K. and Calvin, M. (1977), *Nature, Lond.*, **269**, 725.

Mees, G. (1960), *Ann. Appl. Biol.*, **48**, 601.

Mellor, D. and Maley, L. (1947), *Nature, Lond.*, **159**, 370.

Menger, F. and Portnoy, C. (1967), *J. Amer. Chem. Soc.*, **89**, 4698.

Mercer, F. (1960), *Ann. Rev. Plant Physiol.*, **11**, 1.

Merritt, H. and Putnam, T. (1938), *Arch. Neurol. Psychiat.*, Chicago, **39**, 1003.

Mertz, W. (1975), *Nutrition Reviews*, **33**, 129.

Mertz, W. and Cornatzer, W. (1971), *Newer Trace Elements in Nutrition*, New York: Dekker.

Metcalf, R. and Luckman, W. (eds.) (1975), *Introduction to Insect Pest Management*, New York: Wiley.

Meyer, F., Meyer, H. and Bueding, E. (1970), *Biochim. Biophys. Acta.*, **210**, 257.

Meyer, H. (1899), *Arch. expl Path. Pharmakol.*, **42**, 109.

Meyer, K. and Hemmi, H. (1935), *Biochem. Zeits.*, **277**, 39.

Meyer, M. and Guttman, D. (1968), *J. Pharm. Sci.*, **57**, 895.

Meyers, A., Nolen, R., Collington, E., Narwid, T. and Strickland, R. (1973), *J. Org. Chem.*, **38**, 1974.

Meyers, A. and Shaw, C. (1974), *Tetrahedron Letters*, 717.

Michael, T., Michael, J. and Massell, B. (1967), *J. Bact.*, **93**, 1749.

Michaelis, L. and Hill, E. (1933), *J. Gen. Physiol.*, **16**, 859.

Michaelis, L. and Menten, M. (1913), *Biochem. Z.*, **13**, 333.

Michelson, M. (1969), *Proc. IV Internat. Congress Pharmacol.*, **5**, 103, Stuttgart: Schwabe.

Michelson, M. and Zeimal, E. (1973), *Acetylcholine, an Approach to the Molecular Mechanism of Action*, Oxford: Pergamon Press.

Mietzsch, F., and Klarer, I. (1932), *D. R. Pat.* 607537.

Mihich, E. (ed.) (1973), *Drug Resistance and Selectivity*, New York: Academic Press.

Milanesi, G., and Ciferri, O. (1966), *Biochemistry*, 5, 3926.

Miledi, R., Milinoff, P., and Potter, L. (1971), *Nature, Lond.*, **229**, 554.

Miledi, R. and Slater, C. (1966), *J. Physiol.*, **184**, 473.

Miles, A. and Misra, S. (1938), *J. Hyg. Cambridge*, **38**, 732.

Millardet, A. (1885), *J. Agric. prat., Paris*, **49**, 513, 801.

Miller, A. (1944), *Proc. Soc. Expl Biol. Med.*, **57**, 151.

Miller, E. and Miller, J. (1966), *Pharmacol. Rev.*, **18**, 805.

Miller, E., Miller, J. and Hartmann, H. (1961), *Cancer Res.*, 21, 815.

Miller, G., Doukos, P. and Seydel, J. (1972), *J. Med. Chem.*, **15**, 700.

Miller, J. (1970), *Cancer Res.*, **30**, 559.

Miller, K. and Hildebrand, J. (1968), *J. Amer. Chem. Soc.*, **90**, 3001.

Miller, K., Paton, W. and Smith, E. (1965), *Nature, Lond.*, **206**, 574.

Miller, K., Paton, W., Smith, R., and Smith, E. (1973), *Molec. Pharmacol.*, **9**, 131.

Miller, S. (1961), *Proc. Nat. Acad. Sci., U.S.*, **47**, 1515.

Miller, W., Dessert, A. and Roblin, R. (1950), *J. Amer. Chem. Soc.*, **72**, 4893.

Mirrlees, M., Moulton, S., Murphy, C., and Taylor, P. (1976), *J. Med. Chem.*, **19**, 615.

Mishell, D., Talas, M., Parlow, A. and Moyer, D., (1970), *Amer. J. Obstet. Gynecol.*, **107**, 100.

Misra, A., Hunger, A. and Keberle, H. (1966), *J. Pharm. Pharmacol.*, **18**, 246, 531.

Mitchell, P. (1949), *Nature, Lond.*, **164**, 259.

Mitchell, P. (1961), in *Biological Structure and Function*, (eds. Goodwin, T. and Lindberg, O.), New York: Academic Press, **2**, 581.

Mitchell, P. (1963), in *Structure and Function of Membranes and Surfaces of Cells*, *Biochem. Soc. Symp.*, **22**, 142, Cambridge: Cambridge University Press.

Mitchell, P. and Moyle, J. (1956a), *Biochem. J.*, **64**, 19 P.

Mitchell, P. and Moyle, J. (1956, b), in *Bacterial Anatomy, Symp. Soc. Gen. Microbiol.*, **6**, 150.

Mitchell, P. and Moyle, J. (1957), *J. Gen. Microbiol.*, **16**, 184.

Mitchell, P. and Moyle, J. (1959), *J. Gen. Microbiol.*, **20**, 434.

Mitchison, D. (1962), *Brit. Med. Bull.*, **18**, 74.

Mitscher, L., Bonacci, A. and Sokoloski, T. (1968), *Antimicrob. Agents Chemother.*, 78.

Mitsuhashi, S., Harada, K. and Hashimoto, H. (1960), *Jap. J. Expl Med.*, **30**, 179.

Mitsuhashi, S., Harada, K. and Kameda, M. (1961), *Nature, Lond.*, **189**, 947.

Mittal, K. (ed.) (1975), *Colloidal Dispersions and Micellar Behaviour*, Washington: American Chemical Society.

Miyazaki, H., Tojinbara, I., Watanabe, Y., Osaka, T. and Okui, S. (1970), *Proc. 1st Symp. Drug. Metab. Action*, Chiba (Japan), p. 135.

Molitor, H. (1936), *J. Pharmacol.*, **58**, 337.

Monod, J., Changeux, J.-P. and Jacob, F. (1963), *J. Mol. Biol.*, **6**, 306.

Monod, J., Wyman, J. and Changeux, J.-P. (1965), *J. Mol. Biol.*, **12**, 88.

Moon, R., Grubbs, C., Sporn, M. and Goodman, D. (1977), *Nature, Lond.*, **267**, 620.

Moore, C. and Pressman, B. (1964), *Biochem. Biophys. Res. Commun.*, **15**, 562.

Moore, L., Chen, T., Knapp, H. and Landon, E. (1975), *J. Biol. Chem.*, **250**, 4562.

Morgan, G. and Cooper, E. (1912), *Reports of the 8th International Congress of Applied Chemistry*, **19**, 243.

Morgan, G. and Drew, H. (1920), *J. Chem. Soc.*, **117**, 1456.

Morgenroth, J. and Levy, R. (1911), *Berl. klin. Woch.*, **48**, 1560, 1979.

Mortazani, S., Bari-Hashemi, A., Mozafari, M. and Raffi, A. (1972), *Cancer*, **29**, 1193.

Moss, F. and Lemberg, R. (1950), *Aust. J. Expl Biol. Med. Sci.*, 28, 667.

Moyer, A. and Coghill, R. (1947), *J. Bact.*, **53**, 329.

Mudge, C. and Smith, F. (1935), *Amer. J. Pub. Health*, **25**, 442.

Müller, D., Jaenicke, L., Donike, M. and Akintobi, T. (1971), *Science*, **171**, 815.

Mueller, J. and Vilter, R. (1950), *J. Clin. Invest.*, **29**, 193.

Mueller, P. and Rudin, D. (1967), *Nature, Lond.*, **213**, 603.

Müller, W. and Crothers, D. (1968), *J. Molec. Biol.*, **35**, 251.

Muir, R. (1921), *Proc. Roy. Soc. B*, **92**, i.

Muir, R. and Hansch, C. (1953), *Plant Physiol.*, **28**, 218.

Mullins, L. (1956), in *Molecular Structure and Functional Activity of Nerve Cells*, (eds. Grenell, R. and Mullins, L.), Washington, D.C.: American Institute of Biological Sciences.

Munn, E. (1974), *The Structure of Mitochondria*, London: Academic Press.

Murray, A. (1966), *Biochem. J.*, **100**, 664.

Musajo, L. and Rodighiero, G. (1970), *Photochem. and Biol.*, **11**, 27.

Nachmansohn, D. (1940), *Yale J. Biol. and Med.*, **12**, 565.

Nachmansohn, D. (1959), *Chemical and Molecular Basis of Nerve Activity*, New York: Academic Press.

Nador, K., Herr, F., Pataky, G. and Borsy, J. (1953), *Arch. exper. Path. Pharmakol.*, **217**, 447.

Nagai, K., Yamaki, H., Suzuki, H., Tanaka, N. and Umezawa, H. (1969), *Biochim. Biophys. Acta*, **179**, 165.

Nakatsugawa, T. and Dahm, P. (1965), *J. Econ. Entomol.*, **58**, 500.

Nagasawa, H., Shirota, F. and Mizuno, N. (1974), *Chem. Biol. Interactions, Amsterdam*, **8**, 403.

Nagawa, M. (1960), *Yakugaku Zasshi*, **80**, 761.

Narahashi, T. (1971), *Bulletin WHO*, **44**, 337.

Narahashi, T. and Frazier, R. (1968), *Fed. Proc.*, **27**, 408.

Narahashi, T. and Haas, H. (1968), *J. Gen. Physiol.*, **51**, 177.

Narahashi, T., Moore, J. and Scott, W. (1964), *J. Gen. Physiol.*, **47**, 965.

National Academy of Sciences, U.S. (1967), *Toxicants Occurring Naturally in Foods*, Washington.

Nauta, W. (1977), personal communication.

Navon, G., Ogawa, S., Shulman, R. and Tamane, T. (1977), *Proc. Nat. Acad. Sci. U.S.A.*, **74**, 888.

Nebert, D. and Mason, H. (1963), *Cancer Res.*, **23**, 833.

Nelson, E. (1961), *J. Pharm. Sci.*, **50**, 181.

Nelson, E. and O'Reilly, I. (1960), *J. Pharmacol.*, **129**, 368.

Nelson, E. and O'Reilly, I. (1961), *J. Pharm. Sci.*, **50**, 417.

Nelson, J., Carpenter, J., Rose, L. and Adamson, D. (1975), *Cancer Res.*, **35**, 2872.

Nemethy, G., Scheraga, H. and Kauzmann, W. (1960), *J. Phys. Chem.*, **72**, 1843.

Neumann, P. and Sass-Kortsak, A. (1967), *J. Clin. Invest.*, **46**, 646.

Neurath, H. and Hill, R. (eds.) (1975–   ), *The Proteins*, in 8 Vols, 3rd Edn, New York: Academic Press.

Neville, D. and Davies, D. (1966), *J. Mol. Biol.*, **17**, 57.

Newton, G. and Abraham, E. (1956), *Biochem. J.*, **62**, 651.

Nichol, C. and Welch, A. (1950), *Proc. Soc. Expl Biol. Med.*, **74**, 403.

Nicholson, A., Stone, B., Clark, C. and Ferres, H. (1976), *Brit. J. Clin. Pharmacol.*, **3**, 429.

Nickerson, M. (1957), *Pharmacol. Rev.*, **9**, 246.

Nickerson, W., Falcone, G. and Kessler, G. (1961), in *Macromolecular Complexes* (ed. Edds, M.), New York: Ronald Press, p. 205.

Nielands, J. (ed.) (1974), *Microbial Iron Metabolism*, New York: Academic Press.

Nielsen, F. and Ollerich, D. (1974), *Fed. Proc.*, **33**, 1767.

Nierhaus, D. and Nierhaus, K. (1973), *Proc. Nat. Acad. Sci. U.S.A.*, **70**, 2224.

Nimmo-Smith, R., Lascelles, J. and Woods, D. (1948), *Brit. J. Expl Path.*, **29**, 264.

Nirenberg, M., Jones, D., Leder, P., Clark, B., Sly, W. and Pestka, S. (1963), *Cold Spring Harbor Symp. Quant. Biol.*, **28**, 549.

Nisonoff, A., Hopper, J. and Spring, S. (1975), *The Antibody Molecule*, New York: Academic Press.

Nixon, J., (ed.) (1976), *Microencapsulation*, New York: Marcel Dekker.

Nogami, H. and Matsuzawa, T. (1963), *Chem. Pharm. Bull., Japan*, **9**, 532 (in English).

Noguer, A., Wernsdorfer, W., Kanznetsov, R. and Hempel, J. (1978), *WHO Chromide*, **32**, 9.

Nomura, M., Tissières, A. and Lengyel, P. (1974), *Ribosomes*, New York: Cold Spring Harbor Lab. Press.

Nordbring-Hertz, B. (1955), *Physiol. Planatarum*, **8**, 691.

Northey, E. (1948), *The Sulfonamides and Allied Compounds*, New York: Reinhold.

Northrup, G., Taylor, S., and Northrup, R. (1969), *Cancer Res.*, **29**, 1916.

Norton, S. (1954), *Brit. J. Pharmacol.*, **9**, 494.

Notari, R. (1973), *J. Pharmaceut. Sci.*, **62**, 865.

Notari, R. (ed.) (1975), *Biopharmaceutics and Pharmacokinetics*, New York: Marcel Dekker.

Novak, V. (1966), *Insect Hormones*, London: Methuen.

Nys, G. and Rekker, R. (1973), *Chim. thérap.*, **8**, 521.

O'Brien, I., Cox, G. and Gibson, F. (1971), *Biochim. Biophys. Acta*, **237**, 537.

O'Brien, I. and Gibson, F. (1970), *Biochim. Biophys. Acta*, **215**, 393.

O'Brien, J. (1967), *J. Theoret. Biol.*, **15**, 307.

O'Brien, R. (1967), *Insecticides, Action and Metabolism*, New York: Academic Press.

O'Brien, R., Eldefrawi, M. and Eldefrawi, A. (1972), *Ann. Rev. Pharmacol.*, **12**, 19.

O'Brien, R. and Morris, J. (1972), *Arch. Mikrobiol.*, **84**, 225.

O'Brien, R., Olenick, J. and Hahn, F. (1966), *Proc. Nat. Acad. Sci. U.S.A.*, **55**, 1511.

Östergren, G. (1951), *Colloques internationaux du Centre nationale de la Recherche scientifique (Paris)*, No. 26, *Mécanisme de la Narcose*, p. 77.

Offe, H., Siefken, W. and Domagk, G. (1952), *Naturwiss.*, **39**, 118.

Oker-Blom, N., Hori, T., Leinikki, P., Palosuo, T., Pettersson, R. and Sani, J. (1970), *Brit. Med. J.*, **iii**, 676.

Oki, M. and Urushibara, Y. (1952), *Bull. Chem. Soc. Japan*, **25**, 109.

Oliver, M., Roberts, S., Hayes, D., Pantridge, J., Suzman, M. and Bersohn, I. (1963), *Lancet*, **i**, 143.

O'Malley, B. and Means, A. (1974), *Science*, **183**, 610 (review).

Opitz, K. and Reimann, I. (1973), *Psychopharmacologia*, **28**, 165.

Orloff, J. and Berliner, R. (1956), *J. Clin. Invest.*, **35**, 223.

Ormerod, W. (1961), *Proc. Roy. Soc. Trop. Med. Hyg.*, **55**, 313.

Ortiz, P. (1970), *Biochemistry*, **9**, 355.

Osborn, M., Freeman, M. and Huennekens, F. (1958), *Proc. Soc. Expl Biol. Med.*, **97**, 429.

Osborne, D. (1968), *Nature, Lond.*, **219**, 564.

Osborne, M., Wenger, J. and Zanko, M. (1977), *J. Pharmacol.*, **200**, 195.

O'Sullivan, D. and Sadler, P. (1961), *Nature, Lond.*, **192**, 341.

Overby, L., Duff, R. and Mao, J. (1977), *Ann. N.Y. Acad. Sci.*, **284**, 310.

Overton, E. (1901), *Studien über die Narkosen*, Jena: Gustav Fischer, 195 pp.

Oxford, A., Raistrick, H. and Simonart, P. (1939), *Biochem. J.*, **33**, 240.

Oxford, J. (ed.) (1977), *Chemoprophylaxis and Virus Infections of the Respiratory Tract*, Chemical Rubber Co.: Cleveland, Ohio (2 Vols).

Oxford, J. and Perrin, D. (1974), *J. Gen. Virol.*, **23**, 59.

Ozaki, M., Mizushima, S. and Nomura, M. (1969), *Nature, Lond.*, **222**, 333.

Pachter, I., Raffauf, R., Ullyot, G. and Ribeiro, O. (1960), *J. Amer. Chem. Soc.*, **82**, 5187.

Pagel, W. (1958), *Paracelsus: an Introduction to Philosophical Medicine*, Basel: Karger.

Palade, G. (1952), *Anat. Record*, **114**, 427.

Palade, G. (1959), *Subcellular Particles*, (ed., Hayashi, T.), New York: Ronald Press.

Palaty, V. (1966), *Nature, Lond.*, **211**, 1177.

Papakadjopoulos, D., Nir, S. and Ohki, S. (1972), *Biochim. Biophys. Acta*, **266**, 561.

Pappenheimer, J., Heissey, S. and Jordan, E. (1961), *Amer. J. Physiol.*, **200**, 1.

Paracelsus (v. Hohenheim, T., known as) (1493–1541), *Works* (ed., Peuckert, W.), Basel: Schwabe (1965) in 5 Vols.; *see also* Pagel (1958).

Pardee, A. (1967), *Science*, **156**, 1627.

Pardee, A. and Pauling, L. (1949), *J. Amer. Chem. Soc.*, **71**, 143.

Parham, W. and Wilbur, J. (1961), *J. Org. Chem.*, **26**, 1569.

Park, J. (1954), *Fed. Proc.*, **13**, 271.

Parke, D. and Lindup, W. (1973), *Ann. N.Y. Acad. Sci.*, **226**, 200.

Parke, D. and Rahman, H. (1970), *Biochem. J.*, **119**, 53 P.

Pasqualini, G. (ed.) (1976), *Receptors and Mechanism of Action of Steroid Hormones*, New York: Dekker.

Pasternak, C. and Handschumacher, R. (1959), *J. Biol. Chem.*, **234**, 2992.

Patel, P., Miller, O. and Trendelenberg, U., (1974), *Pharmacol. Rev.*, **26**, 323.

Paton, W. (1960), *Proc. Roy. Soc. Med.*, **53**, 815.

Paton, W. (1961), *Proc. Roy. Soc. B*, **154**, 21.

Paton, W. (1975), *Ann. Rev. Pharmacol.*, **15**, 191.

Paton, W. and Perry, W. (1953), *J. Physiol.*, **119**, 43.

Paton, W. and Zaimis, E. (1948), *Nature, Lond.*, **162**, 810.

Paton, W. and Zaimis, E. (1949), *Brit. J. Pharmacol.*, **4**, 381.

Paton, W. and Zaimis, E. (1952), *Pharmacol. Rev.*, **4**, 219.

Patrick, R. and Barchas, J. (1974), *Nature, Lond.*, **250**, 737.

Patterson, D. and Roberts, B. (1972), *Food Cosmet. Toxicol.*, **10**, 501.

Pauling, L. (1960), *Nature of the Chemical Bond*, 3rd Edn, Ithaca: Cornell University Press (1st Edn, 1939; 2nd Edn, 1940).

Pauling, L. (1961), *Science*, **134**, 15.

Pauling, L. (1967), *The Chemical Bond*, Ithaca, New York: Cornell University Press.

Pauling, P. and Petcher, T. (1973), *Chemico-biological Interactions, Amsterdam*, **6**, 351.

Peacocke, A. and Skerrett, J. (1956), *Trans. Farad. Soc.*, **52**, 261.

Pedersen, C. (1970), *J. Amer. Chem. Soc.*, **92**, 386, 391.

Pedersen, C. (1972), *Organ. Syntheses*, **52**, 66.

Pedersen, P., Greenawalt, J., Chan, T. and Morris, H. (1970), *Cancer Res.*, **30**, 2620.

Penniston, J., Harris, R., Asai, J. and Green, D. (1968), *Proc. Nat. Acad. Sci. U.S.A.*, **59**, 624.

Perkins, E., Wood, R., Sears, M., Prusoff, W. and Welch, A. (1962), *Nature, Lond.*, **194**, 985.

Perkins, J. (1973), *Adv. Cyclic Nucleotide Res.*, **3**, 1.

Perrin, D. (1958), *Nature, Lond.*, **182**, 741.

Perrin, D. (1959), *Reviews of Pure and Appl. Chem. (Australia)*, **9**, 257.

Perrin, D. (1961), *Nature, Lond.*, **191**, 253.

Perrin, D. (1962), *J. Chem. Soc.*, 645.

Perrin, D. (1964), *Organic Complexing Reagents*, New York: Wiley Interscience.

Perrin, D. (1965), *Adv. Heterocyc. Chem.*, **4**, 43.

Perrin, D. (1965a), *Dissociation Constants of Organic Bases in Aqueous Solution*, compiled for I.U.P.A.C., London: Butterworths, (first supplement, 1972).

Perrin, D. (1965b), *J. Chem. Soc.*, 5590.

Perrin, D. (1970), *Masking and Demasking of Chemical Reactions*, New York: Wiley-Interscience.

Perrin, D. and Dempsey, B. (1974), *Buffers for pH and Metal Ion Control*, London: Chapman and Hall; New York: Halsted-Wiley.

Perrin, D. and Hawkins, I. (1972), *Experientia*, **28**, 880.

Perrin, D. and Sayce, I. (1967), *Talanta*, **14**, 833.

Perrin, D. and Sayce, I. (1968), *J. Chem. Soc.*, *(A)*, 82.

Perrin, D., Sayce, I. and Sharma, V. (1967), *J. Chem. Soc.*, *(A)*, 1755.

Perrin, D. and Sharma, V. (1966), *Biochim. Biophys. Acta*, **127**, 35.

Perrin, D. and Sharma, V. (1968), *J. Chem. Soc.*, *(A)*, 446.

Perrin, D. and Sharma, V. (1969), *J. Chem. Soc.*, *(A)*, 2060.

Perry, A., Mattson, A. and Buckner, A. (1953), *Biol. Bull.*, **104**, 426.

Perry, J., McKinney, L. and De Weer, P. (1978), *Nature, Lond.*, **272**, 271.

Pert, C. and Snyder, S. (1973), *Science*, **179**, 1011.

Pert, C. and Snyder, S. (1974), *Molec. Pharmacol.*, **10**, 868.

Perutz, M. (1970), *Nature, Lond.*, **228**, 726.

Perutz, M., Kendrew, J. and Watson, H. (1965), *J. Mol. Biol.*, **13**, 669.

Pestka, S. (1970), *Arch. Biochem. Biophys.*, **136**, 89.

Peters, L. (1960), *Pharm. Rev.*, **12**, 1.

Peters, R. (1936), *Nature, Lond.*, **138**, 327.

Peters, R. (1948), *Brit. Med. Bull.*, **5**, 313.

Peters, R. (1963), *Biochemical Lesions and Lethal Synthesis*, Oxford: Pergamon Press.

Peters, R., Stocken, L. and Thompson, R. (1945), *Nature, Lond.*, **156**, 616.

Peters, R., Wakelin, R., Rivett, S. and Thomas, L. (1953), *Nature, Lond.*, 171, 1111.

Peterson, C. and Edgington, L. (1969), *J. Agric. Food Chem.*, **17**, 898.

Peyronel, G. (1940), *Z. Krist.*, **103**, 139, 157.

Pfeifer, S. (1975 <), *Biotransformation von Arzneimitteln*, Berlin: Veb Verlag, Volk und Gesundheit.

Pfleiderer, W. (cd.) (1975), *Chemistry and Biology of Pteridines*, Berlin: de Gruyter.

Phillips, D. (1966), *Scientific American*, **215**, 78.

Phillips, G., Power, D., Robinson, C. and Davies, J. (1970), *Biochim. Biophys. Acta*, **215**, 491.

Phillips, R. (1966), *Chem. Rev.*, **66**, 501.

Phillips, R., Love, A., Mitchell, T. and Neptune, E. (1965), *Nature, Lond.*, **206**, 1367.

Pietsch, P. (1966), *J. Cell. Biol.*, 31, 86A.

Pigram, W., Fuller, W. and Hamilton, L. (1972), *Nature, New Biol.*, **235**, 17.

Piper, C. (1942), *J. Agric. Science*, **32**, 143.

Pirie, A. and van Heyningen, R. (1954), *Nature, Lond.*, **173**, 873.

Pitts, R. and Alexander, R. (1945), *Amer. J. Physiol.*, **147**, 138.

Pitzer, K. (1959), *Adv. Chemical Physics*, **2**, 59.

Plant, G. (1964), in *Pteridine Chemistry*, (eds. Pfleiderer, W. and Taylor, E.), Oxford: Pergamon Press, p. 443.

Plempel, M., Bartmann, K., Büchel, K. and Regel, E. (1969), *Deutsch. med. Woch.*, **94**, 1356, 1365.

Plimmer, H. and Thompson, J. (1907), *Proc. Roy. Soc. Lond.*, B, **79**, 505.

616   References

Plimmer, H. and Thompson, J. (1908), *idem*, **80**, 1.

Poate, H. (1944), *Lancet*, ii, 238; *Med. J. Aust.*, i, 242.

Poiesz, J., Battula, N., and Loeb, L. (1974), *Biochem. Biophys. Res. Commun.*, **56**, 959.

Poirier, L., Miller, J., Miller, E. and Sato, K. (1967), *Cancer Res.*, **27**, 1600.

Pollak, J. and Woog, M. (1971), *Biochem. J.*, **123**, 347.

Pollock, M. and Perret, C. (1951), *Brit. J. Expl Path.*, **32**, 387.

Pomeranz, B. and Chiu, D. (1976), *Life Sciences*, **19**, 1757.

Pople, J. (1951), *Proc. Roy. Soc.*, *A*, **205**, 163.

Porter, K. and Bonneville, M. (1973), *Fine Structure of Cells and Tissues*, 4th Edn, Philadelphia: Lea and Febiger.

Porter, K. and Bruni, C. (1959), *Cancer Res.*, **19**, 997.

Portoghese, P., Mikhail, A. and Kupferberg, H. (1968), *J. Med. Chem.*, **11**, 219.

Post, L., De Jong, B. and Vincent, W. (1974), *Pest. Biochem. and Phys.*, 4, 473.

Post, R., Merritt, C., Kinsolving, C. and Albright, C. (1960), *J. Biol. Chem.*, **235**, 1796.

Potts, A. (1962), *Investigative Ophthalmol.*, **1**, 522.

Prabhakaran, K. (1973), *Leprosy Rev.*, **44**, 112.

Prasad, A. (ed.) (1976), *Trace Elements in Human Health and Disease*, New York: Academic Press.

Pratesi, P. (1963), *Pure Appl. Chem.*, **6**, 435.

Pratesi, P., La Manna, A., Campiglio, A. and Ghislandi, V. (1959), *J. Chem. Soc.*, 4062.

Pressman, B. (1970), in *Membranes of Mitochondria and Chloroplasts*, (ed., Racker, E.), p. 213. New York: Van Nostrand.

Pressman, B. and Guzman, N. (1974), *Ann. N. Y. Acad. Sci.*, **227**, 380.

Pressman, D., Grossberg, A., Pence, L. and Pauling, L. (1946), *J. Amer. Chem. Soc.*, **68**, 250.

Prestegard, J. and Chan, S. (1970), *J. Amer. Chem. Soc.*, **92**, 4440.

Preston, H. and Steward, J. (1970), *Chem. Commun. Chem. Soc.*, 1142.

Prichard, R. (1970), *Nature, Lond.*, **228**, 684.

Pritchard, N., Blake, A. and Peacocke, A. (1966), *Nature, Lond.*, **212**, 1360.

Prusoff, W. (1967), *Pharmacol. Rev.*, **19**, 209.

Pullman, A. and Pullman, B. (1955), *Cancérisation par les Substances chimiques et Structures moléculaires*, Paris; Masson.

Purcell, W., Bass. G. and Clayton, J. (1973), *Strategy of Drug Design*, New York: Wiley-Interscience.

Purchase, I., Longstaff, E., Ashby, J., Styles, J., Anderson, D., Lefevre, P. and West-Wood, F. (1976), *Nature, Lond.*, **264**, 624.

Putnam, F. and Neurath, H. (1944), *J. Amer. Chem. Soc.*, **66**, 1992.

Putter, I., Barreto, A., Markley, J. and Jardetzky, O. (1969), *Proc. Nat. Acad. Sci. U.S.A.*, **64**, 1396.

Quastel, J. and Wooldridge, W. (1927), *Biochem. J.*, **21**, 1224.

Quastel, J. (1965), *Pharmacol. Rev.*, **17**, 198.

Raa, J. and Goksøyr, J. (1966), *Physiol. Plantarum*, **19**, 840.

Rabaté, E. (1927), *La Destruction des mauvaises Herbes*, Paris: Librairie de l'Academie de l'Agriculture.

Rabinowitch, E. and Govindjee, R. (1969), *Photosynthesis*, New York: Wiley.

Racker, E. and Krimsky, I. (1947), *J. Expl Med.*, **85**, 715.

Radda, G. (1971), *Biochem. J.*, **122**, 385.

Raeymaekers, A., Allewijn, F., Vandenberk, J., Demoen, P., Offenwert, T. and Janssen, P. (1966), *J. Med. Chem.*, **9**, 545.

Raff, R. and Mahler, H. (1972), *Science*, **177**, 575.

Raine, A. and Chubb, J. (1977), *Nature, Lond.*, **267**, 265.

Rajan, K., Davis, J. and Colburn, R. (1974), *J. Neurochem.*, **22**, 137.

Rall, D. and Zubrod, C. (1960), *Fed. Proc.*, **19**, 80.

Rang, H. (ed.) (1973), *Drug Receptors*, New York: Macmillan.

Rang, H. and Ritter, J. (1969), *J. Molec. Pharmacol.*, **5**, 394.

Rang, H. and Ritter, J. (1970), *J. Molec. Pharmacol.*, **6**, 357, 383.

Rapoport, S. (1976), *The Blood-Brain Barrier in Physiology and Medicine* New York: Raven.

Rappaport, C. and Howze, G. (1966), *Proc. Soc. Expl Biol. Med.*, **121**, 1010, 1016.

Rastelli, A., de Benedetti, P., Albasini, A. and Pecorari, P. (1975), *J. Chem. Soc., Perkin II*, 522, (cf. *J. Med. Chem.*, 1978, **21**, 1325).

Rauen, H. (1964), *Arzneimittelforsch.*, **11**, 855.

Raventós, J. (1937), *Quart. J. Expl Physiol.*, **26**, 361.

Rawal, B. (1969), *Med. J. Australia*, **i**, 612.

Rebhun, L. (1975), *Science*, **189**, 1002.

Recknagel, R. and Ghoshal, A. (1966), *Nature, Lond.*, **210**, 1162.

Redi, F. (1684), *Osservazioni intorno agli animali viventi che si trovano negli animali viventi*, Florence: Piero Matini.

Redl, G., Cramer, R. and Berkoff, C. (1974), *Chem. Soc. Reviews, Lond.*, **3**, 273.

Rees, R., Bennett, J., Maibach, H. and Arnold, H. (1967), *Arch. Dermatol.*, **95**, 2.

Reich, E., Goldberg, I. and Rabinowitz, M. (1962), *Nature, Lond.*, **196**, 743.

Reiner, L., Leonard, C. and Chao S. (1932), *Arch. internat. Pharmacodyn. Thér* **43**, 186, 199.

Reiter, M., Cowburn, D., Prives, J. and Karlin, A. (1972), *Proc. Nat. Acad. Sci., U.S.*, **69**, 1168.

Rekker, R. (1977), *The Hydrophobic Fragmental Constant*, Amsterdam: Elsevier.

Remmer, H. (1962), *Proc. First Internat. Pharmacol. Meeting*, **6**, 235.

Rendi, R. and Ochoa, S. (1962), *J. Biol. Chem.*, **237**, 3711.

Reuse, J. (1948), *Brit. J. Pharmacol.*, **3**, 174.

Reuter, H. (1973), *Prog. Biophys. Molec. Biol.*, **26**, 1.

Reyes, P. and Heidelberger, C. (1965), *Molec. Pharmacol.*, **1**, 14.

Reyn, A., Schmidt, H., Trier, M. and Bentzon, M. (1973), *Brit. J. Vener. Dis.*, **49**, 54.

Reynolds, P. (1966), in *Biochemical Studies of Antimicrobial Drugs*, (eds. Newton, B. and Reynolds, P.), Cambridge: Cambridge University Press.

Rich, S. (1954), *Phytopathology*, **44**, 203.

Richards, W. (1970), *Adv. Pharmacol. Chemother.*, **8**, 121.

Richards, W. (1977), *Quantum Pharmacology*, Sevenoaks (U.K.): Butterworth.

Richmond, D. and Somers, E. (1962), *Ann. Appl. Biol.*, **50**, 33.

Richmond, M. and Curtis, N. (1974), *Ann. N. Y. Acad. Sci.*, **235**, 553.

Rickenberg, H., Cohen, G., Butlin, G. and Monod, J. (1956), *Ann. Inst. Pasteur*, **91**, 829.

Ricks, M. and Hoskins, W. (1948), *Physiological Zoology*, **21**, 258.

Rideal, E. (1945), *Endeavour*, **4**, 83.

Riegel, B. and Sherwood, L. (1949), *J. Amer. Soc.*, **71**, 1129.

Rigler, N., Bag, S., Leyden, D., Sudmeier, J. and Reilley, C. (1965), *Anal. Chem.*, **37**, 872.

Rinehart, J., Arnold, J. and Canfield, C. (1976), *Amer. J. Trop. Med. Hyg.*, **25**, 769.

Ringer, S. (1883), *J. Physiol.*, **4**, 29.

Ringold, H. (1961), in *Mechanism of Action of Steroid Hormones*, (eds. Villee, C. and Engel, L.), Oxford: Pergamon Press.

Riou, G. and Delain, E. (1969), *Proc. Nat. Acad. Sci U.S.A.*, **64**, 618.

Ripper, W., Greenslade, R., Heath, J. and Barker, K. (1948), *Nature, Lond.*, **161**, 494.
Ritchie, C. and Sager, W. (1964), *Prog. Phys. Org. Chem.*, **2**, 323.
Ritchie, J, and Greengard, P. (1961), *J. Pharmacol.*, **133**, 241.
Ritchie, J. and Greengard, P. (1966), *Ann. Rev. Pharmacology*, **6**, 405.
Robbins, W., Crafts, A. and Raynor, R. (1952), *Weed Control*, New York: McGraw-Hill.
Roberts, G. (1966), *Biochem. J.*, **100**, 30P.
Roberts, H. (1954), *Nature, Lond.*, **174**, 1178.
Roberts, J. (1968), in *Structural Chemistry and Molecular Biology*, (eds. Rich, A. and Davidson, N.), San Francisco: Freeman & Co.
Roberts, J. and Warwick, G. (1961), *Biochem. Pharmacol.*, **6**, 217.
Roberts, M. and Rahn, O. (1946), *J. Bact.*, **52**, 612.
Robertson, J.D. (1959), in *Biochem. Soc. Symp.*, 16, *Structure and Function of Subcellular Components* (ed. Crook, E.), Cambridge: Cambridge University Press, p. 3.
Robins, R. and Hitchings, G. (1955), *J. Amer. Chem. Soc.*, **77**, 2256.
Robinson, D. and MacDonald, M. (1966), *J. Pharmacol.*, **153**, 250.
Robinson, F. (1971), *Annual Reports in Med. Chem.*, 34.
Robinson, G. (1966), in *Recent Advances in Medical Microbiology*, (ed., Waterson, A.), London: Churchill, p. 254.
Robinson, R. (1946), *Brit. Med. J.*, **i**, 945.
Robinson, R. and Stokes, R. (1959), *Electrolyte Solutions*, 2nd Edn, London: Butterworths.
Roblin, R. (1946), *Chem. Rev.*, 38, 255.
Roblin, R., Lampen, J., English, J., Cole, Q. and Vaughan, J. (1945), *J. Amer. Chem. Soc.*, **67**, 290.
Robson, J. and Stacey, R. (1962), *Recent Advances in Pharmacology*, 3rd Edn, London: Churchill.
Rodgers, P. and Roberts, G. (1973), *FEBS Lett.*, **36**, 330.
Röe, O. (1955), *Pharmacol. Rev.*, **7**, 399.
Roeder, K. and Weiant, E. (1948), *J. Cell. Comp. Physiol.*, **32**, 175.
Roehl, W. (1920), reported in Heymann (1924), *q.v.*
Roehl, W. (1926a), *Archiv. Schiffs. u. Tropenhyg.*, **30**, Beiheft 3, 11.
Roehl, W. (1926b), *Archiv. Schiffs. u. Tropenhyg.*, **30**, Beiheft 1, 103.
Röller, H., Dahm, K., Trost, B. and Sweeley, C. (1967), *Chem. Eng. News*, No. **16**, 48.
Roemer, D., Beuscher, H., Pless, J. and 6 others (1977), *Nature, Lond.*, **268**, 547.
Rogers, E. and 12 others (1960), *J. Amer. Chem. Soc.*, **82**, 2974.
Rogers, H. (1967), *Nature, Lond.*, **213**, 31.
Rogers, H. and Mandelstam, J. (1962), *Biochem. J.*, **84**, 299.
Rogers, H. and Perkins, H. (1968), *Cell Walls and Membranes*, London: Spon.
Rogers, L. (1912), *Brit. Med. J.*, **i**, 1424.
Rolinson, G. and Sutherland, R. (1965), *Brit. J. Pharmacol. Chemother.*, **25**, 638.
Romanovsky, D. (1891), *Vratch*, No. **18**, 438, per *Zbl. Bakt.*, 1892, **2**, 219 (in German). Thesis, St. Petersburg (1891), reprinted in Zasuchin, D. (1951), *Outstanding Investigations of Native Scientists on the Causative Organisms of Malaria*, Moscow.
Roseman, T. and Higuchi, W. (1970), *J. Pharm. Sci.*, **59**, 353.
Rosen, A. (1970), *Biochem. Pharmacol.*, **19**, 2075.
Rosenberg, B. and van Camp, L. (1970), *Cancer Res.*, **30**, 1799.
Rosenthal, S. (1932), *U.S. Pub. Health Reports*, **47**, 933.
Rosenthal, S. and Voegtlin, C. (1930), *J. Pharmacol.*, **39**. 347.
Rosman, M., Lee, M., Creasey, W. and Sartorelli, A. (1974), *Cancer Res.*, **34**, 1952.

Ross, G., Goldstein, D., Hertz, R., Lipsett, M. and O'Dell, W. (1965), *Amer. J. Obstet. Gynecol.*, **93**, 223.
Ross, W. (1953), *Adv. Cancer Research*, **1**, 397.
Ross, W. (1961), *Biochem. Pharmacol.*, **8**, 235.
Ross, W. (1962), *Biological Alkylating Agents*, London: Butterworths.
van Rossum, J. (1966), *Arch. internat. Pharmacodyn. Ther.*, **160**, 492.
van Rossum, J. (1971), *Drug Design*, (ed. Ariëns, E.), **1**, 469.
van Rossum, J. and Ariëns, E. (1959), *Arch. internat. Pharmacodyn. Thér.*, **118**, 418.
van Rossum, J., Cornelissen, M., de Groot, T. and Hurkmans, J. (1960), *Experientia*, **16**, 372.
Roszkowski, A. (1965), *J. Pharmacol.*, **149**, 288.
Roth, B., Falco, E. and Hitchings, G. (1962), *J. Med. Pharm. Chem.*, **5**, 1103.
Roth, B. and Strelitz, J. (1969), *J. Org. Chem.*, **34**, 821.
Roth, G. and Siok, C. (1978), *J. Biol. Chem.*, **253**, 3782.
Roth, H. and Nierhaus, K. (1975), *J. Mol. Biol.*, **94**, 111.
Roth, I., Lewis, C. and Williams, R. (1960), *J. Bact.*, **80**, 772.
Rothschild, J. (1961), *Fed. Proc.*, **20**, 145.
Rothschild, J. and Howden, G. (1961), *Nature, Lond.*, **192**, 283.
Rothstein, A. and Meier, R. (1948), *Fed. Proc.*, **7**, 252.
Rousseau, G., Baxter, J. and Tomkins, G. (1972), *J. Mol. Biol.*, **67**, 99.
Roux, S. and Yguerabide, J. (1973), *Proc. Nat. Acad. Sci. U.S.A.*, **70**, 762.
Rowland, G., O'Neill, G. and Davies, D. (1975), *Nature, Lond.*, **255**, 487.
Rowlands, D. (1973), *Pestic. Sci.*, **4**, 893.
Rowley, D., Cooper, P., Roberts, P. and Lester Smith, E. (1950), *Biochem. J.*, **46**, 157.
Rubbo, S., Albert, A. and Gibson, M. (1950), *Brit. J. Expl Path.*, **31**, 425.
Rubbo, S., Albert, A. and Maxwell, M. (1942), *Brit. J. Expl Path.*, **23**, 69.
Rubbo, S. and Gillespie, J. (1940), *Nature, Lond.*, **146**, 838.
Ruggli, P. (1934), *J. Soc. Dyers and Colourists*, Jubilee Number, p. 77.
Rupp, H., Voelter, W. and Weser, U. (1974), *Fed. Eur. Biochem. Soc. Lett.*, **40**, 176.
Russell, D. and Falconer, M. (1941), *Brit. J. Surg.*, **28**, 472.
Russell, D. and Falconer, M. (1943), *Lancet*, **i**, 580.
Russell, W., Watson, D. and Wildy, P. (1963), *Biochem. J.*, **87**, 26.
Russo, R., Bartošek, I., Villa. S., Guaitani, A., and Garattini, S. (1976), *Xenobiotica*, **6**, 201.
Rye, R. and Wiseman, D. (1966), *J. Pharm. Pharmacol.*, **18**, 114(S).
Ryter, A. and Jacob, F. (1964), *Ann. Inst. Pasteur*, **107**, 384.
Salem, L. (1962), *Canad. J. Biochem. Physiol.*, **40**, 1287.
Salser, J. and Balis, M. (1965), *Cancer Res.*, **25**, 539, 544.
Salton, M. (1951), *J. Gen. Microbiol.*, **5**, 391.
Salton, M. (1964), *The Bacterial Cell Wall*, Amsterdam: Elsevier.
Salton, M., Horne, R. and Cosslett, V. (1951), *J. Gen. Microbiol.*, **5**, 405.
Samuels, H. and Tomkins, G. (1970), *J. Mol. Biol.*, **52**, 57.
Sander, J., Schweinsberg, F. and Menz, H. (1968), *Z. Physiol., Chem.*, **349**, 1691.
Sanger, F. (1963), *Proc. Chem. Soc. Lond.*, 76.
Sarett, L., Patchett, A. and Steelman, S. (1963), *Prog. Drug. Res.*, **5**, 11.
Sarkar, B. and Kruck, T. (1966), in *Biochemistry of Copper*, (eds. Peisack, J., Aisen, P. and Blimberg, W.), New York: Academic Press.
Sarkar, S. and Thach, R. (1968), *Proc. Nat. Acad. Sci. U.S.A.*, **60**, 1479.
Sartorelli, A. and Creasey, W. (1969), *Ann. Rev. Pharmacol.*, **9**, 51.
Sasaki, T. (1954), *Pharm. Bull., Tokyo*, **2**, 104.
Sastry, B., Lasslo, A. and Pfeifer, C. (1960), *J. Pharmacol.*, **130**, 346.
Saunders, J. (1977), *Nature, Lond.*, **266**, 586.

Saunders, L. (1974), *The Absorption and Distribution of Drugs*, London: Ballière Tindall.

Savage, D., Cameron, A., Ferguson, G., Hannaway, C. and Mackay, I. (1970), *J. Chem. Soc. B*, 410.

Savarie, P., Matschke, G., Schafer, E. and Dasch, G. (1973), *Nature, Lond.*, 241, 551.

Sawitz, W. and Karpinski, F. (1956), *Amer. J. Trop. Med. Hyg.*, 5, 538.

Sayce, I. (1968), *Talanta*, 15, 1397.

Sayce, I. (1971), *Talanta*, 18, 653.

Schaeffer, P. (1969), *Bact. Rev.*, 33, 48.

Schaffer, N., May, S. and Summerson, W. (1954), *J. Biol. Chem.*, 206, 201.

Schanker, L. (1959), *J. Pharmacol.*, 126, 283.

Schanker, L. (1961), *Ann. Rev. Pharmacol.*, 1, 29.

Schanker, L. and Jeffrey, J. (1961), *Nature, Lond.*, 190, 727.

Schanker, L., Shore, P., Brodie, B. and Hogben, C. (1957), *J. Pharmacol.*, 120, 528.

Schanker, L., Tocco, D., Brodie, B. and Hogben, C. (1958), *J. Pharmacol.*, 123, 81.

Schatz, A., Bugie, E. and Waksman, S. (1944), *Proc. Soc. Expl Biol. Med.*, 55, 66.

Schazschneider, B., Ristow, H. and Kleinkauf, H. (1974), *Nature, Lond.*, 249, 757.

Scheff, G. and Hasskó, A. (1936), *Zbl. Bakt.*, Abt. I. Orig., 136, 420.

Schellenberg, K. and Coatney, G. (1961), *Biochem. Pharmacol.*, 6, 143.

Scherrer, R. and Howard, S. (1977), *J. Med. Chem.*, 20, 53.

Schettler, G. (ed.) (1973), *Phospholipids in Biochemistry*, 2nd Edn, Stuttgart: Thieme (in English).

Schild, H. (1947), *Brit. J. Pharmacol.*, 2, 189.

Schild, H. (1960), *J. Physiol.*, 153, 26 P.

Schild, H. (1969), *Brit. J. Pharmacol.*, 36, 329.

Schildkraut, C., Mandel, M., Levisohn, S., Smith-Sonneborn, J. and Marmur, J. (1962), *Nature, Lond.*, 196, 795.

Schloerb, P., Blackburn, G., Grantham, J., Mallard, D. and Cage, G. (1965), *Surgery*, 58, 5.

Schmiedeberg, O. (1912), *Arch. Expl Pathol. Pharmakol.*, 67, 1.

Schmitt, H., Schmitt, H. and Fenard, S. (1973), *Arzneimittel Forsch.*, 23, 40.

Schneider, G. (1964), *Naturwiss.*, 51, 416.

Schnitzer, R. (1926), *Z. Immun. Forsch.*, 47, 116.

Schönhöfer, F. (1938), *Medizin u. Chemie*, 3, 62, Berlin: Verlag Chemie.

Schou, M. (1957), *Pharmacol. Rev.*, 9, 17.

Schoenenberger, G. and Monnier, M. (1977),*Proc. Nat. Acad. Sci. U.S.A.*, 74, 1282.

Schrader, G. (1963), *Die Entwicklung neuer insektizider Phosphorsäure-Ester*, 3rd Edn, Weinheim (Germany): Verlag Chemie.

Schramm, M., Orly, J., Eimerl, S. and Korner, M. (1977), *Nature, Lond.*, 268, 310.

Schraufstätter, E. (1950), *Z. Naturforsch.*, 5b, 190.

Schubert, J. (1956), *Methods Biochem. Analysis*, 3, 247.

Schubert, J. (1957), *Chimia*, 11, 113.

Schueler, F. (1953), *Arch. internat. Pharmacodyn. Thér.*, 95, 376.

Schueler, F. (1956), *J. Pharmacol.*, 115, 127.

Schümann, H. (1961), *Arch. expl Path. Pharmak.*, 241, 200.

Schümann, H. and Kroneberg, G. (1970), *New Aspects of Storage and Release Mechanisms of Catecholamines*, Berlin: Springer.

Schulemann, W., Schönhöfer, E. and Wingler, A. (1932), *Klin. Woch.*, ii, 381.

Schulman, J. and Rideal, E. (1937), *Proc. Roy. Soc. B*, 122, 46.

Schultz, F. (1940), *Z. Physiol. Chem.*, 265, 113.

Schultzen, O. and Naunyn, B. (1867), *Arch. Anat. Physiol.*, 349.

Schulz, R., Cartwright, C. and Goldstein, A. (1974), *Nature, Lond.*, 251, 331.

Schwacke, H. (1970), *Deutsch. med. Woch.*, 95, 2437.

Schwarcz, R., Creese, I., Coyle, J. and Snyder, S. (1978), *Nature, Lond.*, **271**, 766.
Schwartz, A., Matsui, H. and Laughter, A. (1968), *Science*, **160**, 323.
Schwarz, K. (1973), *Proc. Nat. Acad. Sci. U.S.A.*, **70**, 1608.
Schwarz, K., Milne, D. and Vinard, E. (1970), *Biochem. Biophys. Res. Commun.*, **40**, 22.
Schwyzer, R. (1958), Ciba Found. Symp., *Aminoacids, Peptides, Antimetabolic Activity*, London: Churchill, p. 171.
Scott, K. and Mautner, H. (1967), *Biochem. Pharmacol.*, **16**, 1903.
Seeger, D., Cosulich, D., Smith, J. and Hultquist, M. (1949), *J. Amer. Chem. Soc.*, **71**, 1753.
Seeman, P. and Roth, S. (1972), *Biochim. Biophys. Acta*, **255**, 171.
Seeman, P., Roth, S. and Schneider, H. (1971), *Biochim. Biophys. Acta*, **163**, 451.
Segal, A., Arnot, R., Thakur, T. and Lavender, J. (1976), *Lancet*, **ii**, 1056.
Sekeris, C. (1971), *Biochem. J.*, **124**, 43 P.
Selbie, F. (1940), *Brit. J. Expl Path.*, **21**, 90.
Selbie, F. and McIntosh, J. (1943), *J. Path. Bact.*, **55**, 477.
Selling, H., Vonk, J. and Sijpesteijn, A. (1970), *Chem. and Indust.*, 1625.
Seven, M. (1960), in *Metal-binding in Medicine*, (eds., Seven, M., and Johnson, L.), Philadelphia: Lippincott, p. 95.
Sexton, W., Slade, R. and Templeman, W. (1941), *Brit. Pat.* 573, 929.
Seydel, J. (1966), *Mol. Pharmacol.*, **2**, 259.
Seydel, J., Ahrens, H. and Losert, W. (1975), *J. Med. Chem.*, **18**, 234.
Seydel, J., Krüger-Thiemer, E. and Wempe, E. (1960), *Z. Naturforsch.*, **15b**, 628.
Seydel, J., Schaper, K., Wempe, E. and Cordes, H. (1976a), *J. Med. Chem.*, **19**, 483.
Seydel, J., Tono-oka, S., Schaper, K., Bock, L. and Wiencke, M. (1976b), *Arzneimittelforschung*, **26**, 477.
Seydel, J. and Wempe, E. (1971), *Arzneimittelforsch.*, **21**, 187.
Shall, S. (1977), *The Cell Cycle*, London: Chapman and Hall; New York: Wiley-Halsted.
Shapiro, H. (1961), *J. Theoret. Biol.*, **1**, 289.
Sharon, N. and Lis, H. (1972), *Science*, **177**, 946.
Shatkin, A. and Tatum, E. (1961), *Amer. J. Bot.* **48**, 760.
Shealy, Y., and Krauth, C. (1966), *J. Med. Chem.*, **9**, 34.
Shefter, E. and Mautner, H. (1969), *Proc. Nat. Acad. Sci. U.S.A.*, **63**, 1253.
Shemyakin, M., Aldanova, E., Vinogradova, E. and Feigina, M. (1963), *Tetrahedron Letters*, **28**, 1921.
Shepherd, R., Bratton, A. and Blanchard, K. (1942), *J. Amer. Chem. Soc.*, **64**, 2532.
Shepherd, R. and Wilkinson, R. (1962), *J. Med. Pharm. Chem.*, **5**, 823.
Sherbert, G. (ed.) (1973), *Neoplasia and Cell Differentiation*, Basel: S. Karger.
Sherlock, E. (1962), *Chem. and Indust.*, 715.
Shiman, R. and Nielands, J. (1965), *Biochemistry*, **4**, 2233.
Shimomura, O. and Johnson, F. (1969), *Biochemistry*, **8**, 3991.
Shin, Y. and Eichhorn, G. (1968), *Biochemistry*, **7**, 1026.
Shindo, H. and Brown, T. (1965), *J. Amer. Chem. Soc.*, **87**, 1904.
Shiota, T., Baugh, C., Jackson, R. and Dillard, R. (1969), *Biochemistry*, **8**, 5022.
Shiota, T., Baugh, C. and Myrick, J. (1969), *Biochem. Biophys. Acta*, **192**, 205.
Shooter, K., Howse, R., Merrifield, R. and Robins, A. (1972), *Chemico-biol. Interactions, Amsterdam*, **5**, 289.
Shoppee, C. (1964), *Chemistry of the Steroids*, 2nd. Edn, London: Butterworths.
Shugar, D. (ed.) (1970), *Enzymes and Isoenzymes*, New York; Academic Press.
Shulman, A. and Dwyer, F. (1964), in *Chelating Agents and Metal Chelates*, (eds. Dwyer, F. and Mellor, D.), New York: Academic Press (Chap. 9).
Shulman, A. and Laycock, G. (1967), *Europ. J. Pharmacol.*, **1**, 295; **2**, 17.

Shulman, A., Laycock, G. and Henry, J. (1965), *Nature, Lond.*, **208**, 568.
Siddall, J., Cross, A. and Fried, J. (1966), *J. Amer. Chem. Soc.*, **88**, 862.
Siegel, M., Sisler, H. and Johnson, F. (1966), *Biochem. Pharmacol.*, **15**, 1213.
Siegel, S. (1962), *The Plant Cell Wall*, Oxford: Pergamon Press.
Siekevitz, P. (1963), *Proc. 5th Internat. Congress Biochem.*, *Moscow (1961)*, **22**, 219, Oxford: Pergamon Press.
Sigel, H. (ed.) (1973<), *Metal Ions in Biological Systems*, New York: Marcel Dekker.
Sih, C. and Takeguchi, C. (1973), in *The Prostaglandins* (ed. Ramwell, P.), Vol. 1, p. 83, New York: Plenum Press.
Sijpesteijn, A. (1970), *World Review of Pest Control*, **9**, 85.
Sijpesteijn, A. and Janssen, M. (1959), *Antonie van Leeuwenhoek*, **25**, 422.
Sijpesteijn, A., Janssen, M. and van der Kerk, G. (1957), *Biochim. Biophys. Acta*, **23**, 550.
Sijpesteijn, A. and Sisler, H. (1968), *Neth. J. Plant. Path.*, **74** (Suppl. I.), 121.
Sillén, L. and Martell, A. (1964), *Stability Constants of Metal-Ion Complexes*, also first supplement (1971), London: The Chemical Society.
Simon, E. (1950), *Nature, Lond.*, **166**, 343.
Simon, E. and Beevers, H. (1951), *Science*, **114**, 124.
Simon, E. and Beevers, H. (1952), *New Phytologist*, **51**, 163.
Simon, E. and Blackman, G. (1949), *Report of 3rd Symposium of the Society of Experimental Biology*, Cambridge: University Press.
Simmons, W. and Zanger, M. (1972), *The Sadtler Guide to NMR Spectra*, Philadelphia: Sadtler Research Laboratories.
Sims, P. (1970), *Biochem. Pharmacol.*, **19**, 285.
Sims, P., Grover, P., Swaisland, A., Pal, K. and Hewer, A. (1974), *Nature, Lond.*, **252**, 326.
Sinclair, J. and Stevens, B. (1966), *Proc. Nat. Acad. Sci. U.S.A.*, **56**, 508.
Sinclair, W. (1965), *Science*, **150**, 1729.
Singer, B. (1976), *Nature, Lond.*, **264**, 333.
Singer, S. and Nicolson, G. (1972), *Science*, **175**, 720.
Sinistri, C. and Villa, L. (1962), *Il Farmaco, Ed. sci.*, *(Italy)*, **17**, 949.
Sinnema, A., Maat, L., van der Gugten, A. and Beyerman, H. (1968), *Rec. Trav. chim. Pays. Bas*, **87**, 1027.
Siperstein, M. and Fagan, V. (1964), *Cancer Res.*, **24**, 1108.
Skipper, H., Schabel, F. and Wilcox, W. (1964), *Cancer Chemotherap. Reports*, **35**, 1.
Skou, J. (1964), *Prog. Biophys. Chem.*, **14**, 131.
Skulachev, V., Yaguzhinsky, L., Jasaitis, A., Liberman, E., Topali, V. and Zofina, L. (1969), *Energy Level and Metabolic Control in Mitochondria*, (eds. Papa, S., Tager, J., Quagliariello, E. and Slater, E.), Bari: Adriatica Editrice, p. 283.
Slade, R. (1945), *Chem. and Indust.*, **40**, 314.
Slater, T. (1966), *Nature, Lond.*, **209**, 36.
Slater, T. and Sawyer, B. (1971), *Biochem. J.* **123**, 815, 823.
Slifkin, M. (1971), *Charge Transfer Interactions of Biomolecules*, London: Academic Press.
Slotboom, A. and Bonsen, P. (1970), *Chem. Phys. Lipids*, **5**, 301.
Smallman, B. and Fiske, R. (1958), *Canad. J. Biochem. Physiol.*, **36**, 575.
Smellie, R. (1970), *Chemical Reactivity and Biological Role of Functional Groups in Enzymes*, London: Academic Press.
Smellie, R. (ed.) (1971), *Biochem. Soc. Symp.*, *Biochem. of Steroid Hormone Action*, London: Academic Press.
Smissman, E. and Steinman, M. (1966), *J. Med. Chem.*, **9**, 455.

Smith, C. (1956), *J. Pharmacol.*, **116**, 67.

Smith, D. (1972), *Muscle*, New York: Academic Press.

Smith, D. and Hanawalt, P. (1967), *Biochem. Biophys. Acta*, **149**, 519.

Smith, E. (1949), *Fed. Proc.*, **8**, 581.

Smith, H. (1925), *Amer. J. Physiol.*, **72**, 347.

Smith, H., Chapman, I. and Marlow, C. (1969), *Nature, Lond.*, **222**, 676.

Smith, J. and Matthews, R. (1957), *Biochem. J.*, **66**, 323.

Smith, L. and Tucker, H. (1977), *J. Med. Chem.*, **20**, 1653.

Smith, M. and Smith, P. (1966), *The Salicylates*, New York: Wiley-Interscience.

Smith, M., Wain, R. and Wightman, F. (1952), *Annals Appl. Biol.*, **39**, 295.

Smith, R. (1973), *The Excretory Function of Bile : the Elimination of Drugs and Toxic Substances in Bile*, London: Chapman and Hall.

Smith, S. and Larson, E. (1946), *J. Biol. Chem.*, **163**, 29.

Smithers, D., Bennett, L. and Struck, R. (1969), *Molec. Pharmacol.*, **5**, 433.

Smyth, D. and Taylor, C. (1957), *J. Physiol., Lond.*, **136**, 632.

Snedecor, G. (1946), *Statistical Methods*, 4th edn, Iowa: State College Press.

Snow, G. (1970), *Bacteriol. Rev.*, **34**, 99.

Sobell, H., Sakore, T., Tavale, S., Canepa F., Pauling, P. and Petcher, T. (1972), *Proc. Nat. Acad. Sci. U.S.A.*, **69**, 2212.

Soloway, S. (1965), *Advances in Pest Contnol*, **6**, 85.

Somers, E. and Pring, R. (1966), *Ann. Appl. Biol.*, **58**, 457.

Somers, I. and Shive, J. (1942), *Plant Physiology*, **17**, 582.

Sompolinsky, D., Zaidenzaig, Y., Schlomowitz, R. and Abramova, N. (1970), *J. Gen. Microbiol.*, **62**, 351.

Sonenberg, M. and Money, W. (1957), *Endocrinology*, **61**, 12.

Speakman, J. (1968), *A Valency Primer*, London: Edward Arnold.

Sperber, I. (1959), *Pharmacol. Rev.*, **11**, 109.

v. Stackelberg, M. (1954), *Z. Elektrochem.*, **58**, 25, 162.

Stamp, T. (1939), *Lancet*, **ii**, 10.

Stanbury, J. and Wyngaarden, J. (1952), *Metabolism*, **1**, 533.

Standen, O. (1963), in *Experimental Chemotherapy*, (eds. Schnitzer, R. and Hawking, F.), New York: Academic Press.

Stearn, A. and Stearn, E. (1924), *J. Bact.*, **9**, 491.

Stedman, E. (1926), *Biochem. J.*, **20**. 719; *Nature, Lond.*, **159**, 194.

Stedman, E. (1929), *Amer. J. Physiol.*, **90**, 528.

Stedman, E. (1947), *Nature, Lond.*, **159**, 194.

Stedman, E. and Stedman, E. (1931), *Biochem. J.*, **25**, 1147.

Steel, C. (1977), *Growth Kinetics of Tumours*, Oxford: Clarendon Press.

Steele, F. and Black, F. (1967), *J. Virol.*, **1**, 653.

Steele, J., Uchytil, T., Durbin, R., Bhatnagar, P. and Rich, D. (1976), *Proc. Nat. Acad. Sci. U.S.A.*, **73**, 2245.

Steidle, H. (1930), *Arch. Exper. Path. u. Pharmakol.*, 157, 89.

Stein, W. (1967), *The Movement of Molecules Across Cell Membranes*, London: Academic Press.

Steinert, M. (1960), *J. Biophys. Biochem. Cytol.*, **8**, 542.

Steinert, M. (1965), *Expl Cell Res.*, **39**, 69.

Steinert, M. and Steinert, G. (1960), *Expl Cell Res.*, **19**, 421.

Stenflo, J., Fernlund, P., Egan, W. and Roepstorff, P. (1964), *Proc. Nat. Acad. Sci. U.S.A.*, **71**, 2730.

Stephens, C., Murai, K., Brunings, K. and Woodward, R. (1956), *J. Amer. Chem. Soc.*, **78**, 4155.

Stephenson, R. (1956), *Brit. J. Pharmacol.*, **11**, 379.

624   References

Sternburg, J., Chang, S. and Kearns, C. (1959), *J. Econ. Entomol.*, **52**, 1070.

Sternburg, J., Kearns, C. and Moorefield, H. (1954), *J. Agr. Food Chem.*, **2**, 1125.

Steuart, C. and Burke, P. (1971), *Nature New Biology*, **233**, 109.

Stewart, D. and Jacobs, M. (1936), *J. Cell. Comp. Phys.*, **7**, 333.

Stockdale, M. and Selwyn, M. (1971), *Eur. J. Biochem.*, **21**, 565.

Stokes, G. and Weber, M. (1974), *Brit. Med. J.*, **ii**, 298.

Stone, J., Mordue, W., Batley, K. and Morris, H. (1976), *Nature, Lond.*, **263**, 207.

Stone, K. and Strominger, J. (1971), *Proc. Nat. Acad. Sci. U.S.A.*, **68**, 3223.

Straub, R. (1956), *Arch. internat. Pharmacodyn. Thér.*, **107**, 414.

Straub, W. (1907), *Pflugers Arch.*, **119**, 127.

Straub, W. and Triendl, E. (1937), *Arch. expl Path. Pharmakol.*, **185**, 1.

Street, J. (ed.) (1975), *Pesticide Selectivity*, New York: Dekker.

Stretton, R. and Manson, T. (1973), *J. Appl. Biol.*, **36**, 61.

Strominger, J., Ito, E. and Threnn, R. (1960), *J. Amer. Chem. Soc.*, **82**, 998.

Strominger, J., Threnn, R. and Scott, S. (1959), *J. Amer. Chem. Soc.*, **81**, 3803.

Strominger, J., Tipper, D., Ensign, J., Ghuysen, J. and Katz, W. (1967), *Biochemistry*, **6**, 906, 921, and 930.

Strugger, S. (1940), *Jenaische Z. Naturwiss.*, **73**, 97.

Sueoka, N. (1961), *J. Mol. Biol.*, **3**, 31.

Sueoka, N. and Quinn, W. (1968), *Cold Spring Harbor Symp. Quant. Biol.*, **33**, 695.

Suki, W., Eknoyan, G. and Martinez-Maldonado, M. (1973), *Ann. Rev. Pharmacol.*, **13**, 91.

Sulser, F. and Sanders-Bush, E. (1971), *Ann. Rev. Pharmacol.*, **11**, 209.

Sulser, F., Watts, J. and Brodie, B. (1962), *Ann. N. Y. Acad. Sci.*, **96**, 279.

Sutherland, E., Øye, I. and Butcher, R. (1965), *Recent Prog. Hormone Res.*, **21**, 623.

Sutherland, K. and Wark, I. (1955), *Principles of Flotation*, 2nd Edn., Melbourne: Australasian Institute of Mining and Metallurgy.

Sutton, L. (ed.) (1947, 1965), *Tables of Interatomic Distances and Configurations in Molecules and Ions*, London: The Chemical Society.

Sutton, L. (1955), in *Determination of Organic Structures by Physical Methods*, (eds. Braude, E. and Nachod, F.), New York: Academic Press.

Suwalsky, M., Traub, W., Shmueli, U., and Subirana, J. (1969), *J. Mol. Biol.*, **42**, 363.

Suzuki, T., Hayashi, K., Fujikawa, K. and Tsukamoto, K. (1964), *J. Biochem., Tokyo*, **56**, 335.

Swain, C. and Lupton, E. (1968), *J. Amer. Chem. Soc.*, **90**, 4328.

Swartz, H., Bolton, J. and Borg, D. (1972), *Biological Applications of Electron Spin Resonance*, New York: Wiley.

Sweatman, W. and Collier, H. (1968), *Nature, Lond.*, **217**, 69.

Sweet, R. and Dahl, L. (1970), *J. Amer. Chem. Soc.*, **92**, 5489.

Swidler, G. (1971), *Handbook of Drug Interactions*, New York: Wiley.

Swintosky, J. (1956), *J. Amer. Pharm. Assoc. Sci. Ed.*, **45**, 395.

Sykes, B., Patt, S. and Dolphin, D. (1971), *Cold Spring Harbor Symp. Quant. Biol.*, **36**, 29.

Szekely, P. and Wynne, N. (1963), *Brit. Heart J.*, **25**, 589.

Szent-Györgi, A. (1960), *Submolecular Biology*, New York: Academic Press.

Taft, R. (1953), *J. Amer. Chem. Soc.*, **75**, 4231.

Taft, R. and Grob, C. (1974), *J. Amer. Chem. Soc.* **96**, 1236.

Taft, R. and Lewis, I. (1959), *J. Amer. Chem. Soc.*, **81**, 5343.

Taft, R., Price, E., Fox, I., Lewis, I., Andersen, K. and Davis, G. (1963), *J. Amer. Chem. Soc.*, **85**, 709.

Tainter, M. (1930), *J. Pharmacol.*, **40**, 43.

Takamiya, K. (1960), *Nature, Lond.*, **185**, 190.

Takamizawa, A., Matsumoto, S., Iwata, T. *et al.* (1975), *J. Med. Chem.*, **18**, 376.

Takasawa, S., Utahara, R., Okanishi, M., Maeda, K. and Umezawa, H. (1968), *Journal Antibiot.*, (Tokyo), **21**, 477.

Takita, T., Maeda, K. and Umezawa, H. (1959), *J. Antibiotics, Tokyo, A.*, **12**, 111.

Tamm, I. and Eggers, H. (1965), *Amer. J. Med.*, **38**, 678.

Tamm, I., Eggers, H., Bablanian, R., Wagner, A. and Folkers, K. (1969), *Nature, Lond.*, **223**, 785.

Tanford, C. (1968), *Accounts of Chemical Research (Amer. Chem. Soc.)* **1**, 161.

Tapley, D. and Cooper, C. (1956), *Nature, Lond.*, **178**, 1119.

Tarshis, I. (1960), *J. Econ. Entomol.*, **53**, 903.

Tashjian, A., Voelkel, E., McDonough, J. and Levine, L. (1975), *Nature, Lond.*, **258**, 739.

Tattersall, M., Jaffe, N. and Frei, E. (1975), in *Pharmacological Basis of Cancer Chemotherapy*, (eds. Cumley, R. and McCay, J.), Baltimore, Maryland: Williams and Wilkins Co.

Tatum, A. and Cooper, G. (1934), *J. Pharmacol.*, **50**, 198.

Taylor, D., Callahan, K. and Shaikh, I. (1975), *J. Med. Chem.*, **18**, 1088.

Taylor, E., Lymn, R. and Moll, G. (1970), *Biochemistry*, **9**, 2984.

Taylor, H. and Burden, R. (1972), *Proc. Roy. Soc., B*, **180**, 317.

Taylor, J., Green, A. and Corgi, G. (1948), *J. Biol. Chem.*, **173**, 591.

Taylor, M. and Storck, R. (1964), *Proc. Nat. Acad. Sci. U.S.A.*, **52**, 958.

Taylor, R. (1959), *Amer. J. Physiol.*, **196**, 1071.

Temin, H. and Mizutani, S. (1970), *Nature, Lond.*, **226**, 1211.

Templeman, W. and Sexton, W. (1945), *Nature, Lond.*, **156**, 630.

Templeman, W. and Sexton, W. (1946), *Proc. Roy. Soc., B*, **133**, 300.

Terenius, L. and Wahlstrom, A. (1978), in *Centrally Acting Peptides* (ed. Hughes, J.), London: Macmillan.

Terracini, B., Testa, M., Cabral, J. and Day, N. (1973), *Internat. J. Cancer*, **11**, 747.

Testa, B. and Jenner, P. (1976), *Drug Metabolism : Chemical and Biochemical Aspects*, New York: Marcel Dekker.

Theodovides, V., Gyurik, R., Kingsbury, W., and Parish, R. (1976), *Experientia*, **32**, 702.

Thoenen, H. (1969), *Bildung u. funktionelle Bedeutung adrenerger Ersatztransmitter*, Berlin: Springer.

Thoenen, H. and Tranzer, J. (1968), *Arch. Pharmacol. Expl Path.*, **261**, 271.

Thomas, H. and Breinl, A. (1905), *Mem. Liverpool School Trop. Med.*, No. 16.

Thomas, H., Herriott, R., Hahn, B. and Wang, S. (1976), *Nature, Lond.*, **259**, 342.

Thomas, R. (1974), *J. Physiol. Lond.*, **238**, 159.

Thomas, R., Boutagy, J. and Gelbart, A. (1974), (a), *J. Pharmacol.*, **191**, 219; (b), *J. Pharm. Sci.*, **63**, 1649.

Thompson, P., Rinertson, J., McCarty, D., Bayles, A. and Cook, A. (1955), *Antibiotics Chemother.*, **5**, 433.

Thorn, G. and Ludwig, R. (1962), *The Dithiocarbamates and Related Compounds*, Amsterdam: Elsevier.

Thorn, M. (1953), *Biochem. J.*, **54**, 540.

Thorne, R. and Bygrave, F. (1974), *Nature, Lond.*, **248**, 351; *Biochem. J.*, **144**, 551.

Thorp, R. and Cobbin, L. (1967), in *Cardiac Stimulant Substances*, (ed. de Stevens, G.), New York: Academic Press.

Tiffany, B., Wright, J., Moffett, R. *et al.* (1957), *J. Amer. Chem. Soc.*, **79**, 1682.

Tilles, J. (1974), *Ann. Rev. Pharmacol.*, **14**, 469.

Tipper, D. and Strominger, J. (1965), *Proc. Nat. Acad. Sci. U.S.A.*, **54**, 1133.

Tisdale, W. and Williams, I. (1934), *U.S. Pat.* 1 972 961.

Tocchini-Valentini, G., Marino, P. and Colvill, A. (1968), *Nature, Lond.*, **220**. 275.

Toft, D., and Gorski, J. (1966), *Proc. Nat. Acad. Sci. U.S.A.*, **55**, 1574.

Tolkmith, H. (1966), *Ann. N.Y. Acad. Sci.*, **136** (art. 3), 59.

Tolmsoff, W. (1962), *Phytopathology*, **52**, 755.

Tomatis, L., Turusov, V., Day, N. and Charles, R. (1972), *Internat. J. Cancer*, **10**, 489.

Topliss, J. (1972), *J. Med. Chem.*, **15**, 1006.

Topliss, J. (1977), *J. Med. Chem.*, **20**, 463.

Topliss, J. and Costello, R. (1972), *J. Med. Chem.*, **15**, 1066.

Towers, N., Kellerman, G. and Linnane, A. (1973), *Arch. Biochem. Biophys.*, **155**, 159.

Traube, J. (1904), *Arch. ges. Physiol.*, **105**, 541.

Tréfouël, J., Tréfouël, Mme. J., Nitti, F. and Bovet, D. (1935), *Compt. rend. Soc. Biol.*, **120**, 756.

Treherne, J. (1956), *J. Physiol.*, **133**, 171.

Treherne, J. (1966), *The Neurochemistry of Arthropods*, Cambridge: Cambridge University Press.

Trevan, J. (1927), *Proc. Roy. Soc. B*, **101**, 483.

Trevan, J. and Boock, E. (1926), Document C. H. 398, Health Organization, League of Nations, Geneva.

Trevan, J. and Boock, E. (1927), *Brit. J. Expl Path.*, **8**, 307.

Triggle, D. and Triggle, C. (1977), *Chemical Pharmacology of the Synapse*, New York: Academic Press.

Trotman, C. and Greenwood, C. (1971), *Biochem. J.*, **124**, 25.

Truffaut, G. and Pastac, I. (1932), *Fr. Pat.* 425 295; cf. *Brit. Pat. App.* 15 446/33.

Truffaut, G. and Pastac, I. (1944), *Chim. et Industr.*, **51**, 79.

Trump, B., Duttera, S., Byrne, W. and Arstila, A. (1970), *Proc. Nat. Acad. Sci. U.S.A.*, **66**, 433.

Tsukamoto, M. and Casida, J. (1967), *Nature, Lond.*, **213**, 49.

Tu, Y. and McCalla, D. (1976), *Chem. Biol. Interactions, Amsterdam*, **14**, 81.

Tuck, L. and Baker, J. (1973), *Chem. Biol. Interactions, Amsterdam*, **7**, 355.

Turnbull, H. (1944), *Aust. N.Z. J. Surg.*, **14**, 3.

Turner, W., Bauer, D. and Nimmo-Smith, R. (1962), *Brit. Med. J.*, **i**, 1317.

Turpaev, T. and Sakharov, D. (1973), in *Comparative Pharmacology*, (ed. Michelson, M.), **1**, 251, Oxford: Pergamon Press.

Uhlenhuth, H. (1907), *Deutsch. med. Woch.*, **33**, 1237.

Umezawa, H. (1973), *Biomédicine*, **18**, 459.

Underwood, E. (1977), *Trace Elements in Human and Animal Nutrition*, 4th Edn, New York: Academic Press.

Underwood, G. (1962), *Proc. Soc. Expl Biol. Med.*, **111**, 660.

Unger, S. and Hansch, C. (1973), *J. Med. Chem.*, **16**, 745.

Unna, K. (1943), *J. Pharmacol.*, **79**, 27.

Unsworth, I., (1861), *St. Mary's Hospital Gazette, London*, **66**, 272.

Usherwood, P. and Machili, P. (1966), *Nature, Lond.*, **210**, 635.

Vallee, B. (1975), *Biochem. Biophys. Res. Commun.*, **62**, 296.

Vane, J. (1971), *Nature New Biology*, **231**, 232.

Vanyushin, B., Belozersky, A., Kokurina, N. and Kadirova, D. (1968), *Nature, Lond.*, **218**, 1067.

Vargha, L., Toldy, L., Feher, Ö. and Lendval, S. (1957), *J. Chem. Soc.*, 805.

Varner, J. and Chandra, G. (1964), *Proc. Nat. Acad. Sci. U.S.A.*, **52**, 100.

Vazquez, D. (1964), *Nature, Lond.*, **203**, 257.

Veldstra, H. (1953), *Ann. Rev. Plant Physiol.*, **4**, 151.

Veldstra, H. (1956), *Pharmacol. Rev.*, **8**, 339.

Veldstra, H. (1956a), in *The Chemistry and Mode of Action of Plant Growth Substances*, (eds. Wain, R. and Wightman, F.), London: Butterworths.

Veldstra, H. (1963), in *Comprehensive Biochemistry*, (eds. Florkin, M. and Stotz, E.), Amsterdam: Elsevier.

Veldstra, H. and van der Westeringh, C. (1951), *Rec. Trav. chim. Pays-Bas*, **70**, 1127.

Veneziale, C., Walter, P., Kneer, N. and Lardy, H. (1967), *Biochemistry* **6**, 2129.

Vermast, P. (1921), *Biochem. Z.*, **125**, 106.

Vianna, G. (1912), *Arch. Brasil. Med.*, **2**, 422.

Vickerman, K. (1962), *Trans. Roy. Soc. Trop. Med. Hyg.*, **56**, 487.

Voegtlin, C. (1925), *Physiol. Rev.*, **5**, 63.

Vogel, H. (1959), *Fed. Proc.*, **18**, 345.

Vonk, J. and Sijpesteijn, A. (1971), *Pest Sci.*, **2**, 160.

Wacker, A., Grisebach, H., Trebat, A., Ebert, M. and Weygand, F. (1954), *Angew. Chem.*, **66**, 712.

Wacker, A., Kirschfeld, S. and Weinblum, D. (1960), *J. Mol. Biol.*, **2**, 72.

Waddell, W. and Butler, T. (1957), *J. Clin. Invest.*, **36**, 1217.

Waddell, W. and Butler, T. (1959), *J. Clin. Invest.*, **38**, 720.

Waddell, W. and Hardman, H. (1960), *Amer. J. Physiol.*, **199**, 1112.

Wade, A. (ed.) (1977), *Martindale, the Extra Pharmacopocia*, 27th Edn, London: Pharmaceutical Press.

Wagner, J. (1961), *J. Pharmaceut. Sci.*, **50**, 359.

Wagner, J. (1967), *J. Pharmaceut. Sci.* **56**, 489.

Wagner-Jauregg, T., Hackley, B., Lies, T., Owens, O. and Proper, R. (1955), *J. Amer. Chem. Soc.*, **77**, 922.

Wain, R. (1955), *Ann. Appl. Biol.*, **42**, 151.

Wain, R. (1956), *Science Progress*, **176**, 604.

Wain, R. (1963), *Nature, Lond.*, **200**, 28.

Wain, R. (1964), in *The Physiology and Biochemistry of Herbicides*, (ed. Audus, L.), London: Academic Press.

Wain, R. and Fawcett, C. (1969), in *Plant Physiology*, (ed. Steward, F.), Vol. 5A, New York: Academic Press.

Walaas, E. (1958), *Acta Chem. Scand.*, **12**, 528.

Wallach, D. and Zahler, P. (1966), *Proc. Nat. Acad. Sci. U.S.A.*, **56**, 1552.

Waller, C., Hutchings, B., Mowat, J. and 13 others (1948), *J. Amer. Chem. Soc.*, **70**, 19.

Waals, L. (1951), *Chem. and Indust.*, 606.

Walshe, J. (1968), *Lancet, London*, **i**, 775.

Wang, J. (1974), *J. Molec. Biol.*, **89**, 783.

War Office, Gt. Britain (1922), *The Official History of the War : Medical Services and Surgery of the War*, Vol. 1., London: H. M. Stationery Office.

Warburg, O. (1927), *Naturwiss.*, **25**, 1.

Warburg, O. and Christian, W. (1943), *Biochem.*, **314**, 149.

Ward-McQuaid, J., Jichlinski, D. and Macis, R. (1963), *Brit. Med. J.*, **ii**, 1311.

Waring, M. (1965), *Molec. Pharmacol.*, **1**, 1.

Waring, M. (1970), *J. Mol. Biol.*, **54**, 247.

Waring, M. and Wakelin, L. (1974), *Nature, Lond.*, **252**, 653.

Warnick, S. and Carter, J. (1972), *Archives Envir. Health*, **25**, 265.

Warren, G., Houslay, M., Metcalfe, J. and Birdsall, N. (1975), *Nature, Lond.*, **255**, 684.

Waser, P. (1960), *J. Pharm. Pharmacol.*, **12**, 577.

Waser, P. (1961), *Pharmacol. Rev.*, **13**, 465.

Watanabe, A., Tasaki, I., Singer, I. and Lerman, L. (1967), *Science*, **155**, 95.

Watanabe, T. (1963), *Bact. Rev.*, **27**, 87.

Watson, J. and Crick, F. (1953), *Nature, Lond.*, **171**, 737.

Watson, W. (1976), *Cell Biology of the Brain*, London: Chapman and Hall; New York: Halsted-Wiley.

Watters, J. and De Witt, R. (1960), *J. Amer. Chem. Soc.*, **82**, 1333.

Webb, E. (ed.) (1972), *Enzyme Nomenclature*, Amsterdam: Elsevier.

Weber, G., Borris, D., De Robertis, E., Barrantes, F., La Torre, J. and Carlin, M. (1971), *Molec. Pharmacol.*, **7**, 530.

Weber, M. and Kinsky, S. (1965), *J. Bact.*, **89**, 306.

Weeks, C., Cooper, A. and Norton, D. (1970), *Acta Cryst. B*, **26**, 429.

Weiden, M. and Moorefield, H. (1964), *World Rev. Pest Control*, **3**, 102.

Weinberg, E. (1954), *Antibiotics Chemother.*, **4**, 35.

Weinberg, E. (1957), *Bact. Rev.*, **21**, 46.

Weinberg, E. (1972), *Ann. N.Y. Acad. Sci.*, **199**, 274.

Weinberg, E. (1974), *Science*, **184**, 952.

Weissberger, A. and Lu Valle, S. (1944), *J. Amer. Chem. Soc.*, **66**, 700.

Weissman, G. and Dingle, J. (1961), *Expl Cell. Res.*, **25**, 207.

Welch, A. (1961), *Cancer Res.*, **21**, 1475.

Welch, A. and Prusoff, W. (1966), *Cancer Chemother. Reports*, **6**, 29.

Wells, P. (1963), *Chem. Rev.*, **63**, 171.

Welsh, J. (1948), *Johns Hopkins Hosp. Bull.*, **83**, 568.

Welsh, J. and Taub, R. (1950), *J. Pharmacol.*, **99**, 334.

Wendel, H. (1964), *Fed. Proc.*, **23**, 387.

Wense, T. (1939), *Archiv. ges. Physiol.*, **241**, 284.

Weres, O. and Rice, S. (1972), *J. Amer. Chem. Soc.*, **94**, 8983.

Werkheiser, W. (1963), *Cancer Res.*, **23**, 1277.

West, T. and Campbell, G. (1946), *DDT, the Synthetic Insecticide*, London: Chapman and Hall.

Westley, J., Oliveto, E., Berger, J. and five others (1973), *J. Med. Chem.*, **16**, 397.

Wettingfeld, R., Rowe, J. and Eyles, D. (1956), *Ann. Int. Med.*, **44**, 557.

Wettstein, F., Staehlin, T. and Noll, H. (1963), *Nature, Lond.*, **197**, 430.

Weyter, F. and Broquist, H. (1960), *Biochim. Biophys. Acta*, **40**, 567.

Wheeler, G. and Alexander, J. (1969), *Cancer Res.*, **29**, 98.

White, G. and Thorn, G. (1975), *Pesticide Biochem. Physiol.*, **5**, 380.

White, J. and Cantor, C. (1971), *J. Mol. Biol.*, **58**, 397.

White, R. and Standen, O. (1953), *Brit. Med. J.*, **ii**, 755.

Whitehouse, M. and Dean, P. (1965), *Biochem. Pharmacol.*, **14**, 557.

Whitley, R., Soong, S., Dolin, R., Galasso, G., Chien, L. and Alford, C. (1977), *New Engl. J. Med.*, **297**, 289.

Whittaker, V. (1951), *Physiol. Rev.*, **31**, 312.

Whittaker, V. (1963), *Biochem. Soc. Symp.*, **23**, 109.

WHO, *see* World Health Organization.

Widmark, E. (1920), *Acta. Med. Scand.*, **52**, 88.

Wiebelhaus, V., Weinstock, J., Maass, A., Brennan, F., Sosnowski, G. and Larsen, T. (1965), *J. Pharmacol.*, **149**, 397.

Wilbrandt, W. (1950), *Arch. expl Path. Pharmakol.*, **212**, 9.

Wilbrandt, W. (1959), *J. Pharm. Pharmacol.*, **11**, 65.

Wilbrandt, W. (1964), *Schweiz. med. Woch.*, **94**, 737.

Wilbrandt, W. and Rosenberg, T. (1961), *Pharmacol. Rev.*, **13**, 109.

Wilhelm, W. and Kuhn, R. (1970), *Pharmakopsychiatrie Neuro-psychopharmakologie*, **3**, 317.

Wilkins, R. (1962), *J. Chem. Soc.*, 4475.
Wilkinson, C. (ed.) (1976), *Insecticide Biochemistry and Physiology*, New York: Plenum.
Wilkinson, J. (1966), *Microbial Physiology and Continuous Culture*, London: H. M. Stationery Office.
Wilkinson, S. and Lowe, L. (1966), *Nature Lond.*, **212**, 311.
Willey, G. (1955), *Brit. J. Pharmacol. Chemother.*, **10**, 466.
Williams, A. (1969), *Chemistry of Enzyme Action*, London: McGraw-Hill.
Williams, A. and Klein, E. (1970), *Cancer*, **25**, 450.
Williams, D. (ed.) (1976), *Bio-inorganic Chemistry*, Springfield, Ill.: Charles C. Thomas.
Williams, L., Jarett, L. and Lefkowitz, R. (1976), *J. Biol. Chem.*, **251**, 3096.
Williams, L., Mullikin, D. and Lefkowitz, R. (1976), *J. Biol. Chem.*, **251**, 6915.
Williams, R. (1952), *J. Chem. Soc.*, 3770.
Williams, R. (1959), *Detoxication Mechanisms*, 2nd Edn, London: Chapman and Hall.
Williamson, D. and Everett, G. (1975), *J. Amer. Chem. Soc.*, **97**, 2397.
Williamson, J. (1959), *Brit. J. Pharm. Chemother.*, **14**, 443.
Williamson, J. and Macadam, R. (1965), *Trans. Roy. Soc. Trop. Med. Hyg.*, **59**, 367.
Williamson, J., Macadam, R. and Dixon, H. (1975), *Biochem. Pharmacol.*, **24**, 147.
Wilson, A. and Schild, H. (1968), *Applied Pharmacology*, 10th Edn, London: Churchill.
Wilson, I. (1962), in *Enzymes and Drug Action*, (eds. Mongar, J. and de Reuck, A.), London: Churchill.
Wilson, I. and Bergmann, F. (1950), *J. Biol. Chem.*, **186**, 682.
Wilson, I. and Cabib, E. (1956), *J. Amer. Chem. Soc.*, **78**, 202.
Wilson, C., Gisvold, O., and Doerge, R. (eds.) (1977), *Textbook of Organic Medicinal and Pharmaceutical Chemistry*, 7th Edn, Philadelphia: Lippincott.
Wilson, I., Harrison, M. and Ginsburg, S. (1961), *J. Biol. Chem.*, **236**, 1498.
Wilson, I. and Meislich, E. (1953), *J. Amer. Chem. Soc.*, **75**, 4628.
Wilson, S. (1949), *Vet. Rec.*, **61**, 395.
Winder, F. and Collins, P. (1970), *J. Gen. Microbiol.*, **63**, 41.
Winkler, A., Green, P., Smith, H. and Pescor, F. (1960), *Fed. Proc.*, **19**, 22.
Winteringham, F. and Barnes, J. (1955), *Physiol. Rev.*, **35**, 701.
Winteringham, F., Loveday, P. and Harrison, A. (1951), *Nature, Lond.*, **167**, 106.
Wintersteiner, O., Stavely, H., Dutcher, J., and Spielman, M. (1949), in *The Chemistry of Penicillin*, (eds. Clarke, H., Johnson, J. and Robinson, R.), Princeton: Princeton University Press, p. 207.
Wipf, H. and Simon, W. (1970), *Helv. Chim. Acta*, **53**, 1732.
Wise, E. and Park, J. (1965), *Proc. Nat. Acad. Sci. U.S.A.*, **54**, 75.
Wiselogle, F. (1946), *A Survey of Antimalarial Drugs, 1941–1945*, Ann Arbor, Michigan: W. Edwards.
Witkop, B. and Foltz, C. (1957), *J. Amer. Chem. Soc.*, **79**, 197.
Wittes, R., Cvitkovic, E., Shah, J., *et al.* (1977), *Cancer Treatment Reports*, **61**, 359.
Wodzicki, K. (1973), *Bull. World Health Org.*, **48**, 461.
Wohl, A. and Glimm, E. (1910), *Biochem. Z.*, **27**, 349.
Wolfe, A. and Hahn, F. (1964), *Science*, **143**, 1445.
Wolfe, A. and Hahn, F. (1965), *Biochim. Biophys. Acta*, **95**, 146.
Wolhoff, J. and Overbeck, J. (1959), *Rec. Trav. Chim.*, **78**, 759.
Wood, G. and Stewart, S. (1971), *J. Pharm. Pharmacol.*, **23**, 248(S).
Wood, J., Wolfe, W. and Irving, G. (1947), *Science*, **106**, 395.
Wood, R., Ferone, R. and Hitchings, G. (1961), *Biochemical Pharmacol.*, **6**, 113.
Wood, R. and Hitchings, G. (1959), *J. Biol. Chem.*, **234**, 2377.

Woodin, A. (1963), *Biochem. Soc. Symp.*, **22**, 126.
Woodroffe, R. and Wilkinson, B. (1966), *J. Gen. Microbiol.*, **44**, 343.
Woodruff, H. (1966), in *Biochemical Studies of Antimicrobial Drugs*, (eds. Newton, B. and Reynolds, P.), Cambridge: Cambridge University Press.
Woods, D. (1940), *Brit. J. Expl Path.*, **21**, 74.
Woods, D. (1962), *J. Gen. Microbiol.*, **29**, 687.
Woodson, B. and Joklik, W. (1965), *Proc. Nat. Acad. Sci. U.S.A.*, **54**, 947.
Woodward, R., Iacobucci, G. and Hochstein, F. (1959), *J. Amer. Chem. Soc.*, **81**, 4434.
Woodward, R., Neuberger, A. and Trenner, N. (1949), in *The Chemistry of Penicillin*, (eds. Clarke, H., Johnson, J. and Robinson, R.), Princeton: Princeton University Press, p. 438.
Woolfe, G. (1965), *Prog. Drug Research, Basel*, **8**, 11 (review).
Woolley, D. (1950), *J. Amer. Chem. Soc.*, **72**, 5763.
Woolley, D. (1952), *A Study of Antimetabolites*, New York: Wiley.
Woolley, D., Strong, F., Madden, R. and Elvehjem, C. (1938), *J. Biol. Chem.*, **124**, 715.
Wong, H., Tolpin, E. and Lipscomb, W. (1974), *J. Med. Chem.*, **17**, 785.
World Health Organization (1970), *Control of Pesticides*, Geneva.
World Health Organization (1971), *WHO Official Records*, **190**, 176.
World Health Organization (1973a), *Pharmacogenetics*, Tech. Report, No. 524.
World Health Organization (1973, b), *Safe Use of Pesticides*, Tech. Report, No. 513.
World Health Organization (1974), *The Work of WHO, 1973*. Annual Report of the Director-General. Geneva (WHO official records, No. 213.).
World Health Organization (1976), *The Work of WHO, 1975. Annual Report of the Director-General*. Geneva (WHO official records, No. 229.).
World Health Organization (1977), *The Work of WHO, 1976–7. Annual Report of the Director-General*. Geneva (WHO official records, No. 243).
Wren, A. and Massey, V. (1965), *Biochim. Biophys. Acta*, **110**, 329.
Wright, S. (1960), *The Metabolism of Cardiac Glycosides*, Springfield, Illinois: Thomas.
Wyatt, G. and Kalf, G. (1957), *J. Gen. Physiol.*, **40**, 833.
Wyss, O., Rubin, M. and Strandskov, F. (1943), *Proc. Soc. Expl Biol. Med.*, **52**, 155.
Wyss, O. and Strandskov, F. (1945), *Ann. Biochem.*, **6**, 261.
Yaeger, J. and Munson, S. (1945), *Science*, **102**, 305.
Yagi, K. (1965), *Adv. Enzymol.*, **27**, 1.
Yamamoto, I. (1970), *Ann. Rev. Entomol.*, **15**, 257.
Yamashita, S. and Racker, E. (1968), *J. Biol. Chem.*, **243**, 2446.
Yendell, A., Tupper, R. and Wills, E. (1967), *Biochem. J.*, **102**, 23P.
Yorke, W., Adams, A. and Murgatroyd, F. (1929), *Ann. Trop. Med. Parasit.*, **23**, 501.
Yorke, W., Murgatroyd, F. and Hawking, F. (1931), *Ann. Trop. Med. Parasit.*, **25**, 351. [*c.f.* Yorke, W., and Murgatroyd, F. (1930), *idem*, **24**, 449].
Youatt, J. (1958), *Austral. J. Expl Biol. Med. Sci.*, **36**, 223.
Youatt, J. (1962), *Austral. J. Expl Biol. Med. Sci.*, **40**, 201.
Youdim, M., Collins, G., Sandler, M., Jones, A., Pare, C. and Nicholson, W. (1972), *Nature, Lond.*, **236**, 225.
Young, A., Zukin, S. and Snyder, S. (1974), *Proc. Nat. Acad. Sci., U.S.*, **71**, 2246.
Yudkin, M. and Davis, B. (1965), *J. Mol. Biol.*, **12**, 193.
Zaffaroni, A. (1974), *Act. Endocrinol.*, Supp. **185**, 423.
Zakharenko. E., and Moshkovski, Y. (1966), *Biofizika*, **11**, 945.
Zanker, V. and Schnith, H. (1959), *Chem. Ber.*, **9**, 2210.
Zbinden, G. and Randall, L. (1967), *Advances Pharmacol.*, **5**, 213.
Zeidler, O. (1874), *Ber. deutsch. Chem. Ges.*, **7**, 1180.

Zeller, E. (1963), *Ann. N.Y. Acad. Sci.*, **107** (Art. 3), 211.

Zentmyer, G. (1944), *Science*, **100**, 294.

Zerahn, K. (1956), *Acta Physiol., Scand.*, **36**, 300.

Ziegler, H. (1970), *Endeavour* (London), **29**, 112.

Zimmerman, P. (1942), *Cold Spring Harbor Symp. Quant. Biol.*, **10**, 152.

Zubay, G. and Watson, M. (1959), *J. Biophys. Biochem. Cytol.*, **5**, 51.

Zuelzer, W. (1964), *Blood*, **24**, 477.

Zwolinski, B., Eyring, H. and Reese, C. (1949), *J. Phys. Colloid Chem.*, **53**, 1426.

Zysk, J., Bushway, A., Whistler, R. and Carlton, W. (1975), *J. Reprod. Fertil.*, **45**, 69.

Subject index

654 · SUBJECT INDEX